The Human Testis

ADVANCES IN EXPERIMENTAL MEDICINE AND BIOLOGY

Volume 1
THE RETICULOENDOTHELIAL SYSTEM AND ATHEROSCLEROSIS
Edited by N. R. Di Luzio and R. Paoletti • 1967

Volume 2
PHARMACOLOGY OF HORMONAL POLYPEPTIDES AND PROTEINS
Edited by N. Back, L. Martini, and R. Paoletti • 1968

Volume 3
GERM-FREE BIOLOGY—Experimental and Clinical Aspects
Edited by E. A. Mirand and N. Back • 1969

Volume 4
DRUGS AFFECTING LIPID METABOLISM
Edited by W. L. Holmes, L. A. Carlson, and R. Paoletti • 1969

Volume 5
LYMPHATIC TISSUE AND GERMINAL CENTERS IN IMMUNE RESPONSE
Edited by L. Fiore-Donati and M. G. Hanna, Jr. • 1969

Volume 6
RED CELL METABOLISM AND FUNCTION
Edited by George J. Brewer • 1970

Volume 7
SURFACE CHEMISTRY OF BIOLOGICAL SYSTEMS
Edited by Martin Blank • 1970

Volume 8
BRADYKININ AND RELATED KININS: Cardiovascular, Biochemical, and Neural Actions
Edited by F. Sicuteri, M. Rocha e Silva, and N. Back • 1970

Volume 9
SHOCK: Biochemical, Pharmacological, and Clinical Aspects
Edited by A. Bertelli and N. Back • 1970

Volume 10
THE HUMAN TESTIS
Edited by E. Rosemberg and C. A. Paulsen • 1970

The Human Testis

Proceedings of the Workshop Conference held at
Positano, Italy, April 23-25, 1970

Edited by

Eugenia Rosemberg, M. D.
Research Director, Medical Research Institute of Worcester, Inc.
Worcester City Hospital
Worcester, Massachusetts

and

C. Alvin Paulsen, M. D.
Professor of Medicine
University of Washington School of Medicine
Seattle, Washington

A SERONO FOUNDATION SYMPOSIUM

PLENUM PRESS · NEW YORK–LONDON · 1970

Library of Congress Catalog Card Number 70-129058

SBN 306-39010-8

A Division of Plenum Publishing Corporation
227 West 17th Street, New York, N.Y. 10011

United Kingdom edition published by Plenum Press, London
A Division of Plenum Publishing Company, Ltd.
Donington House, 30 Norfolk Street, London W.C.2, England

Printed in the United States of America

PREFACE

This volume describes the proceedings of the Workshop Conference on The Human Testis which was held at Positano, Italy, April 23-25, 1970.

The format of the book has been arranged according to topics discussed during the Conference. Each chapter includes individual contributions followed by discussion. Thus, this volume provides a current critical evaluation of the subjects discussed. The Editors assume responsibility for any shortcomings and wish to thank all participants for their unprecedented cooperation in making this publication possible.

The Editors are indebted to Miss Barbara Martin for her able secretarial and administrative assistance and to Mrs. Griff T. Ross who supervised the secretarial staff during the conference. Recognition is also due to Mrs. M. Flack for editorial assistance.

The Workshop Conference could not have taken place but for the Serono Foundation, which supported this Meeting as well as the publication of the Proceedings of this Workshop. The physical as well as the technical arrangements were under the careful direction of Mr. Cesare Florimonte of the Serono Foundation. The support provided by the Serono Foundation is another proof of its generosity in stimulating scientific exchanges and a demonstration of its continuous efforts to support basic and applied studies in the field of human reproduction.

We express our thanks to our Publisher, Plenum Press, for their fine cooperation and for ensuring the rapid publication of this volume.

May, 1970

Eugenia Rosemberg

C. Alvin Paulsen

ACKNOWLEDGMENTS

Individual participants wish to thank Editors and Publishers of journals and books for permission to reproduce previously published figures and tables.

Individual participants desire to express their gratitude to the Endocrine Study Section, National Institutes of Health, USPHS, Bethesda, Maryland, U.S.A., to the National Pituitary Agency, Baltimore, Maryland, U.S.A.; to the Department of Biological Standards, National Institute for Medical Research, Mill Hill, London, and to the Istituto Farmacologico Serono, Rome, Italy, for generous supplies of hormones.

Grants supporting work presented in these proceedings are acknowledged by individual participants and indicated in their respective contributions.

FOREWORD

During the past twenty years many meetings concerning the reproductive process have taken place. Both structure and function of female and male gonads have been major topics at these gatherings. However, in only a few instances has the male gonad, particularly the human, been the main subject of discussion. This Conference was designed to focus attention on the human testis. A group of investigators representing various scientific disciplines was invited to this Workshop to discuss this subject from a morphologic, physiologic, biochemical, genetic and pathologic point of view. In some areas, especially that related to embryology, basic human data are lacking, thus relevant animal studies were also presented. Effort was made in these comparative studies to illuminate rather than complicate the understanding of fundamental phenomena in human reproductive physiology.

This volume contains the Proceedings of this Workshop which served as a forum for interexchange of ideas which have enriched our knowledge of the human testis. If the topics discussed excited our interest for further research and have opened new and original lines of study, then the organization of this gathering was amply justified.

Roberto E. Mancini, M. D.

May, 1970

INTRODUCTORY REMARKS

Roberto E. Mancini, M. D.

Since its creation, mankind has been concerned with problems related to reproduction. Most of the ancient religions clearly exhorted the people to multiply, as this was considered the main if not the only object of marriage. Although this preoccupation seemed from the beginning to involve both the female and male aspects of the pair, a preferential and unbroken thread of attention was paid to the knowledge of the ovary and female genital tract. From the earliest writers to modern researchers, this interest in the female sexual function has also been reflected in the continuous recommendation to seek a reliable method for the control of fertility applicable only to women. In consequence a considerable amount of data has been accumulated on the biology of the ovary as compared with the smaller quantity on the testis. However, the importance and significant symbolism of the untouchable male gonad appeared reinforeed in the ancient Assyrian times, when a woman or even a physician who consciously or unconsciously caused an injury to the testis of a man, could be punished by having their hands cut off. Yet, the shadows of this rather superstitious concept has persisted until today, where in some countries, it is more difficult to get a biopsy of the testis than to perform a similar one on the endometrium or even on the ovary.

It was not before the decade following 1940 that our cognizance of the human testis, thanks to the introduction of surgical biopsies, became a reality and so the mysterious aura which had surrounded the male gonad began to vanish. The biopsy was rapidly incorporated by endocrinologists and urologists as a diagnostic tool. A few years later, studies on the normal and abnormal histology of the different structures of the testis corroborated and amplified previous necropsy findings, and the pathological background of more than one endocrine or non-endocrine disease of this gland was established. A pioneer group of well-known North American, European and Latin American authors have greatly contributed to the opening of this new field of investigation. To all of them, dead or alive, we convey on this special occasion our feelings of sympathy and admiration. Since then, the development of laboratory research and biochemical techniques has led to further progress in important areas of testicular biology. Thus incontestable histophysiological evidence of some basic mechanism operating in the male gonad has been elucidated. This is with special reference to the cellular and subcellular morphology of germinal epithelium and interstitial Leydig cells, and to the final products of both structures, sperm cells and male hormones and the feedback phenomena with the hypophysis.

Apart from the advanced studies on the relationship between Leydig cells and steroidogenesis, we are just at the beginning of our understanding of: a) the dynamics of the human spermatogenic process which is replacing the old wavecycle concept of classical cytologists; b) the sustentacular and nutritional function of Sertoli cells related to germinal cells and spermatozoa; c) the functional significance of the physico-chemical composition of seminiferous tubular wall structures; d) the development and fate of sex chromosomes in the germinal cells; e) some histochemical aspects of spermatogenesis; f) the effects of follicle stimulating and luteinizing hormones and some steroids on the development of germinal and Sertoli cells and interstitial tissue.

Unfortunately, an extension of these approaches is restricted by the small quantity of tissue present in biopsies. However, it is eagerly hoped that more refined instrumentation and methodology will prove rewarding in a more profound analysis of human testicular structure and function, as has occurred with the animal testis. Tissue organ culture techniques, which permit an observation of the direct effect of different agents, molecular biological aspects of cell populations, the metabolic pathway of germinal and Sertoli cell function, the role of tubular wall structures and Sertoli cells in the intratubular diffusion of different molecules, the relationship between Leydig cell steroids and germinal epithelium, cellular and subcellular receptors for the gonadotropic hormones, hypothalamus-hypophyseal-testicular interrelation, radioimmunoassays for FSH and LH, and hemodynamic aspects of testicular function are some of the topics which urgently need the attention of investigators.

This is precisely what this Workshop Conference is intended to do. It is not an exhaustive review of what is known today about the physiology and pathology of the human testis, but is to add a new dimension to our knowledge of this gland by outlining new evidence and provoking additional thoughts and inspiration for further studies. This is the reason why other pathological disorders of the testis, such as inflammation, congenital abnormalities, infections and tumors have been deliberately excluded. On the other hand some other recent approaches which are beginning to contribute to the elucidation of disturbances in the mechanism of spermatogenesis have been added, i.e., immunological factors, chromosomal anomalies of germinal cells, and other topics concerning the significance of seminal plasma chemical composition as an indicator of the adnexal gland function. It was also fully realized that the introduction of a subject related to the assessment of gonadotropin therapy in the still debatable field of male sterility, should be at present of paramount importance. This appears more than justified when it is considered that almost half of infertility in couples is due to the male factor.

It is our intention that all these topics will form a solid guide for present and future fundamental studies, which in turn will provide a better understanding of why and how testicular structure and function may become abnormal. Needless to say the benefit of this view will lead to a rational approach in the study of the heterogenous group of sterile patients, or what today is considered equally important, as a counterpart, to new tools for male contraception.

Finally, the aim of this Workshop Conference was not only to have the pleasure of meeting experts on a subject of common interest, but also to demonstrate that the integrated efforts of embryologists, biologists, geneticists, biochemists, pathologists and endocrinologists will be of great help in substantially increasing the information at present available on the physiology and pathology of the human testis.

LIST OF PARTICIPANTS

Cesar Bergada, M. D.
Director of Research
Department of Endocrinology
Hospital de Ninos
Gallo 1330
Buenos Aires, Argentina

Professor Mario Hector Burgos, M. D.
Instituto de Histologia y Embriologia
Facultad de Ciencias Medicas
Universidad Nacional de Cuyo
Casilla de Correo 56
Mendoza, Argentina

Ann C. Chandley, Ph. D.
Research Scientist
Medical Research Council
Clinical and Population Cytogenetics Research Unit
Western General Hospital
Crewe Road
Edinburgh 4, Scotland

A. Kent Christensen, Ph. D.
Associate Professor of Anatomy
Stanford University
Department of Anatomy
Stanford School of Medicine
Stanford, California 94305

Professor Yves Clermont, Ph. D.
Department of Anatomy
McGill University
Strathcona Medical Building
3640 University Street
Montreal 112, Quebec, Canada

Michel Courot
Maitre de Recherches
Institut National de la Recherche Agronomique
Lab. Physiologie de la Reproduction
37 Nouzilly - France

Joseph R. Davis, M. D., Ph. D.
Professor of Pharmacology
Loyola University Stritch School of Medicine
2160 South First Avenue
Maywood, Illinois 60153

Professor Egon R. Diczfalusy, M. D.
Director, Reproductive Endocrinology Research Unit
Swedish Medical Research Council
Karolinska Sjukhuset
Stockholm 60, Sweden

Piero Donini, M. D.
Director of Research Laboratories
Istituto Farmacologico Serono
Via Casilina 125
Rome, Italy

C. E. Ford, D. Sc., F.R.S.
Head, Cytogenetics Group
Medical Research Council Radiobiology Unit
Harwell, Didcott
Berkshire, United Kingdom

Irving I. Geschwind, Ph. D.
Professor of Animal Science
Department of Animal Science
University of California
Davis, California 95616

Carl G. Heller, M. D., Ph. D.
Director, Division of Reproductive Physiology
Pacific Northwest Research Foundation
1102 Columbia Street
Seattle, Washington 98104

Bryan Hudson, M. D., Ph. D.
Professor of Medicine
Monash University
Prince Henry's Hospital
St. Kilda Road
Melbourne
Victoria 3004, Australia

Jan E. Jirasek, M. D., D. Sc.
Assistant Professor of Obstetrics and Gynecology
University of Minnesota Medical School
Minneapolis, Minnesota 55455

Svend G. Johnsen, M. D.
Hormone Department
Statens Seruminstitut
Copenhagen S., Denmark

Professor Alfred Jost
Director, Laboratory of Comparative Physiology
Faculty of Sciences
9. quai Saint-Bernard
Paris 5e, 75 - France

Marian Jutisz, Ph. D.
Research Director in C.N.R.S.
Laboratoire de Physiologie Cellulaire
College de France
11 Place Marcelin Berthelot
75 - Paris V, France

Juan Carlos Lavieri, M. D.
Chief Laboratory of Andrology
Centro de Investigaciones Sobre Reproduccion
Facultad de Medicina
Paraguay 2155,10° Piso
Buenos Aires, Argentina

Mortimer B. Lipsett, M. D.
Chief, Endocrinology Branch
National Cancer Institute
National Institutes of Health
Bethesda, Maryland 20014

Professor Bruno Lunenfeld, M. D.
Director, Institute of Endocrinology
Tel-Hashomer Government Hospital
Tel-Hashomer, Israel

John MacLeod, Ph. D.
Professor of Anatomy
Cornell University Medical College
Department of Anatomy
1300 York Avenue
New York, New York 10021

Professor Roberto E. Mancini, M. D.
Director
Centro de Investigaciones Sobre Reproduccion
Facultad de Medicina
Paraguay 2155, 10° Piso
Buenos Aires, Argentina

Professor Thaddeus Mann, M. D., Sc. D., Ph. D., F.R.S.
Professor of Physiology of Reproduction
Director, Unit of Reproductive Physiology and Biochemistry
University of Cambridge
Downing Street
Cambridge, England

Luciano Martini, M. D.
Professor of Pharmacology
Institute of Pharmacology
University of Milan
Via Vanvitelli, 32
20129 Milano, Italy

Anthony R. Means, Ph. D.
Assistant Professor
Vanderbilt University School of Medicine
Department of Obstetrics and Gynecology
Nashville, Tennessee 37203

Susumu Ohno, D.V.M., Ph. D., D.Sc.
Chairman, Department of Biology
City of Hope Medical Center
1500 East Duarte Road
Duarte, California 91010

C. Alvin Paulsen, M. D.
Professor of Medicine
Chief, Division of Endocrinology
USPHS Hospital
University of Washington School of Medicine
P.O. Box 3145
Seattle, Washington 98114

Eugenia Rosemberg, M. D.
Research Director
Medical Research Institute of Worcester, Inc.
26 Queen Street
Worcester, Massachusetts 01610

Griff T. Ross, M. D., Ph. D.
Head, Endocrinology Service and
Assistant Chief, Endocrinology Branch
National Cancer Institute
National Institutes of Health
Building 10, Room 10B09
Bethesda, Maryland 20014

Professor Kenneth Savard, D. Sc.
Director, Endocrine Laboratory
University of Miami School of Medicine
Endocrine Laboratory
P.O. Box 875, Biscayne Annex
Miami, Florida 33152

Professor Carl Schirren, M. D.
Leiter der Andrologischen Abteilung
Universitatskrankenhaus Eppendorf
2 Hamburg 20, Martinistr. 52
Germany

Alberto J. Solari, M. D.
Centro de Investigaciones en Reproduccion
Facultad de Medicina
Paraguay 2155
Buenos Aires, Argentina

Anna Steinberger, Ph. D.
Associate Member, Division of Endocrinology and Reproduction
Research Laboratories
Albert Einstein Medical Center
York and Tabor Roads
Philadelphia, Pennsylvania 19141

Emil Steinberger, M. D.
Chairman, Division of Endocrinology and Reproduction
Research Laboratories
Albert Einstein Medical Center
York and Tabor Roads
Philadelphia, Pennsylvania 19141

Philip Troen, M. D.
Physician-in-Chief
Montefiore Hospital
3459 Fifth Avenue
Pittsburgh, Pennsylvania 15213

Oscar Vilar, M. D.
Associate Professor
Centro de Investigaciones en Reproduccion
Facultad de Medicina, 10 ° Piso
Paraguay 2155
Buenos Aires, Argentina

J.-P. Weniger
Docteur de l'Universite de Strasbourg
Maitre de Recherche au Centre National de la Recherche Scientifique
Universite de Strasbourg
rue de l'Universite, No. 12
67 Strasbourg, France

Emil Witschi, M. D., Ph. D.
The Population Council
Bio-Medical Division
The Rockefeller University
York Avenue and 66th Street
New York, New York 10021

CONTENTS

CHAPTER III

CYTOGENETICS OF SPERMATOGENESIS

CHAPTER IV

REGULATION OF TESTICULAR FUNCTION

SECTION 1: ROLE OF THE HYPOTHALAMUS

SECTION 2: TESTICULAR-PITUITARY INTERRELATIONSHIP

SECTION 3: GONADOTROPINS, PURIFICATION AND MEASUREMENT

SECTION 4: METABOLIC EFFECTS OF GONADOTROPINS

SECTION 5: INFLUENCE OF GONADOTROPINS ON TESTICULAR FUNCTION

CHAPTER V

TESTICULAR STEROIDOGENESIS

CHAPTER VI

NON-HORMONAL FACTORS INFLUENCING SPERM PRODUCTION AND TRANSPORT

CHAPTER VII

GONADOTROPIN THERAPY

SECTION 1: TREATMENT OF HYPOPITUITARISM

SECTION 2: TREATMENT OF ADULT SEMINIFEROUS TUBULAR FAILURE

CHAPTER I

EMBRYOLOGY OF THE MALE REPRODUCTIVE TRACT

EMBRYOLOGY OF THE TESTIS

Emil Witschi

The Population Council, Rockefeller University,
New York 10021

Since the gonochoristic higher vertebrates evolved from hermaphrodite ancestors, it seems justified to turn to surviving primitive species in order to gain an understanding of genetic and developmental problems of sex determination. About a hundred years ago it was first realized that rudimentary hermaphrodism still occurs in some local races of the European brown frog (Rana temporaria). The males start out differentiating ovaries which, usually before maturing, transform into testes. It was left to me to find out that in a low percentage the change is still incomplete at the adult stage. Artificial self fertilization and outcrossing of three hermaphrodites to males and females of truly gonochoristic race could be made. As far as I know these are the only reported and proven cases of fully fertile tetrapod vertebrates (1).

Gross differences between X and Y chromosomes, as seen in the human, have not been found in any amphibian species. But in frogs with gonochorism a first step in the evolution of sex chromosomes is taken, showing incomplete conjugation of the fourth largest chromosomes in meiosis and precocious separation in the first meiotic anaphase (2,3). The comparative study of gonad development in hermaphrodite and purely gonochoristic frogs reveals a distinct composite of cortex and medulla. The observation that germ cells of identical constitution become eggs in the cortex and sperms in the medulla led to the assumption of specialized local environments and thus, to the inductor theory of sex differentiation (4). Germ cells, being capable of becoming male or female, evidently carry both female (F) and male (M) genes as do the somatic cells of cortex and medulla. Cortical environment activates F genes; medullary environment activates M genes. Carrying this trend of thought a little further, the cytoplasms of somatic inductor cells appear to produce substances which pass through cell and nuclear membranes and activate the corresponding F or M genes. This will start chains of further reactions resulting next in female differentiation of germ cells and somatic elements of the cortex and correspondingly in male differentiation in the medulla. In hermaphrodites simultaneous differentiation may occur in both systems. In gonochorists prevalence of one or the other is usually determined by genetic factors. The names corticin and medullarin have been given to the cortical and medullary inductor substances. The inductor theory has survived over half a century having adapted to special conditions in mammals, and was only rarely criticized adversely (5).

As to the chemical nature of the inductive substance we know nothing. Evidence, however, demonstrates quite clearly that even before the establishment of indifferent gonads the preprimordia of cortex and medulla are astonishingly active producers of attraction substances, telopherons (possibly telopherases), which guide the migration of primordial germ cells from dorsal endoderm and splanchnopleure to the gonadal site (6). Clever experiments by Dubois (7) show that in chick embryos attraction is at a maximum during the third day (sex differentiation occurs at 5½ days). At this time the presumptive gonad tissues are even able to free and capture germ cells that were already embedded in graft ovaries of 7½ days and in graft testes of an age up to 13 days. In some gonochorists cortex and medulla exhibit separate attraction, as is clearly seen in birds with asymmetric distribution of the germ cells (8). In Triturus the telopherons show sexual differentiation, the male tending to impede germ cell migration in female parabiontic partners (9). Should telopherons be identical with corticin and medullarin which are produced by the same complexes of cells? There is no sure answer to this question, though the experiments of Dubois suggest an end to telopheron production before the stage of sex differentiation.

Since amphibians lend themselves to sex reversal and the African frog Xenopus can readily be bred under laboratory conditions, we have made available male as well as female breeders of either ZZ, SW or WW genetic constitution. This makes it possible to produce all-male and all-female offspring in practically unlimited numbers. Male and female cultures have been challenged with two questions. Firstly, what can you do with offered hormones? Secondly, what can you do with a supply of steroid-precursors? In these investigations I was joined by Giovanni Chieffi, Edward Dale, Heinz Breuer and Kazuya Mikamo (10,11,12). The answers are presented in Tables 1 and 2. Estrogens and androgens are degraded in the livers to less active substances and eventually are completely denatured. This can be done in the early developing livers even before sex glands have become organized (Table 1). On the other hand, labelled precursors remain largely unchanged and no C_{19} and

Table 1. Catabolism of Sex Steroids

INCUBATION WITH C19 AND C18 (4-^{14}C) STEROIDS

Substrates	Xenopus	Metabolites
Dehydroepi-androsterone	Larvae 25c	Δ^5Androstenediol no Δ^4-3Ketosteroids
Testosterone	Larvae 25b to Met. 31 Adult Liver	Androstenedione Androsterone Androstanediol Androstanedione Hxdroxy Compounds Polar Fractions
17 β-Estradiol	Larvae 25a to 25d	Estrone Estriol 6α -Hydroxyestrone 15α -Hydroxyestrone

Met: animals in metamorphosis, Added numbers in second column indicate standard stages of development. Morphologically recognizable sex differentiation occurs at Stage 27.

Table 2. Steroidogenesis from (4-^{14}C) Labelled Precursors

Material	Substrate	Metabolites	%S	Enzymes
L.25c	Acetate	no C19 Steroids		no Desmolases
L.25c	Cholesterin	"		"
L.25c	Pregnenolone	"		"
L.25b	17α-Hydroxy-	Corticoids		Hydroxylases
L.25d	progesterone	Cortisol		"
Testes	17α-Hydroxy-	Androst-		
L.29/30	progesterone	enedione	.030	C17-C20 Desmolase:
Met.31	"	"	.072	17 -Hydroxyproges-
Met.33	"	"	.064	terone C17-C20-lyase
Fr.3mo.	"	"	.065	"
Frog ad.	"	" and Testosterone		
Ovaries	17α-Hydroxy-	Androstene		C17-C20 Desmolase
L.29/30	progesterone	dione	.029	"
Met.31	"	"	.026	"
Met.33	"	"	.035	"
Frog ad.	"	" and 17β -Estradiol		"

L: larvae, Met: animals in metamorphosis, %S: percent substrate radioactivity per animal, mo: months of age, ad: adult, added numbers indicate standard stages of development.Morphologically recognizable sex differentiation occurs at Stage 27.

C_{18} steroids are formed before or during sexual differentiation.

In short, after the supply of 17α-hydroxyprogesterone, which is a likely natural precursor, androstenedione appears near the end of larval life, simultaneously in female and in male cultures. Estradiol and testosterone can be identified only after metamorphosis. Both increase considerably at five to seven months with the approach of sexual maturity. Evidently these findings lend no support to claims that estradiol and testosterone are the chemical inductors of sexual differentiation of the gonads.

The assumption that ovary and testis do not only produce steroid hormones but also start differentiating themselves as a consequence of induction each by its own hormone, still has some strong defenders (13). A review of pertinent literature shows that the search for fetal and embryonic sex hormones in other vertebrates is always based on already differentiated gonads, usually of quite advanced stages. The most valuable series is one on male rats presented by Noumura et al. (14). It starts with testes of 13½ day old rats. They can not be more than half a day beyond initial differentiation. After incubation with tritiated progresterone almost infinitesimal traces of testosterone were found on this (stage 28) and the next day (stage 30). A total of 336 testes yielded 0.1 mμM testosterone and 0.03 mμM androstenedione. After another day (stage 32) conversion rates rose twentyfold and from here until birth there was a steady but only modest increase. Comparison with Xenopus shows that sex differentiation in relation to anatomic body conformation (the basis of standard stages) occurs slightly later (stage 27). Apparently, the first steroid formed is androstenedione but conversion to testosterone follows immediately in the rat, whereas it is delayed considerably in Xenopus. Other reports on mammals (15,16,17,18) give qualitatively similar results but on relatively late fetal stages. Of interest is the failure to find estrogens in ovaries even at midpregnancy (17,18). Since the human fetus is flooded with high concentrations of placental estrogens, this may be a matter of secondary hormonal suppression.

Extensive work on chick embryos by a Paris school has given the remarkable result that female embryos of seven or more days, if explanted in adjusted nutritional media for one to three or more days, release estradiol and estrone in appreciable quantities but no androgens (19). This is surprising for not only in Xenopus but also in other amphibians (20) and in mammals (18) estrogen synthesis very commonly follows that of androgens. The particular pathway for chick embryos has essentially been clarified now by Haffen and Cedard (21). Incubation with radio-labelled dehydroepiandrosterone (DHA) yields estrone and estradiol with female and testosterone with male embryos. The latter also produced minor amounts of estradiol. The females seem to synthesize estrone by short cut aromatisation of DHA.

Morphologic sex differentiation in the chick is recognizable at 5½ days (stage 30). Latent determination must precede this by another half-day (stage 28). Seven-day old embryos (stage 33) correspond developmentally to the metamorphosing Xenopus. However, even at this stage the sex type of gonads in freshly dissected embryos is difficult to assess. This, together with the rapid course of development during the first 10 days, has probably led to certain statements on specific hormone production preceding sexual differentiation (13). Critical consideration of all facts leads to the realization that the chemical nature of corticin and medullarin as also that of the telopherons and of all morphogenetic substances produced by gonad primordia remains unsolved.

As early as 1931 (22) the existence of an antagonism between cortex and medulla had come fully to light. First analyzed in cases of amphibian parabiosis, evidence was soon found throughout the vertebrate classes. Almost forgotten now are the classical experiments of Benoit, Zawadowsky, Padoa and Domm (ably reviewed by the last named) on partial castration of poultry (23). The operations simply remove the cortical repressor which in intact hens prevents hermaphrodite development. Sinistral ovariectomy permits complete testicular organization and growth of the right-side medullary rudiment. But incomplete operation, leaving in situ the left medulla, likewise is followed by development of a testis. Left as well as right "female testes" can fully maintain cock plumage and male-type combs. Spermatogenesis is complete even though the female sex chromosome arrangement is maintained. In some experiments Mintz and Wolff (24) had peeled off the cortices of ovaries of chick embryos aged 9 and 10 days and implanted the medullae into body cavities of indifferent second-day embryos. After 11 to 13 days well developed grafts had assumed a testicular structure.

A spectacular example of medullary-cortical antagonism is presented by freemartinism of cattle. In this case, however, the medulla of the male calf is the dominant system, suppressing the cortical development in the female twin. Contradicting the widely accepted interpretation of the Chicago school, I have early expressed the opinion that the blood-borne principle is not the androgenic steroid but a quite different type of medullary antagonist (25). It gives me great satisfaction that this view is now fully validated by recent experiments of Jost (26). They prove the inability of testosterone to inhibit ovarian development. Recognition of a second principle, a cortex inhibitor released by the testes of the bull twin, is strictly necessary.

The same anti-cortex factor finds application in female to male sex conversion in Xenopus. Testosterone administrations to larvae in no way impede ovarian development. But testis implants almost completely inhibit ovarian differentiation of the cortex. The medullary nodes, however, remain unaffected. Later removal of the implanted testis is followed by compensatory medullary development that often leads to the production of fertile males with testes of female ZW or WW constitution (27).

This now calls for a short consideration of the mechanism by which estrogens feminize genetic males (28). The experiment is successful only during the third week (larvae stage 25, 2.0 - 2.5 cm total length). Later administrations are without effect. The larvae develop like normal females. The medulla nodes do not enlarge but assume the female character. Does the estradiol during the short application stimulate the cortex or inhibit the medulla? We have come to assume the latter. This conclusion is supported by the effect observed after administration of the anti-androgen Cyproterone acetate.[1] If applied during the third week it somewhat irregularly damages the medullar nodules of male larvae which then become irregular hermaphrodites. It seems that here an initial tissue damage is set while with estradiol the genetically favored inductor - the M activating principle - is suppressed.

In 1953 zoologists and medical embryologists were startled by an announcement of Jost (29) that testicular steroids only stimulate male secondary sex characters but do not stop growth of the oviducts nor cause their regression. The possibility was considered that the fetal testis may produce a second, inhibiting, factor. We shall probably hear today more about this from Dr. Jost himself. In the meanwhile, I cannot forsake the opportunity of presenting the amphibian version of the same situation. In Xenopus oviducts develop in males and females immediately following metamorphosis. Left and right ones join in a short unpaired uterine segment before opening into the cloaca. Development continues for 7 months. Then, while the testes start full spermatogenesis, the oviducts regress and soon disappear. If, however, the males are castrated before the seventh month, the oviducts persist indefinitely. Injections of testosterone do not reduce but rather stimulate them. Their reduction can only be brought about by implanted testes. Step by step we have come to realize that testes are not simply manufacturing sperms and testosterone. Exercising their important functions in development and reproduction, they maintain correlations by messengers and receptors, the chemical nature of which is still largely unknown.

I have dwelt largely on amphibian work. In a time when geneticists earn the highest honors occupying themselves with bacteria and molds, an apology should not be expected. Embryology,

1 supplied by Schering AG Berlin, through the courtesy of President K. H. Kimbel, New York.

endocrinology and anatomy of the sex organs remain essentially the same in all tetrapods in spite of complications added in amniotes and particularly in mammals. Why then can we not change sex in mammals as in amphibians? There is no full answer. Certainly a major impediment is the higher evolution of the cytogenetic sex determining mechanisms. However, the defenses are not impregnable as shown by the possibility of full spermatogenesis in poulards with female sets of sex chromosomes; or the permanent masculinization of the mode of secretion of hypophyseal gonadotropins by implantation of a testis in the newborn female rat. A broadened knowledge of existing mechanisms will provide new approaches leading to the control of reproductive processes in the mammalian field.

REFERENCES

1. Witschi, E., J.Exp. Zool., 54: 157, 1929.
2. Witschi, E., J.ind. Abst. Vererb., 29: 31, 1922.
3. Witschi, E. and Opitz, J.M. In Intersexuality, ed. Overzier, Academic Press, 1963.
4. Witschi, E., Arch. mikr. Anat., 86: 1, 1914.
5. Wolff, E., Ann.Fac. Sc. Clermont-Ferrand, 26: 17, 1965.
6. Witschi, E., Carnegie Contr. Embr., 32: 67, 1948.
7. Dubois, R., C. R. Acad. Sci.(Paris), 260: 5108, 1965.
8. Witschi, E., Amer.J. Anat., 56: 119, 1935.
9. Witschi, E. and McCurdy, H.M., Proc. Soc. Exp. Biol. Med., 26: 655, 1925.
10. Rao, G.S., Breuer, H. and Witschi, E., Experientia, 24: 1258, 1968.
11. Rao, G.S., Breuer, H. and Witschi, E., Gen. Comp. Endocr. 12: 119, 1969.
12. Witschi, E. In press.
13. Wolff, E., Haffen, K. and Scheib, D., Ann. Histochim, 11: 353, 1966.
14. Noumura, T., Weisz, J. and Lloyd, C.W., Endocrinology, 78: 245, 1966.
15. Acevedo, J.F., Axelrod, L.R., Ishikawa, E. and Takaki, F., J. Clin. Endocr., 23: 885, 1963.
16. Lipsett, M.B. and Tullner, W.W., Endocrinology, 77: 273, 1965.
17. Bloch, E., Endocrinology, 74: 833, 1964.
18. Jungmann, R.A. and Schweppe, J.S., J. Clin. Endocr., 28: 1599, 1968.
19. Weniger, J.P., C. R. Acad. Sci. (Paris) 261: 809, 1965.
20. Ozon, R., Gen. Comp. Endocr., 8: 214, 1967.
21. Haffen, K. and Cedard, L., Gen. Comp. Endocr., 11: 220, 1968.
22. Witschi, E., J. Exp. Zool., 58: 113, 1931.
23. Domm, L.V., In Sex and Internal Secretions, ed. Allen, E., Williams and Wilkins, Baltimore, p 227, 1939.
24. Mintz, B. and Wolff, E., J. Exp. Zool., 126: 511, 1954.
25. Witschi, E. In Sex and Internal Secretions, ed. Allen, E. Williams and Wilkins, Baltimore, p 145, 1939.

26. Jost, A., Excerpta Medica International Congress Series, 132: 74, 1966.
27. Mikamo, K. and Witschi, E., Genetics, 48: 1411, 1963.
28. Witschi, E., Arch. Anat. Micr. Morph. Exp., 39: 215, 1950.
29. Jost, A., Recent Progr. Hormone Res., 8: 379, 1953.

HORMONAL FACTORS IN THE DEVELOPMENT OF THE MALE GENITAL SYSTEM

Alfred Jost

Laboratory of Comparative Physiology, Faculty of Sciences, Paris, France

During normal development, sex differences appear, in accordance with the initial genetic sex,at the level of many structures, namely the gonads, the genital tract and external genitalia, the mammary glands, the nervous structures in the brain controlling hypophyseal gonadal stimulating function or mediating sexual behavior and many other body secondary sex characteristics. Testicular organogenesis precedes in time any other sex mark and the testes soon take over the control of the other sex characteristics. In female fetuses, ovarian organogenesis lags behind and many fundamental feminine physiological features do not depend upon ovarian development. There is a basic lack of symmetry in the developmental processes in males and in females, and until the age of prepuberal changes, the testis is the active sex differentiator (1,2).

In the frame of the hormonal theory of sex differentiation, it has long been assumed not only that somatic sexual characteristics develop under the control of gonadal hormones, but that the initial sexual differentiation of the gonads themselves is imposed by hormones or diffusible inductors produced inside the gonads. The latter part of the concept originally arose from evidence of partial gonadal sex reversal in freemartins in cattle and in experimental heterosexual combinations in Urodele amphibians. It is noteworthy that in both cases ovarian changes toward testicular organogenesis were imposed secondarily in gonads which were already marked as presumptive ovaries (3).

The present paper will be limited to mammals since basic differences between mammals and for instance, birds, are likely (4).

HORMONAL FACTORS IN GONADAL DEVELOPMENT

The undifferentiated gonadal primordium appears on the internal side of the mesonephros, in the vicinity of the glomeruli. It is made of cells of local origin (their derivation cannot be discussed here) and of primordial germ cells which originate in endodermic organs and migrate toward the gonadal anlage. The primordial germ cells most likely obey a chemotaxis, and are attracted by a substance released by some gonadal cells. The identity of these cells (the presumptive sustentacular or follicular cells which throughout life remain associated with the germ cells are obvious candidates) and the biochemical nature of their effect remain unknown. Neither androgens given to the mother animal during early pregnancy (for instance high dosages of methyltestosterone given to pregnant rabbits from day 7 on (5)) nor the antiandrogen cyproterone acetate given to pregnant rats from day 10 or 11 on (up to 100 mg/day) (6,7) prevented the germ cells from reaching the gonads in seemingly normal numbers. Unless the androgen or the antiandrogen is not transferred from mother to fetus at early stages of pregnancy, it appears that androgens are not likely to play a role in the migration of the germ cells.

The series of organogenetic changes which produce either a testis or an ovary from the early anlage are yet poorly understood, even on purely descriptive bases. A fortiori the mechanisms, especially the humoral or hormonal factors involved, remain conjectural or unknown.

There is a common consensus that testicular organogenesis precedes ovarian organogenesis, and that at first presumptive ovaries are recognized as such mainly because they are not testes. True ovarian organogenesis characterized by follicular formation and delineation of the ovarian stroma is a late event. Some triggering mechanism seems to divert the male gonad from this slow ovarian evolution and to impose a more rapid and early testicular differentiation.

Morphological data. According to a vast literature and to preliminary personal observations in calf, rabbit and rat fetuses some of the first steps in testicular organogenesis can be summarized as follows:

Testicular differentiation becomes first recognizable in the gonadal anlage when a process of cellular differentiation and segregation separates: a)cordlike strands of germ cells and presumptive sustentacular cells which aggregate at a certain distance from the superficial coelomic layer and b) the presumptive intertubular material. In the former, the future seminiferous tubules, the cells soon increase in size and acquire larger cytoplasmic areas whereas the intertubular cells first remain packed and undifferentiated. The superficial layers of the testis (future tunica albuginea) are rapidly deprived of germ cells, perhaps because these cells moved toward the seminiferous tubules. In the inner part of the gonad near the mesonephric glomeruli, the presumptive rete testis is still morphologically undifferentiated but it becomes increasingly distinct.

Some time elapses before true interstitial or Leydig cells appear. In the human fetus separation of seminiferous tubules and intertubular cells begins at the stage of 15-17 mm, whereas Leydig cells showing their distinct characteristics under the electron microscope are just appearing in a 29 mm fetus (8), and they display 3 β-ol-steroid dehydrogenase activity in 30 mm fetuses. Similar time relations between the early appearance of the seminiferous cords and the later cytological and histochemical differentiation of the Leydig cells hold true in several species.

Hormonal factors in gonadal sex differentiation. The existence, the source or the role of hormonal agents governing testicular organogenesis in mammals still remain unknown.

The Leydig cells of the adult type, showing the tubular organization of the agranular endoplasmic reticulum, can hardly be concerned with the early testicular organogenesis since they differentiate at a later stage (8). Moreover, androgens given to pregnant mammals were never seen to impose testicular organogenesis on the primordium of female fetuses. To quote one experiment, androgens given in large amounts to pregnant cows did neither masculinize the ovaries of the female fetuses, nor reduce their ovaries to the freemartin condition, nor prevent premeiosis in the ovocytes, although they masculinized the external genitalia at an early stage (4,9). On the other hand, cyproterone acetate given from day 11 on to pregnant rabbits (80 mg/day) (9) or rats (up to 100 mg/day) (6,7) did not prevent testicular organogenesis. Similarly , in the human syndrome of "testicular feminization", testicular organogenesis occurs despite the admitted insensitivity of the tissues to androgens. Such observations do not favor the hypothesis that conventional androgens play any important role in the initial testicular organogenesis.

A converse question concerning the Leydig cells is: under which influence do they appear in the fetal testis? This has been studied very little so far: interstitial cells were observed to appear and to acquire 3 β-ol-dehydrogenase activity in vitro in rat testes taken from 14.5 day-old rat fetuses, a stage at which they still cannot be detected (10). Leydig cell differentiation thus could occur in the absence of a hypophyseal or extragonadal influence. Nonetheless, the further activity and thriving of the Leydig cells will depend upon the pituitary gland.

Pituitary hormones can hardly be expected to direct the sexual orientation of the gonadal primordium and they do not seem to be necessary for this process. Testes and ovaries are found in infants congenitally deprived of their anterior pituitary in Guernsey calves suffering from hypophyseal aplasia or in mesonephric + gonadal primordium of mice embryos cultivated in vitro (11). In the latter case eventual placental influences are also ruled out.

Another important point concerns intragonadal influences on germ cells. In the testis these cells do not enter into premeiosis until prepuberty, whereas ovocytes display the first premeiotic changes before the definitive ovarian structure is established, and before they are enclosed in primordial follicles and stopped at the diplotene phase (12). Examples of complete sex reversal of germ cells in amphibians or birds suggest an environmental control of their outcome. It is still unknown whether a stimulus for meiosis is acting in the ovary or whether a meiosis-preventing influence prevails in the testis, or both as suggested by Witschi (13). In some invertebrates the ovogenetic evolution is autodifferentiating whereas spermatogenesis is imposed by an extragonadal hormone (14). In the mammalian testes the germ cells are precociously confined in the seminiferous tubules and surrounded by sustentacular cells; it is not unlikely that this leads to their control.

The mechanism of gonadal differentiation remains an open problem. The leading cells in the initial changes are not yet identified. These cells could belong either to the intertubular cells (immature Leydig cells?), to the rete anlage or they could be the sustentacular cells. The role of the germ cells themselves has also to be elucidated. Reciprocal and successive influences can be suspected to exist in the differentiation of the two major types of somatic testicular cells, the Sertoli cells which will impose spermatogenetic metamorphosis upon the germ cells and the Leydig cells which will release androgens.

HORMONAL CONTROL OF THE DEVELOPMENT OF THE GENITAL TRACT

Testicular control of the genital tract. Castration of 19-day old rabbit fetuses in utero showed that in the absence of testes (i.e., in normal or in castrated females and in castrated males) all the body sexual characters become feminine; complementary experiments reinforced the conclusion that the basic developmental trend of the gonadless body is essentially feminine, and that the testes impose masculinity and repress femininity (1, 15, 16,2).

The fetal testes cause the retrogression of the Mullerian ducts (presumptive uteri and tubes which persist in the absence of the testicular influence), stimulate the development of the epididymes, vasa deferentia and seminal vesicles from the Wolffian ducts (these ducts retrogress in the absence of the testes) and impose masculinity on those parts of the genital tract which derive from a common undifferentiated primordium (derivatives of the urogenital sinus, and external genitalia which become feminine if not masculinized by the fetal testes).

These results were confirmed in vivo on mice (17) and in vitro; for instance the Mullerian ducts persist in parts of the genital tract of male fetuses cultivated in vitro unless they are exposed to the action of a fetal testis in mouse or rat experiments (18).

Androgens such as testosterone can replace fetal testes in their masculinizing effects but fail to inhibit the Mullerian ducts (1,16,4). It was surmised that the fetal testis produces two kinds of morphogenetic substances: a Mullerian duct inhibitor, which still has to be uncovered and a masculinizing factor probably similar to androgens. Early testicular synthesis of androgens has been amply demonstrated in rabbit (19) and rat (20) fetuses as well as in other species. The concept of a dual testicular control fits most of the clinical cases of genital abnormalities (2). It also permits one to interpret the prominent effects of the antiandrogen, cyproterone acetate, in rabbit fetuses (21,9). Male fetuses of treated does develop no masculine character probably because cyproterone acetate opposed the fetal androgens. In the meantime their Mullerian ducts retrogress, presumably because the antiandrogen does not oppose the testicular Mullerian inhibitor.

In male rats the effect of cyproterone acetate (C.A.) is not as clear since it does not impair the development of the wolffian ducts and seminal vesicles (6). This lack of effect might be due either to lack of placental transfer of C.A. to the fetus before day 18 or to the inability of C.A. to antagonize the effects of the hormone produced at that stage by the fetal testis (6). In order to further analyze this problem, experiments were carried out in another way (7). Pregnant rats of the Sherman strain were given testosterone propionate (T.P.) alone (2.5 mg/day) or T.P. (2.5 or 10 mg/day) plus C.A. (25 mg/day)and the effects on the female fetuses were studied. In seven female fetuses who received only testosterone, Wolffian ducts and seminal vesicles which were more or less perfect were present. In twelve females who received testosterone (2.5 or 10 mg/day) plus C.A., both the wolffian ducts (excepting inconstant anterior remnants) and the seminal vesicles were absent. Thus at the level of the wolffian derivatives the antiandrogen antagonized high doses of testosterone in females, but it fails to antagonize the secretion of the fetal testis (even if the mother is given 100 mg C.A./day). This difference still has to be explained; it could suggest that the testis of the fetal rat produces on day 18 some hormone which is not antagonized by cyproterone acetate.

Pituitary control of testicular function. Hypophysioprivia affects testicular activity on the genital tract to varying degrees in different species (22).

In rabbits, hypophysectomy by decapitation carried out before the onset of body sex differentiation (on day 19), does not completely stop testicular activity since the anterior parts of the sex ducts are largely normal, but it introduces a definite testicular insufficiency which is conspicuous at the level of the prostate, external genitalia and interstitial cells. Restoration of development is achieved in those fetuses given gonadotropins (23).

In mouse and rat fetuses, absence of the pituitary gland does not prevent masculine organogenesis, nor the multiplication of the germ cells (24), but the synthesis of testosterone has been reported to be reduced at term in the testes of those fetuses who were decapitated on day 16.5 (20). It would appear that during the period covering the major sexual organogenetic processes (days 16 to 19 in rats), and even in the absence of the pituitary, the fetal testes produce enough of their hormone to ensure masculine development.

In human infants congenitally deprived of their pituitary gland, masculinization of the genital tract takes place, but in some instances a small penis or small testicles have been recorded. It is uncertain whether during the period of organogenesis of the genital tract, the human fetal testis needs gonadotropic stimulation or if it is stimulated by the chorionic gonadotropins of the mother which are especially high at that stage of pregnancy. During the second half of pregnancy the fetal testis undoubtedly needs pituitary stimulation for normal functioning (details in 22).

<u>Role of the hypothalamus in hypophyseal gonadal stimulating activity</u>. The fetal hypothalamo-hypophyseal relations have received little attention so far. Experiments performed on fetuses deprived of their hypothalamus by a surgical encephalectomy which leaves the pituitary gland in situ (22,25,26) could be compared with observations made on human anencephalic infants whose anterior pituitary suffers from disturbed or absent hypothalamic connections. In the rat fetus the pituitary corticostimulating activity is more strictly dependent upon the hypothalamus than is the thyrotropic activity. The same situation seems to prevail in the human anencephalic fetuses (26).

In male anencephalic fetuses masculinization is complete. However, hypoplastic testes, reduced number of interstitial cells (27) and inconstant hypoplasia of the penis and scrotum (28) have been observed. The condition of the male genital tract in these infants thus resembles that found in infants without pituitary glands; in both cases sexual differentiation of the genital tract which occurs before the 9th or 10th week is normal. This may be due to testicular stimulation by chorionic gonadotropin. Thus in hypopituitarism and anencephalia, testicular deficiency occurs at a later developmental stage. In the case of the anencephalic fetuses the anterior pituitary might suffer from a lack of hypothalamic influence during the second part of pregnancy (29).

Experiments pertaining to this problem were made on the rabbit since in that species hypophysioprivia produces testicular deficiency (23). Preliminary results (25) will be summarized. Rabbit fetuses were encephalectomized on days 17 to 19 and studied on day 28. Despite the absence of the hypothalamus the pituitary gland differentiated and the genital tract developed almost normally in nine of these fetuses, whereas it was abnormal in three fetuses of the same strain which were decapitated on day 19. The gonadal stimulating activity of the pituitary is not depressed even if the hypothalamus is removed as early as day 17 or 18.

In contradistinction to these experiments the genital tract was of the decapitate type in two spontaneously abnormal male fetuses (anencephaly and otocephaly) collected in another strain of rabbits in which the pituitary gland was present but deprived of hypothalamic connections. Furthermore, the pituitary gland was strikingly congested, and rather small in one of them. It still is difficult to assess whether the difference between the two groups of fetuses can be accounted for by species differences in the onset of functional hypothalamo-hypophyseal relationships or by other factors. These points need further research.

CONCLUSION

We still do not know the hormonal or inductive factors which impose early testicular organogenesis upon the gonadal primordium and appropriate function of the cells within the seminiferous tubules and intertubular spaces. It is obvious that the differentiated testis soon becomes the major source of androgens. But the differentiating testis also releases substances the effect of which cannot be duplicated by conventional androgens. The fetal testis provokes the retrogression of the Mullerian ducts; it inhibits ovarian growth and differentiation when fetal testes and ovaries are grown together either in vitro (30) or in vivo (31). In heterosexual twin calf fetuses, the testis is most likely responsible for the freemartin effect. In the latter case ovarian and Mullerian inhibition begins almost simultaneously. From a chronological point of view it is not inconceivable that both effects might be produced by the same testicular factor (9). Such problems still await solution and it certainly would not be wise to restrict research in fetal testicular endocrinology to testosterone or akin androgens of the adult type.

REFERENCES

1. Jost, A., Arch. Anat. Micr. Morph. Exp. 36: 271, 1947.
2. Jost, A., In Hermaphroditism, Genital Anomalies and Related Endocrine Disorders, ed. Jones, H. W., and Scott, W. W., Williams and Wilkins, Baltimore, 2nd ed. in press, 1969.

3. Jost, A., Phil. Trans. Roy. Soc., in press, 1970.
4. Jost, A., In Organogenesis, eds. De Haan, R. L., and Ursprung, H., Holt, Rinehart and Winston, New York p 611, 1965.
5. Jost, A., Arch. Anat. Micr. Morph. Exp. 36: 242, 1947.
6. Jost, A., Research on Steroids, 3: 207, 1967.
7. Jost, A., Unpublished data.
8. Pelliniemi, L. J., and Niemi, M., Z. Zellforsch., 99: 507, 1969.
9. Jost, A., Excerpta Medica Foundation International Congress Series No. 132, 74, 1966.
10. Picon, R., Arch. Anat. Micr. Morph. Exp., 56: 281, 1967.
11. Wolff, Et., C. R. Acad. Sci. (Paris), 234: 1712, 1952.
12. Ohno, S., and Smith, J. B., Cytogenetics, 3: 324, 1964.
13. Witschi, E., In The Biochemistry of Animal Development, ed. Weber, R., Vol. 2, Academic Press, New York, p 193, 1967.
14. Streiff, W., Ann. Endocr. (Paris), 28: 641, 1967.
15. Jost, A., Gynec. Obstet. (Paris), 49: 44, 1950.
16. Jost, A., Recent Progr. Hormone Res., 8: 379, 1953.
17. Raynaud, A., and Frilley, M., Ann. Endocr. (Paris), 8: 400, 1947.
18. Picon, R., Arch. Anat. Micr. Morph. Exp., 58: 1, 1969.
19. Lipsett, M. B., and Tullner, W. W., Endocrinology, 77: 273, 1965.
20. Noumura, T., Weisz, J., and Lloyd, C. W., Endocrinology, 78: 245, 1966.
21. Elger, W., Arch. Anat. Micr. Morph. Exp. 55: 657, 1966.
22. Jost, A., In The Pituitary Gland, eds. Harris, G. W., and Donovan, B. T., vol. 2, Butterworths, London, p 299, 1966.
23. Jost, A., Arch. Anat. Micr. Morph. Exp. 40: 247, 1951.
24. Creasy, R. K., and Jost, A., Arch. Anat. Micr. Morph. Exp. 55: 561, 1966.
25. Jost, A., Colloque Neuroendocrinologie. Paris: CNRS, in press, 1969.
26. Jost, A., and Geloso, A., C. R. Acad. Sci. (Paris), 265: 625, 1967.
27. Zondek, L. H., and Zondek, T., Biol. Neonat., 8: 329, 1965.
28. Bearn, J. G., Lancet, 2: 464, 1959.
29. Bearn, J. G., Excerpta Medica Foundation International Congress Series No. 157, 21, 1968.
30. Holyoke, E. A., and Beber, B. A., Science, 128: 1082, 1958.
31. MacIntyre, M. N., Anat. Rec., 124: 27, 1956.

THE RELATIONSHIP BETWEEN DIFFERENTIATION OF THE TESTICLE, GENITAL DUCTS AND EXTERNAL GENITALIA IN FETAL AND POSTNATAL LIFE

Jan E. Jirasek

University of Minnesota Medical School, Minneapolis, Minnesota 55455

The purpose of this study is to elucidate the relationship between testicular differentiation, regression of the paramesonephric (Mullerian) duct system and masculinization of the external genitalia in normal human embryos and fetuses and in some male pseudohermaphrodites.

The results described are based on a study of 300 human embryos and fetuses from therapeutic abortions and from 35 male pseudohermaphrodites in which laparotomy was performed and whose testicles were subjected to histological and histochemical study.

1. RELATIONSHIP BETWEEN THE PRIMORDIAL GERM-CELLS (GONOCYTES) AND THE MESONEPHRIC RIDGES

Primordial germ-cells are histochemically recognized by high alkaline phosphatase activity and a considerable quantity of glycogen (1-5). The early entoderm, however, has the same histochemical properties and does not allow identification of germ-cells until the embryos show development of the chordomesodermal process (embryos of about 0.5 mm, 15 to 17 days SH*VII). In embryos showing differentiation of early somites (1.5-5 mm., 17-30 days, SHVIII-XII), the alkaline phosphatase and glycogen disappear from the entodermal cells of the gut, but remain high in primordial germ-cells. These cells begin to migrate from the gut-entoderm into the adjacent mesenchyme in embryos of about 1-2 mm (19 to 20 days, SH IX). Some migrating primordial germ-cells with long cytoplasmic processes are also present in the mesenchyme of the mesentery. Cytoplasmic processes suggest

*SH refers to Streeter's Horizons of differentiation of the human embryo.

the possible ameboid movement of these cells. These findings are in full agreement with the classical concept of Witschi (6).

Primordial germ-cells are regarded as a basic embryonal cell-line (7) and, to date, there is not a single human embryo known showing absence of these cells. Germ-cells were found in embryos of XO or XXY-chromosomal constitution (8) and in embryos showing severe malformations, such as posterior duplication (9). In embryos 5 to 8 mm (32 to 35 days, SH XIV), the primordial germ-cells begin to accumulate in the area of the future genital ridge in the medioventral part of the mesonephric ridge.

Mesonephric ridges in embryos 5 to 8 mm (32 to 35 days, SH XIV) are longitudinal folds on each side of the mesentery related to the development of the mesonephros. The differentiation of the mesonephric (Wolffian) duct has been described (10). Wolffian duct primordia originate from ectodermal material which invaginates from surface ectoderm lateral to somites 8 to 13 as glycogen-rich ectodermal buds which join the pronephric blastema. The epithelium of pronephric and mesonephric ducts is glycogen-rich and the pronephric and mesonephric blastema is glycogen-free (11). The mesenchyme of the mesonephric ridge originates from somites. The lateral surface of the mesonephric ridge is covered by a single-layered epithelium with a distinct basement membrane (mesoderm). The medial surface is covered by a layer of cells which are not separated from the underlying mesenchyme (mesoblast). There is an affinity between the mesoblastic cells of the genital ridge and the primordial germ-cells. A positive chemotropism between the germ-cells and mesoblastic cells has been proposed (12). However, if this chemotropism exists, its chemical nature is unknown.

2. THE INDIFFERENT GONAD (GENITAL RIDGE)

The proliferation of mesoblasts on the medioventral side of the mesonephric ridge gives rise to the genital ridge (embryos 7 to 12 mm, 37 to 42 days, SH XVI). The genital ridge contains mesoblastic cells of coelomic origin, mesenchymal cells penetrating into the genital ridge from the mesonephric mesenchyme, and primordial germ-cells (Fig. 1).

3. DEVELOPMENT OF PARAMESONEPHRIC (MULLERIAN) DUCTS AND THEIR RELATIONSHIP TO MESONEPHRIC (WOLFFIAN) DUCTS

In embryos 14 to 19 mm (44 to 48 days, SH XVIII), cylindrical mesodermal epithelium on the lateral side of the mesonephric ridge invaginates laterally to the cranial part of the genital ridge and approaches the epithelium of the Wolffian duct giving rise to the primordium of the Mullerian duct. The cells of the Mullerian duct grow laterally along the Wolffian duct as a solid cellular cord which gradually becomes luminized and separated from the Wolffian duct by

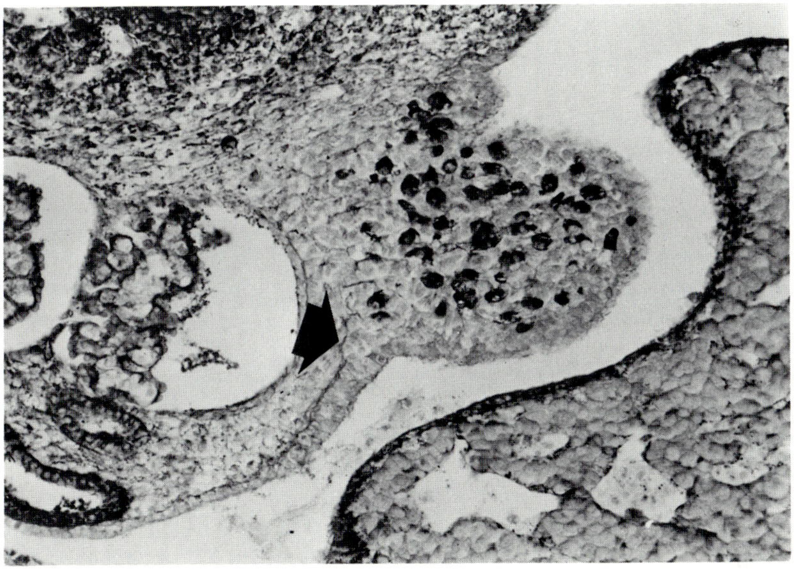

Fig. 1. Indifferent gonad in a 9 mm embryo. The basement membrane underneath the mesodermal epithelium ends lateral to the genital blastema (arrow). Primordial germ cells are rich in glycogen. Colloidal iron - PAS stain. 150x.

mesenchymal connective tissue. Caudal to the mesonephric ridges, the Mullerian ducts cross the Wolffian ducts and approach each other near the midline. Parallel-lying Wolffian and Mullerian ducts contact the dorsal wall of the entodermal urogenital sinus. The Wolffian ducts have previously penetrated into the urogenital sinus. The Mullerian ducts contact only the entodermal epithelium between the Wolffian duct openings and this area becomes the Mullerian tubercle.

Sex-chromosomal constitution is determined at fertilization and sex-chromatin is observed in embryonal tissues beginning the 16th day of development (13,14). In the embryos studied, no sexual differences were observed in the migration of primordial germ-cells, in the formation of the Wolffian and Mullerian ducts nor in the formation of indifferent gonads.

4. CHANGES OF THE GERM-CELLS AND EARLY DEVELOPMENT OF THE TESTICLE

The transformation of the indifferent genital ridge into the testicle is observed in embryos 15 to 19 mm (44 to 48 days, SH XVIII). At this time, the primordial germ-cells temporarily lose their alkaline phosphatase, glycogen and round shape and become incorporated into the testicular cords which differentiate from the blastema of the indifferent genital ridge (Fig. 2). Every testicular cord has a distinct basement membrane. These changes in primordial germ-cells were observed only in normal chromatin-negative embryos. Testicular cords differentiate in situ. No ingrowth of

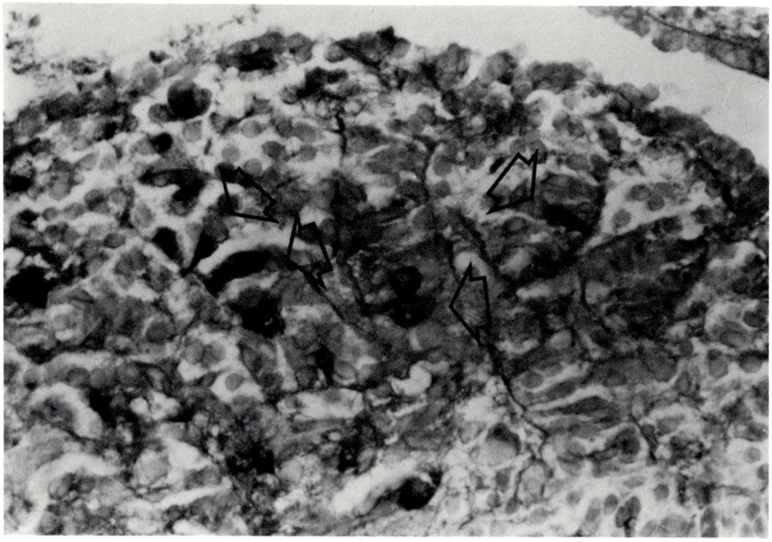

Fig. 2. Differentiation of the testicular cords in a 15 mm embryo. Glycogen-rich germ cells are elongated (arrows) and are attached to the basement membranes of the testicular cords. Colloidal iron-PAS stain, 300x.

cords from the surface epithelium was observed. Four cellular types may be distinguished in the testicular primordium at this time.. Germ-cells and primitive epithelial cells form the testicular cords. Mesenchymal cells of somitic origin fill the interstitial spaces between the testicular cords adjacent to the mesonephros (primordium of the rete testis) and are mixed with mesenchymal cells of mesoblastic (coelomic) origin in the interstitial spaces between the testicular cords. It is believed that the transformation of the genital blasteme into testicular cords takes place only in the presence of germ-cells containing an active XY-chromosomal complex (XY, XYY, XXY, XXXY, XXXXY cell lines).

5. DIFFERENTIATION OF THE TESTICULAR CONNECTIVE TISSUE AND PRIMITIVE TUNICA ALBUGINEA AND REGRESSION OF THE MULLERIAN DUCTS

In embryos 18 to 32 mm (48 to 60 days, SH XIX-XXIII) the reticular connective tissue differentiates between the sex-cords and beneath the surface epithelium. Connective tissue forms a lamina propria of each cord of rete testis and each testicular cord and, finally, a primitive tunica albuginea (embryos 28 to 32 mm, SH XXIII). The development of primitive tunica albuginea ends the period of transformation of the gonadal blastema into the testicular cord. No epithelial cells of the peripheral portion of each cord are slightly PAS-positive and may be called primitive Sertoli cells. The epithelial cells of rete cords are PAS-negative and represent primitive cells lining the rete testis. Strongly PAS-positive, glycogen and alkaline phosphatase-rich germ-cells (spermatogonia) are present among the epithelial cells in both portions of the testicular cords. At the same time as the connective tissue of the tunica albuginea differentiates, the mesenchyme around the Mullerian ducts gives rise to reticular connective tissue. Regression of the Mullerian ducts is first observed at the crossing of the Mullerian ducts and caudal testicular ligament in the area where the Mullerian ducts are nearest to the caudal pole of the testicles (embryos 30 to 35 mm, approximately 60 days). Narrowing of the lumen of the Mullerian duct follows the differentiation of the testicular reticular connective tissue. Release of lysosomal acid hydrolase-acid phosphatase and non-specific esterase is observed in the degenerating Mullerian epithelium. In male fetuses, 45 to 55 mm, as Wolffian ducts grow, the Mullerian ducts fragment and gradually disappear, except at both ends (appendix testis, prostatic utricle). The histogenesis of testicular tunica albuginea and the regression of the Mullerian ducts are closely related. The factors responsible for the regression of the Mullerian ducts as well as for differentiation of the testicular connective tissue, is unknown. The regression of the Mullerian duct is related to the normal development of the ipsilateral testicle. One normal testicle is unable to produce regression of the contralateral Mullerian duct.

6. DIFFERENTIATION OF THE LEYDIG CELLS AND MASCULINIZATION OF THE EXTERNAL GENITALIA

Fetal Leydig cells are epithelioid with acid phosphatase and PAS-positive glycoprotein granules in the paranuclear zone. They contain lipids, high activity of glucose-6-phosphate dehydrogenase and 3 β-hydroxysteroid dehydrogenase (Fig.3). Cells with these characteristics may be found initially in fetuses 32 to 33 mm in the connective tissue between the seminiferous cords under the tunica albuginea (15,16). They originate from the fibroblast-like cells of the testicular interstitium. The differentiation and number of the fetal Leydig cells seem to be under the influence of HCG (15). Incubated in vitro, only testicles containing Leydig cells are able to produce androgens from dehydroepiandrosterone or progesterone. Testicles from fetuses 8 to 9 weeks old are able to convert dehydroepiandrosterone to androstenedione, but not testosterone. Testosterone can be synthesized in vitro by testicular tissue from fetuses 15 to 24 weeks old (17,18,19). Fetal testicles able to produce androgens do not show any maturation of Sertoli cells.

The masculinization of external genitalia begins in fetuses 35 to 40 mm (65 to 70 days old) with the lengthening of the anogenital distance. Shortly after follows the fusion of the labioscrotal swellings developing the scrotum and closing the scrotal rhaphe. Later, in fetuses 70 to 75 days old, this fusion involves the rims

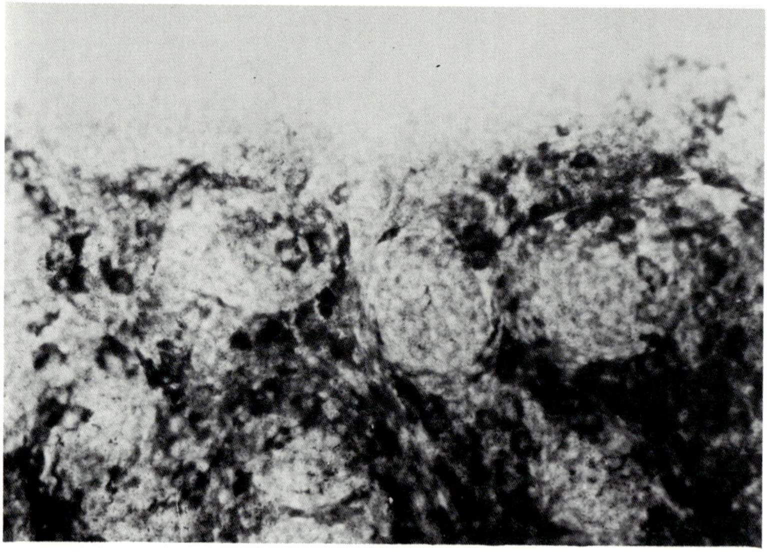

Fig. 3. 3 β-hydroxysteroid dehydrogenase (substrate dehydroepiandrosterone) in the Leydig cells of a 45 mm fetus, 300x.

of the urethral groove. As the penile rhaphe closes, the phallic part of the urogenital sinus gives rise to the cavernous urethra (20). If this fusion does not take place, the external genitalia may feminize or may remain ambiguous, similar to the indifferent stage. If the formation of the scrotal and/or penile rhaphe is incomplete, the external genitalia are hypospadic. Masculinization of external genitalia in normal males depends upon the production of androgens by the testicular Leydig cells. One normal testicle is able to produce complete masculinization of external genitalia.

Female and malformed external genitalia in patients showing androgen-insensitivity suggest that, in addition to androgens, sensitivity of the target tissues forming labioscrotal swellings and a genital tubercle is necessary for normal masculinization of the external genitalia.

7. TESTICULAR DYSGENESIS AND PERSISTENCE OF THE MULLERIAN DUCT IN MALE PSEUDOHERMAPHRODITES

In some male pseudohermaphrodites, a special type of a congenital testicular maldevelopment, testicular dysgenesis, may be recognized (Fig. 4). The following criteria are required for classifying a testicle as dysgenic: 1. Thin insufficiently developed tu-

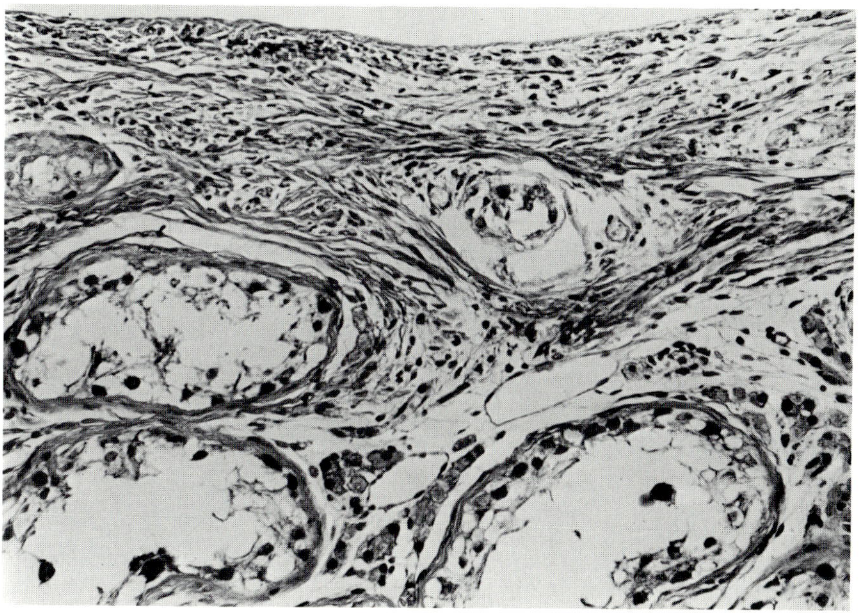

Fig. 4. Testicular dysgenesis. Tunica albuginea is thin and contains cellular connective tissue. Seminiferous tubules underneath are very narrow and degenerating. The other seminiferous tubules are luminized and lined with mature Sertoli cells, spermatogonia and some spermatocytes. Leydig cells are present. Nineteen year old androgen sensitive male pseudohermaphrodite with uterus, bilateral testicular dysgenesis and a normal XY-karyotype. Hematoxylin-eosin, 150x.

nica albuginea; 2. Degenerating, narrow seminiferous tubules underneath the tunica albuginea; 3. Areas of cellular connective tissue resembling ovarian stroma (not always present).

Testicular dysgenesis must be distinguished from gonadal dysgenesis (streak gonads without any germinal elements), from tubular testicular dysgenesis (21) (eosinophilic, enlarged, immature Sertoli cells in some seminiferous tubules of cryptorchic testes), and from tubular, testicular, sclerotizing degeneration found in chromatin-positive males.

Testicular dysgenesis is associated with persistence of the ipsilateral Mullerian duct and is congenital. Before puberty, the dysgenic testicles do not contain Leydig cells. In post-puberal patients, Leydig cells are present and usually hyperplastic and hypertrophic. They contain 3 β-hydroxysteroid dehydrogenase, a high activity of glucose-6-phosphate dehydrogenase and cytoplasmic lipids. The seminiferous tubules are luminized and, in postpuberal patients, lined with mature Sertoli cells. Some are lined with Sertoli cells only. In others, numerous spermatogonia are present. The spermatogonia show a very high activity of alkaline phosphatase. Hyalinization of the basement membranes of the seminiferous tubules is a regular finding. Bilateral and unilateral forms of testicular dysgenesis may be recognized.

In cases showing unilateral testicular dysgenesis, a streak gonad or well-developed cryptorchid, or normal, testicle may be present contralaterally. Unilateral testicular dysgenesis with a streak gonad contralaterally is known under the following names: mixed gonadal dysgenesis; unilateral testicular differentiation or asymmetrical differentiation of gonads (22,23,24).

Patients with unilateral testicular dysgenesis and streak gonad contralaterally and patients with bilateral testicular dysgenesis are phenotypically similar. They show varying degrees of clitoral hypertrophy; they have a vagina and uterus, and they are androgen sensitive. After puberty, their breasts are not developed, although sometimes a slight gynecomastia is present. Cytogenetically, in testicular dysgenesis, XO/XY mosaicism is usual. However, in some patients, only a normal male XY-karyotype has been found. In other cases chromosomal mosaicisms showing, in addition to XO and XY cells, other cell lines such as XXY and XYY-cells have been observed. Patients with unilateral testicular dysgenesis and with a normal or cryptorchid testicle contralaterally are phenotypically males and described as "males with a uterus" (25,26,27). Their external genitalia are male or hypospacid. Fertility may be preserved in some. The uterus is present on the same side as the dysgenic testicle and usually lies in the groin inguinal hernia of the uterus or within the scrotum in a hernial sac.

Dysgerminomas, embryonal dysgerminomas and gonadoblastomas arising from dysgenic testicles are very common. They were present in 7 of our 11 cases of testicular dysgenesis. Embryonal dysgerminomas and gonadoblastomas were observed in three siblings, all showing typical testicular dysgenesis (28).

8. TESTICULAR DIFFERENTIATION IN PATIENTS WITH ANDROGEN INSENSITIVITY

In male pseudohermaphrodites showing androgen insensitivity, some specific histological changes may be recognized. Three clinical syndromes are related to androgen-insensitivity: Complete testicular feminization, incomplete testicular feminization and androgen insensitive form of Reifenstein's syndrome. They differ phenotypically, primarily in the formation of the external genitalia. In complete testicular feminization, the external genitalia are malformed and ambiguous, usually showing a hypertrophied clitoris. In Reifenstein's syndrome the external genitalia are hypospadic. No uterus is found. Female breasts are present in all postpuberal patients insensitive to androgens. Absence of 5 α-androgen reductase, which coverts testosterone to dihydrotestosterone, was observed in skin and sexual hair follicles and is regarded as being related to androgen-insensitivity (29,30). Testicular histology in androgen-insensitive prepuberal patients is normal (16). After puberty, characteristics are testicular tubular adenomas with hypertrophic and hyperplastic Leydig cells. The seminiferous tubules of the adenomas are non-luminized and lined with immature Sertoli cells. The interstitial spaces are either completely filled with hyperplastic Leydig cells or contain only dense collagenous tissue. The discrepancy between the differentiation of Sertoli cells, which are immature, and Leydig cells, which show hypertrophy and hyperplasia, is pathognomonic for patients with testicular tissue insensitive to androgens (Fig. 5). In complete testicular feminization, Sertoli cells do not show maturation. Histochemically, the hypertrophied and hyperplastic Leydig cells in androgen-insensitive patients are similar to the normal ones and contain 3 β-hydroxysteroid dehydrogenase (16, 31). Sertoli cells do not contain any activity of this enzyme. Alkaline phosphatase, suggesting growth activity of spermatogonia, was demonstrated in only one of 12 cases studied histochemically. Nonspecific degenerative changes, such as hyalinization of the basal membranes of some tubules and degeneration of the immature Sertoli cells, are common and develop at puberty or later. Abnormalities of the tunica albuginea were not observed. Testicular tubular adenomas are benign. Malignant tumors originating from non-luminized tubules lined with immature Sertoli cells have not been reported. Malignant tumors of testicular origin in androgen insensitive patients are rare (32).

The regression of the Mullerian ducts in androgen insensitive patients agrees with the normal development of the testicular connective tissue and tunica albuginea observed in the prepuberal patients. The abnormalities of the Wolffian system and the differentiation of the external genitals reflect the complete or incomplete androgen insensitivity of these structures at the time of masculine development.

SUMMARY

Testicular development was studied in material from 300 human embryos and fetuses and 35 male pseudohermaphrodites. The following relationships were observed:

1. In normal chromatin-negative embryos of 15 to 19 mm (44 to 48 days) the primordial germ cells lose their round shape, glycogen and alkaline phosphatase. At the same time, the gonadal blastema

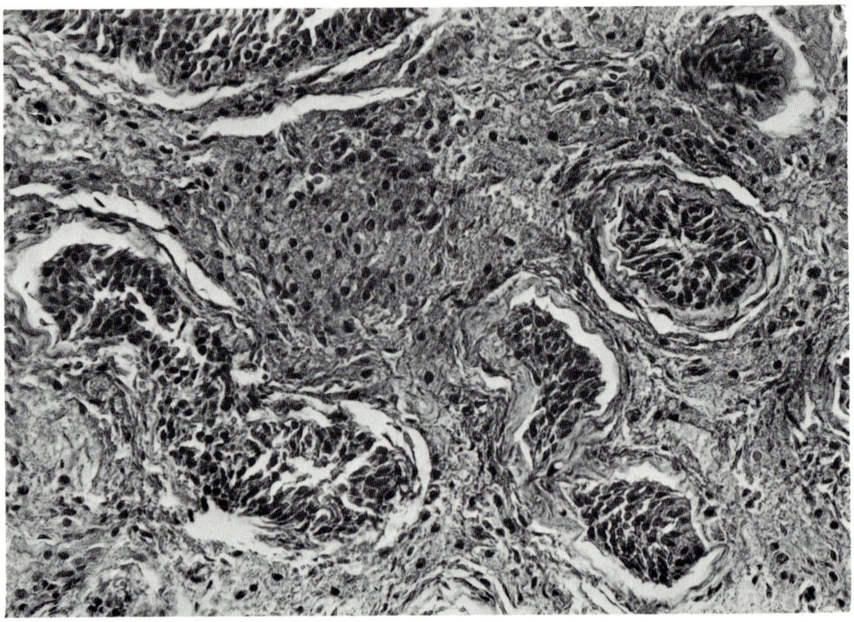

Fig. 5. Biopsy of an intra-abdominal testis showing hyperplastic and hypertrophied Leydig cells and immature Sertoli cells lining non-luminized seminiferous tubules. Discrepancy in the differentiation of the Leydig cells (hyperplasia and hypertrophy) and Sertoli cells (immature) reflects the testicular androgen insensitivity of the patient. Complete testicular feminization in an 18 year old patient, hematoxylin-eosin, 150x.

differentiates into the testicular cords.

2. In embryos of 28 to 35 mm (55 to 60 days) the reticular tissue of the tunica albuginea differentiates ending the transformation of gonadal blastema into testicular cords. At the same time, the regression of the Mullerian ducts begins.

3. In fetuses of 32 to 35 mm (approximately 60 to 65 days) the first Leydig cells showing 3 β-hydroxysteroid dehydrogenase activity are present. No testicular 3β -hydroxysteroid dehydrogenase activity was detected before differentiation of the Leydig cells.

4. Only testicles containing Leydig cells are able to synthesize androstenedione. In vitro, dehydroepiandrosterone is converted to androstenedione by the testicular tissue of fetuses 8 to 9 weeks old. Testosterone was synthesized by testicular tissues of fetuses 15 to 24 weeks old.

5. Masculinization of the external genitalia begins in fetuses of 35 to 40 mm which are 65 to 70 days old. The scrotum and cavernous urethra are formed between days 70 to 75. The presence of Leydig cells is necessary for normal masculinization.

6. In some androgen-sensitive male pseudohermaphrodites, a special type of testicular dysgenesis is present. A dysgenic testicle is characterized by a thin insufficiently developed tunica albuginea, narrow degenerating seminiferous tubules and areas of cellular connective tissue. Dysgenic testicles are unable to produce regression of the Mullerian duct. Tumors arising from seminiferous epithelium of dysgenic testicles were found in 7 of 11 cases studied.

7. In testicular biopsies, the non-luminized testicular tubules with immature Sertoli cells, which are in contrast to the hyperplastic and hypertrophic Leydig cells, suggest the testicular androgen insensitivity of the postpuberal patient.

ACKNOWLEDGMENT

This study presented is a part of Czechoslovakian State research in human reproduction.

REFERENCES

1. McKay, D.G., Hertig, A.T., Adams, E.C. and Danziger, S., Anat. Rec., 117: 201, 1953.
2. McKay, D.G., Adams, E.C., Hertig, A.T. and Danziger, S., Anat. Rec., 122: 125, 1955.
3. McKay, D.G., Adams, E.C., Hertig, A.T. and Danziger, S., Anat. Rec., 126: 433, 1956.
4. Rossi, F., Pescetto, G. and Reale, E., J. Histochem. Cytochem., 5: 221, 1957.
5. Jirasek, J.E., Acta Histochem. (Jena), 13: 220, 1962.
6. Witschi, E., Carnegie Inst., Washington, Contrib. Embryol., 32: 67, 1948.
7. Streeter, G.L., Carnegie Inst., Washington, Developmental Horizons in Human Embryo, Embryology Reprint Vol. II, 1951.
8. Singh, R.P. and Carr, D.H., Anat. Rec., 155: 369, 1966.
9. Jirasek, J.E., Unpublished data.
10. Wenick, M. and McGory, W.W., Birth Defects, 4: 1, 1968.
11. Jirasek, J.E., Unpublished data.
12. Witschi, E., Recent Progr. Hormone Res., 6: 1, 1951.
13. Glenister, T.W., Nature, London, 177: 1135, 1956.
14. Park, W.W., J. Anat., 91: 369, 1957.
15. Niemi, M., Ikonen, M. and Hervonen, A., Ciba Found. Colloq. Endocr., 16: Endocrinology of the Testis, 31, 1967.
16. Jirasek, J.E., Ciba Found. Colloq. Endocr. 16: Endocrinology of the Testis, 3, 1967.
17. Jirasek, J.E., Sulcova, J., Capkova, A., Rohling, S. and Starka, L., Endocrinologie (Dresden), 54: 173-183, 1969.
18. Acevedo, H.F., Axelrod, L.R., Ishikawa, E. and Takaki, F., J. Clin. Endocr., 21: 1611, 1961.
19. Bloch, E., Tissenbaum, B. and Benirschke, K., Biochim. Biophys. Acta., 60, 182, 1962.
20. Jirasek, J.E., Raboch, J. and Uher, J., Amer. J. Obstet. Gynec., 101: 830, 1968.

21. Sohval, A.R., J. Urol, 72: 693, 1954.
22. Sohval, A.R., Amer. J. Hum. Genet., 15: 155, 1963.
23. Bergada, C., Cleveland, W.W., Jones, H.W., Jr. and Wilkins, L., Acta Endocr. (Kobenhavn), 40: 521, 1962.
24. Zourlas, A.P. and Jones, H.W., Jr., Obstet. Gynec., 26: 48, 1965.
25. Young, D., J. Obstet. Gynaec. Brit. Comm., 58: 830, 1951.
26. Prichard, R.W., Arch. Path. (Chicago), 56: 505, 1953.
27. Motyloff, L., Z. Geburtsh. Gynaek., 99: 330, 1931.
28. Jirasek, J.E. and Prem, K.A., Unpublished data.
29. Northcutt, R.C., Island, D.P. and Liddle, G.W., J. Clin. Endocr., 29: 422, 1969.
30. Mauvais-Jarvis, P., Bercovici, J.P. and Gauthier, F., J. Clin. Endocr., 29: 417, 1969.
31. Jirasek, J.E. and Raboch, J., Fertil. Steril., 14: 237, 1963.
32. Hauser, G.A. In Intersexuality, ed. Overzier, C., Academic Press, London, New York, 1963.

HETEROPLASTIC GONADUCT-TESTES COMBINATIONS: A BIOCHEMICAL OUTLOOK

J. P. Weniger

Laboratoire de Zoologie et d'Embryologie experimentale,
Universite de Strasbourg, France

Ten years ago, I performed heteroplastic combinations of embryonic chick and mouse gonads and observed the feminization of the chick testis by the mouse testis (1-3). This result prompted the following experiments with gonaducts.

The question arises as to whether the embryonic chick and mouse testes exert different effects on one and the same gonaduct. This would imply that the hormone secretion of the two kinds of testes is different. Our first consideration is the embryonic mouse wolffian duct.

As shown by Jost (4-8) in his castration and grafting experiments, the testes are essential for the development of the wolffian ducts in the male mammalian embryo. This statement is also valid for in vitro conditions, as shown by Price and Pannabecker (9,10) in their organ culture studies of embryonic rat reproductive tracts. In my own cultures (11), embryonic mouse testes maintained embryonic mouse wolffian ducts and stimulated their growth (Fig. 1). On the contrary, when cultured in combination with embryonic chick testes, the mouse wolffian ducts retrogressed (Fig. 2), just as they do when cultured alone.

Secondly, let us consider the embryonic chick Mullerian duct. This duct is a unique test organ for its responsiveness both to masculinizing and feminizing actions. When subjected to masculinizing influences, it retrogresses (12); feminizing actions produce stimulation of the duct (13).

Experimentally (14), the chick testis brought about the regression of the chick Mullerian duct (Fig. 4), whereas the mouse testis

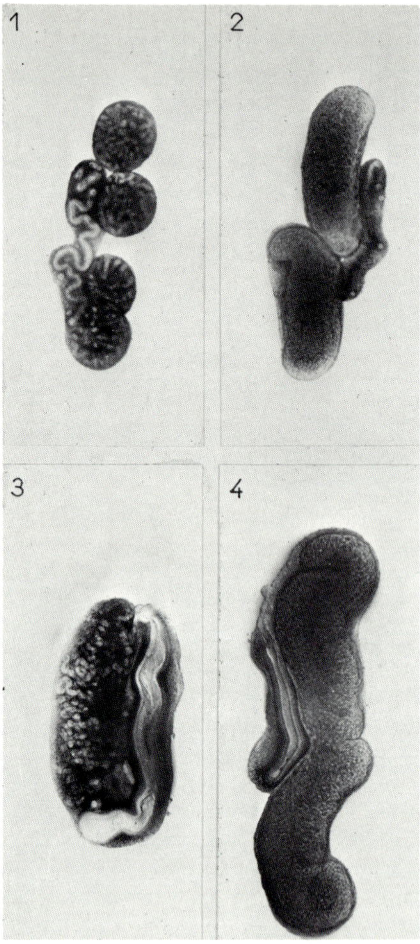

Fig. 1. The left wolffian duct and the testes from a 17-day-old mouse embryo have been grown together in vitro for 3 days: curling of the wolffian duct occurred.

Fig. 2. The right wolffian duct has been cultured for 3 days in combination with the testes from an 8-day-old chick embryo: retrogression occurred.

Fig. 3. The right Mullerian duct from an 8-day-old female chick embryo has been cultured for 5 days in combination with a testis from an 18-day-old mouse embryo: stimulation was observed.

Fig. 4. The left Mullerian duct has been cultured for 5 days in combination with the testes from an 8-day-old male chick embryo: retrogression occurred.

produced stimulation (Fig. 3). Thus, the chick and mouse testes exert opposite effects on the chick Mullerian duct. It may be concluded from this as well as from the foregoing results that there is a difference in the hormone secretion of the embryonic chick and mouse testes. How far do the results of biochemical studies fit this?

Experiments by Jost (4-8) and Price and Pannabecker (9,10) have shown that testosterone prevents the wolffian ducts from degenerating in the castrated male mammalian embryo or in vitro conditions. Indeed, testosterone and androstenedione secretion has been demonstrated in a great variety of embryonic mammalian testes (human: Acevedo et al., (15, 16); Bloch et al., (17); Rice et al., (18); Ikonen and Niemi (19); armadillo: Bloch and Benirschke, (20); rabbit: Lipsett and Tullner, (21); rat: Noumura et al., (22); guinea pig and dog: Bloch, (23); horse: MacArthur et al., (24); mouse:Weniger et al., (25); calf: Weniger et al., (26); sheep: Attal, (27). The question might then be posed as to whether the failure of the embryonic chick testis to promote the development of the embryonic mouse Wolffian duct may be attributed to the lack of testosterone secretion by the chick testis.

Embryonic chick testes were cultured according to the method of Wolff and Haffen (28) in the presence of 1-^{14}C sodium acetate, 4-^{14}C progesterone or 4-^{14}C androstenolone (Table 1). Analysis for radioactive testosterone was carried out in the media, using multiple thin-layer chromatography, derivative formation and recrystallization to constant specific activity, but in no case could it be detected (Figs. 5 and 6, Tables 2 and 3). Thus the lack of testosterone secretion explains the failure of the chick testis to stimulate the mouse wolffian duct.

Table 1. Experimental Conditions for Embryonic Chick Testes Cultures

Experiment	Precursor	Total Activity	Number and Age of Testes (pairs)	(days)	Culture Period (days)
1	Acetate	4.5 mC	889	10	1
2	Acetate	2 mC	373	14	1
3	Pro	5 μC	29	19	1
4	Pro	10 μC	60	12	3
5	Alone	5 μC	103	15	3

Pro: progesterone. Alone: androstenolone.

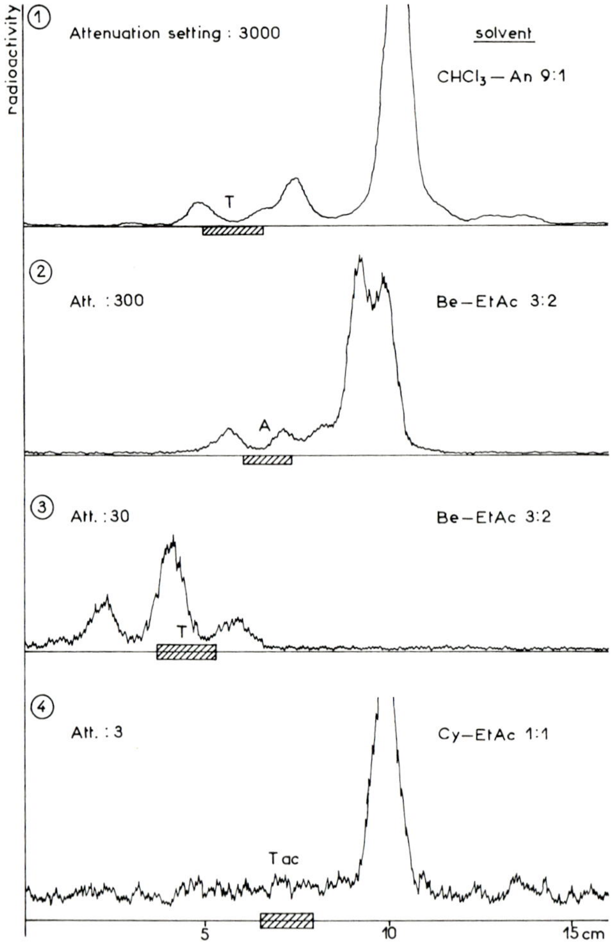

Fig. 5. Radiochromatograms pertaining to the experiment No. 4 (Table 1).

1: Total androgen fraction. There is no definite peak in the testosterone region.

2: Androstenedione obtained by testosterone oxidation.

3: Testosterone obtained by androstenedione reduction. One-fourth was acetylated (radiochromatogram No. 4), the rest recrystallized (Table 2).

4: Background level in the testosterone acetate region. Thus, all the activity was contaminating.

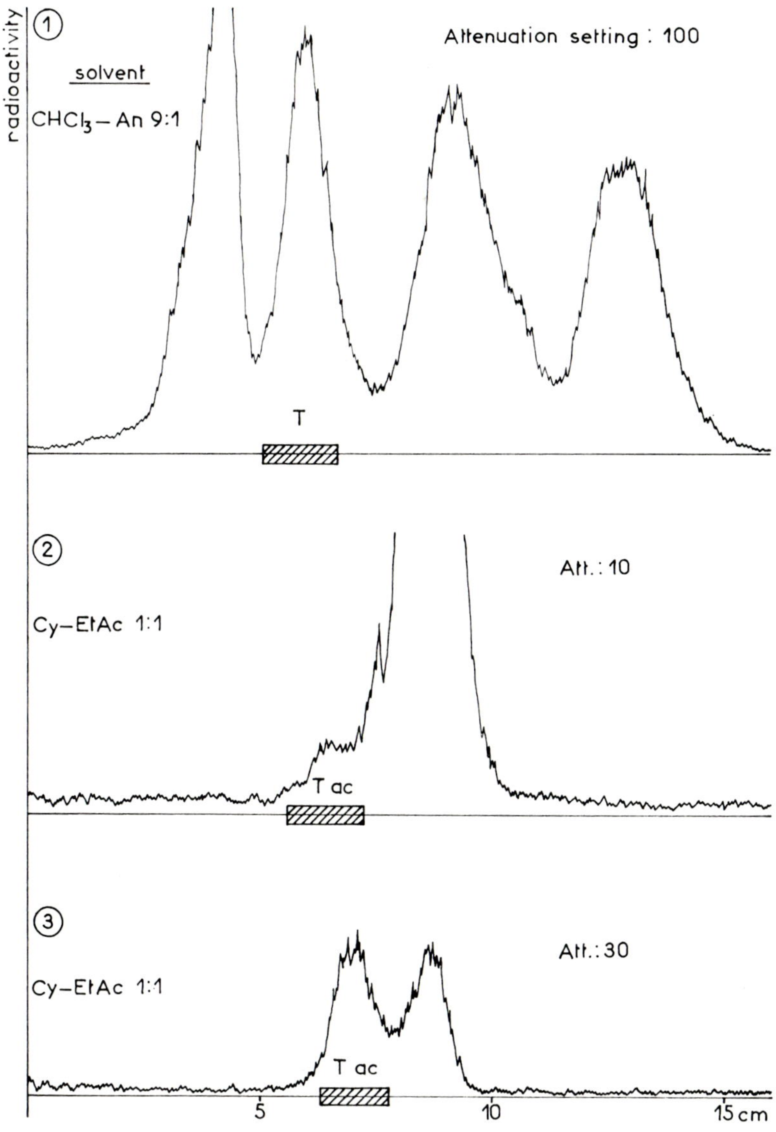

Fig. 6. Radiochromatograms pertaining to the experiment No. 5 (Table 1).

1: Total androgen fraction. A peak seems to be associated with carrier testosterone

2: Testosterone acetate.

3: Rechromatography of testosterone acetate: there is a quite good correspondence with a peak, but recrystallizations will show that all is contaminating activity (Table 3)

Table 2. Recrystallization of Testosterone (Experiment No. 4)

Crystallization	Specific Activity (cpm/mg)	
	Crystals	Mother Liquors
1	258	760
2	83	580
3	74	132
4	58	61

Testosterone was recrystallized (from step 3, Fig. 5) in chloroform-petroleum ether with 20 mg of carrier. Constant specific activity could not be obtained. The background was 30 cpm.

Table 3. Recrystallization of Testosterone acetate (Experiment No. 5)

Crystallization	Specific Activity (cpm/mg)	
	Crystals	Mother Liquors
1	560	1170
2	347	1740
3	170	810
4	124	605
5	83	242
6	-	230
7	36	69

Testosterone acetate (from step 3, Fig. 6) was recrystallized in methanol-petroleum ether with 20 mg of carrier. Constancy of specific activity could not be achieved. The background was 30 cpm.

Table 4. Experimental Conditions for Embryonic Mouse Testes Cultures

Experiment	Precursor	Total Activity	Number and Age of Testes (pairs)	(days)	Culture Period (days)
1	Acetate	1 mC	179	14-19	1
2	Pro	10 μC	28	15-17	3
3	Alone	5 μC	69	14-18	3

Pro: progesterone. Alone: androstenolone.

It has been shown by Weniger, Ehrhardt and Fritig (29) that the embryonic chick ovary secretes estrone and estradiol. Since the embryonic mouse testis exerts on both the embryonic chick testis and Mullerian duct the same feminizing effects as the chick ovary, does this mean that it secretes estrone and estradiol too? Embryonic mouse testes were cultured in the presence of 1-^{14}C sodium acetate, 4-^{14}C progesterone or 4-^{14}C androstenolone (Table 4) but in no case could estrogen formation be demonstrated.

On the other hand, it is unlikely that the secretion of testosterone or androstenedione, or both, would explain the feminizing effects of the mouse testis. Indeed, if it is true that androstenedione feminizes the chick testis, as shown by Wolff, Strudel and Wolff (30) in their injection experiments, both testosterone and androstenedione bring about the retrogression of the chick Mullerian duct. In the same way, the chick Mullerian duct retrogresses when cultured on testosterone propionate-containing media (12).

Thus, the biochemical outlook I ventured upon is strongly negative: The hormone or mechanism responsible for the feminization of the embryonic chick testis and Mullerian duct by the embryonic mouse testis remains to be discovered.

REFERENCES

1. Weniger, J. P., C.R. Acad. Sci. (Paris), 253: 2410, 1961.
2. Weniger, J. P., Arch. Anat. Micr. Morph. Exp., 52: 261, 1963.
3. Weniger, J. P., Ann. Endocr. (Paris), 26: 467, 1965.
4. Jost, A., Arch. Anat. Micr. Morph. Exp., 36: 271, 1947.
5. Jost, A., Arch. Anat. Micr. Morph. Exp., 39: 577, 1950.
6. Jost, A., Recent Progr. Hormone Res. , 8: 379, 1953.
7. Jost, A., Mem. Soc. Endocr., 4: 237, 1955.
8. Jost, A., Mem. Soc. Endocr., 7: 49, 1960.
9. Price, D., and Pannabecker, R., Ciba Foundation Colloquia on Ageing, 2: 3, 1956.
10. Price, D., and Pannabecker, R., Arch. Anat. Micr. Morph. Exp., 48: 223, 1959.
11. Weniger, J. P., Arch. Anat. Micr. Morph. Exp., 54: 909, 1965.
12. Wolff, E., Lutz-Ostertag , Y., and Haffen, K., C. R. Soc. Biol. (Paris), 146: 1793, 1952.
13. Weniger, J. P., Arch. Anat. Micr. Morph. Exp., 50: 269, 1961.
14. Weniger, J. P., Arch. Anat. Micr. Morph. Exp., 52: 497, 1963.
15. Acevedo, H. F., Axelrod, L. R., Ishikawa, E., and Takaki, F., J. Clin. Endocr., 21: 1611, 1961.
16. Acevedo, H. F., Axelrod, L. R., Ishikawa, E., and Takaki, F., J. Clin. Endocr., 23: 883, 1963.
17. Bloch, E., Tissenbaum, B., and Benirschke, K., Biochim. Biophys. Acta., 60: 182, 1962.
18. Rice, B. F., Johanson, C. A., and Sternberg, W. H., Steroids, 7: 79, 1966.
19. Ikonen, M., and Niemi, M., Nature (London), 212: 716, 1966.
20. Bloch, E., and Benirschke, K., Endocrinology, 76: 43, 1965.
21. Lipsett, M. B., and Tullner, W. W., Endocrinology, 77: 273, 1965.
22. Noumura, T., Weisz, J., and Lloyd, C. W., Endocrinology, 78: 245, 1966.
23. Bloch, E., Steroids, 9: 415, 1967.
24. MacArthur, E., Short, R. V., and O'Donnell, V. J., J. Endocr., 38: 331, 1967.

25. Weniger, J. P., Ehrhardt, J. D., and Fritig, B., C. R. Acad. Sci. (Paris), 264: series D, 1069, 1967.
26. Weniger, J. P., Ehrhardt, J. D., and Fritig, B., C. R. Acad. Sci. (Paris), 264: series D,1911, 1967.
27. Attal, J., Endocrinology, 85: 280, 1969.
28. Wolff, E., and Haffen, K., J. Exp. Zool., 119: 381, 1952.
29. Weniger, J. P., Ehrhardt, J. D., and Fritig, B., C. R. Acad. Sci. (Paris), 264: series D, 838, 1967.
30. Wolff, E., Strudel, G., and Wolff, E., Arch. Anat. (Strasb), 31: 237, 1948.

GENERAL DISCUSSION

MANN: Professor Jost referred to the masculinizing effect of the male fetus on the female co-twin, that is, on the freemartin. It is somewhat surprising that in contrast to the enormous amount of work that has been done on the influence of the male on the female, the reciprocal influence of the female on the male co-twin has been largely ignored. An opportunity to investigate this aspect in a quantitative manner arose in conjunction with a recent study of freemartinism by Short et al. (Cytogenetics, 8:,369, 1969). We found that although spermatogenesis was progressing in the testes of the mature bull co-twin, the testes were small and immature with respect to the testosterone/androstenedione ratio. The male accessory organs were also reduced in size. The secretory function of the seminal vesicles, as reflected by the formation of fructose and citric acid, was one tenth of what it should have been in a normal bull. Thus it would seem that the harm inflicted by the male on the female met with vengeance, and that the male twin was unable to develop its own reproductive tract normally.

FORD: Weiss and Hoffman from Giessen in Germany published a paper last year in "Cytogenetics", in which they claimed the presence of XX cells in the bull twin of the freemartin in tissue cultures prepared from testicular material. I do not know which cells grew out from the explants, but it is a very remarkable observation if it is true and I would like to see it confirmed. If the stromal cells grew out, how do the XX cells get there? How do they get into the fixed tissue? And if the germ cells grew out, this is even more remarkable.

JOST: When one studies freemartins after birth, one is studying the sum of all the events which have occurred during the long pregnancy period. In rats, it is obvious that early post-natal treatment with estrogen can have these effects on the testis. It is also known that in the calf fetus the ovary has the capacity to produce estrogens briefly before birth. This would suggest that the estrogenic influence could occur late during pregnancy, when the morphological sex differentiation of the young has long been completed. In our studies and in any others I know of, devoted to sex differentiation in freemartins, i.e. during younger stages, no visible effect of the female twin on the male twin has ever been observed. The physiological significance as to sex and function of the exchange of cells between the male and female twin in cattle, mentioned by Dr. Ford, certainly needs more research.

E. STEINBERGER: We have studied a case of testicular feminization whose testicular biopsy showed masses of Leydig cells and seminiferous tubules with Sertoli cells which appeared immature. The tissue was capable of metabolizing progesterone to testosterone. Both FSH and LH were detected in this patient's urine. Why should these Sertoli cells remain in the immature state in spite of the presence of FSH? Well, if we assume something different from the generally accepted idea that Sertoli cells are under FSH control, and consider the possibility that these cells are under testosterone control, i.e. that their maturation depends on testosterone, then we may have here an example of insensitivity to testosterone not only of peripheral tissues, but also of the Sertoli cells.

JOHNSEN: We have made exactly the same observation as Dr. Steinberger, in the syndrome of testicular feminization.

DICZFALUSY: Could Prof. Jost comment on the nature of the so-called "Mullerian inhibitor"? Could this be the steroid with 21 carbon atoms, or a compound which is non-steroidal?

JOST: A "Mullerian" inhibiting substance has not been isolated so far, and of all the steroids assayed none has shown this effect.

LIPSETT: Was a systematic study made of the human testis in anencephaly? Has the state of the pituitary gland been correlated with the histology of the testis?

JOST: Studies on the testis of anencephalic infants have usually been made at birth. There is no real developmental study, as far as I know, for obvious reasons. It was found by Zondeck and Zondeck that the interstitial cells in this condition were reduced. In some cases the penis was somewhat reduced in size. But it was a true penis showing that masculinization was complete. The condition of the genital tract would suggest that during the early weeks of pregnancy the testis functioned normally. Thereafter, it lacked stimulation. This fits the curve of excretion of chorionic gonadotropins during pregnancy.

LIPSETT: We tend to assume that, in the human, chorionic gonadotropin plays a role in the development of the Leydig cell. We have had the experience of having to abort a woman at four and a half months of pregnancy. This patient presented metastatic choriocarcinoma and rather high titers of HCG. The fetal testis showed Leydig cell hyperplasia.

MARTINI: I would like to know if an attempt has been made to duplicate with crude testicular extracts the effects which are obtained by testicular transplantations.

LUNENFELD: Was an attempt ever made to decapitate or encephalectomize rat embryos prior to the 13th day and assess the fate of oogenesis ?

JOST: First Dr. Martini asked if anyone has tried testicular extracts. This has been attempted in the past but probably not in the best way, and should be repeated. Dr. Lunenfeld asked about meiosis in decapitated rat fetuses. This has been studied recently by Mauleon in France in unpublished experiments. In rat fetuses decapitated on day 16.5, premeiosis occurred in the ovaries. This experiment must be repeated at earlier stages since premeiosis starts between days 17 and 18. Premeiosis was not observed in the sections on day 14. Other authors also state that in the rat premeiosis starts between day 17 and 18. In any case we did not study fetuses decapitated on day 13. In freemartins, if we assume that the effect of the male twin on the female twin is produced by some testicular hormone (this actually has never been demonstrated) then the following chronological events are of great interest: the abnormalities in the ovaries of the female twin begin to appear approximately at, or shortly before the time when the Mullerian ducts are inhibited by the testis both in the male and in the female twin. Chronologically there is a possibility that the same hormone inhibits the Mullerian ducts in both the male and the female partners and the ovarian cortex in the freemartin.

BERGADA: I want to make a brief comment on a human syndrome which resembles very much the unilateral castrated rabbit experiment demonstrated by Dr. Jost. In 1961, in collaboration with Dr. Wilkins, we described this syndrome which we call asymmetrical gonadal differentiation. It is generally induced by an XO/XY chromosomal mosaicism. Surprisingly, the differentiation of the gonads is exactly what their chromosomal constitution would theoretically induce, i.e., a testis on one side and an atrophic or rudimentary gonad on the other side which is similar to the gonadal streak observed in the pure XO cases or Turner's syndrome. This suggests that in the human sexual differentiation is similar to what Dr. Jost and others have showed in experimental animals.

JIRASEK: The Sertoli cells in testical feminization are undifferentiated at least in some portions of the testis. The androgen insensitivity of the individual is reflected in the testis by the lack of maturation of Sertoli cells. With respect to testicular dysgenesis this syndrome was present in all individuals with an XO/XY karyotype. It is possible to distinguish three types of testicular dysgenesis: 1. Bilateral, with dysgenetic testes bilaterally; 2. Unilateral testicular dysgenesis with a dysgenetic testis and a contralateral gonadal streak; and 3. Unilateral testicular dysgenesis with a normal testis on the opposite side. Phenotypically, the cases of the last group are described as males with a uterus. In some such cases the phenotype, including external genitalia, is completely normal male. The uterus is present ipsilaterally to the dysgenic testis. With respect to hypophysial aplasia, it seems that up to the seventh month of fetal development, in the absence of the pi - tuitary, the testes are completely normal.

JOST: I was very interested to see Dr. Jirasek's cases of male pseudohermaphrodites in which there is no inhibition of Mullerian ducts, probably as a result of defective production of the Mullerian inhibitor during fetal life. In these cases there was also an incomplete differentiation of the albuginea. I wonder whether it might be possible to make a parallel between the deficient albuginea differentiation and lack of Mullerian inhibition in the pseudohermaphrodites, on the one hand, and the inhibition of the ovarian cortex and of the Mullerian ducts in freemartins, on the other.

CHRISTENSEN: There has been some discussion of Sertoli cell differentiation this morning. Usually we think of cellular differentiation in terms of the cell's ability to carry out its specific function. Sertoli cells in a normal seminiferous tubule have a very complex relationship with the germinal cells, and probably nurture and support them. I wonder how much we can say about Sertoli cell differentiation where spermatogenesis is not being carried out. I do not know whether the size and appearance of the nucleus is an adequate indication that the cell is capable of carrying out its full rolr in supporting spermatogenesis.

JIRASEK: Infertile patients with Sertoli cells only in the testicular biopsy,show no relationship between the germ cells and Sertoli cells because there are no germ cells. In all these cases, after puberty, the Sertoli cells are fully differentiated or mature. My other remark is just a terminological one. I would be opposed to the use of the term hormone for a substance producing regression of the Mullerian duct because its action in male pseudohermaphrodites is strictly ipsilateral. The dysgenetic testis or the streak gonad is unable to induce regression of the ipsilateral Mullerian duct. However, the regression of the contralateral Mullerian duct may be normal.

MARTINI: Is there any evidence that testosterone can be converted into dihydrotestosterone by the Wolffian and Mullerian ducts?

MANN: There have been several attempts to demonstrate the occurrence of dihydrotestosterone in the mature bull testis but without any success so far.

LIPSETT: I cannot remember whether Jean Wilson found the conversion but she demonstrated the localization of dihydrotestosterone in the

Wolffian duct, similar to the localization found in the prostate and seminal vesicle.

BERGADA: We have studied several patients with different testicular pathology who showed the relationship of interstitial tissue steroid production and tubular development. One was a 19-year-old boy with unilateral cryptorchidism. Another was a 17-year-old boy with hypogonadotropic eunuchoidism and cryptorchidism. In the second case there were no changes in the seminiferous tubules which coincided with an absence of functional interstitial tissue, whereas the first patient demonstrated tubular development. A third type of case is exemplified by sexual precocity and a pseudo-tumor of the testis. We studied a 5-year-old boy with marked hyperplasia of the Leydig cells in one part of the testis, and complete development of the seminiferous tubules with full spermatogenesis within this hyperplasia. In the same testis, away from the area of Leydig cell hyperplasia, the seminiferous tubules were infantile. Finally the testicular biopsy of a 21-year-old patient with a feminizing testis revealed no changes in the seminiferous tubules, which looked infantile. Since all the androgen target organs of these patients do not respond to this hormone, this phenomenon, and the previous situation, support the hypothesis that the seminiferous tubule, independently of gonadotropin action, is a selective target organ for the androgens secreted by the surrounded Leydig cells.

JOST: It may seem strange that the testicular secretion which is responsible for the disappearance of the Mullerian ducts has not been better studied. As a matter of fact, this study is difficult in mammals for technical reasons. In vivo experiments are not easy to make on a large scale. In vitro experiments can be expected to afford better possibilities. But Dr. Weniger in mice and Mrs. Picon in my laboratory in rats observed that inhibition of the Mullerian ducts by fetal testicular tissue grown together in vitro can be obtained only during a very early and limited period of time. In experiments with guinea pig fetuses Dr. Dorothy Price has not succeeded so far in maintaining the Mullerian ducts of male fetuses in vitro. This is probably due to the fact that they disappear at a very early stage. A convenient in vitro system must be devised in order to permit this type of study.

WITSCHI: In my introductory remarks, I attempted to stimulate interest in amphibians. They have not been entering the discussion at all. Possibly they are not well enough known generally, and one does not sufficiently realize that all the essential hormones found in the higher forms, that is in mammals, and in birds, are already present in amphibians. The anatomical situation is often very much clearer, due to more primitive organization of the gonads. I wish again to direct attention to the favorable features for work on primary sexual differentiation and initiation of steroidogenesis in amphibia.

CHAPTER II

HISTOLOGY OF THE TESTIS

DYNAMICS OF HUMAN SPERMATOGENESIS

Yves Clermont

Department of Anatomy, McGill University, Montreal,

Canada

INTRODUCTION

The production of spermatozoa by the seminiferous epithelium of mammals has been and still is the object of numerous cytological and histological investigations (1,2,3). Spermatogenesis in man has not been completely ignored by microscopists, even if it is difficult to obtain properly fixed sections of testis from normal adult individuals for investigative purposes. From the morphological point of view the phenomena occurring within the seminiferous tubules may be classified as being either cytological or histological. Amongst the cytological phenomena there are: the mode of proliferation, renewal and differentiation of spermatogonia, the meiotic divisions of spermatocytes, the metamorphosis of spermatids into spermatozoa, and the release of spermatozoa from the seminiferous epithelium. At the histological level, considering the seminiferous epithelium as a whole, there is a grouping of germ cells into distinct cellular associations. The chronological evolution of these cellular associations is known as the "cycle of the seminiferous epithelium", while the orderly distribution of the cell associations along the seminiferous tubule is referred to as the "wave of the seminiferous epithelium". In the following brief discussion three topics concerning the dynamics of human spermatogenesis will be examined: firstly the steps of spermatogenesis, secondly the cycle of the seminiferous epithelium and its duration, and thirdly, the mode of renewal of spermatogonia.

MATERIAL AND METHOD

Part of the material analyzed consisted of testicular biopsies from healthy prisoners collected by Dr. C.G. Heller of the Pacific

Northwest Research Foundation, Seattle, U.S.A. This material was fixed with Zenker-formol or with Bouin's fluid as modified by Cleland. Following fixation and embedding in paraffin, 5-μ sections were stained with hematoxylin-eosin and with the periodic acid-Schiff-hematoxylin techniques. The best biopsies collected were serially sectioned and stained with hematoxylin-eosin. The topographical arrangement of spermatogonia along the tubular limiting membrane and the distribution of the cell associations formed by spermatogonia, spermatocytes and spermatids along the tubular wall was investigated in reconstructions from these serial sections. The topographical arrangement of spermatogonia was also investigated in dissected tubules, fixed in Bouin's fluid, stained with hematoxylin and mounted "in toto" between glass slide and coverslip.

OBSERVATIONS AND DISCUSSION

Spermatogenesis

Spermatogenesis is the elaborate process whereby spermatogonial stem cells transform into spermatozoa, and involves the production of several types of germ cells that will now be briefly described.

Spermatogonia. With the light microscope the large majority of spermatogonia can be classified into one of the following three categories, respectively referred to as dark type A (Ad), pale type A (Ap) and type B (B) spermatogonia (4,5). The dark type A spermatogonia have an ovoid nucleus containing a deeply stained dust-like chromatin. In the central part of the nucleus a cavity containing a pale stained material is usually present. One or two nucleoli closely applied to the nuclear membrane are also visible (Fig. 1). The pale type A spermatogonia have a discoid or ovoid nucleus containing a pale stained granulated chromatin and show one or two nucleoli attached to the nuclear envelope (Fig. 1). The type B spermatogonia show a spherical nucleus characterized by clumps or granules of heavily stained chromatin distributed along the nuclear membrane, attached to a centrally located nucleolus or floating free in the nuclear sap (Fig. 1). There is some variation in nuclear size and morphology of spermatogonia and some cannot be identified as any one of the three types just described (6,7). These spermatogonia may be either distinct classes of spermatogonia or spermatogonia of the three types described above but at various phases of the cell cycle (i.e. G_1, S or G_2).

When examined under the electron microscope, the various classes of spermatogonia appear difficult to differentiate due to the poor characterization of the chromatin (8,9). However, recently, the three main types of spermatogonia mentioned above have been identified in electron microscope photographs and the existence of a fourth spermatogonial type has been postulated (10).

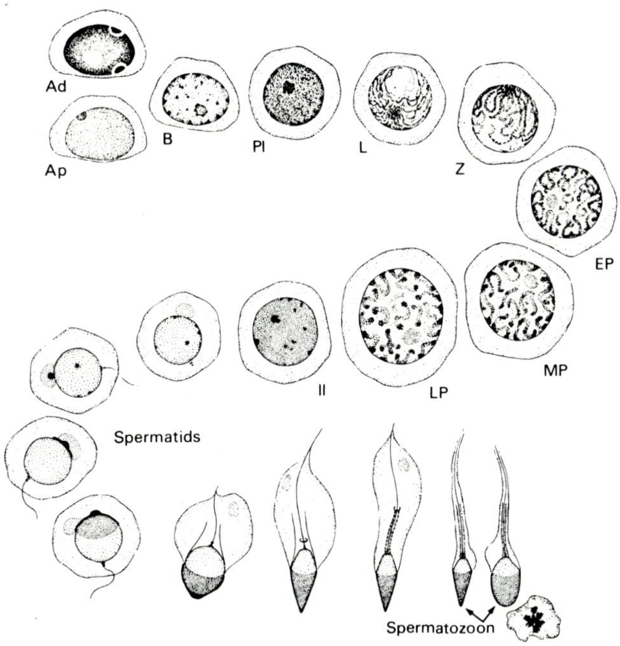

Fig. 1. Series of drawings illustrating the steps of spermatogenesis in man. Spermatogenesis begins with the spermatogonia at the top left and terminates with a spermatozoon at the bottom right. Labels: Ad, dark type A spermatogonia; Ap, pale type A spermatogonia; B, type B spermatogonia; Pl, preleptotene primary spermatocyte; L, leptotene spermatocyte; Z, zygotene spermatocyte; EP, early pachytene spermatocyte; MP, mid-pachytene spermatocyte; LP; late pachytene spermatocyte; II, secondary spermatocytes. Spermatids are shown at various steps of spermiogenesis. A spermatozoon is illustrated as seen from ts lateral (left) and frontal (right aspects. RB, residual body.

Spermatocytes. The preleptotene primary spermatocytes have a spherical nucleus containing a deeply stained granulated chromatin which accumulates on the nuclear membrane and nucleolus. As these primary spermatocytes evolve through the various steps of prophase of the first maturation division, the nucleus undergoes a progressive swelling, and the chromatin assumes the characteristic configurations known as leptotene, zygotene, and pachytene (Fig. 1). Following diakinesis, the primary spermatocytes complete the first maturation division and give rise to secondary spermatocytes. These cells, which because of their short life span are not seen frequently within the seminiferous epithelium, have a spherical nucleus containing a finely granulated chromatin and some larger deeply stained globular masses (Fig. 1). They undergo the second maturation divisions which yield spermatids.

Spermatids and spermiogenesis. Human spermatids embark upon an extraordinarily complex series of cytological changes which have attracted the attention of light and electron microscopists (3,11, 12,13,14). While we will limit ourselves to a brief description of the main steps in spermatid development as seen with the light microscope, it should be remembered that underlying the gross changes to be mentioned, extremely intricate submicroscopical phenomena are taking place. Newly-formed spermatids are characterized by a small spherical nucleus and the usual array of cytoplasmic organelles, among which the Golgi zone, mitochondria, centrioles and chromatoid body are particularly prominent. A well demarcated Golgi zone, which is visible next to the nucleus, soon starts to elaborate small granules which stain vividly with the PA-Schiff technique. These small corpuscles, referred to as proacrosomic granules, coalesce to form a single larger granule, the acrosomic granule, which becomes closely attached to the surface of the nucleus (Fig. 1). The head cap then appears, expanding around the acrosomic granule and growing over the surface of the nucleus. The acrosomic granule and head cap, both well stained by the PA-Schiff technique, together constitute the acrosomic system, which has been shown, with the electron microscope, to be a modified secretory granule and a membrane bound organelle. The Golgi zone, which contributed material to the acrosomic system throughout its formation and development, eventually separates from it to float freely in the cytoplasm (Fig. 1).

At the same time this is going on at one pole of the nucleus, centrioles at the opposite pole have begun to sprout the flagellum. A short time later, a delicate fibrillar structure, the caudal tube or manchette, appears in the cytoplasm, and extends from a close association with the nucleus to surround the flagellum.

As spermiogenesis continues, the acrosomic system rotates toward the limiting membrane of the seminiferous tubule; this reorientation is accompanied by a displacement of the nucleus toward the periphery of the cytoplasm. Following this displacement, the nuclear chromatin starts to condense and becomes more chromophilic. Its shape changes from a sphere to an elongated fusiform body with a conical apex covered with the acrosomic structure (a distinction between acrosome and head cap cannot be made from here on). Around the flagellum, and close to the centriolar apparatus, a delicate "ring" or annulus appears. This ring eventually slides down the flagellum for a short distance and comes to rest at the caudal extremity of the middle piece. The middle piece is that portion of the flagellum between the centrioles and the ring around which the mitochondria will accumulate in a regular covering. The caudal tube disappears soon after the formation of the middle piece.

As spermiogenesis reaches completion, the nucleus condenses further and flattens slightly (front and lateral views are shown in

Fig 1). The anterior two thirds of the nucleus is covered by the delicate acrosomic system, now rather pale staining with PA-Schiff. Much of the cytoplasm, which was seen along the flagellum during the second half of spermiogenesis, flows toward the nucleus and separates from the cell to become the residual body. (The Sertoli cells are actively involved in the process of residual body formation, 15).

Some Characteristics of Spermatogenesis

It is of value at this point to present certain characteristics of spermatogenesis that will serve to introduce the histological phenomenon known as the cycle of the seminiferous epithelium. It is soon apparent to anyone investigating the development of mammalian germ cells, of rodents in particular, that the series of changes taking place during spermatogenesis must be a rigidly programmed and timed process. It has in fact been observed from radioautographic studies on rodents in which ^{3}H-thymidine was used as a label of germ cells that the whole process of spermatogenesis has a constant duration (9,16,17,18). The same can be said for each individual step of spermatogenesis. Thus, the duration of spermatogenesis or of any of its component steps for a given species and strain of animal has a given and fixed duration.

In various mammals, including man, it appears that several spermatogonial stem cells form a group and enter spermatogenesis simultaneously. Moreover, topographical analyses on spermatogonial stem cells of the rat (20), bull (21), monkey (22) and man (4) have clearly indicated that when these cells divide, they do so synchronously in groups. Thus, clusters of germ cells evolve through the entire spermatogenic process synchronously, and as a consequence, large numbers of cells all at the same step of development are seen in the seminiferous epithelium. One such group of cells will be referred to as a "generation" in the following discussion.

New groups of spermatogonial stem cells are periodically entering into spermatogenesis before the previous generations have completed their transformation into spermatozoa. Because of this, the seminiferous epithelium is composed of several generations of germ cells, the youngest generations being close to the limiting membrane of the tubule and the more mature germ cells being closer to the lumen of the tubule (Fig. 3).

THE CYCLE OF THE SEMINIFEROUS EPITHELIUM

It has long been recognized that the various generations of germ cells are not associated at random, but form cellular associations of fixed composition (1,23). Thus for example, spermatids at a given step of development are always associated with the same types of spermatocytes and spermatogonia. Consequently, only a limited number of cell associations can be seen in various cross sections of the seminiferous tubules. This characteristic arrangement of the germ cells implies that in any one area of the seminiferous epithelium, the aforementioned cellular associations follow each other in time. The resulting orderly sequence gives rise to the so-called "cycle of the seminiferous epithelium" (23).

Each typical cell association which may then be considered as a "stage of the cycle" can be classified and identified using various arbitrary cytological or histological criteria. Our previous studies of the seminiferous epithelium in several mammals identified the stages by making use of the steps of development of the spermatids stained with the periodic acid-Schiff-hematoxylin technique; the periodic acid-Schiff component demonstrated particularly well the changes taking place in the acrosomic structure of the spermatids (23).

The remarkable arrangement of the germ cells described for most mammals was more difficult to demonstrate in the human testis. Some authors, impressed by the poor organization of spermatogonia, spermatocytes and spermatids in the seminiferous tubules of man, concluded that in contrast to other mammals there was little, if any, correlation between the developmental steps of the germ cells (24,25,26). The author (27), following an investigation of serially sectioned human testicular biopsies fixed in Zenker-formol, found that man was not fundamentally different from other mammals in that germ cells formed typical cell associations. A classification of these typical cell associations into six stages of a cycle was then proposed. The cellular composition of these stages is illustrated in Fig. 2. For a detailed description of the cycle the reader is referred to the original publication (27). In the course of this study it was emphasized, however, that the typical cell associations were frequently obscured by irregularities resulting from the following features. Firstly, in man (unlike most other species where cell associations occupy large segments of tubule), each typical cell association occupies small areas of the tubular lining, such that in tubular sections usually more than one cell association can be identified (Fig. 3). Thus, cells at the interface of two adjacent cell associations usually intermix to produce groupings which are difficult to classify. Secondly, cellular associations are often incomplete due to the absence of one or two generations of germ cells. Thirdly, even a slight pressure on the delicate seminiferous tubules at the time of collection of the biopsy displaces germ cells, disorganizes the seminiferous epithelium and makes the identification of the stages of the cycle impossible. All these factors and possibly others contribute to a disorderly appearance in human tubular histology.

The frequency with which the various stages of the cycle in man appear in tubular sections was taken to be an index of their

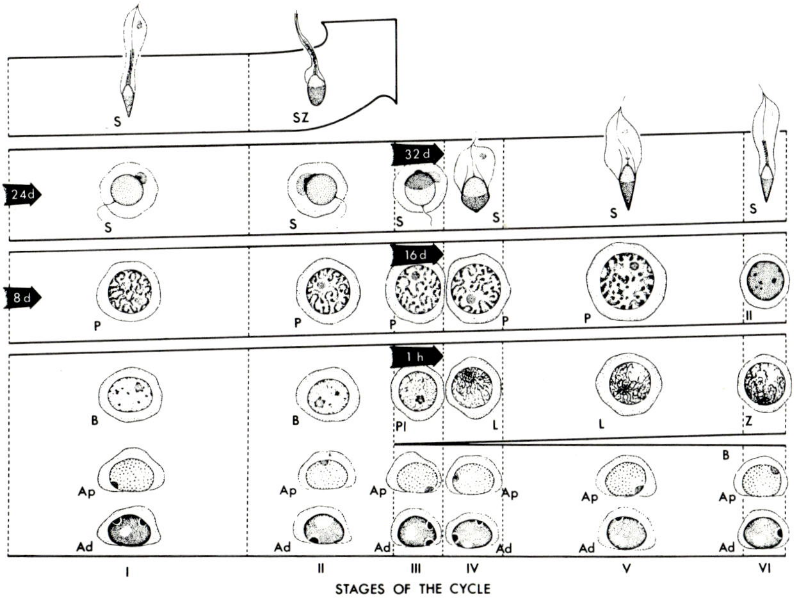

Fig. 2. Diagram illustrating the cellular composition of the six stages of the cycle of the seminiferous epithelium in man. The stages of the cycle are labelled with Roman numerals (I-VI) and correspond to cell associations which succeed one another in time in any given area of the seminiferous tubule according to the sequence from left to right. Following stage VI, stage I reappears and the sequence starts over again. The space allotted to the stages of the cycle are proportional to their relative duration. Lettering: Ad, Ap, B, respectively dark type A, pale type A, type B spermatogonia; Pl, L, Z, P, respectively preleptotene, leptotene, zygotene, pachytene primary spermatocytes; II, secondary spermatocyte; S, spermatids; SZ, spermatozoon, illustrated from its ventral aspect. The arrows correspond to the most advanced labelled cells at various time intervals (indicated on the arrows) after an intratesticular injection of ^{3}H-thymidine (modified from Heller and Clermont, 28). See discussion in the text.

relative duration (27). The stages were of unequal duration, so the space allotted to each stage of the cycle in Fig. 2 was made to correspond approximately to its relative duration.

The duration of the cycle of the seminiferous epithelium in man was estimated by using ^{3}H-thymidine and radioautography (28,29). The radioactive label was injected locally in the testis and biopsies were collected from the sites of injection at various intervals thereafter. Some observations that were made on the radioautographs

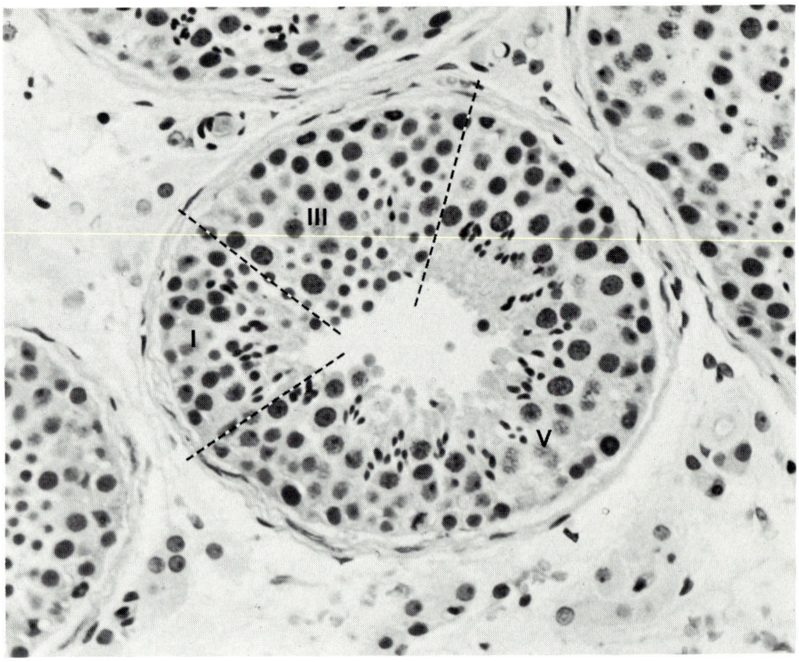

Fig. 3. Low power microphotograph of a tubular cross section showing side by side three typical cell associations (numbered by Roman numerals) as well as their approximate demarcation lines. Fixation: Zenker-formol; staining: hematoxylin -eosin. Magn. x 40.

are shown in Fig. 2. One hour after ^{3}H-thymidine injection some spermatogonia and many preleptotene spermatocytes were labelled as they were duplicating their DNA in preparation for mitosis or meiosis. No other germinal elements showed a radioautographic reaction. Therefore, the preleptotene spermatocytes, the oldest germ cells to be labelled one hour after injection, were considered as the "most advanced labelled cells". This group of cells was followed through the cycle of the seminiferous epithelium at various time intervals after ^{3}H-thymidine injection. Arrows in Fig. 2 give the stages of the cycle in which the most advanced labelled cells, obviously derived from the labelled preleptotene spermatocytes at one hour, were seen at 8, 16, 24 and 32 days after ^{3}H-thymidine administration. At one hour, 16 and 32 days after injection, the most advanced labelled cells, i.e. the preleptotene, pachytene spermatocytes and spermatids respectively, were located in stage III of the cycle. Therefore, it took 16 days for the preleptotene spermatocytes to go through a complete series of six stages (i.e. IV, V, VI, I, II, III) and reappear in stage III as pachytene spermatocytes. Similarly, it took another 16 days for these pachytene spermatocytes to go through another complete series of six stages to become spermatids in stage III. The duration of a complete series of six stages or of one cycle of the seminiferous epithelium would thus be close to 16 days. This estimate was confirmed by observations made at 8 and 24 days after injection. At these two time intervals, the most advanced labelled cells were pachytene spermatocytes and early spermatids, both found at the onset of stage I of the cycle (Fig 2). In this case again it took 16 days for the stage I - pachytene spermatocytes to go through the complete series of six stages to reappear in stage I as newly-formed spermatids.

MODE OF RENEWAL OF SPERMATOGONIA

It is obvious that the continuous production of spermatozoa by the seminiferous tubules, production which in quantitative terms is astronomical over the life span of a normal individual, requires not only an active proliferation of spermatogonia but a maintenance or renewal of the stock of spermatogonial stem cells. While the mode of renewal of spermatogonia has been extensively analyzed in several mammalian species (1,3) the kinetics of the human spermatogonial population has been the object of relatively few investigations. Roosen-Runge and Barlow (26) were the first to tackle the problem systematically by means of a quantitative analysis of the spermatogonial population. From their study they proposed the existence of seven classes of spermatogonia; they regarded the apparent existence of seven differently sized groups of dividing spermatogonia in metaphase as confirmation of this conclusion. They also suggested that new spermatogonial stem cells were produced by any one of the first three or four spermatogonial divisions.

We have re-examined the problem (4,5) following a quantitative analysis of spermatogonia and preleptotene spermatocytes at the various stages of the cycle and a study of the topographical distribution of the dark and pale type A spermatogonia along the tubular limiting membrane. From these data it was found that for each dark type A spermatogonium, there is one pale type A cell at all times during the cycle of the seminiferous epithelium, an observation that was confirmed by the quantitative data of Steinberger and Tjioe (30). It was also calculated that the proportion of either of these two classes of type A spermatogonia to type B cells was 1:2 and finally that the ratio of dark type A or pale type A spermatogonia to preleptotene spermatocytes was 1:4. In summary, the proportions of the various cells counted was as follows: Ad:Ap:B:Pl = 1:1:2:4:. It was also observed that the dark and pale type A spermatogonia, seen in maps which show their topographical arrangement along the tubular wall, were arranged in homogeneous groups and that within these groups the spermatogonia formed pairs of identical cells. This arrangement of the dark and pale type A spermatogonia throughout the duration of the cycle was taken to indicate that the mitoses of spermatogonial stem cells are "equivalent" in nature (i.e. mitoses giving rise to two morphologically identical cells); therefore, the possibility of having "differential" mitoses (i.e. divisions giving rise to two morphologically distinct spermatogonia) to explain the renewal of spermatogonial stem cells should be abandoned. A similar finding was made in several other mammals (19,20,21). These various data (i.e. quantitative and topographic) were used to build a tentative model to illustrate the mode of renewal of spermatogonia in man (Fig. 4). In this model the dark type A spermatogonia were considered as stem cells and according to this scheme one member of a pair of type Ad spermatogonia would give rise to a pair of new stem cells while the other member would produce a pair of the more differentiated type Ap spermatogonia. These in turn would produce type B spermatogonia which would give rise to spermatocytes (Fig. 4).

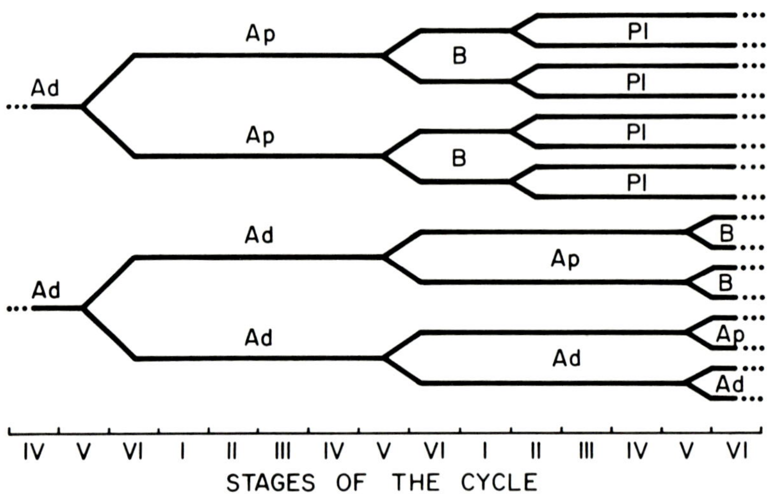

Fig. 4. Model illustrating the development and renewal of spermatogonia in man. Lettering: Ad, Ap, B, respectively dark type A, pale type A, type B spermatogonia; Pl, preleptotene spermatocytes. Roman numerals indicate the stages of the cycle. This model (taken from Clermont, 4) was mainly based on the following two observations: a) spermatogonial mitoses are equational in nature; b) the ratios of cell counts were the following: Ad:Ap:B:Pl = 1:1:2:4. This model is considered only as a tentative illustration of spermatogonial renewal (see discussion in the text).

Although supported by the counts, this model is based on a number of assumptions that remain to be confirmed by additional experimental data. These assumptions are: 1) There is only one generation in each class of spermatogonia; 2) Spermatogonia of each type divide once but only once during each cycle of the seminiferous epithelium; 3) The dark type A spermatogonia constitute the most primitive spermatogonial elements and a class of renewing stem cells; the pale type A spermatogonia would be differentiated elements which arise from the dark type A and in turn give rise to type B cells; 4) Once spermatogonia embark on their course of differentiation into spermatocytes (Ap onward) their evolution is unidirectional and irreversible; they do not revert back to the stem cell condition; 5) The incidence of spermatcgonial degeneration is not important enough to alter the cell ratios. Since so many assumptions remain to be confirmed, it is clear that the model proposed should not be considered as being definitive but, on the contrary, as a first approximation suggested by the data collected so far.

SUMMARY

In man, as in other mammals, spermatogenesis is a long and elaborate process which involves several distinct classes of germinal elements. There are the spermatogonia of which there are at least three main types in human tubules, the dark type A, the pale type A and the type B spermatogonia. Spermatogonia proliferate to give rise to primary spermatocytes. These go through a long prophase which shows characteristic morphological configurations of the chromosomes (leptotene, zygotene, pachytene). This prophase is followed by the subsequent steps of the first maturation division that yields secondary spermatocytes. These cells, after a short interphase, go through the second maturation division which results in the formation of spermatids. In turn, spermatids metamorphose through an extremely complex series of morphological changes into spermatozoa.

The timing of the various steps of spermatogenesis appears to be rigidly fixed and since several spermatogonial stem cells enter spermatogenesis simultaneously, large groups of germinal cells evolve through spermatogenesis synchronously. One such group is referred to as a "generation" of germ cells. The seminiferous epithelium is composed of four or five distinct generations of germ cells. In man, as in other mammals, such generations are not randomly arranged, but form cellular associations of fixed composition. These cell associations, six in man, follow each other chronologically in a regular sequence in any given area of the seminiferous tubule, to form the cycle of the seminiferous epithelium. Such cell associations are often overshadowded by irregularities mainly resulting from the mixing of germ cells. The cycle of the seminiferous epithelium lasts approximately 16 days.

The mode of renewal of spermatogonia was investigated by means of a quantitative and topographical analysis on the various types of spermatogonia; from this, a tentative model to illustrate the development of spermatogonia was proposed. According to this model the dark type A spermatogonia would divide to produce equal numbers of new dark type A spermatogonia and of pale type A spermatogonia.

Each one of the latter would give rise to two type B spermatogonia which in turn would produce four spermatocytes. This model, based on several assumptions not yet verified by observation, should be considered only as a preliminary approximation; the problem of spermatogonial renewal in man remains an open question.

ACKNOWLEDGEMENTS

This work was supported by the Population Council, Inc. The help of Dr. Claire Huckins in the preparation of the manuscript is acknowledged. The drawings were prepared by Mrs. M. Oeltzschner.

REFERENCES

1. Roosen-Runge, E.C., Biol. Rev., 37: 343, 1962.
2. Leblond, C.P., Steinberger, E. and Roosen-Runge, E.C. In Mechanisms Concerned with Conception, Pergamon Press, New York, 1963.
3. Clermont, Y., Arch. Anat. Micr. Morph. Exp. (Suppl.), 56: 7, 1967.
4. Clermont, Y., Amer. J. Anat., 118: 509, 1966.
5. Clermont, Y., Fertil. Steril., 17: 705, 1966.
6. Barr, A., M.Sc. Thesis, McGill University, Montreal, Canada, 1967.
7. Mancini, R.E., Narbaitz, R. and Lavieri, J.C., Anat. Rec., 136: 477, 1960.
8. Tres, L.L. and Solari, A.J., Z. Zellforsch., 91: 75, 1968.
9. Vilar, O. and Paulsen, C.A., Anat. Rec., 157: 336, 1967 (Abstr.)
10. Rowley, M.J., Berlin, J.D. and Heller, C.G., Proceedings of the Society for the Study of Reproduction, 1969.
11. Gatenby, J.B., Beams, H.W. and Woodger, J.H., Quart. J. Micr. Sci., 65: 137, 1921.
12. Clermont, Y. and Leblond, C.P., Amer. J. Anat., 96: 229, 1955.
13. Fawcett, D.W. and Burgos, M.H., Ciba Foundation Colloquium on Ageing, 2: 86, 1956.
14. Fawcett, D.W., Int. Rev. Cytol., 7: 195, 1958.
15. Fawcett, D.W. and Phillips, D.M., J. Reprod. Fertil. (Suppl.), 6: 405, 1969.
16. Clermont, Y., Leblond, C.P. and Messier, B., Arch. Anat. Micr. Morph.Exp ., 48: 37, 1959.
17. Clermont, Y. and Harvey, S.C., Endocrinology, 76: 80, 1965.
18. Desclin, J. and Ortavant, R., Ann. Biol. Anim. Bioch. Biophys., 3: 329, 1963.
19. Clermont, Y. and Leblond, C.P., Amer. J. Anat., 104: 237, 1959.
20. Clermont, Y. and Bustos-Obregon, E., Amer. J. Anat., 122: 237, 1968.
21. Hochereau, M.T., Proceedings VI Cong. Intern. Reprod. Anim. Insem. Artif., Paris 1: 149, 1968.
22. Clermont, Y., Amer. J. Anat., 126: 57, 1969.
23. Leblond, C.P. and Clermont, Y., Ann. N.Y. Acad. Sci., 55: 548, 1952.

24. Branca, A., Arch. Zool. Exp. Gen., 62: 53, 1924.
25. Roosen-Runge, E.C., Fertil. Steril., 7: 251, 1956.
26. Roosen-Runge, E.C. and Barlow, F.D., Amer. J. Anat., 93: 143, 1953.
27. Clermont, Y., Amer. J. Anat. 112: 35, 1963.
28. Heller, C.G. and Clermont, Y., Science, 140: 184, 1963.
29. Heller, C.G. and Clermont, Y., Recent Progr. Hormone Res., Academic Press, 20: 545, 1964.
30. Steinberger, E. and Tjioe, D.Y., Fertil. Steril., 19: 960, 1968.

DISCUSSION

SOLARI: Several years ago we stated that different bodies can be identified in the nuclei of human spermatogonia (Tres, L. and Solari, A.J., Z. Zellforsch mikr. Anat., 91: 75, 1968). One kind of spermatogonium has a type of nuclear body which we called type 1; identified by histochemical methods and ultrastructural techniques as a typical nucleolus. Other spermatogonia have another kind of nuclear body, which is not a characteristic nucleolus, but is attached to the nuclear membrane. It is not chromatin, hence it cannot be a sex chromosome. We have called it type II body. The type B spermatogonium has chromatin bodies which are never closely associated with the nuclear envelope, so again here we have no evidence of a heteropyknotic sex chromosome. We have some histochemical reactions on another kind of nuclear body, which we called number 4; the fifth kind of nuclear body is the only one which is chromatin in nature, but is too small to be a sex chromosome. In summary, we have five types of nuclear bodies in human spermatogonia, and these facts relate to what Prof. Clermont has said, that human spermatogonia must have several steps in their evolution, and these steps in evolution are probably expressed by the characteristic nuclear structures.

CLERMONT: Since I have not studied these cells with the electron microscope I have no comments to make on this point.

VILAR: Among the prepuberal spermatogonia one cannot see the typical adult A pale or A dark spermatogonia. They appear during puberty.

PAULSEN: Dr. Clermont, what is the status of the so-called Ao spermatogonia in human beings? I believe that you have described the Ao spermatogonia in the rat. Also, would the Ao spermatogonia correspond to the A_1 spermatogonia of the monkey?

CLERMONT: The type A_1 spermatogonia, which we have described in the monkey, are probably the equivalent to what we have called the type Ao spermatogonia in the rat, judging from their proliferative activity. As far as the human is concerned, we still do not know of course, but it is quite possible that the A dark spermatogonia would be the equivalent of the type Ao spermatogonia of the rat and the type A_1 of the monkey.

E. STEINBERGER: Dr. Clermont, I was particularly interested in your expression of ambiguity concerning the question of which is the stem cell - the dark or the pale type A spermatogonia. You have proposed in your publications that it is the dark type A although no definite evidence is available for this. I would like to suggest that the type A pale spermatogonium may be the stem cell, at least in the mature type of spermatogenesis. This suggestion is made on the basis of two lines of evidence: 1) that in culture, gradually, the more mature cell types degenerate, and the ratio between the dark and pale changes and shifts towards the pale. In other words, with time, we have numerous pale type spermatogonia which keep dividing, while the dark disappear. 2) the observation on two biopsies from oligospermic individuals, in which no spermatocytes or spermatids were present and the seminiferous tubules were lined with type A pale spermatogonia. I feel that these observations provide some evidence that it is the pale spermatogonia that may be the stem cells.

CLERMONT: What was the age of the testicular tissue that you used for your culture?

E. STEINBERGER: The age varied anywhere between 20 and 30 to 60 days.

CLERMONT: As I said in my presentation, most of the spermatogonia that we see in the human seminiferous tubules could be classified amongst the three classes of cells that were mentioned, i.e. the dark and the pale type A spermatogonia and the type B spermatogonia, but there is still the possibility that other classes of spermatogonia exist. Dr. Heller's group, from their electron microscopic studies, postulated the presence of a fourth type of spermatogonium, so it is not impossible that other spermatogonia with type A pale characteristics would be present along the limiting membrane and could serve as stem cells. We still know too little about the human spermatogonial stem cells.

JIRASEK: I would like to know what is the metabolic significance of the dark or clear spermatogonia. I always thought that the clear spermatogonia were related to the accumulation of glycogen in these cells. The spermatogonia containing glycogen in the cytoplasm appear in the sections as clear. I do not know what cell type begins to accumulate glycogen.

CLERMONT: I should say first, that when I talk of dark or pale type A spermatogonia, I always refer to the staining of the chromatin. What we observed in PA-Schiff stained preparations is that glycogen is present within the cytoplasm of dark type A spermatogonia, while the pale type A have a rather pale cytoplasm. The significance of this observation remains to be clarified.

JOHNSEN: I would like to know if one germinal cell association is associated with one particular Sertoli cell, so that one Sertoli cell and its germ cell association form a unit.

CLERMONT: I do not think so; the area occupied by the given cell association is extremely variable. In some tubules, a given association may occupy a large area, and in this case many Sertoli cells will be seen in it. In other tubules, the same cell association many occupy a small and narrow area of the seminiferous epithelium, and in this case one or a few Sertoli cells will be seen in it. I would say, however, that generally, there are many Sertoli cells per typical cell association.

BURGOS: In favor of a metabolically low active type of spermatogonium in the human testis, the electron microscope shows some cells which contain cytoplasmic crystalloids of Lubarsch and clusters of closely packed mitochondria. These cells usually have a dark nucleus and sometimes contain a portion of clear nucleoplasm which appears under the light microscope as a vacuole.

JOST: Dr. Clermont, you emphasized the fact that the chronology of all the events during spermatogenesis is very rigid. I would like to know if you have any evidence that this is controlled by some other cells, as for instance the Sertoli cells, or if the germ cells do it by themselves?

CLERMONT: We have no evidence favoring one or the other possibility. I do not really know what could control the timing of spermatogenesis.

ELECTRON MICROSCOPY OF THE HUMAN SEMINIFEROUS TUBULES

Oscar Vilar, C. Alvin Paulsen and Donald J. Moore

Centro de Investigaciones sobre Reproduccion, Facultad de Medicina, Buenos Aires, Argentina and Department of Medicine, Washington State University, Seattle, Wash.

The germinal epithelium of the testis is composed of different cell types which constantly undergo changes through a complicated combination of proliferation, differentiation and renewal. Clermont has postulated (1-3) that human germ cells are systematically arranged into six basic stages, and has proposed models for the development and renewal of spermatogonia in man. On the other hand other authors have stated that the cellular division and combinations in the human testis lack the synchronism and steadiness which is seen in other mammals (4-6).

With the development of the electron microscope, certain ultrastructural characteristics of the human testis have been investigated. Data have been accumulated with respect to the testicular connective tissue (7,8), the Sertoli cells (9-13) and the spermatids (14-16).

The present paper is directed towards obtaining information which would provide a basis for more detailed investigation into the histophysiology and histopathology of the germinal epithelium. In recent years research in cellular pathology has emphasized the importance of cytoplasmic(17) rather than nuclear changes, as these appear to be the earliest cellular modifications following diverse types of injury. Therefore, identification and description of the normal germinal cell ultrastructural characteristics are essential to the understanding of morphological events following injury or disease processes.

MATERIAL AND METHODS

For these studies biopsy specimens were obtained from 10 healthy men who had no record of former testicular disease. Biopsy was performed by a modification of Charny's technique (18). The material was prepared for electron microscopy following the method already reported (19).

RESULTS

Tubular Wall

Electron microscopical studies of the wall of the human seminiferous tubules clearly showed two main components: a) The internal one, attached to the germinal epithelium is the basal membrane presenting a lamellar structure, the lamellae are separated by spaces of low electron-density(18). This structure presented infoldings which appeared simple or rather labyrinthic and included some collagen fibers or cytoplasmic processes of the wall cells. The depth of indentation reached one or two microns. b) The external layer showed an alternate arrangement of collagen fibers oriented at different angles together with cells. The cells are extremely elongated, their endoplasmic reticulin was poorly developed and was mainly in the form of lamellae. Fine filaments aggregated in bundles are seen in the cytoplasm of the cells which were found to be somewhat similar to smooth muscle fibers (20).

Germinal Epithelium

The germinal epithelium is composed of spermatogenic or germinal cells and Sertoli cells. It is now a widely accepted belief that there are two independent cell lines in the mammalian testis.

The Sertoli cells are most conspicuous in this epithelium. The germinal cells, with the exception of the earlier spermatogonia are dispersed amongst the Sertoli cells and are separated from the basement membrane by the cytoplasmic processes of the Sertoli cells, which in many cases are not wider than 200Å.

Sertoli Cells. These showed a well developed endoplasmic reticulum which appeared as flat and parallel aggregated cisternae, with associated ribosomes arranged on the membranes in single strands. This type predominated in the cytoplasmatic processes surrounding the germinal cells. In the basal portion of the cell, which contains its characteristically lobulated nucleus with a prominent nucleolus, ribosomes were arranged in membrane-free clusters, and the endoplasmic reticulum appeared in Caufield's solution-fixed preparations as numerous empty smooth-surfaced vesicles of about 600 to 1800Å in diameter. Fixation with glutaraldehyde changes this appearance into a rather tubular form: short, tortuous, interconnected tubules averaging 240-300Å in diameter with localized dilatations were seen in the central portions of these cells, while in the periphery they formed arrays of long, flat membranous profiles. The ground substance of the cytoplasm appeared as a dense material made of granules smaller than ribosomes. As the density of the ground substance is higher than that of the germinal cells, the body of the Sertoli cells and their processes clearly stood out over the surrounding elements. Regarding the density of the ground substance, two types of Sertoli cells can be distinguished; dark and light. At present we are not able to relate these two types to any functional stage or ascertain if they correspond to the two different types of cells demonstrated by Johnsen at light microscopical level (21). Ground substance also included bundles of microtubules of about 300Å. Microfibrils with diameter averaging 35Å were particularly numerous around the nuclear membrane. They were prominent near the head of the spermatids where they appear in bundles parallel to the axis of the spermatid (12). Sertoli cells show wide attachment to the lamellar basement membrane, whose characteristic "pegs" protrude into these cells (7,8).

Spermatogonia. Different types of spermatogonia can be demonstrated with the electron microscope. In the following description we are going to avoid identification by using the alphabet. There are two reasons for this: first, there is more than one paper dealing with spermatogonia where similar letters refer to different cells (1,22). Secondly, when following alphabetical order it could be assumed that this order is related to the sequence of the cells in the spermatogenic line.

The flat type spermatogonium appeared as a rather small, oval-shaped cell. Its larger diameter was parallel to the basement membrane to which it was attached. The nucleus contained one or two conspicuous nucleoli composed of coarse, dense strands which branched and anastomosed in an irregular network. The ground substance of the cytoplasm contained disseminated microtubules and very abundant, uniformly scattered fine granules, 120Å in diameter, which made these cells appear darker than other spermatogonia and spermatocytes, although lighter than Sertoli cells. The endoplasmic reticulum was poorly developed and consisted of a few flat membranous profiles, while occasional scattered clusters of four or five larger and denser ribosomal granules were seen. The round or ovoid mitochondria were relatively large and contained a dense matrix with clearly marked parallel cristae; they tended to aggregate close to the poles of the nucleus. The unremarkable Golgi apparatus also appeared in the vicinity of the nucleus.

Following glutaraldehyde fixation some of the flat spermatogonia showed a circular rarefaction in the center of the nucleoplasm, which appeared as a "vacuole" of less density, but without any limiting membrane or special structure within it. This characteristic was not exclusive to flat spermatogonia as similar "vacuolizations" could also occasionally be seen in round spermatogonia, preleptotene spermatocytes and in spermatids.

The round type spermatogonium, a larger, circular cell, was also attached to the basement membrane. Its round, homogeneous nucleus was lighter and contained a small nucleolus which frequently did not show up in the ultra-thin sections. The ground substance of the cytoplasm was less dense and contained no microtubules, although the Golgi apparatus was more conspicuous. While the mitochondria were smaller, they showed well-developed cristae in a dense matrix. In contrast to the flat type spermatogonia, they were scattered throughout the cytoplasm. Small crystal like structures were seen. They presented an irregular shape and were formed of bundles of fibrils or tubules aligned in the long axis. The nucleus of human spermatogonia has been studied recently by Tres and Solari (23). Five different types of nuclear bodies were observed in type A (flat) spermatogonia. Type I bodies are typical nucleoli. Types II, III and V are considered to be atypical nucleoli. Type IV bodies are small chromatin condensations. These authors stated that they could not establish a valid criterion for distinguishing the different kinds of A gonia at the ultrastructural level although they suggested the existence at least 2 types of A gonia. In these authors' criteria the different nuclear bodies probably reflect different metabolic activities.

A third type of cell was noted which seemed to correspond to the usual descriptions for preleptotene primary spermatocyte. The cytoplasmic subcellular characteristics of this cell were very similar to those of round spermatogonia and showed little resemblance to those of primary spermatocytes. They differed from the round type spermatogonia in that they were separated from the basement membrane, as well as from neighboring cells, by the previously described ramifications of the Sertoli cell cytoplasm. It was frequently noted that intercellular bridges existed between these preleptotene cells and round spermatogonia.

Although in the course of meiosis primary spermatocytes underwent remarkable changes in size as well as in the characteristics of the nucleus, the subcellular features of the cytoplasm remained stable. These changes in the nucleus will be presented later on by Dr. Solari. The numbers of polyribosomes dispersed throughout the ground substance were greater than in any other germ cell type. But since the ground substance contained little else, the primary spermatocytes were the lightest cells in the germinal epithelium. Short and very flat membranous profiles were scattered throughout the cytoplasm, and flat saccules were located throughout the nucleus. The prominent Golgi apparatus, round and rather compact in form, was situated at one of the poles of the nucleus. The cristae mitochondriales did not show the straight parallel pattern which was seen in the spermatogonia; instead, they followed an irregular course and frequently coalesced with the outer membrane, giving the mitochondria a "vacuolated" appearance (24). Microtubules were scattered throughout the cytoplasm, and although their appearance was undistinctive, they seemed to be unrelated to the microtubules of the spindle during the first meiotic division.

The earliest modification of primary spermatocytes, which enabled those cells to be distinguished from spermatogonia, was the appearance of very fine single leptotene threads. These were always present even in the youngest spermatocytes. We were, therefore, unable to find a "resting" stage that could be interposed between the spermatogonial mitosis and the meiotic prophase.

The secondary spermatocytes were relatively small cells, slightly larger than young spermatids, and obviously smaller than the neighboring spermatocytes. They were seen infrequently and appeared close to or partially in the lumen of the seminiferous tubules. The nucleus was round with a rather homogeneous aspect; the nucleolus was very inconspicuous and was absent much of the time. The endoplasmic reticulum was made of rosaries of small flat saccular profiles which were arranged concentrically in relation to the nucleus. The limiting membranes of these saccules were agranular and tortuous. Scattered among the endoplasmic reticulum,round mitochondria were found,which present the same vesiculization seen in the primary spermatocytes and spermatids. Resting and dividing secondary spermatocytes were generally seen co-existing in the same portion of the tubule.

During the course of spermiogenesis, the spermatids showed changes in the configuration of the acrosome which did not differ from those classically known (14,15). Five different stages of progressive change in the morphology of the spermatid were easily characterized.

In Stage A, corresponding to the beginning of spermiogenesis, the spermatids were round, with a round homogeneous nucleus. Toward the end of this phase the acrosome granule, as well as the acrosome vesicle, could be seen.

The cap finally became established during Stage B, and the nucleus could be seen starting its elongation, although the appearance of the nucleoplasm remained unchanged. During this stage the microtubule of the manchette first appeared, while within the cytoplasmic branches of the Sertoli cell similar microtubules became arranged parallel to the axis of the spermatid.

Elongation proceeded during Stage C, but the most remarkable change occurred in the nucleoplasm where chromatin-like material became condensed in flocs or large irregular granules, which gave the nucleus a "tigroid" appearance.

During Stage D, progressive reduction in nuclear size could be observed, the chromatin flocs formed wider clusters, and the nucleus became more and more compact until all the interstices among the flocs were obliterated and the nucleus again presented a homogeneous appearance.

In the final phase, Stage D2, most of the cytoplasm of the spermatid became eliminated, and residual bodies could be seen; either partially free in the lúmen of the tubule, or in the process of being "phagocytozed" by the Sertoli cells.

DISCUSSION

Each cell in the human germinal epithelium shows, in both the cytoplasm and the nucleus, particular subcellular characteristics which allow its identification in electron micrographs. For the cytologic study of the testis, electron microscopy offers undoubted advantages over light microscopy. The distinctive features of the germinal cell types that can be established with the light microscope, either in normal or pathological conditions, represent primarily morphological configuration of the chromatin and the nucleolus, since the cytoplasmic details are poor and the cellular limits are difficult, or impossible to determine. Furthermore, different fixatives give diverse chromatin patterns, and it is sometimes difficult to classify spermatogonia or correlate the different classifications which appear in the literature (3,22).

Clermont (1) recognized two types of A spermatogonia (A dark and A pale), the first one having a large vacuole-like cavity in the nucleus. He gave a ratio of Ad:Ap of 1:1. We were not able to establish with the electron microscope the same discrimination among spermatogonia. Following fixation with glutaraldehyde, we observed in some nuclei a rarefaction of the nucleoplasm which might appear as a vacuole-like structure, but since procedures in the preparation of the specimen are different, it is difficult to affirm that this "vacuole" corresponds to that described by light microscopists. On the other hand, our ratio between the "vacuolated" and "non-vacuolated" flat spermatogonia is not 1:1, but closer to that of Roosen-Runge and Barlow (5) who found vacuoles in 96 of 1000 nuclei. We observed in the fragments fixed in glutaraldehyde, that similar "vacuoles" could be found in other types of germinal cells (gonovytes, spermatogonia, round spermatids, etc.). Thus it appears that this "vacuole" is not a distinctive characteristic of any type of cell, or of any specific stage, but a kind of modification of the nucleus of the germinal cells due to the aldehyde fixation. Its significance we are not yet able to evaluate.

We did not find an identifiable resting stage of primary spermatocyte that would be interposed between the last spermatogonial mitosis and the meiotic prophase. The youngest spermatocyte seemed to be already in meiosis. Sotelò and Trujillo-Cenoz (25) reported the same finding in other species, and stated that "the appearance of very fine chromosome threads (leptotene threads) seems to be the better mark to recognize the transformation of spermatogonia into spermatocytes. The preleptotene cell, here described, presented subcellular characteristics, which corresponded to those of B spermatogonia rather than spermatocytes, except for the fact that they were not attached to the basement membrane but were surrounded by Sertoli cells and so separated from the other cells and the basement membrane. The existence of cellular bridges between these cells and B spermatogonia unquestionably indicates their origin. The preleptotene stage probably represents a more differentiated type of B spermatogonia moving into the core of the germinal epithelium.

It could be speculated that the establishment of the above mentioned relationship between the Sertoli and the preleptotene cell is an unavoidable determining factor that induces, after the last spermatogonial division, the transformation of the spermatogonium into a primary spermatocyte, which in time will be able to accomplish meiotic division. The function of the Sertoli cells is not yet known, but it was suggested long ago that the products of the secretion of these cells could supply nutrition to the germinal cells (26). Also, it has been shown that they can act as an active transporting system as labelled substances injected into adult rats leave the circulation in the intertubular spaces and rapidly move into the seminiferous tubules, diffusing through the cytoplasm of the Sertoli cells (10). Christensen and Fawcett(27) have advanced the idea that the site of hormone production in steroid producing cells is in the agranular endoplasmic reticulum. The agranular endoplasmic reticulum of the Sertoli cell could be considered a morphological base to support the claim that these cells produce steroid hormones, but no consistent proof has been found at the present time. As was also speculated by Christensen (8) the parallel microtubules in the Sertoli cytoplasm could be related to the mechanism of the release and holding of the spermatids.

The supporting cells reach maturity at pubertal ages, simultaneously with the beginning of spermatogenesis, and an obvious regulation by the hypophysis occurs. We can only conjecture as to whether gonadotropins act upon both germinal and Sertoli cells or whether the primary target is the supporting cells (Sertoli) which then could influence the germinal ones. Courot (28) injected gonadotropic preparations into lambs whose testes were not yet showing spermatogenic activity and observed that while no important evolution of the gonocytes was seen, a fairly constant stimulation of precursors of Sertoli cells was observed.

Mancini et al. (22) have described additional types of spermatogonia in the adult human testis; binucleated, hypertrophic and pyknotic. While binucleated spermatogonia, as well as other binucleated types, are seen frequently and merely indicate a delay of the cytokinesis as Fawcett and Burgos (14) have reported, hypertrophic and pyknotic cells are seen rather seldom, and in our opinion have little significance. Large spermatogonia have been interpreted as polyploid cells (5), and pyknosis probably indicates failure of isolated cells to pursue the complete evolution toward spermatozoa.

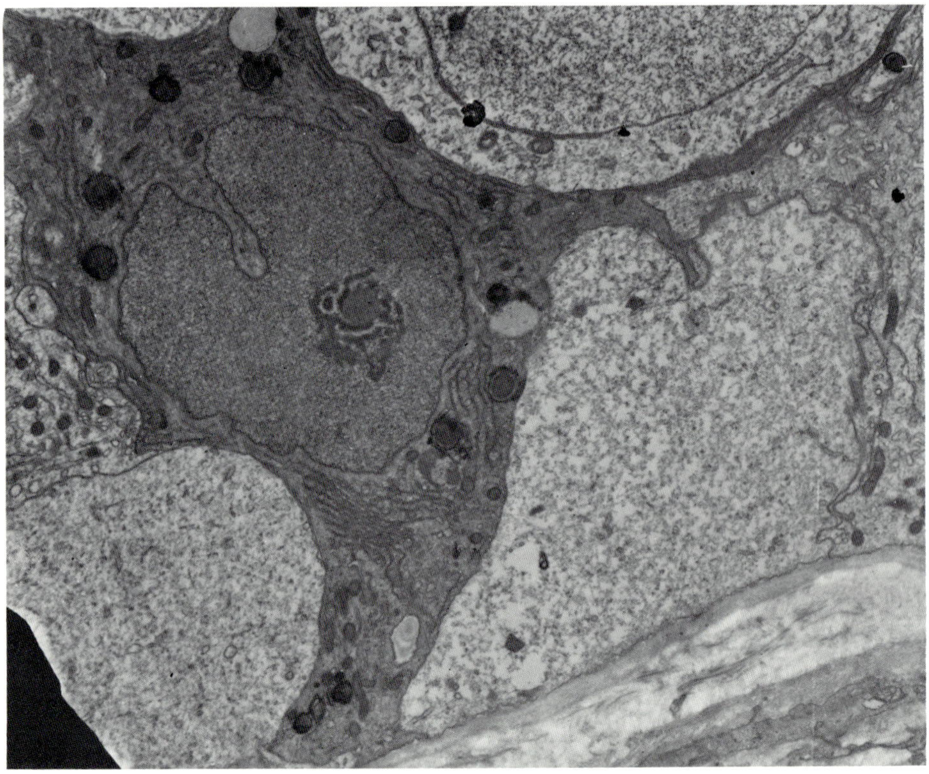

Fig. 1. Human Sertoli cell. Note the well developed nucleolus. x 17,000

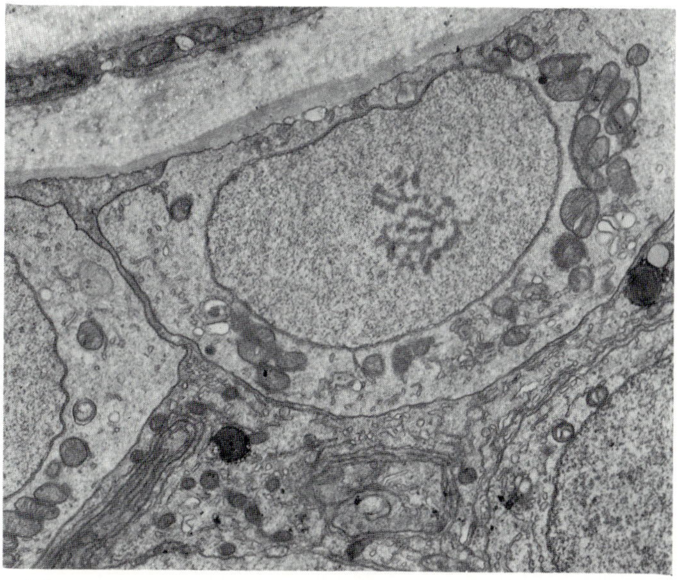

Fig. 2. Flat spermatogonium in contact with the basal lamina. x 30,000.

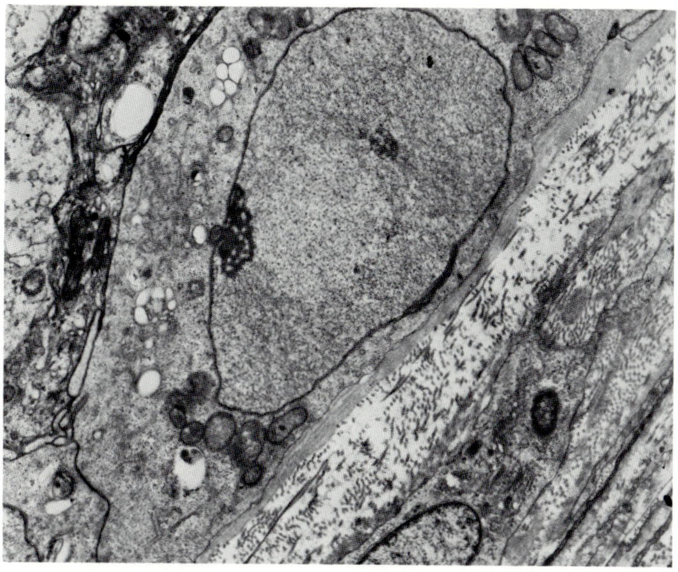

Fig. 3. Flat spermatogonium. Note the "vacuolization of the nucleus" x 27,300.

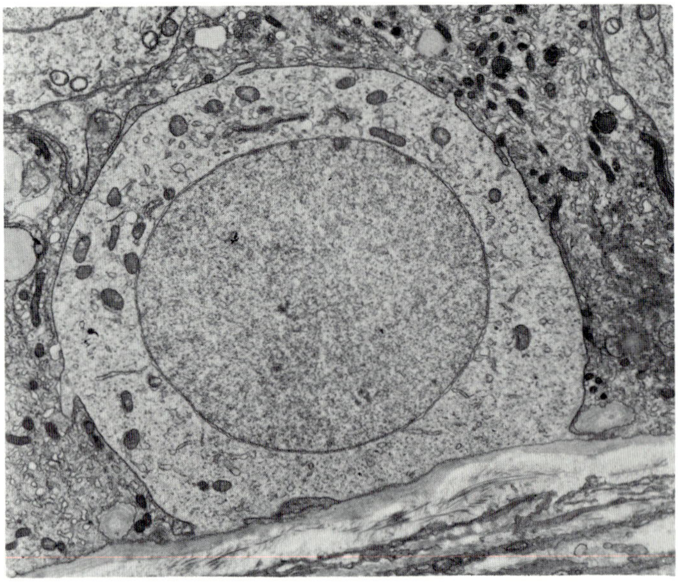

Fig. 4. Round spermatogonium. Note that the basal lamina forms "pegs" which project into the Sertoli cells. x 18,000.

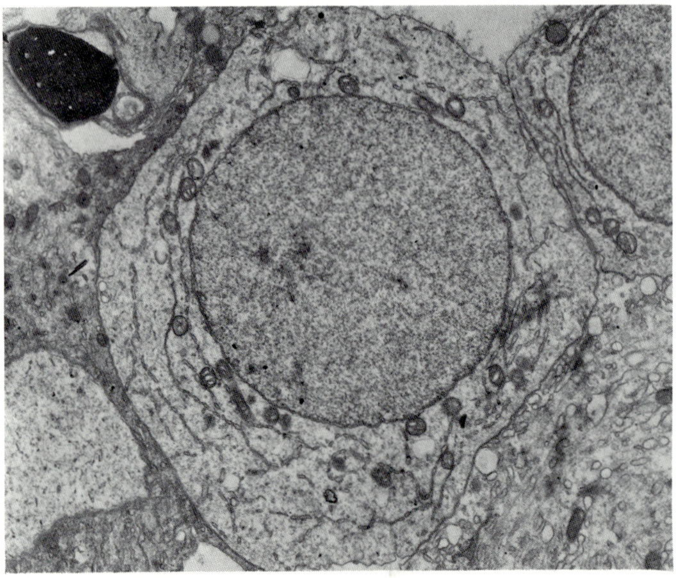

Fig. 5. Spermatocyte II. x 17,000.

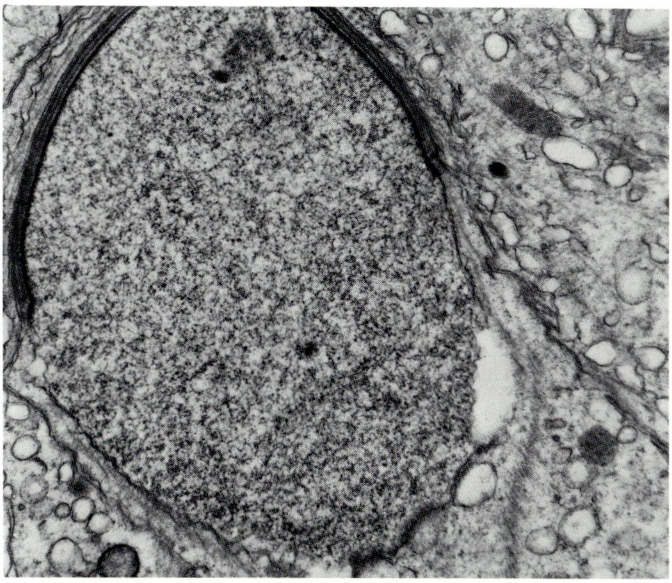

Fig. 6. Spermatid B. Note the tubules of the "manchette" as well as those in the cytoplasm of Sertoli cell. x 40,000.

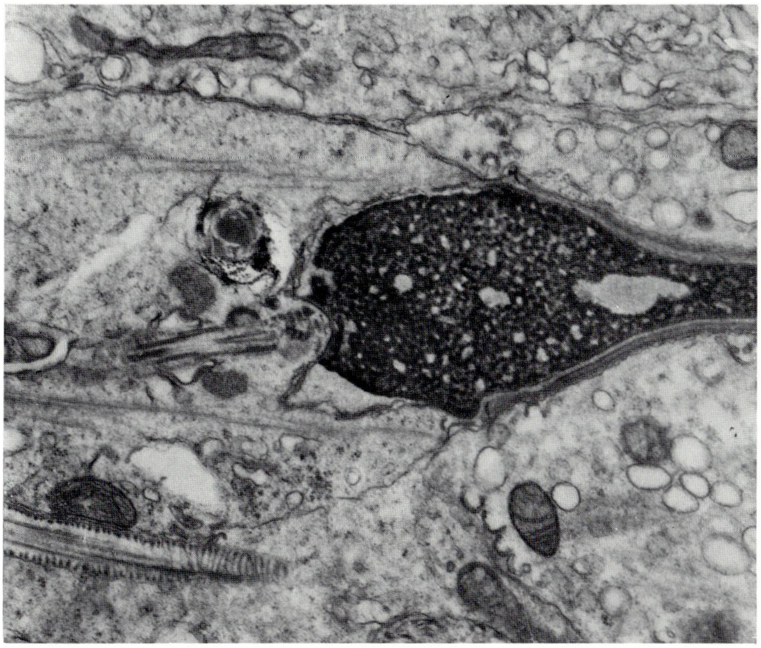

Fig. 7. Spermatid D. Note condensed nuclear material and the connecting piece. x 27,300.

ACKNOWLEDGEMENTS

Supported by the National Research Council (Argentina) and by AEC contract No. At (45-1) - 2225.

REFERENCES

1. Clermont, Y.,Amer.J. Anat. 112: 35, 1963.
2. Clermont, Y.,Amer.J. Anat. 118: 509, 1966.
3. Clermont, Y., Fertil. Steril. 17: 705, 1966.
4. Branca, A., Arch. Zool. Exp. et Gen. 62: 53, 1924.
5. Roosen-Runge, E.C. and Barlow F.B.,Amer.J. Anat. 93: 143, 1953.
6. Markewitz, M., Veenema, R. and Fingerhut, B., Int. J. of Fertil., 14: 22, 1969.
7. Burgos, M.H., Rev. Soc. Argent. Biol. 35: 309, 1959.
8. Mancini, R.E., Vilar, O., P. del Cerro, M. and Lavieri, J.C., Acta Physiol. Lat. Amer., 14: 382, 1964.
9. Fawcett, D.W. and Burgos, M.H., Anat. Rec. 124: 401, 1956.
10. Vilar, O., Perez del Cerro, M.P. and Mancini, R.E., Exp. Cell Res., 27: 158, 1962.
11. Bawa, S.R., J. Ultrastruct.Res., 9: 459, 1963.
12. Nagano, T., Z. Zellforsch., 89: 39, 1968.
13. Nagano, T., Z. Zellforsch., 73: 89, 1966.
14. Fawcett, D.W., Burgos, M.H., Ciba Colloquia on Aging of Transient Tissues, 2: 86, 1955.
15. Horstmann, E., Z. Zellforsch., 54: 68, 1961.
16. De Kretser, D.M., Z. Zellforsch., 98: 477, 1969.
17. Trump, B.F., Goldblatt, P.J. and Stowell, R.E., Lab. Invest. 14: 1969, 1965.
18. Paulsen, C.A., In Textbook of Endocrinology, ed. Williams, R.H. R.E. Saunders, Philadelphia, p. 405, 1962.
19. Vilar, O., Steinberger, A. and Steinberger, E., Z. Zellforsch. 74: 529, 1966.
20. Clermont, Y., Exp. Cell Res. 15: 438, 1958.
21. Johnsen, S.G., Acta Endocr. (Kobenhavn) 61: 111, 1969.
22. Mancini, R.E., Narbaitz, R. and Lavieri, J.C., Anat. Rec. 136: 477, 1960.
23. Tres. L. and Solari, A.J., Z. Zellforsch., 91: 75, 1968.
24. Andre, J., J. Ultrastruct. Res. Suppl. 3: 1, 1962.
25. Sotelo, J.R. and Trujillo-Cenoz, O., Z. Zellforsch., 51: 243, 1960.
26. Regaud, C., Arch. Anat. Micr. Morph., 4: 231, 1901.
27. Christensen, A.K. and Fawcett, D.W., J. Biophys. Biochem. Cytol. 9: 653, 1961.
28. Courot, M., Ann. Biol. Anim. Bioch. Biophys. 5: 145, 1965.

FINE STRUCTURE OF TESTICULAR INTERSTITIAL CELLS IN HUMANS

A. Kent Christensen

Department of Anatomy, Stanford School of Medicine

Stanford, California 94305

It is now well established that the interstitial or Leydig cells are the principal site of androgen production in the mammalian testis. In rats, the interstitial tissue can be separated from the seminiferous tubules and shows considerably more activity than the tubules in synthesizing androgen from cholesterol in vitro (1,2). Proof that the interstitial cells are indeed the source of this activity within the interstitial tissue comes from histochemical studies in which the reaction product of 3β -hydroxysteroid dehydrogenase appears mainly in these cells. This approach has been applied to a variety of vertebrate species with consistent results, although it appears somewhat more difficult to demonstrate in the human testis (3).

For a number of years we have been interested in the fine structure and correlated function of testicular interstitial cells, especially in guinea pigs (4-6), rats (7), mice (8) and opossums (9). In the present paper I will summarize the fine structure of human testicular interstitial cells, based on the literature and on recent electron microscopy done in this laboratory on human testes fixed by perfusion.

There is already a considerable literature on the light and electron microscopy of human interstitial cells. Observations with the light microscope have been reviewed by Stieve (10), Ito and Oinuma (11), and Sniffen (12). The most useful general descriptions of human interstitial cells as seen by electron microscopy are those of Fawcett and Burgos (13), Yamada (14) and de Kretser (15,16); papers by Nishimura and Kondo (17), Schmidt (18), Hatakeyama (19) and Nagano (20) are also available. Pelliniemi and Niemi (21) have followed the development of interstitial cells with the electron microscope in the human fetus. The fine structure of interstitial cells in the testicular feminization syndrome (22) and in an androgen-producing tumor (23) have been described. Restricted topics have been dealt with by Desolle (24) Sisson and Fahrenbach (25) and Yasuzumi et al. (26).

With all these papers available on the fine structure of human interstitial cells, why publish another one here? Aside from whatever use a brief review may serve, the main justification lies in the improved preservation for electron microscopy obtained by perfusion-fixation in the present material. Steroid-
are notoriously difficult to fix for electron microscopy, and this has led to considerable dispute about some important aspects of their fine structure. The most notable uncertainty concerns the normal structural organization of the smooth endoplasmic reticulum (ER), which is characteristically abundant in steroid-secreting cells. Most of the enzymes of androgen biosynthesis from small precursors are probably either attached to the smooth ER or lie in the cytoplasm near it (see (7) for an extensive review of the fine structure and cell fractionation literature on steroid-secreting cells). It is of considerable functional interest to know whether this reticulum is a continuous system of interconnected membrane tubules, which would allow transport within a stable closed system, or whether it is a discontinuous system of membrane vesicles, posing very different functional problems. The evidence one obtains from electron micrographs on questions such as this depends on how the tissue was preserved for electron microscopy.

The method of preservation used in all the previous studies on human interstitial cells is to cut the testis tissue into small pieces in a drop of fixative. Aside from the mechanical damage as the tissue is diced, the slow penetration of the fixative gives ample time for degenerative change and a differential response by cells to the gradual increase in fixative concentration around them. As a result, the quality of fixation may vary markedly from one place to another in a single small piece of tissue. In contrast, fixation by perfusion supplies fixative rapidly and uniformly to all parts of the testis without disturbing structural relationships, and the preservation obtained is of consistent high quality throughout the whole organ. Perfusion-fixation has been used previously in this laboratory to study testicular interstitial cells in guinea pigs (4) and rats (7).

In the present paper I will describe the fine structure of testicular interstitial cells from human testes that have been fixed by perfusion with a formaldehyde-glutaraldehyde-picric acid fixative (27), used 2/3 strength). One testis came from a 64-year old man undergoing orchiectomy because of prostatic cancer. The man had otherwise been healthy and active, and the testes appeared relatively normal by light microscopy. The other testis used in this study was from a 22-year old man, and was removed because it had become lodged under the skin above the external inguinal ring. This testis appeared cryptorchid by light microscopy. In both cases the testes were received from surgeons within a minute or so after the blood supply had been clamped off, and the stubs of two main branches of the testicular artery in the spermatic cord were then cannulated with blunted 20 gauge needles. Details of the perfusion apparatus and method have been published previously (4). Perfusion continued for about an hour, after which the testes were allowed to remain another hour before being sliced and were then left in fixative for another two or three hours. The material was stored in the refrigerator overnight or longer in 0.1M sodium cacodylate buffer. Small pieces of tissue were postfixed in 1.3% osmium tetroxide buffered with s-collidine (28), and were then dehydrated and embedded in Epon (29). The material was stained in block with 1% uranyl acetate in ethanol during the dehydration. Pale gold sections were stained with lead citrate and were viewed in an RCA EMU-3F or a Siemens Elmiskop 1A electron microscope. Sections 2μ in thickness for light microscopy were cut from the Epon blocks and were stained by the method of Richardson et al. (30).

In the rest of this chapter I will first catalogue and briefly describe the various structures seen in human interstitial cells, basing the description on the electron micrographs of perfused material that illustrate the paper,with supplemental information from the literature. I will then attempt to correlate functional information with these fine structure observations to the modest extent that is possible at present, and will also compare the organelles as seen in humans with those in steroid-secreting cells of other species. A more extensive description of the interstitial tissue in the human testis fixed by perfusion is being prepared for publication elsewhere.

GENERAL DESCRIPTION OF THE INTERSTITIAL CELLS

In a light micrograph of perfusion-fixed testis from a 64-year old man (Fig. 1), the dark interstitial cell clusters are seen between lighter seminiferous tubules. Small blood vessels, appearing white and somewhat swollen here because of the perfusion, often have a few interstitial cells associated with them or may pass through interstitial cell clusters. The white rectangle in Fig. 1 encloses an area similar to that shown in a very low power electron micrograph in Fig. 2.

The large cluster of interstitial cells in Fig. 2 lies in the interstitial tissue outside the tunica propria, a sheath of flattened (and perhaps contractile) cells surrounding the seminiferous tubule. A capillary (cap) receives hormone produced by the cluster. Below the capillary is an adventitial macrophage (mac). Three interstitial cell nuclei are visible at the top of the cluster. The white circles in the interstitial cells are lipid droplets whose content

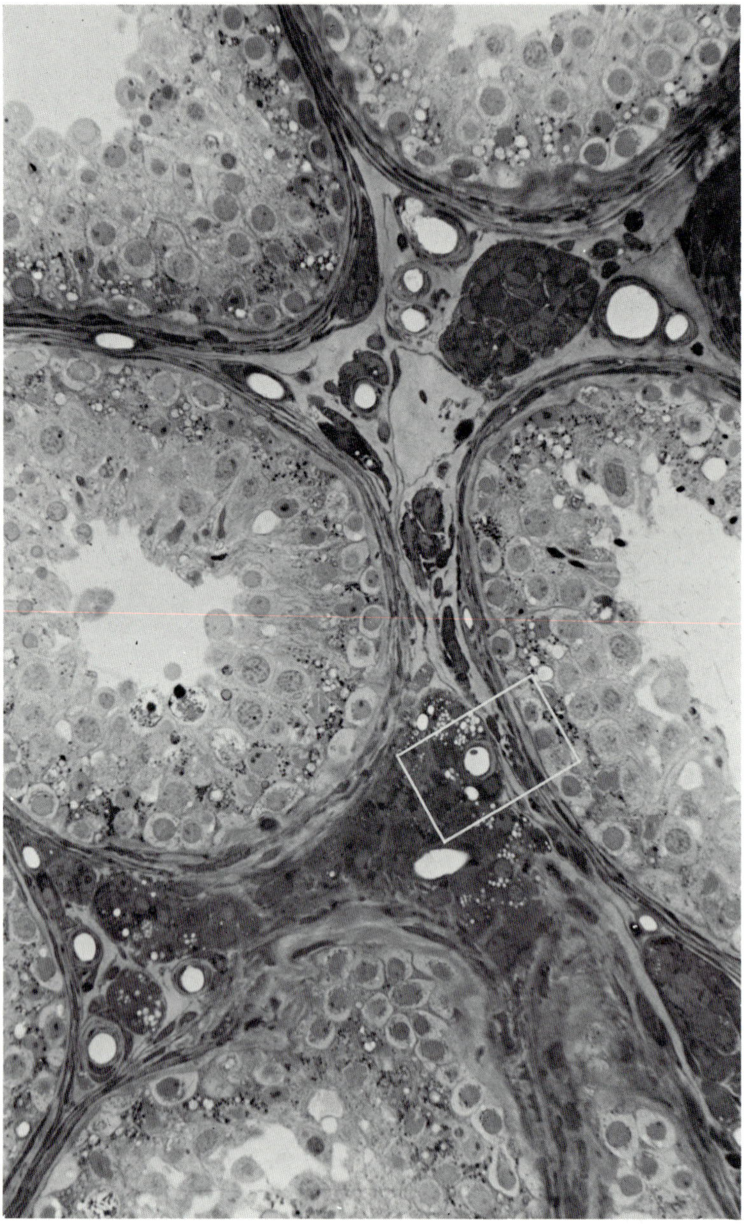

Fig. 1. Light micrograph of human testis fixed by perfusion. Dark clusters of interstitial cells lie between the seminiferous tubules. The area enclosed by the rectangle is similar to that shown in a low power electron micrograph in Fig. 2. From 64-year old man; 2μ Epon section of material fixed and embedded for electron microscopy. x 450.

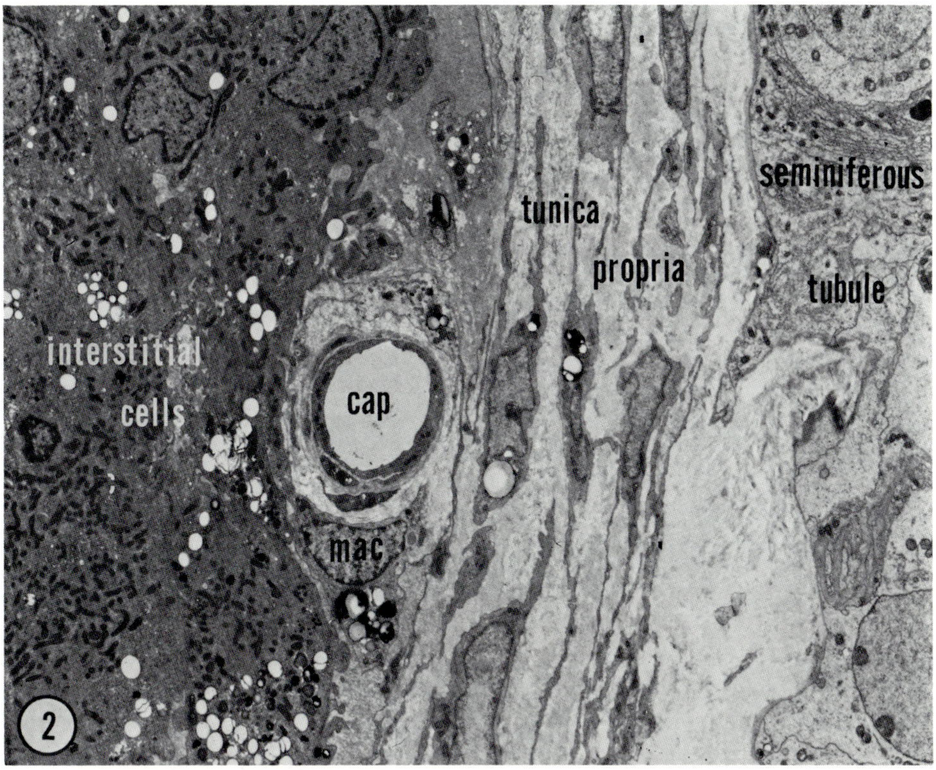

Fig. 2. Edge of a seminiferous tubule and adjacent interstitial cells, showing general level of preservation in perfused material. This very low power electron micrograph shows an area resembling that enclosed in the rectangle in figure 1. A capillary (cap) and adventitial macrophage (mac) are included in the field. The white circles in the interstitial cells are extracted lipid droplets. From a 64-year old man. x 2400.

has been extracted by the solvents used for electron microscopy. The dark gray structures scattered throughout the cytoplasm are mitochondria, while the black granules, especially evident at lower right in the cluster, are lipofuscin pigment granules. Note the uniform texture of the cytoplasm in the interstitial cells of this perfused material. There are no "dark" and "light" cells, as have been described in human testis fixed by routine methods (for example, 15,16). There is also no indication that the smooth endoplasmic reticulum is vesiculated in any of the cells. The preservation shown here is typical of that seen in all the sections that have been examined from both perfused testes.

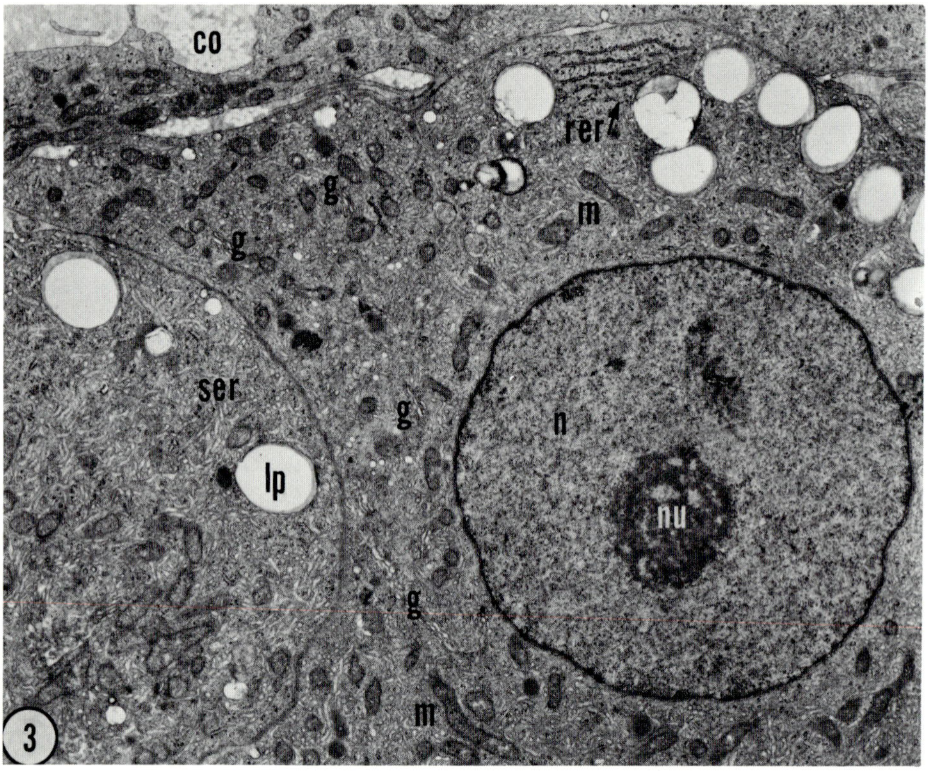

Fig. 3. Human interstitial cells, showing general cellular organization. See text for description and abbreviations. Ectopic testis from 22-year old man; perfusion-fixed. x 7,100.

Fig. 3 is an electron micrograph showing most of one interstitial cell and parts of two others, still at fairly low magnification. The nucleus (n) is large and round, and contains a prominent nucleolus (nu) made up of a network of nucleolonemata. There is little heterochromatin in the nucleus, except for a scanty layer, here almost lacking, just inside the nuclear envelope (it is more prominent in the nuclei of Fig. 2). The cytoplasm contains a few large, partially extracted lipid droplets (lp) and many mitochondria (m), generally rod-shaped and about 0.3μ in diameter, that are cut in various planes of sections. The cytoplasm between the mitochondria is filled with smooth endoplasmic reticulum (ser), which will be better seen in subsequent electron micrographs. The cell contains an unusually large patch of rough endoplasmic reticulum (rer), consisting of five flattened cisternae; isolated small cisternae are scattered here and there in the cytoplasm. Elements of the Golgi complex (g) are seen in various parts of the cell. No basal lamella is visible on the outer surface of the plasma membrane. Small white spots in the extracellular space are negative images of collagen fibers (co) cut in cross section.

A view of the cytoplasm at higher magnification is seen in Fig. 4. The most striking feature of the interstitial cell cytoplasm, as in most steroid-secreting cells, is the abundant smooth endoplasmic reticulum (ser) composed of interconnecting tubules extending throughout the available cytoplasmic space. The tubules are generally 600-700 Å in diameter and branch and anastomose freely in three dimensions, although in this two-dimensional view many are seen only in cross or oblique section. At upper left are small profiles of rough endoplasmic reticulum (rer) which connect (arrow) with the smooth reticulum. Free ribosomes (r) lie between the tubules of the smooth ER, but are not attached to them. Some of these ribosomes occur in clusters that probably constitute polysomes (ps). The mitochondria (m) are generally rod-shaped but here are mostly cut in cross or oblique section. Their internal structure will be seen to better advantage in Fig. 5. A large partially extracted lipid droplet (lp) is present in the lower part of the field. An element of the Golgi complex (g) consists of two (usually more) flattened sacs lying parallel to one another. At right is part of a crystal of Reinke (cr), showing one of the several crystal patterns seen as this structure is cut in various ways relative to its three crystal axes. Within the nucleus at the bottom of the micrograph is scanty heterochromatin (h) and a fibrous lamina (fl) lining the inner surface of the nuclear envelope, which is penetrated by occasional pores (p). The surface of the cell at upper left is thrown into irregular folds which lie against processes from adjacent cells; in one area the adjacent plasma membranes have fused as a tight or gap junction (tj).

Fig. 5 is a thinner section at higher magnification to give further detail of some structures seen previously. The tubules of the smooth ER are cut in longitudinal (ser) and various oblique or cross sections. No content can be made out within these tubules. The mitochondria are generally rod-shaped, of variable diameter, and may branch in complex ways (m). It is difficult to interpret the three-dimensional form of the cristae. In some cases they appear to be lamellar, extending across the mitochondrion, while others seem to be tubular. These profiles can be explained if one assumes that most of the cristae are fenestrated lamellae. The cristae presumably arise from the inner membrane of the mitochondrion, but only occasionally can a direct connection be found (arrow). The usual mitochondrial granule (mg) is often seen, and it is not uncommon to find what appear to be intramitochondrial lipid droplets (not shown here). Within the mitochondria shown in Fig. 5

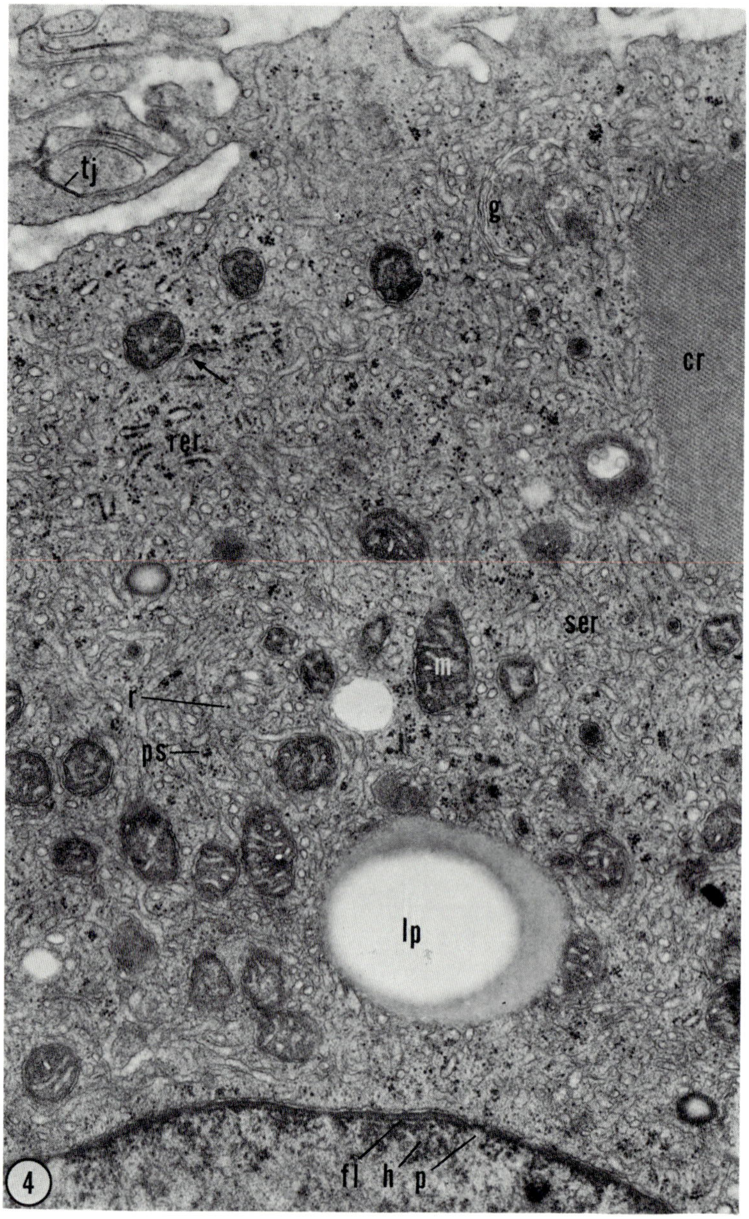

Fig. 4. Cytoplasm of human interstitial cell, showing abundant smooth endoplasmic reticulum (ser) and crystal of Reinke (cr). See text for other abbreviations. Ectopic testis from 22-year old man; perfusion-fixed x 24,000.

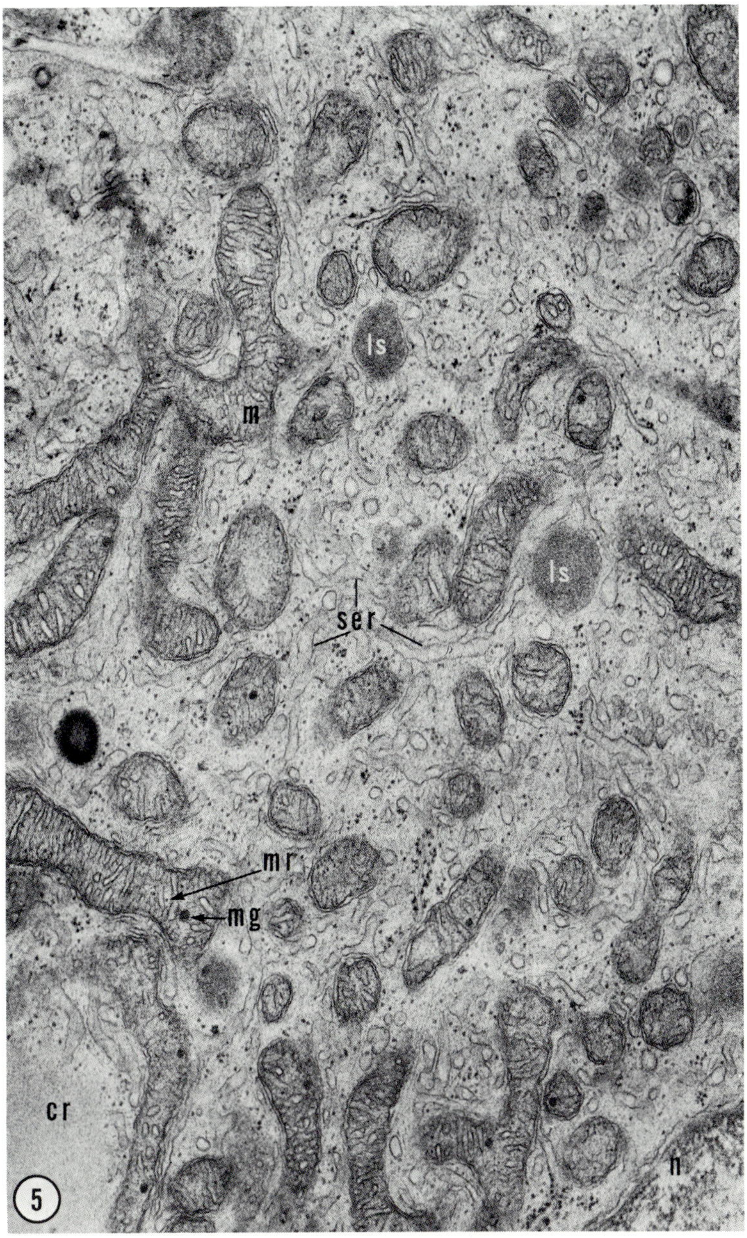

Fig. 5. Detail of cytoplasm in human interstitial cell. The mitochondrial cristae are probably in the form of fenestrated cisternae. Occasional cristae clearly arise from the inner mitochondrial membrane (arrow). The mitochondria also contain conventional matrix granules (mg) and presumptive mitochondrial ribosomes (mr). Ectopic testis from a 22-year old man; perfusion-fixed. x 33,000.

are also numerous small particles of a size and appearance one would expect for mitochondrial ribosomes (mr). A nucleus (n), a crystal of Reinke (cr) and presumptive lysosomes (ls) are also present in the field. Lysosomes may allow the development of residual bodies, in which the polymerization products of autoxidized unsaturated fatty acids may accumulate to produce a pigment, giving rise to lipofuscin pigment granules (shown only at low magnification in Fig. 2).

In this description I have emphasized the structures whose preservation is improved by perfusion-fixation, and have not pretended to cover the extensive literature on Reinke's crystals and their precursors, on cytoplasmic filaments, on lipofuscin pigment or on some other topics of interest in the fine structure of human interstitial cells.

COMPARATIVE AND FUNCTIONAL CONSIDERATIONS

In conclusion I will summarize briefly how the organelles of human testicular interstitial cells compare with those seen in the steroid-secreting cells of other mammals. In addition, I will outline some of the correlations that might be made between structure and function in human interstitial cells, if one is allowed to supplement the meager evidence from human material with data from animal studies on steroid-secreting tissues. Such extrapolations are hazardous because of possible tissue and species differences, but they may at least give a heuristic functional outlook to the fine structure that has been presented. To attempt either of these summaries with full documentation would be cumbersome and would surpass the bounds allowed for this brief chapter. Those who desire the complete references are referred to our review (7) describing the fine structure and cell fractionation studies on steroid-secreting cells in mammals.

Human interstitial cells are moderate steroid-secreting cells from several points of view. The cells average about 15μ in diameter and are thus larger than interstitial cells of rats (about 10μ), but considerably smaller than those of the boar (about 35μ). The smooth ER is more abundant than that seen in rat interstitial cells (certainly more than rat adrenal cortical cells), but is not as voluminous as that of guinea pig or opossum interstitial cells, or guinea pig granulosa lutein cells. Human interstitial cells have less rough ER than many other steroid-secreting cell types. The mitochondria resemble morphologically those of the guinea pig interstitial cell, and are very different from the larger mitochondria with tubular cristae seen in mouse interstitial cells. Even these are unimpressive compared to the very large mitochondria with vesicular cristae that dominate the cytoplasm of adrenal fasciculata cells in the rat adrenal. The development of adrenal mitochondria reflects their additional role in carrying out the 11β-hydroxylase and (in the glomerulosa) 11β -hydroxylase reactions. Interstitial cells have very large mitochondria in the human fetus. The Golgi complex has a sameness about it throughout steroid-secreting cells, being somewhat concentrated at one pole of the nucleus, around the centrioles, but also sending arms out to other parts of the cell. Reinke's crystals are supposedly unique to man, although Stieve (10) says they occur in dogs. The human lipofuscin granule resembles that seen in mouse interstitial cells, but that found in guinea pigs is organized differently- rat and opossum interstitial cells lack lipofuscin granules. Human interstitial cells are moderate in their content of lipid droplets. They contain considerably fewer than adrenal fasciculata cells of rats, but do contain some, in contrast to the interstitial cells of mature rats, opossums and boars, where lipid droplets are uncommon.

Fig. 6 summarizes the probable movements of substrates within a cell over the course of steroid biosynthesis, according to the cell fractionation literature. Cholesterol biosynthesis seems to take place on or near the smooth endoplasmic reticulum. The wide variation in the amount of smooth ER in steroid-secreting cells led to the suggestion (4) that the amount of smooth ER reflects the extent to which the cell makes its own cholesterol rather than taking it in from the plasma, and some correlations with biochemical literature were cited. One interesting example is the insect prothoracic gland, source of the steroid ecdysone, where cells almost entirely lack a smooth ER. It turns out that their cholesterol is derived entirely from the diet (31).

Whether or not human interstitial cells make their own cholesterol, the question arises of how the cholesterol is supplied to the mitochondria for side chain cleavage. A glance at an electron micrograph like that shown in Fig. 4 immediately makes it obvious that this involves a logistic problem How does cholesterol get from its site of synthesis (or uptake from the plasma) to the mitochondria? The smooth ER usually occupies a much larger percentage of the cytoplasmic volume than the mitochondria, and yet it appears that to enter steroid synthesis the cholesterol must be funneled through the mitochondria. Cholesterol is a normal constituent of biological membranes and tends to be taken up by membranes, so it seems unlikely that cholesterol could pass by simple diffusion across a field of smooth ER. It has been suggested that the newly synthesized cholesterol may be sequestered in the smooth ER, and that this organelle may constitute a vast reservoir of cholesterol for steroid synthesis (32). One could imagine a membrane "circulation" that would bring ER membranes into contact with mitochondria, although we see little indication of this in static electron micrographs. The smooth ER in most steroid-secreting cells is abundant enough so the mitochondria must be constantly jostled by it, but the problem still remains how to channel cholesterol from a large volume of

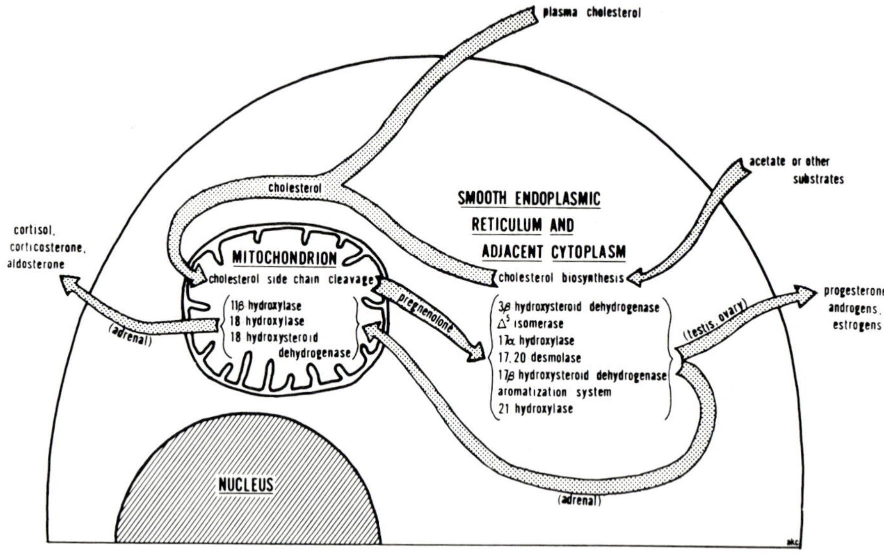

Fig. 6. Summary diagram of intracellular substrate movements during steroid biosynthesis, according to the cell fractionation literature. Cholesterol is either synthesized in the smooth ER and adjacent cytoplasm, or taken up from the plasma. Cholesterol then passes to the mitochondria for cleavage of its side chain. Pregnenolone emerges from the mitochondrion and is then transformed to androgens by enzyme systems in the smooth ER. Used by permission from A.K. Christensen and S/W. Gillim, in The Gonads, ed. McKerns, K.W., Appleton-Century-Crofts, p. 415, 1969.

smooth endoplasmic reticulum to mitochondria that may constitute a much smaller volume. The egress of pregnenolone from the mitochondria presents similar problems, although it is possible that the subsequent steps of androgen biosynthesis are not equally distributed throughout the smooth ER.

If the cholesterol side chain cleavage system is present on the inner membranes of human interstitial cell mitochondria, as seems to be the case in mitochondria of hog adrenal (33), this means that cholesterol must pass the outer membrane on its way in, and pregnenolone must do the same on its way out. The large globules sometimes seen in mitochondria of human interstitial cells, and whose fine structure suggests they are lipid droplets, may well be pools of either cholesterol or pregnenolone within the mitochondrion.

The function of the Golgi complex in steroid-secreting cells is unknown. In cells that make protein for export, such as the pancreatic acinar cell (34), the newly-synthesized proteins are transported to the Golgi complex within the endoplasmic reticulum, and in the Golgi complex are dehydrated to form secretory granules to be secreted from the cell. It is unknown whether any similar function takes place in steroid-secreting cells, although the Golgi complex is often well developed in these cells and there is some evidence that it hypertrophies during times of heightened steroid production (35,36). Other suggestions as to possible functions for the Golgi complex in steroid-secreting cells have been made, but are rather tenuous at the present stage of our understanding.

Our meager knowledge of the pathways and time-course by which substrates and products move through steroid-secreting cells underscores the need for a means of localizing steroids within cells at the electron microscope level. This is extremely difficult because the conventional techniques of electron microscopy that might permit autoradiography involve solvents that would either remove or displace the steroids from their original positions. It has been shown by Stumpf and Roth (37) that stringent requirements must be met to localize steroids by autoradiography even at the light microscope level: 1) The tissue must be frozen without fixation, 2) The tissue must be kept at a temperature of below -60° throughout cutting and freeze-drying of frozen sections, and 3) no solvents of any kind can contact the tissue throughout the whole process. Over the last few years we have been developing a means of cutting frozen thin sections that will satisfy these criteria at the electron microscope level (38,39), and we are just beginning experiments that we hope will allow us to follow radioactive steroid substrates through the cells after a pulse-label in vitro. If successful, this should allow us to chart the path of substrates through the cell and also to show whether or not these substrates accumulate in the mitochondria at any time period or in the Golgi complex, and how long it takes the materials to clear the cell. Through the use of specific inhibitors it should be possible to show where individual steps occur.

ACKNOWLEDGEMENTS

I am indebted to Dr. Norris Finlayson, of the El Camino Hospital, Mountain View, California, and to Drs. Gilbert LeBlanc, Lynn Frary and Richard Weinstein of the Oakland Naval Hospital for their cooperation in obtaining the material used in this study.

This work was supported by research grant HD-01512 from the U.S. Public Health Service.

REFERENCES

1. Christensen, A.K., and Mason, N.R., Endocrinology, 76: 646, 1965.
2. Hall, P.F., Irby, D.C. and de Kretser, D.M., Endocrinology, 84: 488, 1969.

3. Baillie, A.H., Ferguson, M.M. and Hart, D.McK., Developments in Steroid Histochemistry, Academic Press, London, 1966.
4. Christensen, A.K., J. Cell Biol., 26: 911, 1965.
5. Frank, A.L. and Christensen, A.K., J. Cell Biol., 36: 1, 1968.
6. Black, V.H. and Christensen, A.K., Amer. J. Anat., 124: 211, 1969.
7. Christensen, A.K. and Gillim, S.W., In The Gonads, ed. McKerns, K.W., Appleton-Century-Crofts, New York, p 415, 1969.
8. Christensen, A.K. and Fawcett, D.W., Amer. J. Anat., 118: 551, 1966.
9. Christensen, A.K. and Fawcett, D.W., J. Biophys. Biochem. Cytol., 9: 653, 1961.
10. Stieve, H., Mannliche Genitalorgane, Handbuch der mikroskopischen Anatomie des Menschen,ed. v. Mollendorf, W., vol 7 (Harn- und Geschlechtsapparat), part 2, Julius Springer, Berlin, 1930.
11. Ito, T. and Oinuma, S., Okajimas Folia anat. Jap., 18: 497, 1939.
12. Sniffen, R.C., Arch. Pathol., 50: 259, 1950.
13. Fawcett, D.W. and Burgos, M.H., Amer. J. Anat., 107: 245, 1960.
14. Yamada, E., Gunma Symposia on Endocrinology, 2: 1, 1965.
15. de Kretser, D.M., Z. Zellforsch, 80: 594, 1967.
16. de Kretser, D.M., Z. Zellforsch, 83: 344, 1967.
17. Nishimura, R. and Kondo, I., Urologia Internationalis, 18: 1, 1964.
18. Schmidt, F.C., Z. Zellforsch, 63: 707, 1964.
19. Hatakeyama, S., Acta Path. Jap., 15: 155, 1965.
20. Nagano, T., Gunma Symposia on Endocrinology, 2: 19, 1965.
21. Pelliniemi, L.J. and Niemi, M., Z. Zellforsch, 99: 507, 1969.
22. Gordon, G.B., Miller, L.R. and Bensch, K.G., Lab. Invest., 13: 152, 1964.
23. Cervos-Navarro, J., Tonutti, E. and Bayer, J.M., Endokrinologie, 47: 23, 1964.
24. Dessolle, N., Comptes Rendus Acad. Sci., 264: 2018, 1967.
25. Sisson, J.K. and Fahrenbach, W.H., Amer. J. Anat., 121: 337, 1967.
26. Yasuzumi, G., Nakai, Y, Tsubo, I, Yasudo, M. and Sugioka, T., Exp. Cell Res., 45: 261, 1967.
27. Ito, S. and Karnovsky, M.J., J. Cell Biol., 39: 186A, 1968.
28. Bennett, H.S. and Luft, J.H., J. Biophys. Biochem. Cytol., 6: 113, 1959.
29. Luft, J.H., J. Biophys. Biochem. Cytol., 9: 409, 1961.
30. Richardson, K.C., Jarett, L. and Finke, E.H., Stain Technol., 35: 313, 1960.
31. Osinchak, J., Z. Zellforsch, 72: 236, 1966.
32. Fawcett, D.W., In Intracellular Membraneous Structure, eds. Seno, S. and Cowdry, W.V., Japan Soc. for Cellular Chem., Okayama, Japan (supplement for Symposia of the Society for Cellular Chemistry, vol 14), p. 15, 1963.
33. Yago, N. and Ichii, S., J. Biochem., 65: 215, 1969.
34. Jamieson, J.D. and Palade, G.E., J. Cell Biol., 34: 577, 1967.

35. McDonald, D.M., Seiki, K., Prizant, M. and Goldfien, A., Endocrinology, 85: 236, 1969.
36. Rouiller, G. and Schimmer, B., Anat. Rec., 163: 342, 1969.
37. Stumpf, W.E. and Roth, L.J., J. Histochem. Cytochem., 14: 274, 1966.
38. Christensen, A.K., In Autoradiography of Diffusible Substances, eds. Roth, L.J. and Stumpf, W.E., Academic Press, New York, p. 349, 1969.
39. Christensen, A.K., Proceedings 7th International Congress of Electron Microscopy (Grenoble, France), in press, 1970.

DISCUSSION

LUNENFELD: Dr. Vilar, did you ever find cellular bridges between Sertoli and germinal cells, which could explain how information or substances could be directly transferred from the Sertoli to the germinal cells, or do you think that information has to be transferred to germinal cells by diffusion?

VILAR: If you mean real intercellular bridges, not at all. But some authors have described pinocytocis vesicles either in the cytoplasm of the Sertoli or germinal cells close to the plasma membranes. Whether or not this means any kind of transmission or transference of substances, I do not know. The possibility has been mentioned.

HUDSON: I would like to ask a question that could be directed either to Dr. Vilar or to Dr. Christensen. Do they believe that the secretions of the interstitial cells pass across the rather thick lamina propria that surround the tubule and so nourish the germinal cells?

VILAR: I cannot tell specifically about the transference of the secretion of the interstitial cells, but we have studied the transference into the seminiferous tubule of different substances. For instance, if you put isolated seminiferous tubules in a medium containing 20% of a mixture of sodium and potassium ferrocyanide, you can see, after ten minutes, with the prussian blue reaction that the ferrocyanide is able to pass through the structures of the tubular wall to the germinal epithelium via the Sertoli cells. This experience could be repeated in vivo either with ferrocyanide or with labelled albumin. For example, when the testis of a rat was injected with rat albumin labelled with a fluorescent dye, the fluorescence diffused well in the intertubular spaces, and by way of the germinal epithelium passed into the lumen of the tubules. This means that the albumin is able to pass through the complicated tubular wall. When we used labelled globulins, they apparently did not go through the tubular wall. When albumin labelled with iodine 131 was injected into the testis, the albumin was accumulated around the tubular wall and in the lumen of the seminiferous tubule. The same phenomenon can be seen with the electron microscope, labelling the proteins with ferritine. After 30 minutes ferritine labelled albumin appears in pinocytosis vesicles and also in lysosomal bodies of the Sertoli cells which apparently act as an extracellular compartment for the germinal cells, (Vilar and Mancini, Acta Europea Fertilitatis, 1970, in press).

CHRISTENSEN: The work of Waites and Setchell has shown that the seminiferous epithelium and its tunica propria may be rather selective about what they allow to pass. But I see no a priori reason why steroids could not penetrate the cellular layers of the tunica propria, each of which is no thicker than a capillary endothelium.

MANCINI: I would like to mention that the data reported by Dr. Vilar as regards the origin of seminiferous tubule fluid are in contrast with those of Shetler et al. (J. Physiol. 189: 63, 1967) who have worked with rams. They collect a fluid at the level of the rete testes and they assume that this fluid is not a consequence of displacement or diffusion from the intertubular vessels to the seminiferous tubules, but a product of an active process inside the tubules. However, they do not provide direct evidence of such a process.

A. STEINBERGER: I would like to ask Dr. Vilar, and perhaps Dr. Christensen as well, whether they had the opportunity to examine testicular tissue under the conditions of gonadotropic stimulation, as well as gonadotropic deprivation? And, if so, what were the ultrastructural changes, particularly in the smooth endoplasmic reticulum and mitochondria of the Sertoli cells and Leydig cells?

CHRISTENSEN: I have not studied the human testis after gonadotropin stimulation, but the literature on mammals (including humans) indicates that the changes are mostly quantitative rather than qualitative. In other words, the organelles become more abundant, but their appearance remains much the same.

PAULSEN: I should like to expand Dr. A. Steinberger's point relative to changes in the interstitial cells following gonadotropin stimulation. Dr. de Kretser has shown that there is an increase in the smooth endoplasmic reticulum, mitochondria and lysosomes. These changes were quantitative rather than qualitative. With respect to the crystalloids of Reinke, Dr. de Kretser has demonstrated that these may be found in the nucleus as well as in the cytoplasm of the interstitial cells. This is in contrast to our previous beliefs using light microscopy studies that the crystalloids were present only in the cytoplasm. If the crystalloids of Reinke are both in the cytoplasm and nucleus of two cells of the body that secrete testosterone, i.e. the interstitial cells of the testis and the hilar cells of the ovary, they may have some function.

CHRISTENSEN: I do not think anyone has much of an idea of what the crystals are doing. Dr. Yamada (Gunma Symp. on Endocr. 2 : 1-17) described intranuclear crystalloids in 1965, so it has been known for some time that they and what appear to be their precursors occur in the nucleus, as well as in the cytoplasm. However, it is well known from early work (reviewed by Stieve 1930 and others) that the crystals vary greatly in abundance from person to person, and it has not been possible to correlate this variation with any functional condition. Crystals seem to be all but lacking in some men of normal fertility. Also, they do not seem to occur in any other mammal besides man, although the testes of all mammals presumably secrete androgens. I therefore find it difficult to believe that they play an essential role in androgen synthesis or secretion in human interstitial cells.

SOLARI: I want to add to what has just been said about the Reinke crystals. Dr. Vilar found that the optical diffraction pattern of the crystals is almost hexagonal; this pattern was repeated in crystals from several individuals.

JOHNSEN: We would think that the crystals of Reinke may have some bearing on the functional state of the Leydig cells. We have found that they are absent in Leydig cell hyperplasia, whatever the cause. They are absent in Klinefelter's syndrome, in testicular feminization, and it would appear that they are, in fact, absent in any kind of poor testis.

PAULSEN: I should like to remind Dr. Johnsen that we presented data at the Laurentian Hormone Conference in 1955 which showed that crystalloids of Reinke were evident in patients with Klinefelter's syndrome. Also Dr. de Kretser demonstrated these crystalloids in his hypogonadotropic patients before as well as after gonadotropic therapy.

DAVIS: Dr. Vilar, are smooth muscle cells present in the tunica propria surrounding the seminiferous tubule?

VILAR: I personally think they are not, but I know that Dr. Clermont considered these cells myoepithelial cells related to contraction, and responsible for the movements of the seminiferous tubules.

CLERMONT: We have seen cells of the limiting membrane pulsating in the rat, so there must be contractile elements in this location. Dr. M. Ross working with the electron microscope also demonstrated that similar cells in man have characteristics of smooth muscle fibers, and were considered as contractile cells. Dr. Fawcett now calls them myoid cells, I think. So he must be convinced that they have characteristics of smooth muscle cells.

MANN: It is now fairly clear that testosterone is secreted by the testes along three routes, namely, spermatic vein blood, lymph and rete testis fluid. The concentrations seem to be of the same order of magnitude. The concentration of testosterone is only a little lower in the lymph than in the spermatic vein blood; and only a little lower in the rete testis than in the lymph. One would think that there must be some common mechanism which regulates the movement of testosterone from the interstitial cells by all three avenues. Much has been learned already, particularly from Dr. Mancini's work, on the permeability of testicular blood capillaries, and from the recent work by Fawcett on the testicular lymphatic sinusoidal vessels, that makes it possible to visualize how testosterone enters the blood and lymph. But what is the mechanism of testosterone entry into the seminiferous tubules? Dr. Vilar showed us in his electron micrographs how parts of the Sertoli cell protoplasm fill the spaces between the interstitial cells and the membranes around the seminiferous tubules. Is it possible that the Sertoli cells are actually able to transport testosterone?

CHRISTENSEN: It is always possible that the Sertoli cells may transport steroids from the interstitial tissue into the seminiferous epithelium, but this would be difficult to prove. Certainly the descriptive fine structure would not allow us to settle this question. But if we are eventually successful in following steroids by autoradiography on frozen thin sections of fresh tissue, then it should be possible to demonstrate whether or not labelled steroids are taken up by the Sertoli cells.

MANCINI: We have been successful in injecting intratesticularly a very small amount of labelled homologous albumin. Provided there was no disruption or rupture of seminiferous tubules by the needle, this labelled albumin goes in large part into the intertubular lymphatic vessels and only a small part diffuses into the seminiferous tubules through the Sertoli cell cytoplasm.

OHNO: Mitochondria have their own ribosome which is a bacterial type. So translation by the mitochondrial ribosome is inhibited by cycloheximide. Therefore, I would like to ask two questions: first, are the ribosomes inside the mitochondria of the interstitial cell? And, second, regarding messenger RNA for steroid enzymes, are they translated by mitochondrial ribosome, and therefore sensitive to chloramphenicol? Or does the translation actually occur outside the mitochondria, and the enzymes get in afterwards?

CHRISTENSEN: It is a very interesting question about which I have no information. We do see what could be interpreted as mitochondrial ribosomes inside the mitochondria. However, I know of no evidence as to whether mitochondrial steroidogenic enzymes (20-, 22-, 11- and 18-hydroxylases) are coded by mitochondrial DNA.

LUNENFELD: Dr. Christensen, have you formed any working hypothesis on the sequential transportation of such traits and products from the different particulate fractions in interstitial tissue and on the regulation of this transport?

CHRISTENSEN: As you know, cholesterol forms an important component of biological membranes, and may be taken up by membranes; consequently, it seems unlikely that cholesterol could diffuse across an extensive field of smooth endoplasmic reticulum. The membranes of smooth reticulum may constitute an extensive reservoir of cholesterol, as has been suggested by Fawcett, and movements of the reticulum may serve to bring fresh cholesterol to the mitochondria for side-chain cleavage. One would look in electron micrographs for a very close association between the smooth ER and mitochondria. This is sometimes seen, but not with a frequency that would be expected if this means of transport were a basic mechanism.

HISTOLOGY OF THE HUMAN TESTIS FROM NEONATAL PERIOD TO ADOLESCENCE

Oscar Vilar

Centro de Investigaciones sobre Reproduccion. Facultad de Medicina. Buenos Aires, Argentina

The history of the testicular structures from birth to the end of the adolescence period is to be discussed, from the histological point of view, with the consideration that this gonad contains three fundamental structures: a) the stroma, including albuginea, the intertubular connective tissue and the seminiferous tubule wall; b) the Leydig cells and c) the germinal epithelium. All these three structures show definite morphological, histochemical and ultrastructural changes which can be interrelated as well as correlated with the age of the individual.

Few data are available regarding the human prepuberal testes. Information given in the literature is often fragmentary since it is very difficult to obtain material of different ages with a satisfactory sequence. Our material was obtained either from biopsies according to the technique of Charny and Meranze (1) or from fresh necropsy material. We are deeply indebted to Dr. Sebastian Rosasco and Dr. E. Carpaneto who kindly provided us several biopsies. Preparation of the tissue for light microscopy, histochemistry and electron microscopy is reported elsewhere (2-6).

A. THE STROMAL CONNECTIVE TISSUE

Some authors have shown that the tunica albuginea has the typical appearance of juvenile connective tissue in the fetal gonad (7). During the post-natal ages maturation of this tissue takes place (8). This structure shows progressive changes from the new-born to the 8-year-old child. During the first two months of life, the thickness of the albuginea is about 300 μ. Its histological features match those corresponding to a juvenile connective tissue arranged in three layers: 1) the outer one, beneath the vaginal tunic, contains young fibroblasts, very fine collagen and reticulin fibers and few blood vessels; 2) the middle layer shows a similar structure but less collagen fibers; positive reactions for mucopolysaccharides are observable in the interfibrillar spaces; 3) the inner layer is richer in cells, mucopolysaccharides and blood vessels, but only reticular fibers are seen. During the first year of age some changes occur in the cells and fibers. Fibroblasts diminish in number and undergo a slight maturation; collagen fibers become thicker, more abundant and oriented; reticular fibers are scarcer, reactions for mucopolysaccharides gradually disappear and vascularity diminishes. These changes take place mainly in the outer and middle layers since the deeper one preserves most of the characteristics of the juvenile connective tissue. From then, thinness of the albuginea accentuates with age, with an increase in collagen fibers, reaching its peak between six and eight years when the width of the albuginea is close to 230 μ.

At early puberty the main feature in the albuginea is an increase in the thickness (about 380 μ). The middle layer appears edematous and numerous blood vessels and hypertrophied fibroblasts are present; the collagen fibers and bundles are swollen with rather diffuse limits. The inner layer shows less striking changes since a very loose network of reticulin fibers predominates and the presence of edema is very difficult to assess.

In the following stages corresponding to the middle and late phases of puberty, the thickness of the albuginea gradually increases. Numerous collagen fibers are arranged in parallel, edema disappears and fibroblastic cells now show the features of the so-called fibrocytes. Reticular fibers as well as interfibrillar mucopolysaccharides progressively diminish. The most prominent feature in the outer layer is the coalescence of collagen fibers in a similar way as that seen in dense connective tissue. At the end of puberty the albuginea is 450 μ thick.

The previously described histological modifications also develop in the connective tissue of the septae.

Intertubular spaces. From birth to the fourth year of age, juvenile fibroblasts are predominant in these areas, but later decrease in number and become of a more mature type. The intertubular spaces are filled by a homogeneous mass of an amorphous plasma-like substance which is eosinophilic and PAS positive. Reticulin fibers are abundant in the testes of the new born, but diminish progressively thereafter while the intertubular spaces widen and the cellular population becomes more mature and scarcer.

At the beginning of puberty, proliferation of juvenile fibroblasts again takes place; congestion of blood vessels and an increase in the amorphous plasma-like intercellular substance are striking changes. A very loose network of reticulin fibers persists.

At the end of puberal maturation there is a reduction in the degree of hyperemia; mucopolysaccharides are no longer detected histochemically and the whole cell population decreases; the juvenile fibroblasts almost disappear whereas the mature ones persist although in reduced number. These cells have a slender fusiform shape with the cytoplasm forming a narrow rim around the nucleus. The nucleus is relatively large, showing scarce invaginations and rather uniform karyoplasm, except for the periphery, where dense granules attached to the nuclear membrane sharply define the boundaries of the nucleus. The Golgi apparatus is not particularly outstanding and the endoplasmic reticulum is represented by a few vesicles with ribosomes attached to them. Inclusion bodies, myelin-like figures and lipids are also present. Light and electron microscopical studies show changes in the <u>wall of the seminiferous tubules</u> which proceed from birth to maturity.

The basement membrane is very thin in the newborn. It is PAS positive, pale blue with Azan's stain; silver impregnation reveals a delicate net of reticulin fibers. The electron microscope shows that it is composed of two parts: the internal and the external. The former, a continuous band about 1100 Å thick (lamina basalis), shows a rather homogeneous structure consisting of electron-dense material with discernible and regularly distributed fine granules.

Surrounding the basement membrane is an external layer composed of cells with multiple expansions. The endoplasmic reticulum shows dilated cisternae studded with ribosomes which are also seen free in the cytoplasmic matrix; fibrils are abundant in the cytoplasm; the intercellular spaces are occupied by dense bundles of typical protofibrils and collagen fibers with characteristic periodicity. No elastic fibers were seen.

This structure presents no striking changes until the beginning of puberty. At this time the tubular wall increases in thickness as well as in complexity. At early puberty the continuous internal lamina basalis preserves the same characteristics mentioned above but pronounced changes soon develop. The following striking features are seen: a) a lamellar structure separated by low electron-dense spaces replaces the original homogeneous band; b) infoldings of this lamina basalis develop and are preferentially located in between the spermatogonia and Sertoli cells. These processes appear simple or rather labyrynthic, including some collagen fibers and fine cytoplasmic branches of the underlying connective cells (9). The depth of indentation of these infoldings reaches one or two microns in some cases and can be seen with the light microscope.

The external arrangement of collagen fibers and cells is more complex. Collagen fibers appear abundant and alternately stratified with cells considered either fibrocytes (5,9,10) or smooth muscle fibers (11,12). When techniques for elastic fibers are applied, they show that during the development of puberty, short and fine elastic fibers appear. Nevertheless no evidence of them could be shown with the electron microscope (5,13).

B. THE LEYDIG CELLS

These cells originate from fibroblasts during fetal life (14, 15), puberty or adult stage (16-18). Different types of cells, with special distribution according to age were seen in the intertubular spaces and were designated as type A, B, C and D fibroblast-like cells, fetal and adult Leydig cells and degenerating cells. These different types of cells represent progressive steps in the transformation from the juvenile fibroblast of the mesenchyme (fibroblast A) to the fetal or adult Leydig cell. This differentiation means changes in size and shape, as well as modifications in histochemical reactions. Loss of basophils, appearance of lipids, especially those grouped as 3-beta steroids, increased activity for oxidative enzymes, lipases, esterases (4) and hydroxy-steroid dehydrogenases (19) are characteristics which appear progressively in all these transitional stages. Leydig cells are fully differentiated about the 12th week of fetal life (20). They are present in the testes of the newborn (they reach a peak just before birth) and several weeks after birth Leydig cells have disappeared completely. No evidence of transformation of Leydig cells into other cell types is found; on the contrary cell degeneration seems to be the rule. The ultrastructural characteristics of the fully mature fetal Leydig cells are much like their adult counterparts except that no crystals of Reinke are visible. These cells show a number of histochemically demonstrable enzyme activities and such a gradual development of some of them has been demonstrated in the human(19,20). These enzyme activities strongly suggest that steroids are actively produced in the fetal Leydig cells. Parallel with the depletion of fetal Leydig cells at birth, a proliferation of less differentiated fibroblasts begins and increases during infancy. Although the juvenile type of fibroblast predominates, there are also more mature cells having a tendency to be located close to the tubular wall.

When puberty begins there is a decrease in the number of juvenile fibroblasts and an increase in more mature fibroblasts and immature Leydig cells as well as transitional and degenerating elements.

When puberty is complete, only mature fibroblasts and Leydig cells remain. Leydig cells of the more mature type increase with the development of puberty whilst degenerating forms decrease.

The differentiation of fibroblasts into mature Leydig cells is characterized not only by modification in the light and electron microscopical features (18) but also because a number of histochemical characteristics develop. Cytochemical methods give positive reactions for lipids, cholesterol, ascorbic acid, lipases, esterases, leucylaminopeptidase, oxidative enzymes and for a wide variety of hydroxysteroid dehydrogenases including 3-α, 6-β, 11-β, 16-β, 17-β, 20-α and 20-β hydroxysteroid dehydrogenases. Most of these enzymes can be fitted into a broad biochemical pattern (19,21) but several have not been satisfactorily integrated. Most of these enzyme activities are present not only in the mature Leydig cells but also in the precursor fibroblast-like cells.

C. THE GERMINAL EPITHELIUM

There is at present general agreement sustaining the hypothesis that the cell population of the germinal epithelium consists of two different lines and that the early segregated cells (primordial germ cells) in the yolk sac are the only source of the definite sex cells while Sertoli cells are originated in the so-called supporting cells derived from the coelomic epithelium. But this theory is based on personal interpretation of morphological findings and it is quite obvious that more work is needed to establish precisely what happens (22-24). The available literature on the human developing testis is incomplete (16,17,25). The migration of gonocytes in the human embryo seems to have been demonstrated (26) but not their future destiny.

Newborn to 2-month-old baby. The seminiferous epithelium of the newborn human testis is composed of solid cords about 50 μ in diameter where two main types of cells are easily differentiable. The most numerous are the precursors of Sertoli cells (supporting or indifferent cells) which are cuboidal or columnar, forming a multilayer tissue which is attached to the basement membrane. These cells have a round or elongated nucleus sometimes with deep indentations surrounded by a thin rim of cytoplasm. One, two or more dense bodies are recognized as possessing nucleolar structure without the complexity seen in the adult Sertoli cell. Mitochondria are elongated, small in diameter and possess a dense matrix and short cristae oriented transversally. Polyribosomes, fibrils and few lysosomal bodies are contained in the ground substance. The "intercellular spaces" between neighboring supporting or immature Sertoli cells narrow from time to time while there is accumulation of dense material beside the plasma membrane. These are the junctional structures already described in the mouse (27). Either after stain with polychrome blue or under the electron microscope (EM), the supporting cells were of two types: dark and light. The last ones are more frequently seen. The significance of these two types of Sertoli cells is uncertain. Our data differ from that reported by Johnsen (28) in that we find differences not only in the nucleus but in the cytoplasm as well.

The second type of cells found at this age are those belonging to the germinal line. Among them we can first describe the gonocyte or primordial germ cell which is large and posesses basophilic cytoplasm. They are the most striking cells of the seminiferous cord. They are sometimes found in the center of the cord, sometimes laterally, but always isolated from the basement membrane by the supporting cells. They show one or two large and quite characteristic nucleoli, the rest of the nucleoplasm being clear and homogeneous (28). In the cytoplasm sparse endoplasmic reticulum and scattered clusters of free ribosomes are seen. In the light ground substance the mitochomdria are characteristically large, with well-defined cristae without a definite pattern. They show a tendency to polarization. The so-called A-bodies (29,30) are not present in our human testes, but multilamellar figures and residual bodies are not an unusual finding.

A second type of germinal cell is already present in the two month old testis. They are smaller, more irregular in shape and show attachment to the basal membrane. These cells, which are still large and have many similar nuclear and cytoplasmic characteristics, could be identified with the "transitional" (29) or primitive type A spermatogonia (31) of the rat. They have a higher number of more spread mitochondria.

A halo or clear zone can appear in the nucleus of some of these "transitional cells" and this change is also frequently associated with vacuolization. While the proportion of cells which have established contact with the lamina basalis increases, those unattached cells diminish progressively.

Infancy and childhood. The following changes take place at this stage. Supporting cells divide actively, especially during infancy and then remain stationary until the beginning of puberty. Consequently they appear more numerous than in the younger animals, forming a palisade-like layer. The diameter of the tubules remains unchanged. Big gonocyte cells occupy the center of the tubule and become less numerous with age. Some of them appear "swollen" (20 μ) but the size of the nucleus is not modified; branches of them are interposed among the supporting cells. These cells are called hypertrophic spermatogonia (2) and show in their structure evidence of cellular degeneration. Some of them also appear as bi-or multinucleated cells.

The so called intermediate cells divide,especially during childhood, and originate smaller round cells, attached to the basement membrane, frequently showing intercellular bridges. Their cytoplasm is light, with few flat membranous profiles, big mitochondria with defined cristae and a moderately dense matrix. The nucleoli are well-developed. These cells have been considered both in animal and human as spermatogonia (29,32). By the observation of multiple sections it is evident that numerous intermediate forms exist between the transitional large cell and the smaller spermatogonium. It is also a fact that the number of these spermatogonial cells diminishes until the beginning of puberty. There are two possible reasons for this fact: 1) the rate of mitosis of these cells is very low; 2) the cells degenerate.

Puberty. At the onset of puberty the germinal epithelium is lined with numerous palisade supporting cells, scarce spermatogonial cells and occasional gonocyte-like cells (hypertrophic spermatogonia). When puberal development starts changes in the germinal epithelium take place very rapidly. With the fragmentary material which it is possible to obtain in humans, the precise interpretation of the facts is very difficult.

Spermatogonial proliferation is the first histological evidence of puberty, and it proceeds generally after the clinical features of the age are present. These are growth of pubic and axillary hair, change in voice, etc. which are indicators of the presence of circulating androgens. When spermatogonial proliferation is present, all adult types can be seen simultaneously. We were not able to find one single biopsy in which spermatogonial cells correspond in toto to a unique generation of cells.

Almost at the same time the supporting cells start their transformation into adult Sertoli cells. They stop dividing and increase in size but remain attached to the basal membrane. The cytoplasm contains an increased amount of tubular and vesicular agranular endoplasmic reticulum. Lipids become frequent inclusions. The nuclei become more irregular and the nucleolus develops the characteristics of the adult type with three components: amorphous, granular and fibrillar. When the lumen becomes evident, the cytoplasm sends numerous lateral expansions between the neighboring germinal cells which also interdigitate with those of the Sertoli cells. Numerous intermediate forms (immature Sertoli cells) are present at the beginning of puberty. At this time, spermatocytes in the leptotene and pachytene stages are present and are followed by spermatids which complete their development at the end of puberty.

COMMENTS

From the results presented here it is evident that all the structures of the testes show changes from birth to puberty, which is the moment when the final and full organization of the gonad takes place. The existence in the Leydig cells of a definite cycle of growth and differentiation during the fetal life followed by a period of involution after birth is evident. The connective tissue structures show two developmental phases, the first one during infancy which is characterized by a progressive fibrogenesis and parallel reduction of the mucopolysaccharides.

The definite organized maturation of the human testes starts at puberty which cannot be matched with any chronological age. The proliferation of the connective cells, precursors of the future Leydig cells, is the first step and it is followed by the proliferation of spermatogonial cells and maturation of Sertoli cells. Spermatogenesis will be complete thereafter.

Although it is generally believed that the genesis of Leydig cells occurs later than spermatogenesis (16,32), it is also accepted that the proliferating interstitial cells provide the source of androgens throughout the puberal period (34) even without achieving the characteristic morphology of the adult Leydig cells.

Also, apparently under the influence and control of hormones, the connective tissue structures go through their second developmental phase which begins at the onset of puberty and extends throughout adulthood.

The history of the germ cells after birth is more difficult to explain. From the observation of many authors it is evident that two different cellular lines exist. The Sertoli cell line passes during infancy and childhood through a period of cellular proliferation. Then at puberty proliferation stops and they differentiate into mature types. The germinal line is derived from the primary gonocyte. During the course of infancy and childhood a series of changes takes place which leads to the development of several intermediate types of spermatogonial cells.

At this moment several questions arise: 1) Which one of these cells is a "definite spermatogonium" and what are the features that make it different from the preceding cells? (This question has been posed before (35). 2) Could this definite spermatogonium be considered as the stem cell of the seminiferous tubules? 3) Which cell of the seminiferous tubules of the adult testes could be identified with this cell?

It is very difficult to answer this question properly. What we have in hand is an incomplete set of static histological observations. Therefore the explanation of the dynamics of the renewal of this cell population in the human testes is based on subjective interpretations.

ACKNOWLEDGEMENTS

This work was supported by the Consejo Nacional de Investigaciones Cientificas y Tecnicas, Argentina.

The technical assistance of Miss Lourdes Farinati is most appreciated.

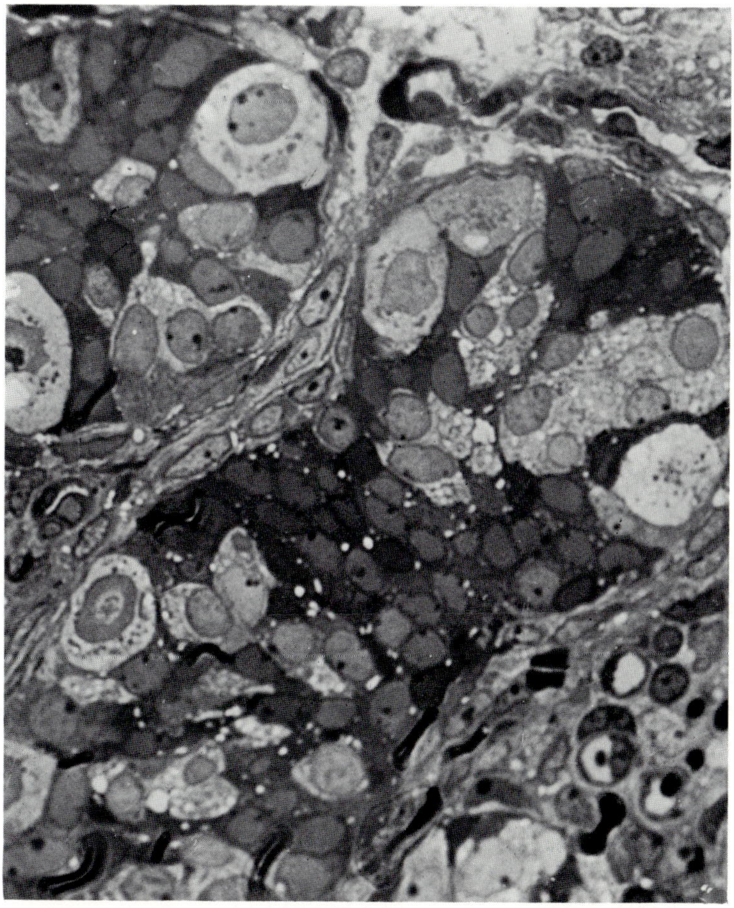

Fig. 1 Testis of a 2-month-old boy. Maraglas embedded section stained with blue polychrome. Numerous gonocytes and spermatogonial cells (some vacuolated) are seen in the seminiferous cords. x 760.

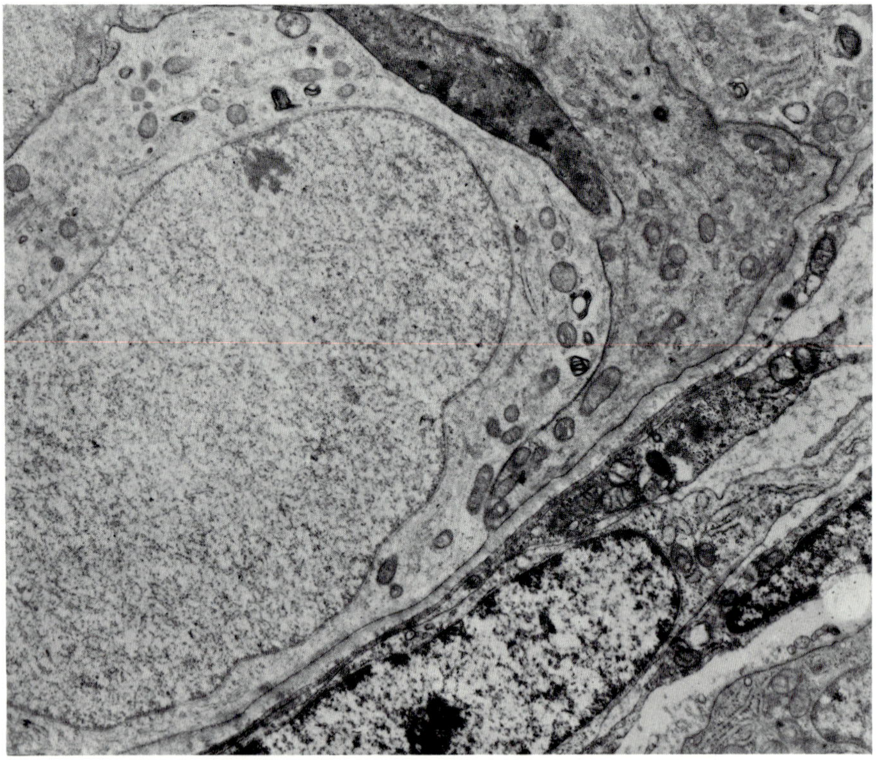

Fig. 2 Testis of a 2-month-old boy. Electron microscopical picture of a "transitorial" cell showing broad attachment to the basement membrane. It is surrounded by light and dark supporting cells. x 9200

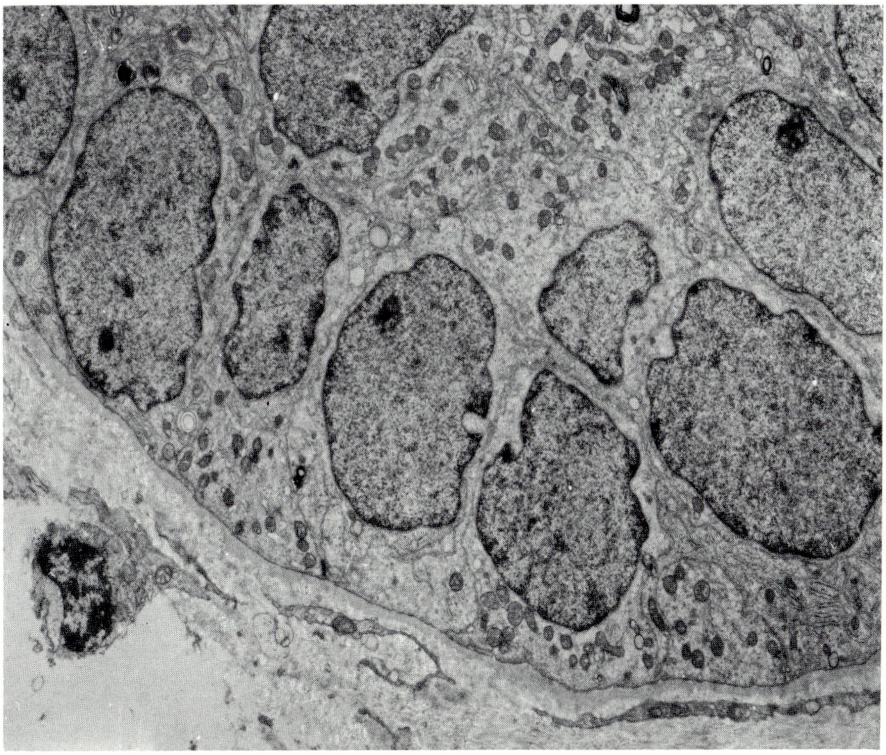

Fig. 3 Testis of an 11-year-old boy. Only supporting cells can be seen. x 2600.

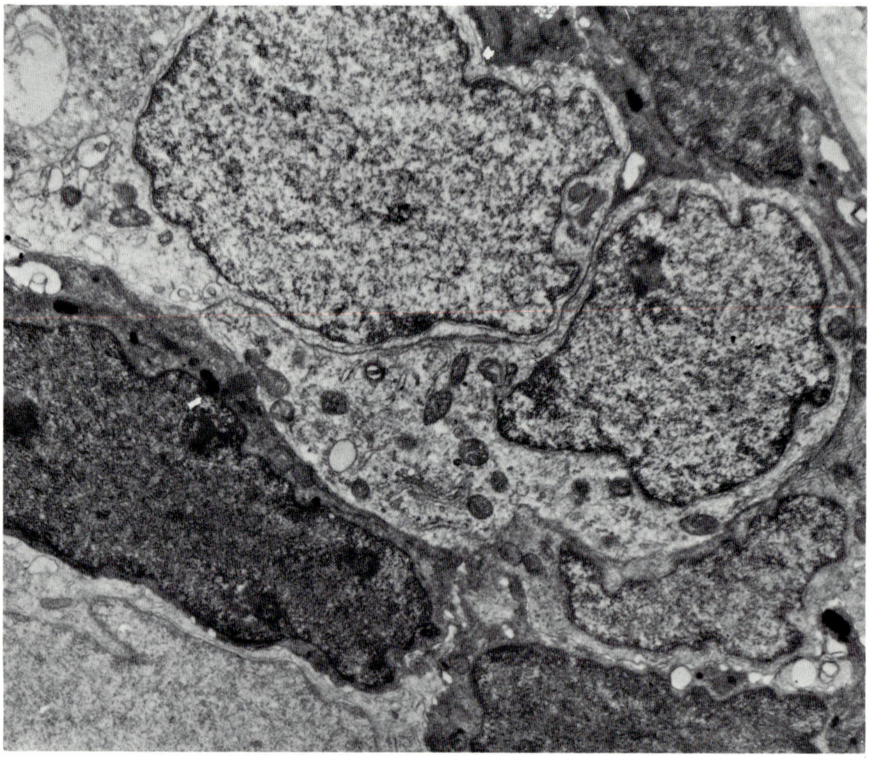

Fig. 4 Testis of an 11-year-old boy showing supporting cells (dark and light). x 8500.

REFERENCES

1. Charny, C.W. and Meranze, D.M., Surg. Gyn. and Obst., 74: 836, 1942.
2. Mancini, R.E., Narbaitz, R. and Lavieri, J.C., Anat. Rec., 136: 477, 1960.
3. Vilar, O., Perez del Cerro, M. and Mancini, R.E., Exp. Cell Res., 27: 158, 1962.
4. Mancini, R.E., Vilar, O., Lavieri, J.C., Andrada, J.A. and Heinrich, J.J., Amer. J. Anat., 112: 203, 1963.
5. Mancini, R.E., Vilar, O., Perez del Cerro, M. and Lavieri, J.C., Acta Physiol. Lat. Amer., 14: 382, 1964.
6. Vilar, O., Steinberger, A. and Steinberger, E., Z. Zellforsch., 74: 529, 1966.
7. Gillman, J., Contributions to Embryology, Carnegie Inst., 32: 83, 1949.
8. Savoie, J.C. In Evolution morphologique et histochimique du testicule chez le nourrisson et l'enfant, Masson et Cie, ed. Paris, p. 19, 1957.
9. Burgos, M., Rev. Soc. Argent Biol., 35: 309, 1959.
10. Vilar, O., Steinberger, A. and Steinberger E., Z. Zellforsch, 78: 221, 1967.
11. Clermont, Y. Exp. Cell Res., 15: 438, 1958.
12. Ross, M.H. and Long, I.R., Science, 153: 1271, 1966.
13. de la Balze, F.A., Bur, G., Scarpa Smith C. and Irazu, J., J. Clin. Endocr., 14: 626, 1954.
14. Bouin, P. and Ancel, P., C.R. Soc. Biol. (Paris), 55: 1682, 1903.
15. Esaki, S., Z. Mikr Anat. Forsch, 15: 368, 1928.
16. Charny, C.W., Conston, A.S. and Meranze, D.M., Fertil. Steril., 3: 461, 1952.
17. Sniffen, C., Ann. N.Y. Acad. Sci., 55: 609, 1952.
18. Fawcett, D.W. and Burgos, M.H., Amer. J. Anat., 107: 245, 1960.
19. Baillie, A.H., Fergusson, M.M. and McK Hart, D., Developments in Steroid Histochemistry, Academic Press, N.Y., 1966.
20. Niemi, M., Ikonen, M. and Hervonen, A., In Ciba Found. Colloq. Endocr., Vol. 16. Endocrinology of the Testis., eds. Wolstenholme, G.E. and O'Connor, M., J.A. Churchill Ltd. London, p.31, 1967.
21. Seilicovich, A. y A. Perez Lloret, Actas de la XIV Reunion Anual, Soc. Arg. Inv. Clinica. Bariloche, Argentina 1969, p 97.
22. Gier, H.T. and Marion, G.B., Biol. Reprod. Suppl., 1: p. 1, 1969.
23. Clermont, Y. and Perey, B., Amer. J. Anat., 100: 241, 1957.
24. Sapsford, C.S., Aust. J. Zool., 10: 178, 1968.
25. Stieve, H., Der Hoden in Hand. der mikros. Anat. des menschem., W. von Mollendorf, 7(2). 1930.
26. Witschi, E., Contributions to Embryology, 32: 69, 1948.
27. Flickinger, Ch. and Fawcett, D.W., Anat. Rec., 158: 207, 1967.
28. Pierce, G.B. and Beals, D.F., Cancer Res., 24: 1553, 1964.

29. Franchi, L.L. and Mandl, A.M., J. Embryol. Exp. Morph., 12: 289, 1964.
30. Roosen-Runge, E. and Leik, L., Amer. J. Anat., 122: 275, 1968.
31. Steinberger, E., Steinberger, A. and Perloff, W.H., Anat. Rec., 148: 581, 1964.
32. de Kretzer, D.M., Virchow Arch. (Zellpath) 1: 283, 1968.
33. Wershub, L.P., The Human Testis: A Clinical Treatise. Charles C. Thomas, Springfield, Illinois, 1962.
34. Segal, S.J. and Nelson, W.O., In Recent Progress in Endocrinology of Reproduction, ed. Lloyd, C.W., Academic Press, New York, 1959,p107.
35. Roosen-Runge, E., In Charny, C.W., Conston, A.S. and Meranze, D.R., Ann. N.Y. Acad. Sci., 55: 543, 1952.

DISCUSSION

JOHNSEN: I would like to comment upon Dr. Vilar's statement that the first puberal step is proliferation of Leydig cell precursors which are producing androgens. Dr. Vilar stated that these events are followed by development of spermatogenesis. I am willing to accept that we get Leydig cell precursors early and also that such cells do contain steroid enzymes, but I am not willing to accept that in man, Leydig cell function occurs before initiation of tubular development. This in fact contradicts the clinical sequence of events observed at puberty. Tanner has shown in his book "Growth at Adolescence" (2nd ed., Oxford, 1962) that puberty starts with growth of the testes which reflects tubular development. This continues for two years and when pubic hair appears, the testes are at least half adult size and the development of the tubular system is far advanced with near complete spermatogenesis. Development of spermatogenesis before Leydig cell function is shown beautifully in fertile eunuchs. In 1967, we (Johnsen, S.G.: Acta Endocr. (Kobenhavn) 1967, Suppl. 124, 17) showed some such cases. One was a completely infantile patient of 20 years with no pubic hair and an androgen level 15 times lower than in normal men but nevertheless with advanced tubular development.

Pubic hair is a very sensitive index and responds quickly as an indicator of androgen level. Pubic hair can be seen in any pre-puberal boy two or three weeks after administration of HCG. Presence of pubic hair is no proof of Leydig cell function. But its absence proves that there can be no more than an extremely small androgen production. Hence, in man, advanced development of the tubules and the germinal epithelium occurs first followed by Leydig cell function, and not vice versa.

VILAR: Sorry, Dr. Johnsen, but I do not agree with you. The microphotograph I showed you which corresponds to the first stage of puberty belonged to a child having pubic hair but no growth of the testis. The histology showed, as you say, no histological puberal development. I would like Dr. Lipsett to comment on the secretion of androgens by the prepuberal and puberal testis.

LIPSETT: I think one problem is that Dr. Vilar is referring only to morphology whereas Dr. Johnsen is referring not only to morphology but also to a clinical effect of a hormone which we might be able to relate to secretion. I think that one should try to utilize both parameters: secretion and morphology, in trying to clarify such problems. Recently,working with Dr. Vanha Pertula from Finland, we studied development of the testis in rats from 20 to 70 days of age. In the immature rat there were a few Leydig cells present and, as Dr. Mancini showed some time ago in the human, most of these cells had perinuclear basophils and the rate of testosterone secretion was very low. However, as the perinuclear basophils decreased, the rate of testosterone secretion increased to adult levels. Here, at least, perinuclear basophils seemed to be a morphologic feature which correlated with Leydig cell function. In other similar situations, I feel that some of the discrepancies may be resolved when we are able to follow several parameters.

JOST: Dr. Vilar showed us very well developed interstitial cells in the two month old baby. These well developed Leydig cells later disappear. Could Dr. Vilar tell us how the system of intracytoplasmic tubules,which characterize the adult type of Leydig cell, disappear, or do all the differentiated Leydig cells degenerate during childhood before being replaced by another set of Leydig cells at puberty? My second question relates to the correlation between the degenerating germ cells of the final stages of spermatogenesis and the immaturity of the Leydig cells; could you comment upon that?

VILAR: The disappearance of Leydig cells after birth is due to cell degeneration, i.e. they do not involute again into fibroblast type cells. The Leydig cells degenerate very soon after two months of age, so in a very young child, say three years old, there are no interstitial cells at all except fibroblasts.

MANN: I do not think we should exclude the possibility that in the course of the sexual development of the male, there is an early phase when testosterone is produced, followed by a second stage when the testosterone production diminishes and a third stage when testosterone production increases again. In support of that concept two examples may be given. In the bull calf, at birth and during the first few months of life, androstenedione but very little testosterone is present in the testes. This high androstenedione/testosterone ratio is maintained until five months of age. Only later does testosterone become the dominant androgen. However, in the bovine fetal testis, there is more testosterone than androstenedione. Thus, the ratio of testosterone to androstenedione is high before birth, low during the first few months of life, and then it goes up again. The second example is derived from the work by Attal (Endocrinology, 85: 280, 1969) who has shown that in the fetal testis of the ram there is a high testosterone/androstenedione ratio early in pregnancy, but during the later stage of fetal development that ratio decreases. Towards the end of pregnancy it increases once more.

BERGADA: With regard to pubic hair development after HCG treatment, we have a wide experience in the treatment of cryptorchidism in children, and we have never seen pubic hair development after HCG treatment with doses of 1000 IU weekly given for 2 to 8 months. However, congestion and erections of the penis have been noted.

MANCINI: I fully agree with Dr. Lipsett that until we are able to measure, in the same individual, different parameters which must be integrated, we will not be able to reach a definite conclusion regarding puberal development. Second, it is difficult to accept what Dr. Johnsen has said. Our studies showed that proliferation and appearance of different types of spermatogonial cells and partial maturation of Sertoli cells may develop in the absence of morphologically identifiable Leydig cells, but in the presence of fibroblast like cells. Moreover, the beginning of meiosis may be present in the absence of the Leydig cells, but completion of meiosis, development of spermatids and spermatozoa and maturation of Sertoli cells were observed when fully mature Leydig cells were present.

JOHNSEN: Dr. Mancini, I would say that I think we will have to accept the existence of the fertile eunuch. We have described several such patients, and Faiman and Ryan from the Mayo Clinic have described another patient with measurable FSH, but undetectable LH, no Leydig cells, and undetectable testosterone. Dr. MacLeod showed in a hypophysectomized male that when FSH is administered, development of spermatogenesis without Leydig cells, and without a rise in plasma testosterone occurred. I think we will have to accept that advanced development of the germinal epithelium in the absence of Leydig cells can happen in normal puberty.

E. STEINBERGER: A few weeks before this meeting, we saw a patient who may shed some light on the discussion here. He was a 6-year-old boy with a Leydig cell tumor of one testicle. He showed some penile enlargement and very early pubic hair. The tumor showed typical microscopic characteristics of a Leydig cell tumor. The tumor tissue avidly converted progesterone to testosterone in vitro. The testicular tissue on the tumor side showed spermatogenesis up to early spermatids while the contralateral testicle was small (normal for the age) and microscopic study revealed small tubules lined with Sertoli cells and gonocytes, as expected in the testicle of a 6-year-old boy.

JIRASEK: According to my experience, using the 3-β-hydroxysteroid dehydrogenase reaction, I was able to demonstrate that the transformation of the fibroblast-like cells into the Leydig cells containing the 3-β-hydroxysteroid dehydrogenase, precedes the onset of spermatogenesis. I would like to inquire if the luminization of the seminiferous tubules precedes or follows the differentiation of Leydig cells.

VILAR: In our biopsies, the formation of the lumen apparently coincides with the appearance of few mature Leydig cells.

WENIGER: Dr. Vilar, in the human, do the Leydig cells originate in the interstitial tissue? It has been shown by Dr. Sheib in the chick embryo that the Leydig cells grow out from the germ cords.

VILAR: In the human testis, either in the fetal or in the puberal period, progressive transformation is seen from very juvenile fibroblasts to fully mature Leydig cells.

CHAPTER III

CYTOGENETICS OF SPERMATOGENESIS

MORPHOLOGICAL ASPECTS OF MEIOSIS AND THEIR GENETICAL SIGNIFICANCE

Susumu Ohno

Department of Biology, City of Hope Medical Center

Duarte, California

The ultimate aim of meiosis is to segregate four haploid cells from a single diploid cell as a result of two successive cell divisions. The prerequisite for this segregation of haploid sets is the exact longitudinal pairing between two homologous chromosomes which takes place during early phases of first meiosis. Furthermore, peculiar behavior of the centromere at first meiotic anaphase is required for this segregation. In ordinary mitosis, the centromere of each chromosome splits, and, during anaphase, two chromatids move away from each other toward opposite division poles. As a result, two diploid daughters are produced from one diploid cell. In the case of first meiotic anaphase, on the other hand, two chromatids of each chromosome are held together by the unsplit centromere, and the repulsive movement is between one whole chromosome against the whole of its homologous counterpart. As a result, two haploid daughters result from a diploid mother cell. Inasmuch as each chromosome thus produced and included in the haploid nucleus is already made of two chromatids, new DNA replication does not take place between first and second meiosis. The second meiosis is purely mechanical in that it merely serves to separate one chromatid of each chromosome from the other.

Either coincident with or immediately following the longitudinal pairing of homologous chromosomes (synapsis), an event of genetic importance takes place. This is recombination which is due to exchanges of pieces of chromatids between paired homologues. The consequence of such exchange is seen in the form of visible chiasmata between homologues at later phases of first meiosis, i.e., diplotene and diakinesis. Such intrachromosomal recombination between the maternally derived and paternally derived homologues, as well as the random nature of segregation of haploid sets, insures that the finally produced gametes are of many different genetic constitutions and represent mixtures of varying degrees of parental genetic material.

Deviations from the above described norm of meiosis do occur in certain exceptional species. For example, no crossing-over (recombination) takes place during meiosis of the male fruit fly (Drosophila), and the male mealybug (hemipteran insect) transmits only the maternally derived haploid set to its gametes. Human male meiosis, however, faithfully follows the norm of meiosis. There is nothing exceptional about the process.

Various stages of male meiosis are described below with emphasis on underlying functional significance.

COMMITMENT TO MEIOSIS AND THE SYNTHETIC PHASE

Primary spermatocytes are direct derivatives of spermatogonia. The mitotic cycle of spermatogonia must be interrupted at some point and a commitment made by their daughter cells to go into meiosis instead of returning to the mitotic cycle. According to Monesi (1) in the laboratory mouse, such commitment is automatically made when type A (dusty) spermatogonia differentiate into type B (crust-like). The type B spermatogonia divide just once before becoming primary spermatocytes.

It is of interest to note that certain abnormal sex chromosome constitutions appear to preclude differentiation from spermatogonia to spermatocytes. The fertile human XYY-male is expected to produce four types of gametes; normal X- and Y-bearing, as well as abnormal XY- and XY-bearing spermatozoa. As a result, he should sire three times more sons than daughters and two-thirds of his sons should again be abnormal; XYY and XXY. Yet the available records show that only normal XY sons and XX daughters are found among his progeny. Melnyk and his colleagues (2) have recently shown that spermatogonia of the XYY man exhibit considerable mitotic instability. Consequently, the normal XY-constitution is restored to some of the spermatogonia, and only those with the normal constitution differentiate into spermatocytes and complete meiosis. The situation found in the XYY man is reminiscent of that normally found in a particular rodent species (Microtus oregoni). In this species, the female is normally XO, and this remarkable feat is accomplished by selective elimination of the X from spermatogonia of the XY male (3).

After commitment, primary spermatocytes do not proceed immediately into first meiotic prophase. Necessary preparations for meiosis must first be made. The intervening period between the last spermatogonial telophase and the leptotene stage of first meiotic prophase is commonly referred to as the premeiotic resting stage which is an unjustifiable misnomer for this most metabolically active stage. During this stage, primary spermatocytes replicate their DNA. There appears to be a subtle but very important difference between premeiotic S-phase and premitotic S-phase. On plant materials, Stern and Hotta (4) have shown that a small but significant DNA component of the chromosomes, about 0.3% of the total DNA, fails to replicate by the termination of the premeiotic S-phase. Its replication is delayed to the zygotene stage of first meiotic prophase. This delayed DNA synthesis may be an essential prerequisite for synapsis of homologous chromosomes which begins at the zygotene stage.

Aside from DNA replication, premeiotic primary spermatocytes engage in intense transcriptional and translational activities. Analysis of the enzyme phenotype of mature sperm produced by genetic heterozygotes suggests that most of the enzymes contained in mature spermatozoa were specified by the diploid nucleus of primary spermatocytes and have been stored in the cytoplasm either in the form of messenger RNA or already made enzyme molecules. The haploid nucleus of secondary spermatocytes does not appear to direct spermiogenesis. It has been shown that the elimination of a number of chromosomes from secondary spermatocytes does not affect subsequent spermiogenesis. Functional and fertile nullosomic spermatozoa are produced. (5).

SYNAPTIC PHASES

When chromosomes are seen for the first time as individual entities inside the nuclear membrane, primary spermatocytes are said to have entered the "leptotene" stage of first meiotic prophase. By definition, at this earliest prophase stage, all the chromosomes (46 in the case of man) should be distributed at random with no hint of homologous pairing. Thus, there is no foolproof criterion which enables us to distinguish the leptotene nucleus of primary spermatocytes from the early prophase nucleus of spermatogonia. It is probable that the "leptotene" stage, as such, does not exist in a strict sense in that necessary preparations for homologous pairing have already been made in the interphase-like nucleus of the premeiotic stage.

Longitudinal pairing between two homologous chromosomes, which is accomplished in primary spermatocytes, is very exact as witnessed by the formation of a quadrivalent by an individual heterozygous for a reciprocal translocation. When one chromatid of a metaphase chromosome is completely stretched out, it should become a single strand of DNA double helix hundreds of microns long. The uniqueness of an individual chromosome no doubt lies in its DNA base sequence. Proteins associated with DNA are too short in variety to be homologue specific. It then follows that the exact pairing between two homologues must be based on the near identity of their

DNA base sequences. However, unless many parts of two homologous chromosomes are first placed in close vicinity of each other either by chance or by design, such attraction cannot become sufficiently powerful to accomplish exact longitudinal pairing of homologues.

Viewed in this light, "bouquet" orientation of individual chromosomes seen at the "zygotene" stage of the first meiotic prophase gains added significance. Furthermore, if the "leptotene" stage does not exist, as I am inclined to believe, "zygotene" marks the beginning of the first meiotic prophase.

At zygotene, individual chromosomes are still in an extremely fine, thread-like state, but both ends (telomeres) of all the chromosomes are oriented toward one point in the nuclear membrane; thus giving the appearance of a "bouquet". Because of this orientation, the chromosomes of like size tend to be placed in close proximity to each other along their length. Indeed, homologous pairing has already begun in parts wherever two homologous segments happen to lie near each other. What is the force which induces partial homologous pairing at zygotene? DNA replication, transcription of DNA base sequence to messenger RNA base sequence, and, in fact, life itself, owes its existence to the inherent complementality that exists between two purine and pyrimidine base pairs; adenine and thymine as well as guanine and cytosine. Therefore, the attraction to form a double helix exists only between a single uncoupled DNA strand and its complementary single strand; there is no attraction between two identical strands of DNA double helices. If the DNA replication has already been 100% completed during the premeiotic interphase-like stage, each zygotene chromosome, being made of two complete DNA double helices, is already equivalent to two sister chromatids. No attraction is left between two satisfied homologous chromosomes. However, it should be recalled that Stern and Hotta (4) have shown that about 0.3% of the DNA fails to replicate. If parts of a zygotene chromosome contain uncoupled single DNA strands not yet replicated, such single strands can form stable double helices with their complementary counterparts contained in its homologue. In fact, this appears to be the most likely mechanism by which the exact longitudinal pairing between two homologous chromosomes is initiated during zygotene. Subsequent completion of longitudinal pairing appears to be aided by a sort of protein cement formed between homologous chromosomes. The presence of such protein cement was first noted by Moses (6) with the use of an electron microscope and termed "synaptonemal complex".

When the process of longitudinal pairing is completed, primary spermatocytes are said to have entered the pachytene stage. Thus, the human pachytene nucleus contains 22 autosomal bivalents and the XY-bivalent (Fig. 1). An autosomal bivalent of pachytene has the appearance of a rather thick thread showing a more or less distinct transverse banding pattern. The position of a centromere

Figures 1 and 2 are pachytene and diakinesis or first meiotic metaphase figures obtained from testicular biopsy of a normal human male subject. The air-dry preparation is shown courtesy of Dr. John Melnyk of this institute.

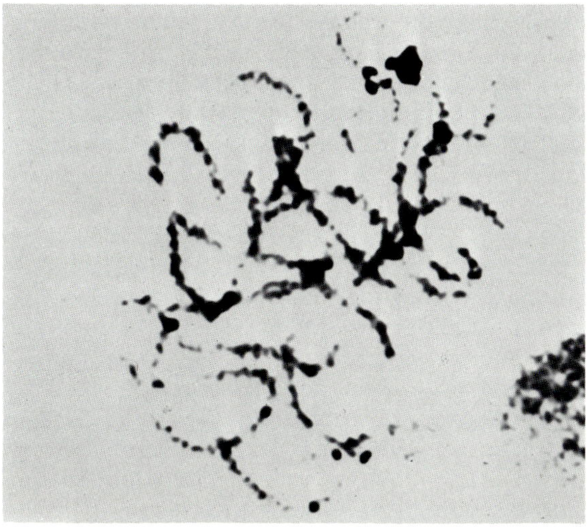

Fig. 1. Pachytene. An intensely stained sex vesicle enclosing the X and the Y is seen at 12:30 o'clock.

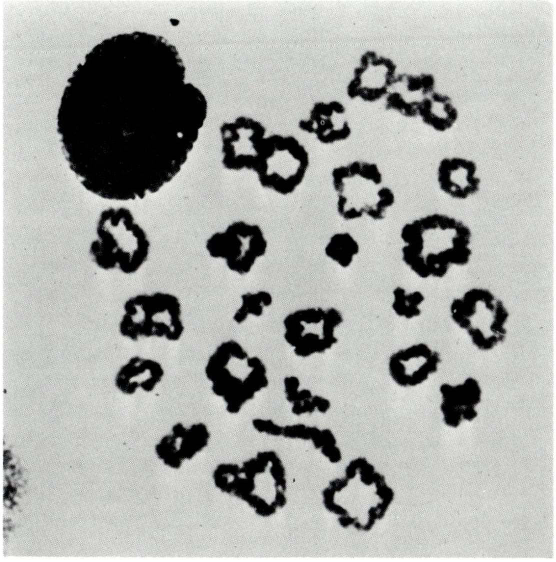

Fig. 2. Diakinesis or 1st meiotic metaphase. 22 autosomal bivalents and the X and the Y in typical end-to-end association are seen. The XY-bivalent is at 6 o'clock inside.

is, as a rule, marked by an adjacent knob of heavily stained heterochromatin (centromeric heterochromatin). In sharp contrast to the thread-like autosomal bivalents, the XY-bivalent exists as a conspicuous mass of heterochromatin embedded in the sex vesicle (7) which is rich in RNA (8).

Unlike autosomes, which always exist as a pair in diploid organisms, the X and the Y of mammalian males are the determiners of the opposite sexes, and there is very little homology between the X and the Y. The Y carries none of the many structural genes unrelated to the act of sex determination carried by the X. Although an extremely short arm of the acrocentric human Y may be homologous to the distal end of the short arm of the metacentric X (9,10) and genuine longitudinal pairing appears to occur within the sex vesicle between the extremely short homologous segments of the X and the Y (11), the presence of such a short homologous segment appears to offer insufficient attraction to bring the X and the Y together during zygotene and pachytene. Yet, the segregation of the X against the Y at the end of first meiosis can be assured only if the largely nonhomologous X and Y form a respectable bivalent. The formation of a peculiar sex vesicle in male pachytene nuclei apparently reflects the special device mammalian species invented to bring the X and the Y together. Heteropyknosis (condensation) may be the means employed to deemphasize the great difference that exists between the DNA base sequences of the X and the Y. Indeed, two X-chromosomes during female meiosis b have in exactly the same manner as any other autosomal pairs (12). From the end of last spermatogonial telophase to the end of the pachytene stage is a period of long duration. From what is known in the mouse(1) it may be inferred that in man nearly 10 days would be taken up by this period.

FROM DIPLOTENE TO THE END OF FIRST MEIOSIS

Genetic recombination (crossing-over) which is due to exchange of parts of chromatids between paired homologous chromosomes is most likely to occur either during the process of homologous pairing (zygotene) or immediately after the completion of longitudinal pairing (pachytene). First, breaks must occur at corresponding positions of the DNA strands of paired homologues; subsequent rejoining of broken ends by a repair enzyme may unite the broken end of one with that of its homologue thus accomplishing an exchange. Although we have no way of catching the process of recombination "in the act" under the microscope, the consequence of crossing-over becomes evident at the stage following pachytene which is referred to as the "diplotene" stage.

At the beginning of "diplotene", homologous autosomes which in pachytene were paired side-by-side along their entire length fall apart from each other except at certain places where chiasmata have been formed. As expected, more chiasmata are seen on larger bivalents. The largest autosomal bivalent seen in the human diplotene nucleus may show as many as five chiasmata; three interstitial and two terminal. Although diplotene chiasmata most likely represent the consequence of crossing-over events which took place in the preceding stages of first meiotic prophase, the position of a chiasma does not appear to coincide with the precise point of an actual exchange. Our genetic knowledge tells us that crossing-over occurs essentially at random along the entire length of an autosome. In sharp contrast, diplotene chiasmata tend to be positioned with remarkable regularity in a given autosomal bivalent. Furthermore, the mean number of chiasmata exhibited by a large autosomal bivalent appears to be too small to equal the number of genetic crossing-overs expected of so large a genetic unit (linkage group). If falling apart of pachytene homologues is due to the repulsion between pairs of centers located along the length of a bivalent, all actual points of crossing-over contained in the region between two adjacent repulsive centers would move away toward the middle as a result of the repulsive movement and be seen as a single chiasma. This would account for the relatively small number of chiasmata actually seen and also for the tendency of chiasmata to occur at fixed sites of a given bivalent.

Soon diplotene bivalents begin rapid condensation, and primary spermatocytes reach the "diakinesis" stage, which marks the end of the first meiotic prophase. This progressive condensation is accompanied by further terminalization of chiasmata. Two or three interstitial chiasmata of diplotene can now be seen as a single terminal chiasma. Thus, many of the autosomal bivalents of diakinesis assume an O-shape (two terminal chiasmata) and some small ones an X-shape (a single terminal chiasma) as shown in Fig.2. It is my opinion that counting the number of chiasmata on diakinesis bivalents is a rather futile endeavor, for it will tell us about the degree of chiasma terminalization, rather than the frequency of genetic crossing-over. At diakinesis, the X and the Y are clearly seen in a characteristic end-to-end association. Chen and Falek (10) have recently presented rather convincing evidence that this association in man is between the extreme short arm of the acrocentric Y and the terminal end of the short arm of the X.

Diakinesis is the best stage in which to count the number of bivalents and detect the presence of a quadrivalent expected in an individual heterozygous for a translocation. Some of the translocations which cannot be detected by examination of somatic diploid metaphase figures can be detected at diakinesis.

At the end of diakinesis, disappearance of the nuclear membrane is followed by the alignment of already condensed bivalents on the equatorial plate of the first meiotic spindle. The difference between diakinesis and first meiotic metaphase is in the alignment and not in the appearance of individual bivalents.

At anaphase of ordinary mitosis, the centromere of each chromosome splits, and two sister chromatids move away from each other toward the opposite division poles. Thus, in man, each daughter cell receives 46 chromatids as a result of mitosis. In the case of first meiotic anaphase, on the other hand, two sister chromatids of each chromosome are held together by the unsplit centromere, and the repulsive movement is between one whole chromosome against the whole of its homologous counterpart. Thus, as a result of first meiosis, each daughter cell receives 22 autosomes and the X or the Y. The segregation of two haploid sets from a diploid set is therefore accomplished.

SECOND MEIOSIS

The stage between the first meiotic telophase and second meiotic prophase is called "interkinesis". On a pair of daughter secondary spermatocyte nuclei, the condensed X can clearly be seen on one and the condensed Y on the other. Interkinesis is a rather inert stage. There is no need for S-phase (DNA replication), since each chromosome in the haploid nucleus is already made of two chromatids. Furthermore, most of the enzymes and proteins needed for the ensuing stage of spermiogenesis have already been synthesized and stored in their cytoplasm by the mother cell during the premeiotic stage. Thus, after the interkinesis stage which is of short duration, secondary spermatocytes merely go through the motion of haploid mitosis, which is the true nature of second meiosis. At the end, each daughter cell receives 23 chromatids including an X-chromatid or a Y-chromatid. It can be said that the spermatozoa are in the G-1 stage of haploid interphase.

A major cause of known types of chromosome anomalies should be sought in meiotic errors occurring either during spermatogenesis or oogenesis. Analysis of second meiotic metaphase figures is the only way to accurately estimate the frequency of errors committed by first meiosis. Unfortunately, the morphology of second meiotic metaphase chromosomes is such that they are not readily amenable to analysis. Sister chromatids of each chromosome which are loosely held together at the centromere do not attain the fully condensed state; instead they remain stringy in appearance.

ACKNOWLEDGEMENTS

This work was supported in part by a grant (CA 05138) from the National Cancer Institute, U.S. Public Health Service.

REFERENCES

1. Monesi, V., Amer.Zool., 1: 374, 1961.

2. Melnyk, J., Thompson, H., Rucci, A.J., Vanasek, F., and Hayes, S., Lancet. ii: 797, 1969.
3. Ohno, S., Jainchill, J., and Stenius, C., Cytogenetics, 2: 232, 1963.
4. Stern, H., and Hotta, Y., Genetics, 61: 27, 1969.
5. Lindsley, D.L., and Grell, E.H., Genetics, 61: 69, 1969.
6. Moses, P.B., Ann. Rev. Genet., 2: 364, 1968.
7. Sachs, L., Ann. Eugen., 18: 255, 1954.
8. Ohno, S., Kaplan, W.D., and Kinosita, R., Exptl. Cell. Res., 11: 520, 1956.
9. Ferguson-Smith, M.A., Lancet, ii: 475, 1966.
10. Chen, A.T.L., and Falek, A., Science, 166: 1008, 1969.
11. Solari, A.J., Genetics, 61: 113, 1969.
12. Ohno, S., Klinger, H.P., and Atkin, N.B., Cytogenetics, 1: 42, 1962.

DISCUSSION

CLERMONT: Dr. Ohno, you said that it was possible to prevent meiosis experimentally. Could you explain how this could be done?

OHNO: This of course was done on a plant, by Hatta and Stern, where the cells in the same step of meiosis can be recovered in mass. By increasing the temperature, nucleic acid synthesis is completed and the cells go into mitosis instead of meiosis.

E. STEINBERGER: I would like to emphasize the fact that most of these studies have been performed in a plant (lily). If I recall correctly these plant cells are capable of going through meiosis and completing the reduction division in vitro with no difficulty. In cultures of mammalian testis meiotic division fails to take place suggesting that conditions necessary for completion of meiotic process in a plant spermatocyte must differ greatly from those which occur in the mammalian testis.

OHNO: I have to disagree with you on this point. What we learned from comparing the sequences of direct gene products is the amazingly conservative nature of natural selection. Really important things have never really changed in evolution, the examples being transfer RNA and histone IV. Exchange of genetical information is based on the complementality of base sequences. Such a process must have begun at the very beginning of life. For this reason, I believe that the principle of meiotic process must be the same in all living creatures.

E. STEINBERGER: I want to apologize to Dr. Ohno. I did not mean to imply that the basic mechanisms involved in the lily are not necessarily similar to those of higher species. However, there are also basic differences. For example, bacteria may reproduce sexually, but still we cannot compare this with mammalian sexual reproduction, particularly with regard to the various regulatory mechanisms which in higher species are obviously highly developed.

FORD: Dr. Ohno, I was a little surprised at your opposition to the chiasma-type hypothesis, that is the assumption of a direct 1 to 1 relationship between chiasmata observed in the spermatocyte and genetic cross-over. I would like to ask how you explain the classic experiments of Beadle, for example, which showed a very close correlation? We have unpublished information in the mouse making use of overlapping translocations, and correlating our chiasma counts with the position of the break points on the genetic map. We find extremely good agreement.

OHNO: Well, I believe that one has to distinguish the intergenic crossing-over from intragenic crossing-over and what has traditionally been measured is the crossing over between the genes. There is a reason to explain the fact that intergenic-crossing over should not happen as often as intragenic crossing-over. This is because if you think of a chromosome as a single strand of DNA double helix, there has to be a number of signals which say "here is the beginning of one structural gene, and there is a beginning of the other." Such a signal might be a promoter base sequence which is inserted between structural gene base sequences. Thus, evolution has to reduce the number of intergenic crossings-over in order to avoid too many unequal crossings-over which would be lethal. For this reason I think that there are far more frequent intragenic crossings-over than intergenic crossings-over.

FORD: This may be, but the fact remains that there is extremely good agreement between cytologically observed chiasmata and genetically identified cross-overs. One can estimate the total genomic length of the mouse chromosomes and estimate it fairly accurately. I have been watching my predictions over a number of years, and at one stage the genetic map of one of the mouse chromosomes was much longer than I had anticipated any mouse chromosome could be. True enough, two or three years ago it was found that there were two separate linkage groups involved and now the map again is consistent with chiasma counts.

OHNO: Within the H2 locus of the mouse the intragenic crossing-over occurs at the rate of 3×10^{-3}. And the rate of crossing-over between the H2 locus and the next TL-locus is, I believe, considerably less.

FORD: I do not deny, of course, what you are saying. We must find some means of reconciling that with the counts of chiasmata in diplotene and diakinesis.

SOLARI: I think that there is a lot of evidence about the relationship between chiasmata and genetic crossing-over. For instance, Taylor's experiments strongly support these relationships, but this refers to intergenic crossing-over. The intragenic crossing-over is a rather open problem and I find Dr. Ohno's suggestion a very interesting one. I think that there may be two mechanisms for intragenic and intergenic crossing-over during meiosis and this would be perfectly in agreement with some models of the molecular structure of the synaptonemal complex.

ULTRASTRUCTURE AND HISTOCHEMISTRY OF THE NUCLEUS DURING MALE MEIOTIC PROPHASE

Alberto J. Solari and L. L. Tres

Centro de Investigaciones sobre Reproduccion, Facultad de Medicina - Paraguay 2155, Buenos Aires, Argentina

The life of the human first spermatocyte lasts about 23 days (1). During this period predetermination of meiosis, synapsis. chiasmata formation and segregation of homologues occurs; it is also possible that some abnormal phenomena such as meiotic non-disjunction occur during this time.

These processes are accompanied by ultrastructural and histochemical changes that will be reviewed here, with attention focused on human cells.

THE PROPHASE STAGES

Preleptotene. If incomplete replication of DNA is a prerequisite for meiosis, as it seems to be in the lily (2), then meiosis determination begins in the preleptotene stage, during the synthesis phase of DNA (S-phase). In the lily, meiosis determination is completed later, in the post-synthetic (G-2) phase (2).

However, from the ultrastructural viewpoint, we do not have any morphological basis for identification of the human preleptotene stage. The suspected cells can be considered either as leptotene, because of the presence of chromatin threads, or they cannot be distinguished from type B spermatogonia. Recent work by Lima-de-Faria et al. (3) attempts to explain this. These authors found that DNA synthesis continues in leptotene and leptotene-zygotene spermatocytes in culture. It could be that true preleptotene is a short-lived stage which rapidly evolves to nuclear condensation which is characteristic of the leptotene stage, while continuing with the functions usually associated with the preleptotene, the main one being the premeiotic synthesis of DNA. The peculiar transformation of mitochondria from the regular morphology observed in the spermatogonia to the swollen aspect seen in spermatocytes (produced by the dilation of the intracristal space) is observed only in cells which have lost all connection with the base membrane by the interposing cytoplasm of Sertoli cells. As similar mitochondrial changes have been related with functional stages (4), a relatively abrupt metabolic change may be associated with preleptotene and meiosis determination.

Leptotene. Leptotene nuclei are characterized by the condensation of chromatin, which forms many thread-like patches (Fig. 1). Axial condensations or single cores 300 Å wide may be observed in some cells which are more advanced in development. A small granular, horseshoe shaped nucleolus is present in leptotene and in zygotene.

Zygotene. The beginning of zygotene is marked by the appearance of synaptonemal complexes (SC) inside the nucleus. The number of SC increases up to the end of zygotene. The sex pair ("sex vesicle") appears during zygotene as a homogeneous zone of chromatin fibrils containing single cores.

Pachytene. This stage occurs most frequently in the sections (Fig. 2). Early pachytene nuclei contain long stretches of SC associated with densely packed chromatin fibrils. During mid and late pachytene the chromatin becomes gradually less packed with the exception of the "basal knobs" (5) and the sex pair (6). Nucleoli grow during mid-pachytene and attain their maximum volume at late pachytene (Fig. 2), when the whole nucleus is swollen and the sex pair appears as a prominent dense mass attached to the nuclear envelope (Fig. 2).

Diplotene. The diplotene stage is marked by the virtual disappearance of SC inside the nucleus. Single cores are observed in the loose masses of chromatin fibrils. A special tripartite and convoluted structure has been observed in one human bivalent during prometaphase and metaphase (7).

THE SYNAPTONEMAL COMPLEX

This is the most distinctive structure found in meiotic nuclei, (8,9) and its occurrence during synaptic stages in meiosis seems to be universal (10). The SC is a plane, tripartite structure composed of two lateral elements flanking a third, central element (Fig. 3) The SC lies in the axis of each bivalent during zygotene and pachytene, that is, it is located at the place where the two homologues face each other. The lateral elements of the SC are rods denser and wider (about 400 Å wide) than the central element which is about 150 Å wide. In frontal sections the central element appears to be formed of three longitudinal filaments 40 Å thick. Transverse

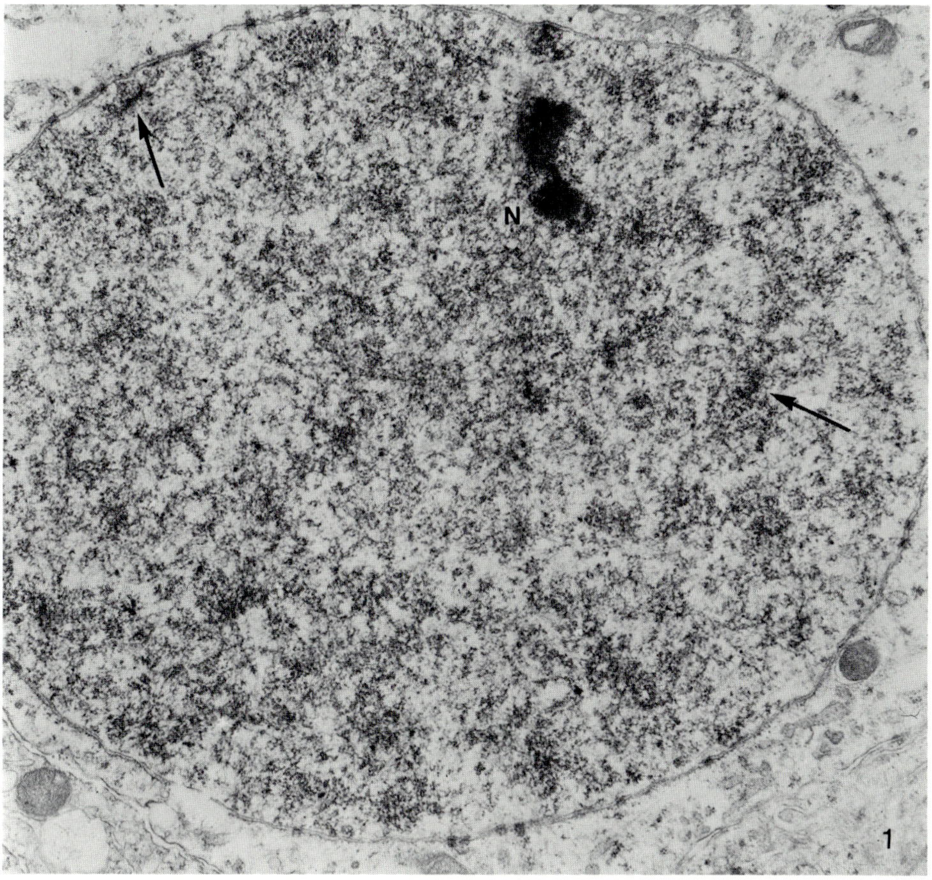

Fig. 1. Human leptotene spermatocyte. Chromatin threads with axial condensations (arrows). N, nucleolus. X 24,500 (without reduction).

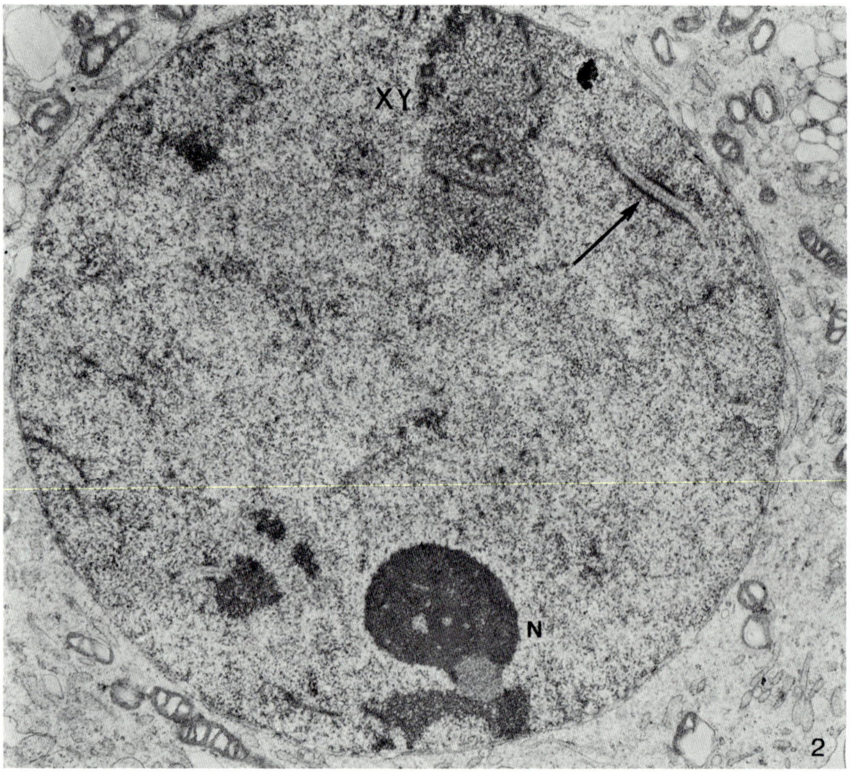

Fig. 2. Human pachytene spermatocyte. XY, XY pair; N, nucleolus. Synaptonemal complex (arrow). X 20,000 (without reduction).

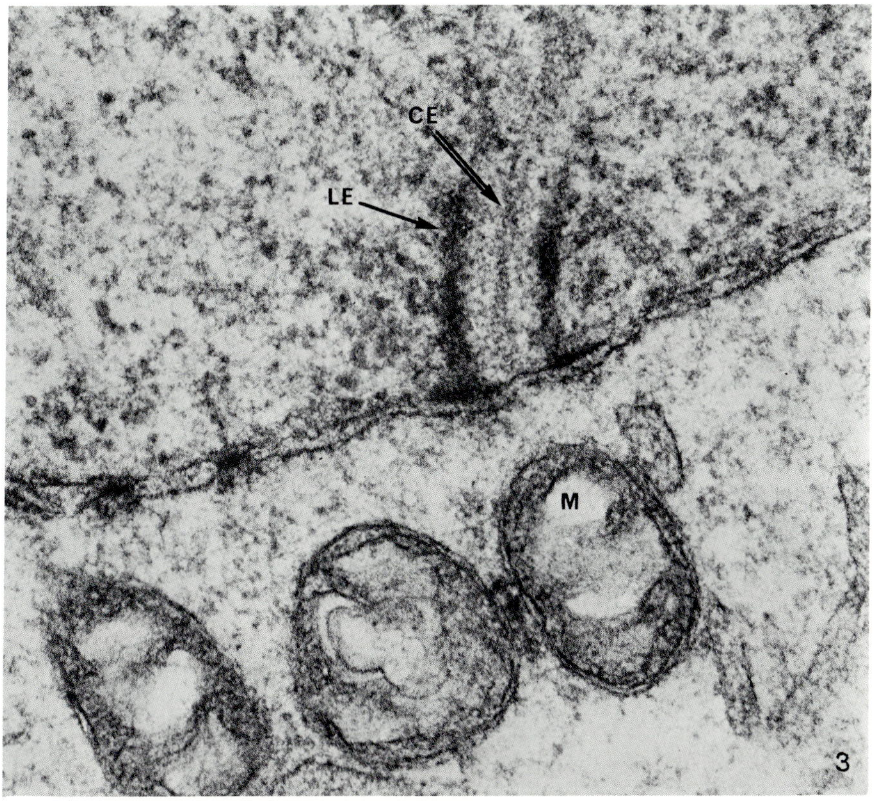

Fig. 3. High magnification micrograph of a human pachytene nucleus. LE, lateral element of a synaptonemal complex. CE, central element. M, dilated intracristal space of mitochondria. X 152,000.

fibrils cross from the lateral to the central element. Each lateral element is surrounded by chromatin fibrils of one homologue, except at the medial side. The SC is present all along the synapsed homologues (11) and its two ends are attached to the nuclear membrane (12). Histochemical tests have shown that DNA is not present except in the narrow inner layer of the lateral elements (13). Thus, the main components of the SC must be different from those of chromatin fibers. Sheridan and Barrnett (14) have shown that in the lily the lateral elements contain a basic component, probably a lysine-rich protein, which is stained with alcoholic phosphotungstic acid, and which is probably different from common histones. Thus, the main mass of the SC is formed by the deposition of a special substance on specific parts of zygotene chromosomes (9). However, small amounts of DNA can exist in the transverse fibrils (8) and perhaps in the central element.

The formation of the SC has been studied with serial sections in a few cases only (11,15). These show that leptotene chromosomes bearing single cores pair to form the SC. Thus, each lateral element pertains to each homologue, while the central element seems to result from the condensation of the transverse fibrils. The fate of the SC at diplotene varies with different species. In the human the SC disappears while the homologues come apart from each other forming chromatin patches which bear single cores, that is, lateral elements remain, at least for a time, joined to single chromosomes.

Recent evidence indicates that at least two biochemical events may be related to the SC formation. In the lily, 0.3% of the total DNA does not replicate during the premeiotic S-phase, but it is replicated specifically during zygotene (2). If this delayed DNA synthesis is inhibited, the SC formation is also inhibited (16). Certain non-histone proteins are synthesized at zygotene; if this synthesis is inhibited with cycloheximide the arrest of nuclei at zygotene results.

It has been assumed that the presence of the SC expresses the synapsis of homologous segments of chromosomes (10) and that it is a prerequisite for chiasma formation (8). A number of observations contradicting these assumptions have been recorded (17,9) but they generally refer to stages different from zygotene and early pachytene. Thus, zygotene synapsis is accompanied by formation of the SC.

THE SEX PAIR IN HUMAN SPERMATOCYTES

The XY pair is formed at zygotene as a dense body often called the "sex vesicle." This heteropyknotic sex pair is formed by chromatin fibrils with a special degree of packing (6,18,19). This special condensation of the human sex chromosomes is present in the leptotene stage, but it is absent in the human spermatogonia (20).

The XY pair forms an oblong mass associated with the nuclear envelope (Fig. 2). Inside the chromatin mass, 400 Å wide sections of single cores are observed. The pattern of the cores in the human XY pair has been studied with serial sections and model building of whole, reconstituted, XY pairs (21). Two cores are present at all times in the XY pair, and they have constant features (Figs. 4 and 5). They are the long and the short cores, corresponding to the axes of the X and the Y chromosomes respectively. Both cores begin and end on the nuclear envelope, but they have a common end (Fig. 5)

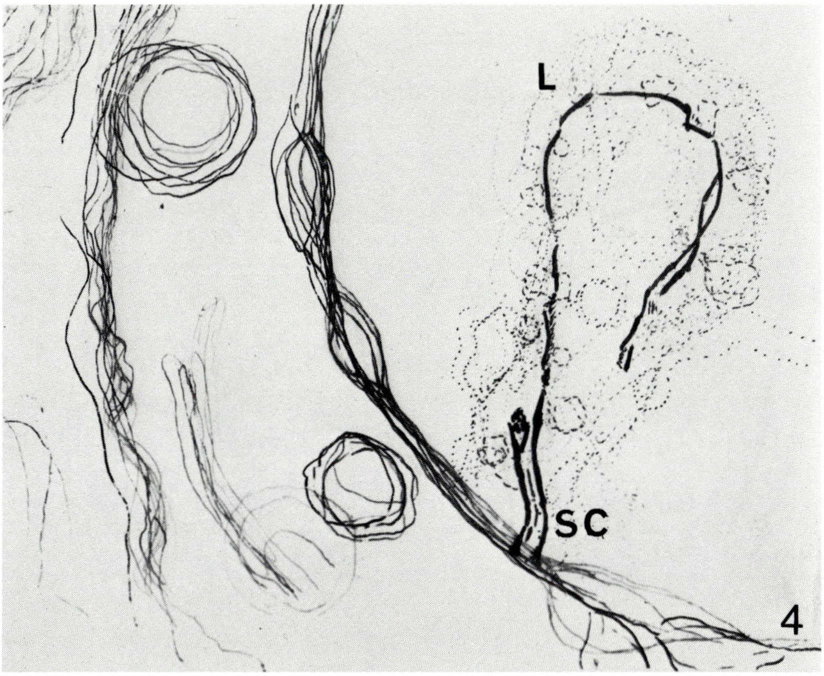

Fig. 4. Photograph of a partially reconstructed XY pair from human spermatocyte. L, long core. SC, synaptonemal complex formed at the common end of both cores.

formed by the union of the two cores. In that region a synaptonemal complex is formed which measures 0.4 to 0.8 microns in length. This SC is formed in zygotene and early pachytene and it shortens and becomes unrecognizable during mid and late pachytene. A similar pattern of the cores has been observed in the mouse and in the rat (22).

The remaining length of the cores, especially the long core, is convoluted at some places; this coiling is exaggerated during mid and late pachytene, forming the ring bodies (6). As the centromeres have not been identified with the electron microscope, no evidence is provided that is associated with one of the two extremes of each sex chromosome. However, from the optical picture of the human XY pair, it has been assumed that the short arm of the X chromosome is involved in the end-to-end joining with the Y (23). From the data cited above, which agree with those concerning other mammals, it is concluded that in the human there is partial synapsis between the X and the Y chromosomes. Pairing is restricted to a small part of both chromosomes, involving the tip of the X chromosome. Chiasmata and crossing-over might be possible in that region, and the latter would be reflected in the partial X-linkage of genes located in that segment.

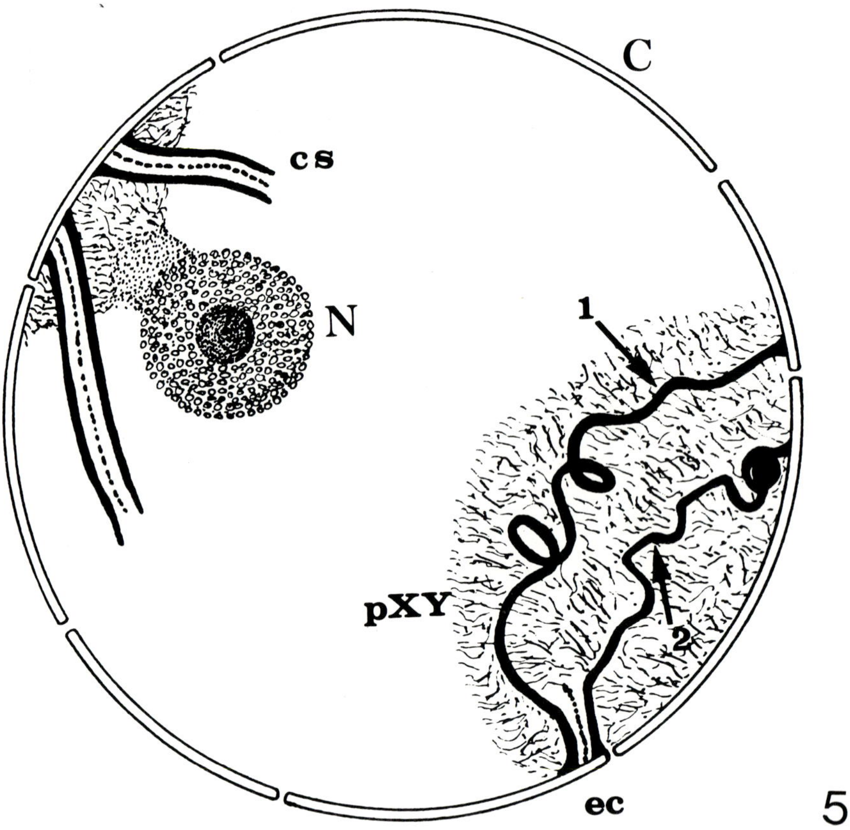

Fig. 5. Schematic drawing of a human spermatocyte during pachytene. cs, synaptonemal complex ending on a basal knob associated with the nucleolus (N). pXY, XY pair; ec, common end; 1, long core; 2, short core. C, nuclear envelope.

NUCLEOLI OF HUMAN SPERMATOCYTES

It has been proved (24,6) that in human spermatocytes, nucleoli are not regularly associated with the sex pair, but are regularly associated with "basal knobs". These basal knobs are centered by one or more SC that end immediately on the nuclear envelope (Fig. 5). Thus, nucleoli are associated with the heteropyknotic tips of some autosomes (6). In the human these autosomes must be the satellited acrocentrics, that is, the members of groups 13-15 and 21-22.

The ultrastructure of the main and secondary nucleoli shows two clear-cut regions: a granular, outer region and a central, dense and fibrillar region(there is also a connecting region associated with the basal knob).

Thus, a sort of natural segregation of zones occurs in the pachytene nucleoli of humans as well as other mammals (19).

Histochemical tests show that the human XY pair does not contain RNA (6). In the main nucleolus, RNA is found in the granular zone. The inner dense zone gives negative reaction for RNA as well as for DNA tests (7).

CONCLUSION AND SUMMARY

During meiotic prophase special structures are formed which are intimately related to synapsis and chiasmata formation. The synaptonemal complex is formed at zygotene by the union of single homologues on which a deposition of SC material,including basic protein,forms definitive lateral elements. The SC material is deposited on a small part of each homologue, as the main mass of the chromosome is formed by chromatin fibrils which form loops at the sides of each lateral element. It is assumed that this linear part of each homologue associated to SC material is the one involved with synapsis and crossing-over. The cores of the sex pair behave like the lateral elements of the SC, and are collinear to the axes of the X and Y chromosomes. The spatial reconstruction of the human XY pair shows the presence of a small SC formed by both chromosomes. It is concluded that effective partial synapsis exists in the XY pair. The tip of the short arm of the X chromosome is probably involved in that pairing. Crossing-over and partial sex-linkage of some genes may exist.

Nucleoli of spermatocytes show a segregation of their regions and a zone without detectable RNA.

ACKNOWLEDGMENTS

We thank Prof. R. E. Mancini for his support and Dr. J. C. Lavieri for providing the human biopsies. The authors are Members of the Scientific Career, Consejo Nacional de Investigaciones Cientificas y Tecnicas. This work was partially supported by a Grant of the Population Council.

REFERENCES

1. Heller, C. G. and Clermont, Y ., Recent Progr. Hormone Res., 20: 545, 1964.
2. Stern, H. and Hotta, Y. Genetics, Suppl., 61: 27, 1969.
3. Lima-de-Faria, A., German, J., Ghatnekar, M., McGovern, J. and Anderson, L., Hereditas, 60: 249, 1968.
4. Hackenbrock, C.R., Proc. Nat. Acad. Sci. U.S.A., 61: 598, 1968.
5. Woollam, D.H., and Ford, E.H., J. Anat., 98: 163, 1964.
6. Solari, A.J. and Tres, L., Chromosoma , 22: 16, 1967.
7. Tres, L., Thesis. Facultad de Medicina, Univ. de Buenos Aires, 1970.

8. Moses, M.J., Genetics, Suppl. 61: 41, 1969.
9. Moses, M.J., Ann. Rev. Genet., 2: 363, 1968.
10. Moses, M.J. In Cytology and Cell Physiology, ed. Bourne, G., Academic Press, New York, p. 423, 1964.
11. Wettstein, R. and Sotelo, J.R., J. de Microsc., 6: 557, 1967.
12. Woollam, D.H., Ford, E.H. and Millen, J., Exp. Cell Res., 42: 657, 1966.
13. Coleman, J.R. and Moses, M.J., J. Cell Biol., 23: 63, 1964.
14. Sheridan, W.F. and Barrnett, R.J., J. Ultrastruct. Res., 27: 216, 1969.
15. Moens, P.B., Chromosoma, 23: 418, 1968.
16. Roth, T.F. and Ito, M., J. Cell Biol., 35: 247, 1967.
17. Sotelo, J.R. and Wettstein, R., Chromosoma, 15: 389, 1964.
18. Solari, A.J., Exp. Cell Res., 38: 160, 1964.
19. Solari, A.J., J. Ultrastruct. Res., 27: 289, 1969.
20. Tres, L. and Solari, A. J., Z Zellforsch., 91: 75, 1968.
21. Solari, A.J. and Tres, L., J. Cell Biol. (in press).
22. Solari, A.J., Genetics Suppl. 66: 113, 1969.
23. Hulten, M., Lindsten, J., Ming, P.M. and Fraccaro, M., Ann. Hum. Genet., 30: 119, 1966.
24. Ferguson-Smith, M.A., Cytogenetics, 3: 124, 1964.

DISCUSSION

CLERMONT: Dr. Solari, you have indicated that in the nuclei of pachytene spermatocytes there are many nucleoli. Could you tell us if all these nucleoli are identical, or different morphologically when examined with the electron microscope?

SOLARI: The nucleoli in human spermatocytes are generally three or four. One is a main nucleolus. The others are secondary nucleoli. This fact has been observed independently by Ferguson-Smith (Cytogenetics 3: 124, 1964) and in our laboratory. Secondary and main nucleoli are identical in their ultrastructure, and all of them are related to acrocentric chromosomes.

FORD: I would like to ask Dr. Solari how he distinguishes between a terminal chiasma and a terminal association which is not a terminal chiasma.

SOLARI: I would like to interpret your question as referring to the XY pair. In the human and in the mouse, the XY pair as seen by the light microscope has no non-terminalized chiasmatic relationship. What we have seen is that there is an ultrastructural basis for synapsis, that is, a synaptonemal complex, and thus it points to the possibility of the existence of a chiasma. We have not said that there are chiasmata in the XY pair. We have demonstrated synapsis. We think that we are on the road to demonstrating chiasmata.

FORD: All the evidence that I have seen of association between X and Y, in man, either of my own or published by other workers, does not exclude the possibility that there was an earlier chiasma which terminalized by the time that observation was made. Equally, I have not hitherto encountered evidence on the other side for parasynaptic pairing, chiasma formation and terminalization. I contend that the issue is still an open one.

SOLARI: This is a point of disagreement. I think that our evidence of synapsis points to the possible existence of chiama. Your evidence and the evidence of other authors of the end-to-end relationship meaning chiasma terminalization has been opposed by other authors who thought that the relationship could be explained by a joining of the X and Y by the remaining material of the sex vesicle. This was one interpretation different from a chiasmatic mechanism, so I would say that the question merits more proof, but that our results strongly suggest chiasma formation between the X and the Y.

E. STEINBERGER: Dr. Solari, have you observed any extrusion of nucleoli in spermatocytes?

SOLARI: I have observed extrusion of nuclear material which I have not identified histochemically in secondary spermatocytes. I could not positively say that nucleoli are extruded.

JOST: Dr. Solari, you emphasized several times the fact that, in humans, there is no relation between the nucleolus and the sex chromosomes, whereas there is such a connection in the mouse. What is the significance of this difference?

SOLARI: Dr. Ohno (Ohno S., Kaplan W. and Kinosita, R., Exp. Cell. Res. 13: 358, 1957), proved that nucleolus organizers are on the X-chromosome of the mouse, and that in the human, nucleolus organizers are not in the sex chromosomes.

JIRASEK: There is an association between the nucleolus and sex chromatin in mammalian ganglionic cells. It was described in the original paper by Barr in cats, and by others, including myself in the human. Could you comment on this association?

SOLARI: I cannot comment on human ganglionic cells, of which I have no experience. But I would say that there is a close approachment between a secondary nucleolus and the XY pair in the human spermatocyte. This occurs with a low frequency and we have explained this fact by the use of serial sections. (Solari, A. J. and Tres, L., J. Cell Biol., April, 1970). The formation of the nucleolus is related to a heterochromatic knob, and the sex chromosomes are also formed by heterochromatin. Also, as Dr. Ohno said, there is affinity between the different heterochromatic parts of the chromosomes. Thus, the hypothetical explanation of the infrequent proximity but absence of structural continuity between the sex chromosomes and some secondary nucleoli is based on the fact that the heterochromatin of the nucleoli can be associated to some heterochromatin of the sex chromosomes, but not the nucleolus itself.

THE CYTOGENETICS OF THE MALE GERM CELLS AND THE TESTIS IN MAMMALS

C. E. FORD

Medical Research Council, Radiobiology Unit,
Harwell, Didcot, Berkshire, England

INTRODUCTION

The testis was the classical source of material for chromosome study in mammals. The first objectives were the determination of chromosome number, the identification of the sex chromosomes and the characterization of the normal course of meiosis in spermatocytes. Later, chiasma counts, the analysis of meiotic behavior in structural heterozygotes and mapping the distribution of chromomeres in pachytene with a view to the recognition of individual bivalents were all attempted. These latter tasks are barely more than begun even today. However, cytogenetic methods can contribute in a different way to an understanding of some aspects of testicular biology, the main operational theme being the identification of specific cell types in a mixed population by specific features of the karyotype. Four of these aspects are considered below.

Determination of the Gonads in Embryogenesis

The question of whether the nature of the mammalian gonad is determined during embryogenesis by germ cells or by cells of the mesenchymal stroma is still not answered satisfactorily. A cytogenetic study of some mosaics and chimeras may contribute to the solution in a unique way. The point can be made by reference to results from a study of two human 45,X/ 46,XY (i.e. XO/XY) mosaic cases. Both were children with ambiguous external genitalia raised as boys, and at laparotomy both were found to have a testis one side and a streak gonad the other. Cultures were set up from biopsy specimens taken from all four gonadal structures and eventually preparations were made and samples of mitotic cells identified as XO or

XY (1). In the one case 30 percent of the cells in the sample from the testis culture were XY compared with 10 percent from the streak gonad, the difference being formally significant at the 1 percent level. The proportions of XY cells were in the second case 20 per cent from the testis and again 10 percent from the streak gonad. This time the difference bordered on significance at the 5 percent level. If it may be assumed successively that these data were representative of the explants, that the explants were representative of the stromata of the whole structures from which they were taken, and that the stromata were derived from the original mesenchymal cells of the gonadal ridges, then they suggest three conclusions. First, that the nature of the primitive gonad is influenced by the somatic cells of the gonadal ridge. Second, that relatively few XY cells in a mixture with XO cells are sufficient to initiate testicular differentiation of the gonad primordium. And third, that there is a threshold proportion of XY cells below which testicular development fails and ovarian development takes its place. Singh and Carr (2) have demonstrated the presence of normal or nearly normal ovaries in 45,X fetuses and there is therefore good reason to suppose that streak gonads are derived from pre-existent ovaries, at least in subjects with a 45,X cell line. A corollary would be that cells of the gonadal ridge that contain a Y chromosome can influence the morphogenetic behavior of neighboring cells that do not contain a Y chromosome.

Before firm conclusions can be drawn it will be necessary to assemble more information of the same kind from other 45,X/46,XY human mosaics and to test the validity of the assumptions carefully. Meanwhile, some support for the basic idea that a minimal proportion of mesenchymal XY cells in the gonad primordium is necessary for testicular differentiation is provided by information obtained from cultures of gonadal tissue from human 46,XX/46,XY chimeras. The noteworthy feature is that XY cells were not recognized in either of two cultures from ovarian biopsies but were present in all three cultures established from testicular explants. Original references have been given elsewhere (1).

Most informative of all could be the intensive study of experimental 40,XX/40,XY chimeras in the mouse as begun by Mystkowska and Tarkowski (3). In such animals it should eventually be possible to relate the proportion of XX to XY in both germ cells and in cultures grown from gonadal explants to the histological nature of each gonad.

Competition between Germ Cells

Mystkowska and Tarkowski (3) studied in detail a series of nine mice obtained subsequent to embryo fusion. The inbred stocks used, CBA-p and CBA-T6T6, differed in both coat pigment and karyotype. Seven were overt chimeras as determined by inspection of the coat and retinae. Examination of the chromosomes in direct preparations from bone marrow of six of them showed that three were 40, XX/40,XY chimeras; two phenotypic males and a hermaphrodite. Breeding tests with the two males showed that only one of the two components had contributed to the functional spermatozoa, and, as the progeny included males, that component must have had an XY sex chromosome constitution. Subsequent direct examination showed that the spermatocytes in the testes of these two animals, and in the one testis of the hermaphrodite, were all XY.

The important point is that all the germ cells detected in the testes of these three animals were 40,XY cells, whether identified directly or inferred from the breeding data. To account for this result it might be postulated that the primordial germ cells arise from a relatively small number of precursors and, in a chimera, are therefore commonly all derived from the one component or all from the other. But if this is so it may be supposed that in an XX/XY chimera the probability that they will all be XY is approximately 1/2 and the probability that they are all XY in three successive XX/XY animals is $(\frac{1}{2})^3$ or 1 in 8. In a 39,X/41,XYY mosaic mouse studied in this laboratory it was found that although both cell types were present in bone marrow, all the germ cells were XYY (4). If now the cell types compared are taken as those with one or more Y chromosomes and those that lack a Y chromosome, the probability that the germ cells of the testis will all be of the first type in four out of four animals is 1 in 16. Although this is insufficient for outright rejection of the hypothesis of "purity" of the primordial germ cell population, it renders it somewhat unlikely.

The alternative is to suppose that the initial population of primordial germ cells may be mixed and that in the developing testicular environment germ cells that contain a Y chromosome are favored over those that do not. The idea of a mixed initial germ cell population is favored by data assembled by Russell (5) on mosaic mutant mice. She showed that mice with mosaic coat phenotypes attributable to presumptive gene mutation very early in development are almost invariable germ cell mosaics as well. But the most telling evidence is again provided by Mystkowska and Tarkowski (3). A further two animals in their series of seven were 40,XY/40, XY chimeras and their breeding records showed quite decisively that both components were present in the germ cell population. The evidence as a whole therefore strongly favors the view that XX germ cells may not be able to multiply in the testicular environment of the mouse, and if they are able to multiply, that they are eliminated by the time the animals are of breeding age. This could be by differential proliferation or differential survival or both and could be regarded as a form of competition.

It is appropriate now to mention observations made on germ cells in testicular preparations from human 47,XYY males. Results have been reported from 11 subjects (6-10). Despite the absence of any hint of mosaicism in blood cultures, the vast majority of spermatocytes are of the constitution of 46,XY; they have lost one of the two Y chromosomes. Only in one of the 11 subjects have a few presumptive 47, XYY cells been identified. These were cells with a univalent X and an apparent YY bivalent (9).

A special elimination mechanism for one of the two Y chromosomes has been suggested (7). But there is no precedent in mammalian cytogenetics for such a special mechanism and the alternative view is therefore preferred that once a Y chromosome had been lost by chance lagging or non-disjunction, the resultant cell with a normal 46,XY complement would enjoy selective advantage in proliferation or survival or both.

Clonal Proliferation of Germ Cells in the Irradiated Mouse Testis

The preparations are made from the testes of mice after recovery from exposure to ionizing radiation some of the spermatocytes are found to contain a quadrivalent configuration indicative of the presence of a reciprocal translocation. Other spermatocytes may contain two or more quadrivalents or multivalent configurations of a higher order. In some preparations from single testes several cells were found to exhibit the same unique multivalent configuration or set of configurations and were interpreted to be clones produced by the multiplication of single spermatogonia in which translocations had been induced by the irradiation (11). Two spermatocytes from one clone are shown in Figs. 1 and 2.

Figs. 1 and 2.

Two spermatocytes from one testis of a mouse killed nine months after exposure to 600 R 250 kVp X-rays. Both contain a chain of eight chromosomes and are members of the same clone. The uniqueness resides in the relative lengths of the successive chromosomes in the chain. Variation in the position and number of the chiasmata are irrelevant but can modify its gross appearance. Accordingly other spermatocytes of the same clone might be expected with, for example, a ring of eight or two chains of four.

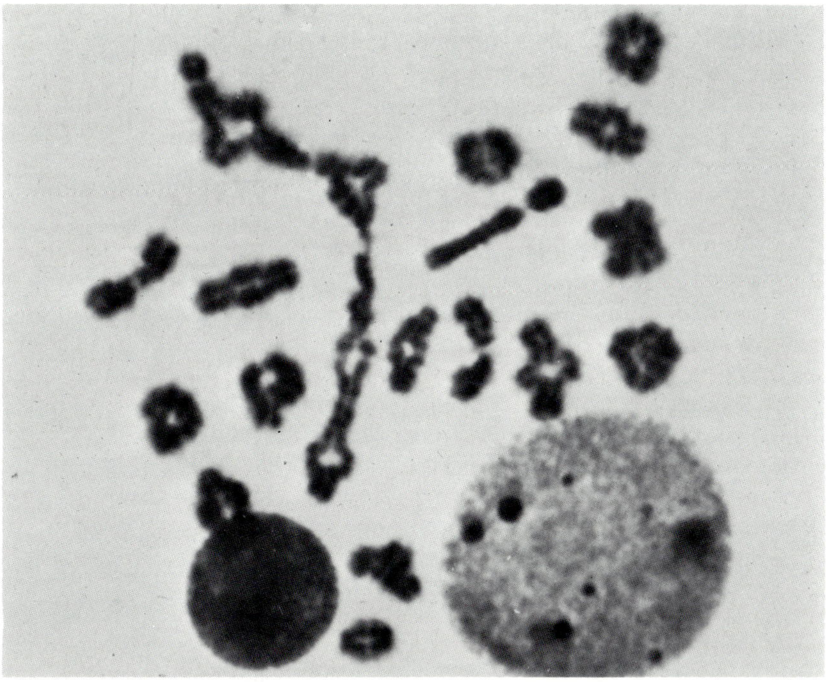

Fig. 1.

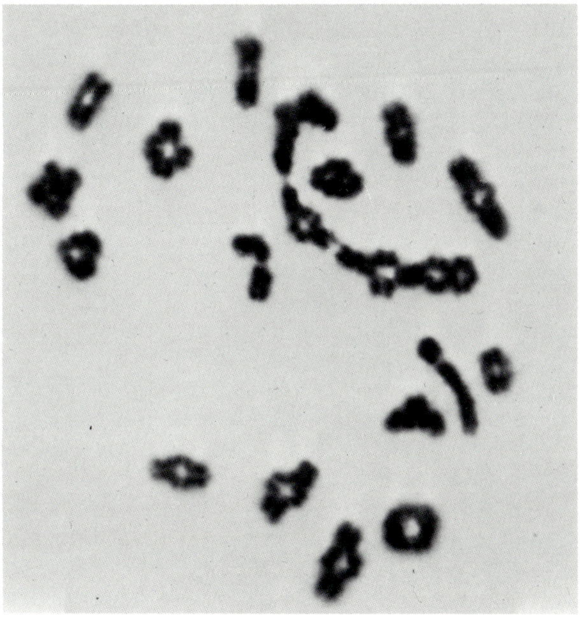

Fig. 2.

In further unpublished work on mice exposed to an acute X-ray dose of 600 R the occurrence of such clones has been repeatedly confirmed, some of them making up three or four percent of the whole sample. It is assumed that the samples of cells analyzed are drawn randomly from the spermatocyte population since a separate cell suspension is made from each whole testis as the initial step in the preparative schedule. Oakberg (12) has reported that only some three per cent of type A spermatogonia in the mouse survive acute exposure to 600R X-rays. If the conservative assumption is made that there are 5×10^5 type A spermatogonia in the normal mouse testis, there should still be 10^4 survivors. If all contributed equally to the regeneration of the seminiferous tissue, the probability of identifying members of the same clone in the samples of 200 or 400 spermatocytes normally examined would be negligibly low. It follows either that the numbers of surviving spermatogonia that contribute to regeneration must be very much less than Oakberg's estimate of the proportion of survivors would suggest or that there is very strong differential proliferation as between different clones. Or both could be responsible in part.

Clermont and Huckins (13) have shown that there are some 30 tubules in the normal rat testis that have connections to the rete testis but not to one another. If the mouse testis has a similar structure and if type A spermatogonia cannot move from one tubule to another, the maximum clone size expected if the whole of a tubule were repopulated by the descendants of one surviving spermatogonium would be four or five per cent, allowing for some variation in size between tubules. The observation of clones constituting three to four percent of the sample suggests that repopulation of a tubule by descendants of a single spermatogonium may indeed occur.

It is hoped that careful squash preparations of separate short lengths of tubule will confirm the validity of the clone interpretation and also give direct information about the length of tubule that may be occupied by a single clone.

Genetic Information and Spermatogenesis

Mice of either sex that are heterozygous for a reciprocal translocation between autosomes (as opposed to a Robertsonian translocation) are normally semi-sterile. That is to say, in matings to normal, litter size is reduced to about 50 per cent of that recorded for parallel matings of their structurally homozygous sibs. However, Lyon and Meredith (14) reported five stocks in which the heterozygous males were completely sterile. These stocks were established from semi-sterile daughters of irradiated males and were maintained through the female line. In another experiment, Cattanach et al (15) treated males with ethane methane sulphonate and found seven completely sterile sons out of 17 that were heterozygous for autosomal reciprocal translocations.

Semi-sterility of reciprocal translocation heterozygotes is satisfactorily explained by segregation of unbalanced haploid gametic genomes. Full sterility, however, cannot be accounted for in these terms. The supposition is that it is a direct consequence of the presence of the translocation itself and so should be attributed to one of the classical three alternatives of position effect, or gene mutation associated with one of the break points, or minor duplication or deletion associated with one of the break points. But to demonstrate that the translocation itself is responsible (through whichever of these mechanisms) would require proof that sterility remained associated with the translocation on further breeding, i.e. could not be separated from it by crossing over. Given this proof, the inference follows that genetic information located at or near to one or both of the break points is in some way concerned with spermatogenesis. And the fact that the break points of the mouse translocations that have been mapped are widely scattered over many of the chromosomes suggests that many different genetic loci may be involved. Specific supporting evidence is provided by the persistent association of male sterility with the translocation on further breeding of four of the five translocation stocks reported by Lyon and Meredith. (The fifth was lost). Furthermore, three of the eight break points have now been located on different chromosomes (Lyon, personal communication).

The alternative formal explanation that has been advanced by some; that sterility is a consequence of the disturbance of the meiotic process by the rearrangement _as_ a rearrangement, can be dismissed. Apart from the great difficulty of envisaging a causal sequence initiated by a mechanical factor and terminating in physiological failure there are two specific reasons for rejection: the property of male heterozygote sterility is shown by some translocations but not by others that are mechanically equivalent, and in two of the cases reported by Cattanach and his colleagues meiotic cells were reported to be absent, the presence of a presumptive reciprocal translocation having been established by observations of chromosomes in mitosis. Meiosis not begun cannot be disturbed by abnormalities of pairing.

The proportion of all reciprocal translocations between autosomes in the mouse that bring about sterility in male heterozygotes has not yet been estimated and may not be great. Lyon and Meredith's five stocks were established from 46 F_1 daughters with significantly reduced fertility. Translocations were inferred to be present in 36. Heterozygotes of both sexes were semi-sterile in 26 and in the remaining five some of the male heterozygotes were semi-sterile and some completely sterile.

In contrast to the purely autosomal translocations it is remarkable that heterozygous males are sterile in eight of the nine X-autosome translocations recorded in the mouse (16,17). Most are proved or assumed reciprocal translocations with the distal and proximal portions of the X chromosome physically separated from one another. It may therefore be significant that the one exception with some semi-sterile male heterozygotes is a 3-point rearrangement with a segment of the chromosome bearing linkage group I inserted into the X chromosome, which otherwise preserves its structural integrity (18). Merely to suppose that the X chromosome is rich in loci that are in some way concerned with spermatogenesis would not readily account for the exception. A somewhat more plausible explanation, however, could be provided if the physical separation into two parts of the X chromosome in the reciprocal translocations should interfere with the normal development of the sex vesicle at early prophase in the primary spermatocyte and thereby disturb later events in spermatogenesis.

SUMMARY

Cytogenetic study of certain natural human mosaics and chimeras and experimentally produced XX/XY chimeras of the mouse may eventually provide a decisive answer to the question whether the testicular or ovarian nature of the embryonic gonad is determined by the germ cells themselves or by somatic cells of the mesenchymal stroma.

There is evidence from experimental mouse chimeras and from a natural mosaic mouse that in the testicular environment, germ cells containing at least one Y chromosome are favored over germ cells that lack a Y chromosome. In human 47,XYY male subjects, one of the two Y chromosomes is eventually lost from the overwhelming majority of the cells of the germ line. Strong selective proliferation of karyotypically normal 46,XY cells after accidental loss of one Y chromosome could account for this observation.

Clones of spermatocytes characterized by specific chromosome rearrangements can be identified in the testes of mice that have recovered after radiation - induced depletion of the seminiferous epithelium. Numerical considerations suggest either that fewer surviving A-type spermatogonia contribute to the regeneration of the seminiferous tissue than had hitherto been supposed, or that there is a strong proliferative differential between different clones, or both.

Considerations arising from the association of male sterility with heterozygosity for certain specific reciprocal translocations between autosomes in the mouse suggest that many autosomal loci may be concerned in some way with spermatogenesis. All males heterozygous for a reciprocal translocation between an autosome and the X chromosome yet reported are sterile. This suggests either that the X chromosome is particularly rich in loci concerned in spermatogenesis or that a special unitary explanation, possibly disturbance of the formation of normal sex vesicle in early meiotic prophase, may apply.

REFERENCES

1. Ford, C.E. J. Biosocial Science Supplement 2: 7, 1970.
2. Singh, R.P. and Carr, D.H., Anat. Rec. 155: 369, 1966.
3. Mystkowska, E.T. and Tarkowski, A.K., J. Embryol. Exp. Morph. 20: 33, 1968.
4. Evans, E.P., Ford, C.E. and Searle, A.G., Cytogenetics 8: 87, 1969.
5. Russell, L.B., In The Role of Chromosomes in Development. ed. Locke, M. Academic Press, N.Y. p 153, 1964.
6. Thompson, H., Melnyk, J. and Hecht, F., Lancet, (ii): 831,1967.
7. Melnyk, J., Thompson, H., Rucci, A.J., Vanasek, F. and Hayes, S., Lancet (ii): 797, 1969.
8. Hulten, M., Lancet (i): 717, 1970.
9. Evans, E.P., Ford, C.E., Chaganti, R.S.K., Blank, C.E. and Hunter, H., Lancet (i): 719, 1970.
10. Tettenborn, U., Schwinger, E. and Gropp, A. Deutsche Med. Wschr. 95: 158, 1970.
11. Searle, A.G., Evans, E.P., Ford, C.E. and West, B.J., Mutat. Res. 6: 427, 1968.
12. Oakberg, E.F., Jap. J. Genet., 40 (Suppl.): 119, 1965.
13. Clermont, Y. and Huchins, C., Amer. J. Anat., 108: 79, 1961.
14. Lyon, M.F. and Meredith, R., Cytogenetics, 5: 335, 1966.
15. Cattanach, B.M., Pollard, C.E. and Isaacson, J.H., Mutat. Res., 6: 297, 1968.
16. Russell, L.B. and Montgomery, C.S., Genetics 63: 103, 1969.
17. Lyon, M.F., Searle, A.G., Ford, C.E. and Ohno, S., Cytogenetics, 3: 306, 1964.
18. Ohno, S. and Cattanach, B.M., Cytogenetics, 1: 129, 1962.

DISCUSSION

ROSS: Dr. Ford, do you accept the evidence that apparently morphologically normal testicular differentiation can occur in the absence of a demonstrable Y chromosome, and if you accept this evidence, how do you rationalize it in relation to the possible role of the Y chromosome in testicular differentiation?

FORD: I think the best answer in man is the hypothesis of Ferguson-Smith, that in instances of testicular differentiation in the human species, in the absence of the Y chromosome, more specifically in the presence of two X chromosomes, as in the majority of true hermaphrodites and the so-called "XX male", this can be accounted for by exchange of material between the X chromosome and the Y during spermatogenesis in the father of the exceptional individual. The evidence favoring this interpretation is mounting, and is derived from the study of the Xg blood group system in the parents and in the exceptional children by Race and Sanger. There are three instances on record out of the small number of families that have been analyzed in which the mother was Xg negative and the father Xg positive, yet the child, XX, true hermaphrodite or XX male was Xg negative like the mother, implying that there had been no contribution of the Xg locus from the father to his exceptional child. Now, when two exceptional events occur together like that, it is reasonable to suppose that there may be some association between them, and that the association is an actual exchange of material between the X-chromosome and the Y, which at the same time could be associated with the transference of male-determining genetic information. Now, we need the further background of the Lyon hypothesis. Given the presence of active male-determining material on some of the X-chromosomes, not on others, then depending on the proportion of the two types of cell in the early gonads, one could, in theory, get either ovarian or testicular development.

PAULSEN: With respect to those phenotypic males having testes but where only a single stem-cell line, namely XX, has been found, is it not possible, Dr. Ford, that in vivo or in vitro cellular selection may play a role in this finding? Dr. Gartler has published data which emphasize the importance of these phenomena.

FORD: I agree, it is a formal possibility, and it is one that I think de la Chapelle favors. On the whole, though, although I am prepared to accept the existence of cryptic mosaics, I do not think that it can be sufficient to account for the considerable number of these XX males and XX true hermaphrodites, in whom none but XX cells have been identified.

PAULSEN: I agree that there may be several explanations. One study of a phenotypic male with scrotal testes revealed only an XX line examining the chromosomes from tissue culture of testes, skin and blood (Hecht, F., et al. Pediatrics, 38: 982, 1966). These studies were repeated by obtaining additional material from each tissue. Two stem cell lines including one with XXY sex chromosomes were demonstrated.

A. STEINBERGER: Does Dr. Ford, or any of the other speakers, have information regarding the duration of G1, S and G2 periods in the spermatogonial cells, and how they compare with the somatic cells in the human?

SOLARI: There is information but not in humans. In some mammals, the duration of the S phase before the last division of type B spermatogonia is much longer than somatic S phase, and this seems to be an indication of the transition between the classic S phase of the mitotic cycle to the very long S phase of the preleptotene.

WENIGER: In relation to the first point discussed by Dr. Ford, it has been shown by L. Bounours that the chick embryo, the germinal crescent of which has been destroyed by x-irradiation, develops sterile testes or ovaries, in accordance with its genetic sex.

OHNO: Dr. Ford, may I ask you two questions. One, Beatrice Mintz has her own idea which can be expressed as an "all or none" theory to explain why so few of her allophenic mice are hermaphrodites. She believes that most of the XX/XY mosaics develop either as normale males or normal females. What do you think of her explanation? And another question is that in your spermatogonial clone, the clone is presumably heterozygous for a translocation or translocations, so presumably you get two types of viable gametes produced. Do you recover these two gametic types in expected one-to-one frequency among the progeny?

FORD: In reply to the first question, I had not seen Beatrice Mintz's own interpretation, but I am aware that her data appeared to differ very strongly from the data obtained by Mystkowska and Tarkowski on the one hand, and McLaren and Bowman on the other. Mintz obtains almost equal numbers of apparent females and apparent males with very few true hermaphrodites, whereas Mystkowska and Tarkowski and McLaren and Bowman obtain very great excesses of males and a greater proportion of hermaphrodites. I think that the only satisfactory resolution to this problem will be when all these chimeras are identified chromosomally. With respect to the second question, let me say that after irradiation of the testis and following recovery, there are very many clones of spermatocytes, some carrying one, some two, some three reciprocal translocations and some none at all. So the sperm population produced by such an individual will be a very complex one indeed, and the problem of working out what its constitution would be is quite difficult. Nevertheless, we have attempted it, and our conclusion is that only about half the expected number of semi-sterile offspring are produced by such males as would be expected from the chromosome observations. Now to the specific question as to the number of types of viable gametes or of gametes that would give viable individuals. Assuming two-by-two segregation of the association of four, there are ten possible gametic types of which two will give fully viable individuals, one homozygous normal, the other carrying the translocation. That is, of course, when a single translocation is segregating.

CHROMOSOME STUDIES ON TESTICULAR CELLS OF SUBFERTILE MEN

Ann C. Chandley

Medical Research Council, Clinical and Population Cytogenetics Unit, Western General Hospital, Edinburgh, 4

GENETIC CAUSES OF INFERTILITY

Infertility in man is recognized as a reduced capacity for producing live offspring.

The causes of this reduction may be many and varied, but in a proportion of cases, the infertility can be brought about by genetic factors which may not directly harm the individual carrying them, but which may produce defects in gametogenesis. Such defects are known in other species. For example, spermatogenic depression or arrest has been reported in mutant strains of *Mastomys* (1), and the guinea pig (2), and mutants which affect synapsis and disjunction at meiosis are well known in several plant species and in *Drosophila* (3,4,5). In the bull, a change in sperm morphology resulting in loss of reproductive function is known to be brought about through a recessive gene acting in spermiogenesis (6) and it is possible that gene action is also responsible in man for producing abnormalities of this kind. For example several reports have been made of infertile patients whose infertility is attributable to a defect in sperm morphology (7,8,9) and recently an example of what may be a desynaptic mutant in man has been reported by Pearson (10). Among the patients attending a subfertility clinic in Oxford, England, Pearson found an azoospermic male in whom the mitotic karyotype was normal, but in which many of the chromosomes at diakinesis were present as unpaired univalents. (Fig. 1) The average number of chiasmata per cell was four compared with the normal mean frequencies of 55.9 and 52.7 per cell which have been reported by Ford and Hamerton (11) and Kjessler (12). The fact that some chiasmata at least were present in the cells at diakinesis suggests that the chromosomes had been paired in early prophase but had later undergone desynapsis, and the presence of some pairs of univalents of approximately equal

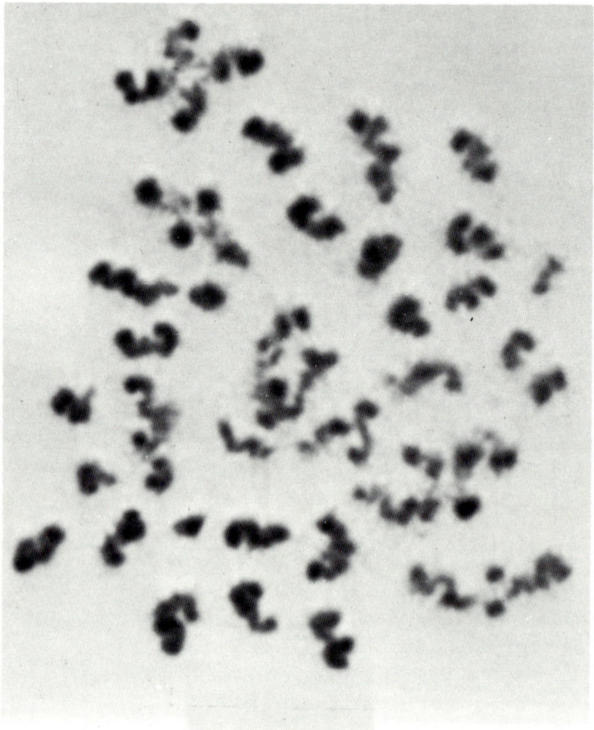

Fig. 1. Diakinesis in a desynaptic male showing many chromosomes present as univalents and a very low number of chiasmata. (Reproduced by kind permission of Dr. P. Pearson).

size lying in juxtaposition gave further support to this idea.

CHROMOSOME ABERRATIONS IN SUBFERTILE PATIENTS

More information is available regarding the association between infertility and chromosome aberrations in men, and much of it has been obtained through systematic surveys of patients attending subfertility clinics. One of the earliest surveys, carried out by Ferguson-Smith et al. (13) in Glasgow, revealed that 11% of all patients having a sperm count of less than 1 million sperm per ml. of seminal fluid were sex chromatin positive on a buccal smear. In a later survey, carried out in Sweden, Kjessler (12) found the incidence of such males to be 16%, a figure in agreement with that reported earlier by Ferguson-Smith et al. (13). Mitotic chromosome studies in the four sex chromatin positive males found by Kjessler (12) out of a total of 25 patients having sperm counts of <1 mill. sperm/ml. revealed that two had the usual XXY sex chromosome complement of an uncomplicated Klinefelter while the other two were mosaics of the XY/XXY type. Meiotic studies were not possible since all four males lacked histological signs of spermatogenesis in the seminiferous tubules.

Among 131 sex chromatin negative subfertile individuals, Kjessler found six patients with abnormal mitotic karyotypes. (A further two patients with Y chromosomes of unusual size were also found but variations in the size of the Y chromosome are known to occur in about 3% of the normal male population (14) and these latter two patients will therefore not be considered further.) All but one of the six patients with abnormal karyotypes belonged to classes with less than 40 million sperm per ml., and no individuals with an abnormal karyotype were found among patients with more than 80 million sperm per ml. (Table 1).

In a similar survey on subfertile males carried out in Edinburgh by McIlree et al. (15), abnormal mitotic karyotypes were found in three sex chromatin negative individuals out of a total of 50 patients having sperm counts of less than 20 million sperm per ml. and in addition, two patients were found in which the mitotic karyotype was normal but in which a multivalent was thought to be present at diakinesis in the primary spermatocytes. In a current Edinburgh survey, one patient with an abnormal mitotic karyotype has so far been found out of a total of 45 sex chromatin negative individuals with sperm counts of less than 20 million per ml.

TYPES OF CHROMOSOME ABNORMALITIES FOUND IN SUBFERTILE PATIENTS

Sex Chromosome Mosaicism

Among the six patients with abnormal karyotypes reported by Kjessler, four were sex chromosome mosaics. Three patients were 45,X/46,XY mosaic. The testicular histology on these patients was apparently normal and primary spermatocytes from two of the XO/XY mosaics showed some cells at diakinesis which Kjessler claimed had an XO sex chromosome constitution. In addition other cells were chromosomally normal and had a normal XY bivalent.

Autosomal Abnormalities

Among the subfertile patients reported by Kjessler was one azoospermic male, whose testicular histology showed the typical appearance of germinal cell aplasia and whose mitotic karyotype showed 47 chromosomes. The extra chromosome was approximately the size of a G group chromosome but was apparently metacentric. In our current Edinburgh survey, we have found an oligospermic male with a similar abnormality, and it is of interest that the patient's brother has now also presented at the infertility clinic and he too has been found to show the same abnormality in blood. A testicular biopsy has not yet been performed, however. The patient was a 30 year old

TABLE 1

CYTOGENETIC DATA ON SEX CHROMATIN NEGATIVE SUBFERTILE PATIENTS FROM THREE INDEPENDENT SURVEYS

Survey	Total Patients	Abnormal Karyotypes	Sperm Count	Mitotic Chromosomes	Meiotic Chromosomes
	21	1	Azoospermic	47,XY,mar+	Extra univalent present at diakinesis.
	24	2	1-20 mill./ml.	45,XY,D-,D-,t(DqDq)+	Trivalent present in most spermatocytes.
			"	46,XY/47,XXY	Normal
Kjessler 1966	21	2	21-40 mill./ml.	45,X/46,XY	XO spermatocytes present
			"	45,X/46,XY(?)	"
	14	0	41-60 mill./ml.		
	20	1	61-80 mill./ml.	45,X/46,XY	Not studied
	31	0	>81 mill./ml.		
	131	6			
	34	2	Azoospermic	46,XY,Gr	Two univalents present at diakinesis.
McIlree 1966			"	45,X/46X,Ydic	X and Y present as univalents in most cells.
	16	3	<20 mill./ml.	45,X/46,Xinv(Yp+q-)	Normal
			"	46,XY	Multivalent present at diakinesis.
			"	"	"
	50	5			
Chandley 1969	45	1	<20 mill./ml.	47,XY,mar+	Extra univalent at diakenesis

male who had counts of 7 and 3 million sperm respectively on two separate occasions and on each occasion, less than 30% of the sperm were morphologically normal and no more than 30% were motile. The mitotic karyotype showed a small extra chromosome, slightly smaller than a G group chromosome which was apparently metacentric (Fig. 2)

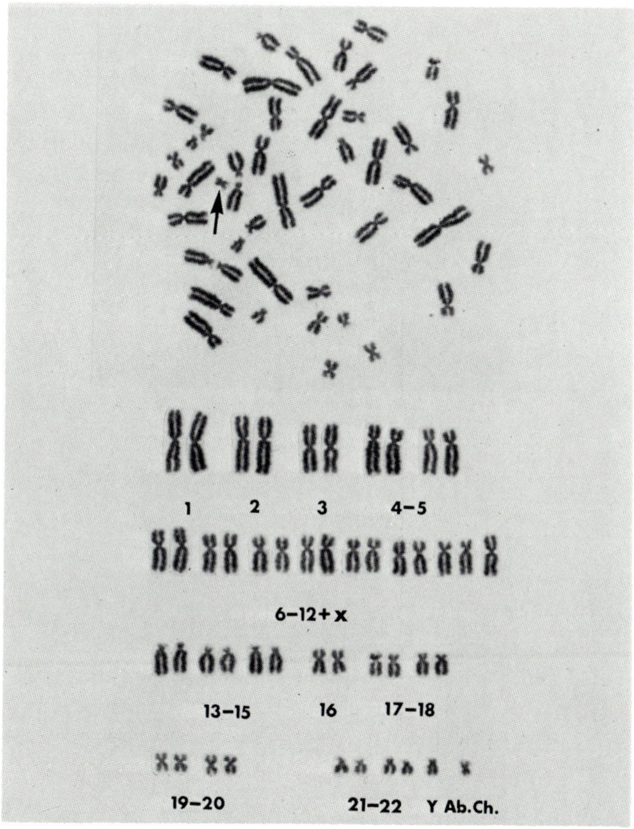

Fig. 2. Mitotic karyotype from an oligospermic patient with a small extra centric chromosome.

Meiotic preparations made by the method of Evans et al. (16) showed many cells in diakinesis I but very few second meiotic divisions. At diakinesis, the small extra chromosome could be seen in most cells as a univalent lying free from the other bivalents, and no abnormal configurations were seen (Fig. 3). It was also observed in a few cells in Metaphase II as a small dot-like chromosome.

Many diakineses showed degenerative changes in the bivalents and it appeared that meiotic arrest was occurring in many cells between the first and second meiotic divisions.

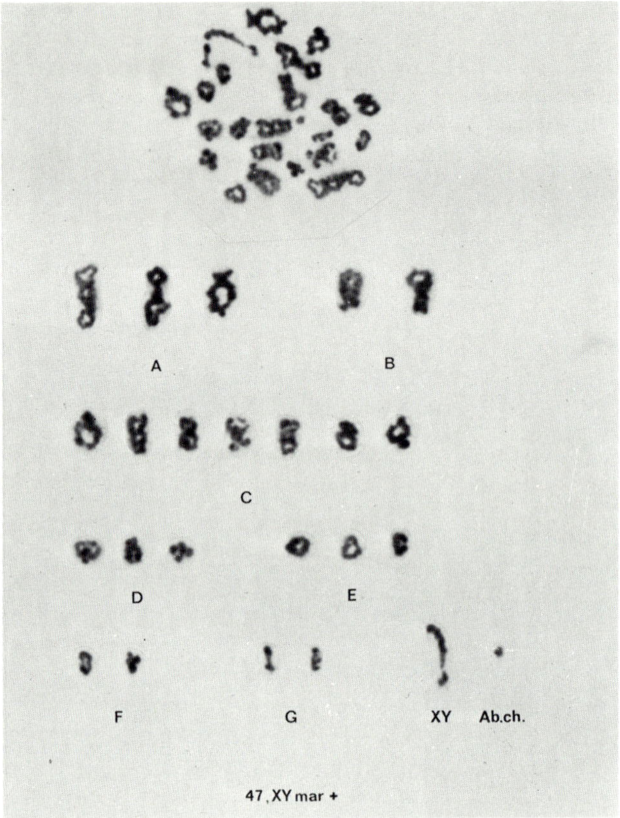

Fig. 3. Diakinesis and meiotic karyotype from the patient with a small extra centric chromosome. The extra chromosome is seen as a univalent in most primary spermatocytes.

The presence of supernumary chromosomes in oligospermic males has also been reported by Smith et al. (17) and by Hulten et al. (18), but their origin is not known, and direct evidence that the infertility is in any way related to the presence of the extra chromosome is lacking. Supernumary chromosomes have been reported, for example, in many apparently normal individuals as well as in patients showing a variety of pathological conditions (19,20).

The sixth patient with a mitotic chromosome abnormality, reported by Kjessler, was an oligospermic male who was the carrier of a heterologous D/D translocation and whose testicular histology showed spermatogenic arrest of many gametes at the spermatid level.

We have also had the opportunity to study meiosis in an oligospermic male with a translocation of this kind.

The patient did not originally present at the infertility clinic but was found through his sister, also a carrier of a D/D translocation, who reported with secondary infertility and a history of several abortions. He was found to have a sperm count of 17 million per ml., only 30% of which were morphologically normal, and his testicular histology showed reduced spermatogenic activity, but all stages of maturation up to mature sperm were present in the tubules.

The karyotype in mitotic cells from the blood showed 45 chromosomes including 4 D group chromosomes and a large metacentric chromosome similar in size to a No. 3 chromosome (Fig. 4). This was interpreted as consisting of the major parts of the two missing D group chromosomes joined together by translocation of a centric fusion type.

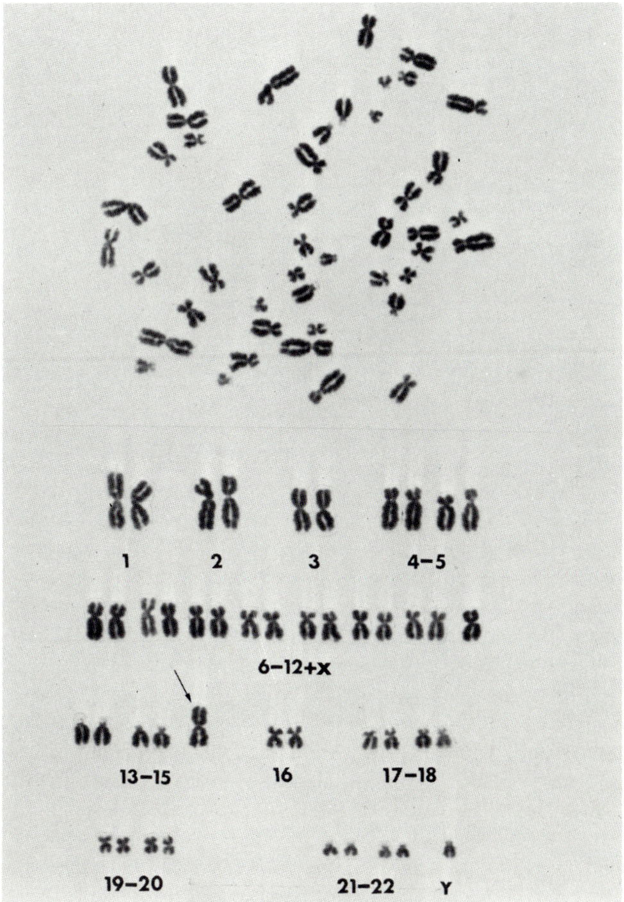

Fig. 4. Mitotic karyotype in an oligospermic patient with a heterologous D/D translocation.

At meiosis, a large trivalent representing the pairing configuration of the two translocated D chromosomes with their normal homologues was seen in most cells at diakinesis (Fig. 5). The number of cells in second meiotic metaphase was approximately equal in number to those in diakinesis and there was no evidence of meiotic arrest at this stage.

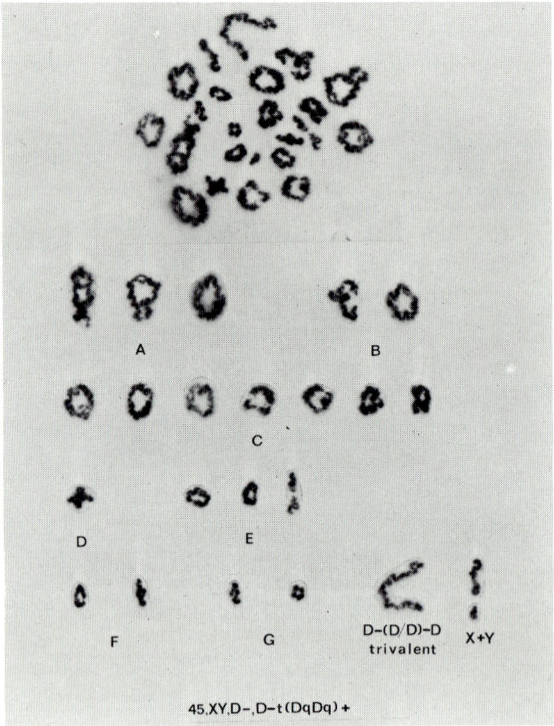

Fig. 5. Diakinesis and meiotic karyotype from the carrier of the D/D translocation. Twenty-two structures are present in the primary spermatocyte including a trivalent formed by the pairing of the two translocated D chromosomes with their normal homologues.

The various types of trivalent configuration found are shown in Fig. 6. Various numbers of chiasmata were found ranging from 2 to 5.

Segregation from a trivalent of this kind is expected on theoretical grounds to produce gametes of two main types: one type carrying a genetically balanced set of chromosomes and another type carrying an unbalanced set. However, the observations from known

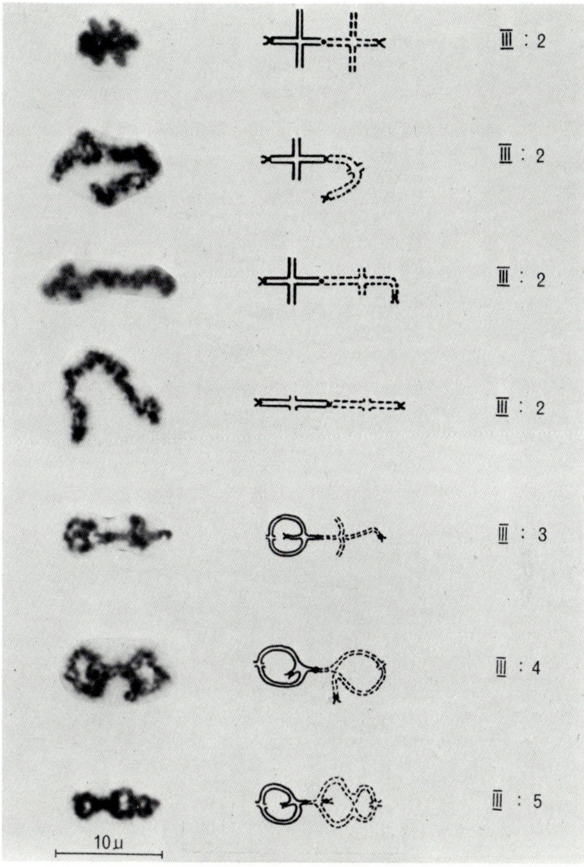

Fig. 6. Cut-out trivalents from primary spermatocytes of the D/D translocation heterozygote and suggested interpretations of the configurations observed.

carriers of D/D translocations suggest that only sperm which are balanced with regard to their D chromosomes are efficient at fertilization. Aneuploid offspring with the D trisomy syndrome are rare among D/D carriers and the frequency of spontaneous abortions in unions involving a D/D translocation carrier is no higher than the levels found for the population as a whole (21,22).

Hamerton (22) has suggested that preferential segregation at Anaphase I and selective fertilization of the egg by euploid sperm may both be factors which favour the production of balanced offspring. Another possibility is that eggs fertilized by aneuploid sperm are lost as preimplantation zygotes and therefore go undetected. Kjessler (12) has suggested that the reduction in numbers of sperm observed in his D/D translocation carrier reflects the elimination, during spermiogenesis, of unbalanced sperm and this may also account for the oligospermy observed in our D/D translocation carrier.

Multivalent associations at diakinesis of the type expected in carriers of a balanced translocation were also reported in two oligospermic males by McIlree et al. (15). The chromosomes involved in these cases could not however be identified in mitotic cells from peripheral blood. Both patients showed meiotic arrest in some cells between diakinesis and metaphase II. Meiotic arrest at this stage was also observed by McIlree et al. in an oligospermic male showing a ring 21/22 chromosome in mitotic cells from blood and skin (Fig. 7). Cells at diakinesis showed 22 bivalents, including the XY bivalent, plus two G group chromosomes which were present as univalents. In some cells the X and Y chromosomes were also present as univalents (Fig. 8), and many of the bivalents showed degenerative changes and a reduced number of chiasmata.

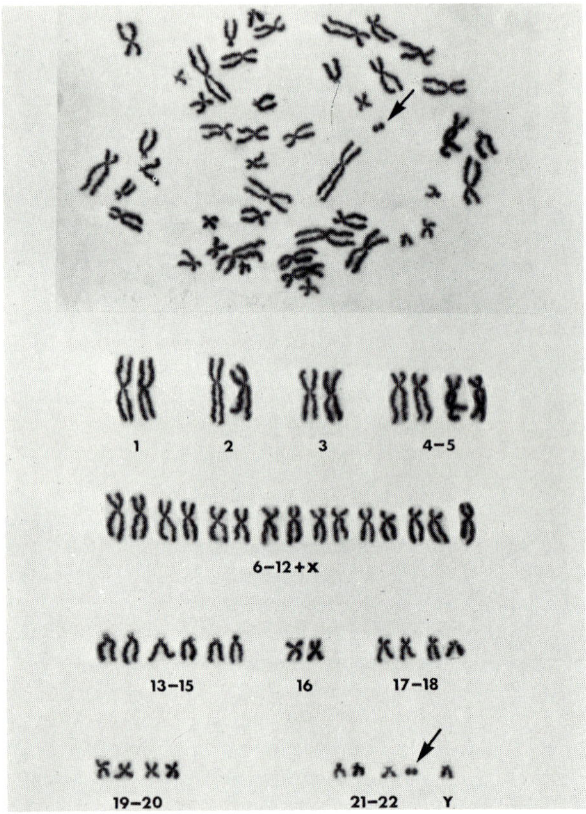

Fig. 7. Mitotic karyotype from an oligospermic male showing a ring chromosome replacing a Group 21-22 autosome. (From: McIlree et al. Lancet, Mar. 26, 679-682, 1966).

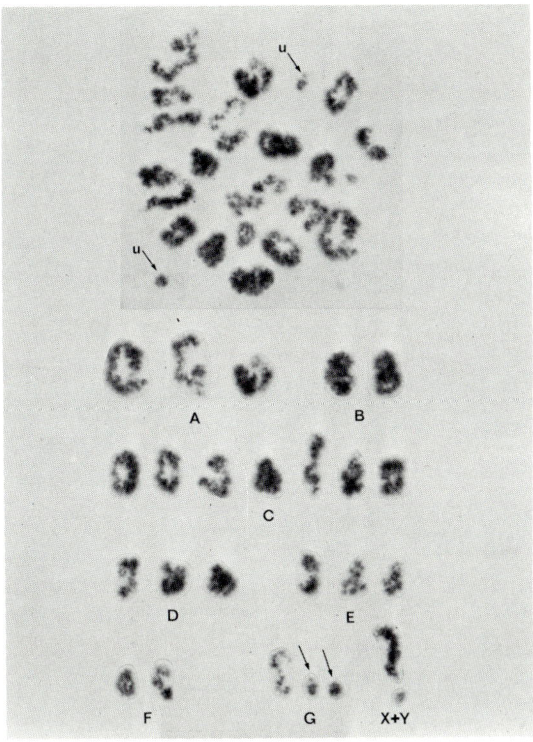

Fig. 8. Diakinesis and meiotic karyotype from the oligospermic male with a ring 21/22 chromosome in the blood, showing degenerative changes in the bivalents, very low numbers of chiasmata and two small chromosomes present as univalents. (From: McIlree et al. Lancet, Mar. 26, 679-682,1966)

McIlree has suggested that the failure to pair of the two homologues in this case may be due to one of these being a ring chromosome, and the pairing failure has led in some way to the development of degenerative changes in the chromosomes and the breakdown of spermatogenesis.

Structural Alterations of the Y Chromosome

Degenerative changes in the bivalents at diakinesis and meiotic arrest between diakinesis and metaphase II were also observed by McIlree et al. (15) in an azoospermic male showing a Y chromosome with a dicentric appearance in mitotic cells from peripheral blood (Fig. 9). The Y chromosome of the patient's father was normal. The blood of the patient also showed a 45, X cell line (14/100 cells) which may have some relevance to the finding of infertility. At

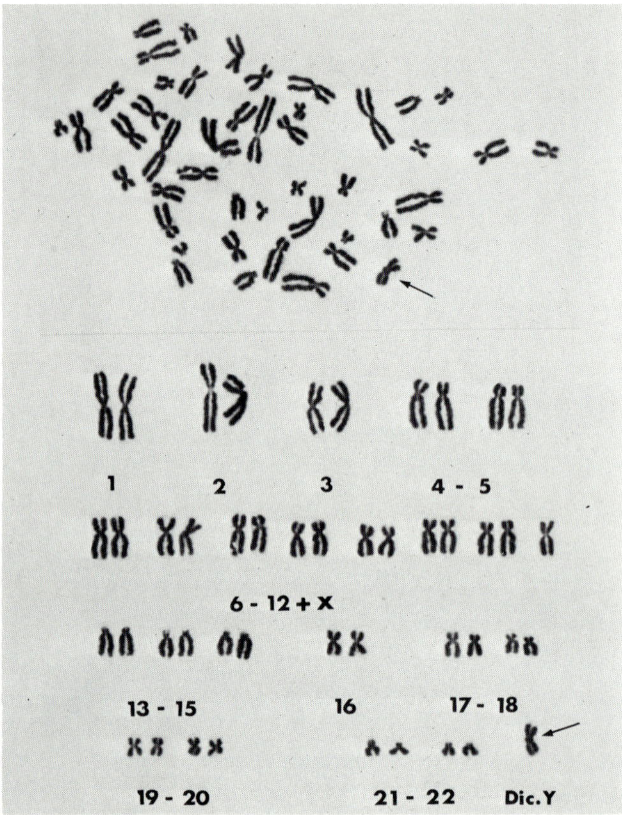

Fig. 9. Mitotic karyotype in an oligospermic male with a dicentric Y chromosome. (From: McIlree, M.E., et al. Lancet, 2: 69, 1966.)

diakinesis, the X and Y chromosomes were present as univalents in many cells and it is possible that here also, the failure to pair has led in some way to the degenerative changes and meiotic arrest observed.

Another structural alteration of the Y chromosome, possibly due to a pericentric inversion (23) was reported by McIlree et al. (15) in an oligospermic male who also showed a 45,X cell line in peripheral blood. The Y chromosome was a metacentric similar in size to a 19-20 group chromosome and was also found in the patient's father and all his male relatives. As none of the patient's male relatives were subfertile, it seems unlikely that the abnormality is related to the patient's subfertility. However, the patient was the only member of the family in whom a 45,X cell line was demonstrated and it may well be that this bears some relationship to his subfertility.

At diakinesis, primary spermatocytes from this patient showed a normal end-to-end association.

The study of meiosis in subfertile men is of great value both to the clinician in diagnosing the cause of the infertility and also in providing basic information on meiosis in the human male. However, it is still not possible to say with certainty whether any particular chromosome abnormality is a cause of infertility, although there is sometimes strong evidence that this may be so.

Further studies should, however, lead to a greater understanding of the processes involved and may eventually lead to a recognition that a specific group of abnormalities are associated with a particular chromosome aberration.

ACKNOWLEDGEMENT

The present investigations were carried out in collaboration with Dr. Melville Kerr and Mr. Peter Edmond of the Edinburgh Royal Infirmary who kindly supplied the biopsies and Dr. N. MacLean of the Department of Pathology, Western General Hospital, Edinburgh, who provided the pathological reports. The technical assistance of Mrs. Sheila Christie and Miss Judy Dennison is gratefully acknowledged.

REFERENCES

1. Menzies, J.I., Nature, 179: 1142, 1957.
2. Sinks, J., Anat. Rec., 121: 367, 1955.
3. Blakeslee, A.F., Yearbook Carnegie Institute (Washington), 27: 42, 1928.
4. Beadle, J.W., Cornell Univ. Agriculture Experiment Station Mem., 129: 1, 1930.
5. Sandler, L., Lindsley, D., Nicoletti, B. and Trippa, G., Genetics, 60: 525, 1968.
6. Donald, H.P. and Hancock, J.L., J. Agric. Sci., 43: 178, 1953.
7. Williams, W.W., J. Urology, 64: 614, 1950.
8. Kagan, C.A. and Kirov, S.M., Urologica, 28: 34, 1963.
9. Ross, A. and Kerr, M., Personal communication, 1969.
10. Pearson, P.L., Personal communication, 1969.
11. Ford, C.E. and Hamerton, J.L., Nature, (London), 178: 1020, 1956.
12. Kjessler, B., Monographs in Human Genetics, 2: Ed. Karger, S., Basel, 1966.
13. Ferguson-Smith, M.A., Lennox, B., Mack, W.S. and Stewart, J.S. S., Lancet, ii: 167, 1957.
14. Court Brown, W.M., Jacobs, P.A. and Brunton, M., Lancet ii: 561, 1965.
15. McIlree, M.E., Price, W.H., Court Brown, W.M., Selby Tulloch, W., Newsam, J.E. and MacLean, N., Lancet, ii 69, 1966.

16. Evans, E.P., Breckon, E. and Ford, C.E., Cytogenetics, 3: 289, 1964.
17. Smith, K.D., Steinberger, E., Steinberger, A. and Perloff, W. H., Cytogenetics, 4: 219, 1965.
18. Hulten, M., Lindsten, J., Fraccaro, M., Mannini, A., and Tiepolo, L., Lancet, ii: 22, 1966.
19. Armendares, S., Buentello, L., Cuevos-Sosa, A. and Cantu-Garza, J., Cytogenetics, 8: 177, 1969.
20. Mukerjee, D. and Burdette, W.J., Amer. J. Hum. Genet., 18: 62, 1966.
21. Walker, H. and Harris, R., Brit. Med. J., 2: 25, 1962.
22. Hamerton, J.L., Cytogenetics, 7: 260, 1968.
23. Jacobs, P.A. and Ross, A., Nature, (London), 210: 352, 1966.

DISCUSSION

LUNENFELD: In the last five years, quite a number of laboratories have become interested in studying mitosis and meiosis in testicular biopsies. Now I wonder whether you could speculate, based on available data today, what is the percentage of genetic factors in infertility?

CHANDLEY: By genetic factors, you mean gene mutation, the kind of case I was showing in the desynaptic male. Well, to my knowledge, this is the only one which has been found in human meiosis. Perhaps Dr. Ford or Dr. Ohno know of others?

OHNO: Speaking of this achiasmate mutant, I assume that he was a homozygote. It follows then that both parents are obligatory heterozygotes. I wonder if you looked at his father to see what the heterozygous condition was like.

CHANDLEY: I am not sure whether the parents were looked at but I do not think they were.

E. STEINBERGER: Dr. Chandley, you have shown a karyotype 46 plus extra metacentric chromosome in a patient with oligospermia. About 5 years ago we published a case almost identical to yours, and interestingly enough in our case the patient's mother had an identical karyotype. My question is, have you examined the parents of this patient? Since in our case the patient's mother has this extra chromosome and obviously was fertile, the presence of this extra chromosome cannot interfere with fertility, at least in the female. Could the oligospermia in this patient be simply coincidental to the cytogenetic finding? An as a follow-up to this question how many individuals with perfectly normal sperm count and fertility did you examine and look for abnormalities in the meiotic metaphase?

CHANDLEY: In reply to the first question, as far as I can recall, neither of the parents of this patient have been examined, but as

I said, the brother of the patient showed it. Now whether this has any relationship to the infertility is certainly not clear at all, because there have been reports of supernumary chromosomes in a variety of patients who have been perfectly normal and others who showed a variety of pathological conditions.

E. STEINBERGER: Was the brother oligospermic?

CHANDLEY: Yes, the brother was also oligospermic, but we have not yet taken a testicular biopsy; in fact, he would not allow us to do so.

PAULSEN: Sergovich from Toronto has published a survey which indicates that D/D translocation is one of the most common chromosomal abnormalities, appearing in one-tenth percent of the general population. Thus, it is important for us who are not geneticists to understand the relationship or relevance of D/D translocation to the pathogenesis of oligospermia. We recently studied a patient with oligospermia. His sperm count ranged from three to fifteen million/ml. His serum and urinary FSH levels were normal. In his testis we found D/D 13-15 translocation in mitotic and meiotic chromosomes. Histologically the testis revealed a decrease in numbers of late pachytene spermatocytes and spermatids. I would assume from what has been said that this represents an unbalanced chromosomal abnormality which has led to a loss of germ cells during meiosis. Would this be a correct interpretation?

CHANDLEY: Kjessler suggested in his D/D translocation that the oligospermia which he detected was in fact due to the loss of the unbalanced sperm in spermiogenesis, but whether this is so, we do not know. Dr. Ford would argue that unbalanced sperm are perfectly capable of fertilizing eggs but they may then cause a breakdown in the zygote. Perhaps Dr. Ford would like to comment at this point.

FORD: For 15 years or so I have been testing all information that came my way for the possibility that unbalanced sperm were not capable of functioning in fertilization and I have not encountered any contrary information. Now the fact that I have never encountered any does not exclude the possibility that in certain circumstances if may occur. The next point I would like to make is that Robertsonian translocations, like the human D/D translocations, would appear to have played a major part in karyotype evolution of the mammals. Indeed there are several species in which there is a balanced polymorphic system involving translocations of that form. A common shrew in Europe, for example, may be heterozygous for as many as four of these changes at one time and such individuals must obviously have a nearly normal fertility or the selection pressure operating against them would be enormous. Now this is not to deny the information from our own species. I would appear to be a matter of what specific genetic material is involved and what the nature of the genetic lesion is.

ROSS: Is it not true that the male may be the carrier of these D/D translocations, transmitting them to his progeny? If this is true then certainly not all spermatozoa containing the abnormal chromosomes can be eliminated.

CHANDLEY: Well, transmitting the translocation to his progeny does not mean that the progeny are unbalanced. If the progeny are carrying the translocations, then they themselves are balanced. Is that what you meant?

ROSS: No, the sperm necessarily must have carried the translocated chromosomes, if he transmitted it to his offspring.

CHANDLEY: But in a balanced form. If the offspring is a carrier himself, this is a balanced condition. The offspring of D/D translocations occur in the ratio of 1:1 normal to balanced, in those few cases in which offsprings have been shown. In fact, very few carriers of D/D translocations have been shown to have live offspring.

JIRASEK: I would like to refer to the pairing between X and Y chromosomes. In the karyotypes it seemed to me that X and Y chromosomes were paired end to end.

CHANDLEY: From a meiotic preparation, it really is not possible to say exactly what the nature of the X-Y pairing is. If you want to know whether you can see a chiasma configuration or anything like that, you certainly can not.

SOLARI: I think that from light microscopic evidence, we cannot be certain about the existence of a chiasma between the X and the Y. But from our electron microscopic studies, we can say that there is strong evidence for normal, partial synapsis between the X and Y chromosomes, in the rat, in the mouse and in the human. If there is a chiasma, this is now an open question to be really proved with strong evidence which I think will be provided very soon.

BERGADA: I just want to emphasize what Dr. Chandley said about the incidence of chromatin positivity in man. In an article published in Acta Helvetica Paediatrica last year, we indicated that one in every 80 boys with cryptorchidism is chromatin positive; and this is really a very high incidence. Furthermore, in a recent survey performed in Buenos Aires during medical examination of candidates for military service, approximately one in every 500 normal men was chromatin-positive. So this is something that we have to bear in mind when we study the infertile patient.

CHANDLEY: I should like to present two more cases worthy of note. The first was a 37-year-old male who presented at the subfertility clinic and who was found, on a semen analysis, to be completely azoospermic. His mitotic karyotype showed no obvious abnormality. His testicular histology showed numerous dividing cells but a deficiency of spermatids and a complete absence of mature sperm.

Meiotic investigations, however, revealed that he was the carrier of a balanced translocation between a C group chromosome and either an E or an F group chromosome (since E and F bivalents often appear alike in size in meiotic preparations it was difficult to reach a decision on this point).

An examination of 35 spermatocytes at diakinesis showed that 21 normal bivalents, including the XY bivalent, plus a quadrivalent, were present in the majority of cells. Few 2nd metaphases were observed, and it seemed that meiotic arrest was occurring in most cells after diakinesis.

The second case was a 39-year-old azoospermic male who was found to be the carrier of a reciprocal translocation between a C and a G group chromosome. His mitotic karyotype, and that of his mother showed 46 chromosomes including three normal G chromosomes and an abnormal chromosome about the size of a G group chromosome. His testicular histology showed that the tubules contained a high proportion of dividing cells, but in most tubules, the end stages of spermiogenesis were deficient, and few mature sperm could be seen .

Meiotic studies revealed that the majority of spermatocytes at diakinesis had 21 normal bivalents, including the XY bivalent, and either a quadrivalent, which was in the form of a long chain, or a trivalent plus a univalent. Chiasma counts were made on 20 diakineses and showed a mean chiasma frequency of 41.5 compared with a frequency of 50-55 for normal males. The breakdown of meiosis and azoospermia in these two patients is undoubtedly related to the presence of the translocations.

CHAPTER IV

REGULATION OF TESTICULAR FUNCTION

SECTION 1: ROLE OF THE HYPOTHALAMUS

MECHANISM OF ACTION OF FSH AND LH RELEASING FACTORS

Irving I. Geschwind

Department of Animal Science

University of California, Davis

The mechanism of action of the hypothalamic releasing factors has been a subject of intense study during the past three years. For such studies, either crude hypothalamic or stalk-median eminence extracts or more purified releasing factors have been employed. Pure releasing factors for the pituitary gonadotropins, FSH and LH, in which we are interested, have not as yet been isolated, and indeed there is some question whether separate releasing factors exist (see, for example, White [1]).

Initially, the approach to the study of mechanism of action reflected contemporary involvement with inhibitors of peptide bond synthesis or of DNA-dependent RNA synthesis. The particular parameter investigated was gonadotropin release. Subsequently, limited explorations were made of the metabolic or energetic requirements for hormone release, but by far the greatest effort in this area has gone into investigations of the roles which various cations play in the process. The other major parameter which has been the subject of experimentation is gonadotropin synthesis. Whereas the isolated rat pituitary incubated for a few hours in appropriate medium has been the substrate of choice for demonstrating modifications of gonadotropic hormone release, longer term incubations and organ culture of the pituitary have been widely employed for studies of the control of pituitary hormone synthesis. In order to demonstrate hormone release, a specific assay for the gonadotropin in question must be employed. Generally, bioassays have been used, but more recently immunoassays have come to the fore and are increasingly replacing bioassays due to the considerable advantages of the former. Immunological techniques are also employed in the study of hormone synthesis, with specific antibodies being used to selectively precipitate the desired hormone after a gland has been incubated in the presence of a radioactive amino acid or monosaccharide (the gonadotropins are glycoproteins). However, most of the evidence purportedly demonstrating de novo synthesis of hormonal protein has been acquired by bioassay of the total amounts of hormone in experimental and control systems (gland plus incubation medium). When the amount of hormone in the experimental system significantly exceeds that present originally in the gland or in the control system, de novo synthesis has been assumed. The limitations of these assumptions will be discussed below.

The purpose of this paper is to present a review of our knowledge of the mechanism of action of LH- and FSH-releasing factor(s). Much of the information has already been analyzed and compared with what is known of the mechanism of action of the other hypothalamic hypophysiotropic factors and of secretagogues for other endocrine and exocrine glands (2,3). The comparisons effected have stressed the details of the release process. In this paper greater attention will be given to the synthetic process.

For reasons of economy no references will be given for studies of non-gonadotropic hormones or proteins which have been previously reviewed. The reader is referred to two reviews (2,3) for the appropriate references to the original literature.

HORMONE RELEASE

It is now accepted that a primary action of the hypophysiotropic factors is modification of release of anterior pituitary and intermediate lobe hormones. There is also general agreement that the modification imposed on the release of gonadotropins is a stimulatory one, as is evident from the increases in circulating gonadotropins found in man and other animals after administration of the factors, and from the increases in the amounts of hormone released into the medium upon incubation of pituitary glands in the presence of the factors. The mechanics of the release process have not been elucidated specifically for the gonadotropins, but there is no reason to believe that they differ from what has been described for other proteins in involving a process of reverse pinocytosis, emiocytosis. The most recent studies of this process are those of Amsterdam et al. (4) on the secretory cycle of the rat parotid gland. Only a limited number of ultrastructural studies of releasing factor action have been reported, and all have been restricted to the action of the growth hormone releasing factor.

The Role of De Novo Protein and RNA Synthesis in the Release Process.

A number of studies have been carried out in which the effects on the release process of the administration of puromycin, an inhibitor of protein synthesis, or actinomycin D, an inhibitor of DNA-dependent RNA synthesis, have been determined (Table 1). When

Table 1. Dependence of In Vitro Releasing Factor-Stimulated Pituitary Gonadotropin Release on Continuing Protein or RNA Synthesis in the Rat Anterior Pituitary

Hormone Released	Inhibitor	Effect on Release	Reference
1. LH	Puromycin (100)*	46% Normal	(5)
	" (200)	Normal	(6)
	" (80)	"	(7)
	Actinomycin D (10)	"	(5)
	" " (80)	"	(7)
	" " (1-2)**	"	(8)
2. FSH	Puromycin (100)	61% Normal	(9)
	" (10)	Prevented	(10)
	Actinomycin D (10)	79% Normal	(9)
	" " (2)	"No block"	(11)
	" " (10)	Prevented	(10)
	" " (1)**	Unaffected	(11)

*Concentration expressed as μg per ml medium. ** In vivo, rather than in vitro. Dose expressed as μg per g body weight.

no effects of inhibitor administration are to be found, one can state with reasonable certainty that continuing protein or RNA synthesis is not required for the release process. When modification of release does occur in the presence of inhibitor one must consider the possibility that the inhibitor is not restricted in its action to the process being studied. Nevertheless, because most of the experiments reported are for the in vitro situation, and because the experiments with LH and FSH, although frequently performed under essentially similar conditions, lead to different results, the results of the experiments can be accepted as consequences of the effects which the inhibitors have on the two synthetic processes. LH release from pituitaries incubated with hypothalamic extract or purified LRF plus an inhibitor is obviously not affected by the inhibitors, and similar results have been found for TSH release. On the other hand, FSH release is extensively, if not completely inhibited. In a kinetic study Jutisz and de la Llosa have demonstrated that in the presence of cycloheximide, an inhibitor of protein synthesis, FSH release is essentially normal for the first half hour, and thereafter little release takes place (12). A similar partial inhibition has been seen in studies of antibody and of insulin release. It would seem most reasonable to assume that the continuing protein synthesis required for release of FSH, as for these other two non-pituitary proteins, involves synthesis of the secreted proteins. If indeed FSH synthesis is required, the fact that the considerable amount of preformed or storage hormone present in the gland could not be released would indicate that this latter hormone is not part of a readily-releasable pool, but instead turns over much more slowly than hormone that can be released. It is not apparent, however, why the control of FSH release should differ from that of LH release in this important aspect.

The Role of Metabolic Energy in the Release Process

Earlier experiments (2,3) carried out on the release of several proteins, especially enzymes from exocrine glands, had suggested that inhibitors of oxidative phosphorylation inhibit release. However, more recently it has been reported that in catecholamine release from perfused bovine (13) and cat (14) adrenals either glycolysis or oxidative phosphorylation could supply the energy required for release. Both processes had to be inhibited to prevent release of the hormone in response to stimulation, and carbamyl - choline-induced chymotrypsinogen release from the incubated rat pancreas was unaffected by the presence of 8 μg/ml oligomycin, an inhibitor of oxidative phosphorylation (15). Only a single study has been reported on the effect of metabolic inhibitors on release of LH, as stimulated by crude hypothalamic extract (16). Neither 2×10^{-4}M dinitrophenol nor 1×10^{-3}M cyanide affected release, whereas 0.1 μg/ml of oligomycin produced a partial inhibition. An inhibitory effect of oligomycin has also been observed by others studying TSH release, but the reported effects of dinitrophenol on TSH release have been variable. Insensitivity of the release process to the presence of cyanide has also been found for TSH, as well as for catecholamines (13,14). In all other systems investigated, however, both dinitrophenol and cyanide have been found to inhibit release, and we have no idea why the process in the pituitary should be so different in its sensitivity to these inhibitors.

A partial list of those sites in the release process which may be energy-dependent is found in Table 2. The background for each of these suggestions has been given elsewhere (3), and I would like to add some information about two points only now. One is that although others had found that ATP itself promoted release of catecholamines, vasopressin, and oxytocin from their respective isolated secretory granules, it has failed to promote insulin release from isolated β -cell granules (17). The other concerns adenyl cyclase and its product 3', 5'-cyclic adenylic acid (cAMP). The latter, and its derivative 0', N-dibutyryl cyclic AMP (DBC), have been demonstrated to promote the release of parotid and pancreatic amylases, insulin, growth hormone, TSH, and ACTH. Moreover, TRF had been shown to elevate pituitary cAMP levels. Although none of these early (i.e., 1 to 3 years old) reports dealt with gonadotropins, there was no reason to believe that what had been found for the other pituitary hormones would not apply to the gonadotropins as well.

Table 2. Steps in the Release Process Which May be Energy-Dependent.*

1. De novo protein synthesis, when required (e.g., for FSH release).

2. Protein transport between rough endoplasmic reticulum and Golgi complex.

3. Fission-fusion of cell and granule membranes.

4. Modification of cell membrane structure, brought about by a phospholipase upon activation of the latter.

5. Conformational change in cell membrane promoted by the interaction of ATP and membrane-bound ATPase.

6. Postulated microtubular, microfilamentous system, which links secretion granules to the cell membrane and which upon contraction promotes fusion of the granule and cell membranes.

7. Membrane-associated adenyl cyclase.

*The reader is referred to ref. 3 for a more extended discussion of each of these suggestions.

Within the past year we have seen reports that both cAMP and DBC stimulate FSH release from the isolated rat pituitary (18), that theophylline, an inhibitor of the phosphodiesterase which hydrolyzes cAMP, while ineffective by itself at a 2.5 mM concentration, did potentiate the effect of FSH-RF on release (18), and that a hypothalamic extract which promoted a 3-fold increase in LH release during a 6-hour incubation of rat anterior pituitary glands, concomitantly stimulated a two-fold increase in cAMP and adenyl cyclase levels in the gland (19). Such extracts were specific for the anterior pituitary, and the increases in cAMP levels could be observed within three minutes of incubation of the glands and increased with the duration of incubation. Moreover, the effect of extract on adenyl cyclase levels was already marked one minute after its addition to pituitary homogenates (19). These latter results of course do not prove a cause-effect relationship between elevated cAMP levels and LH release, since a crude hypothalamic extract and entire anterior pituitary glands were employed. Nevertheless, the results are consistent with the developing hypothesis that the releasing factors stimulate adenyl cyclase activity, and the cAMP formed thereby acts as a "second messenger" for release. Similar increases in incubated pituitary adenyl cyclase and cAMP levels have been reported after addition of a stalk-median eminence extract which stimulated TSH and growth hormone secretion (20). In these experiments the extract was shown to have no effect on phosphodiesterase activity.

Finally, it should be emphasized that if this is an energy-requiring step in the release process, it is not the only one, for dinitrophenol can block the exogenous cAMP-induced release of parotid amylase.

The Role of Cations in the Release Process

We are all indebted to Douglas for the initiation of studies on the part cations play in the release process. The many experiments which he and his co-workers performed on the release of catecholamines and of vasopressin established the following: Elevated $[K^+]$ itself induces release, with an optimum $[K^+]$ reached at between 10 and 15 times the normal medium concentration, and for that release and for specific secretagogue-stimulated release Ca^{++} is required: in the presence of normal concentrations of the latter, Mg^{++} in elevated concentrations acts as an inhibitor of release, but the antagonism can be reversed by elevating the $[Ca^{++}]$: the response to a secretagogue increases with $[Ca^{++}]$ up to a certain optimum concentration of the latter; and depolarization of cell membranes by secretagogues is not a sufficient stimulus for the extrusion process. A theory of "stimulus-secretion coupling" was advanced. The theory, which has found many advocates, postulates that a secretagogue modifies the cell membrane so as to make it more permeable to Ca^{++} and Na^+ , thereby leading to the depolarization, but it is the entry of Ca^{++} which triggers the release process.

Limited studies of the anterior pituitary have established that elevated $[K^+]$ stimulates release of LH, FSH, TSH, ACTH, and growth hormone; that for LH a five-fold increase in $[K^+]$ does not stimulate release (22), but that for both LH and FSH an optimum effect is found with 60 mM K^+; that the high $[K^+]$ effect is additive with the effects of releasing factors on gonadotropin release (12,16,22); that in the absence of Ca^{++}, both high $[K^+]$- and releasing factor-induced release of LH and FSH are inhibited; and that elevated $[Mg^{++}]$ also inhibits release of the gonadotropins (Table 3). Table 3 also records the effects of the absence of Na^+, K^+, or Mg^{++} from the medium. Except for the lack of an effect of Mg^{++}-deficiency, which is consistent with what has been found for other secretory processes, it is difficult to comment on the effects produced by deficiencies of the other two cations, since 0 mM K^+ has been found to stimulate insulin and catecholamine release, and to inhibit parotid amylase release, while a Na^+-free medium has been found to inhibit insulin release, and by one group of investigators, catecholamine release (26), while another group has found it to potentiate catecholamine release.

The theory of "stimulus-secretion coupling" does not account for the varied effects of Na^+ and K^+ deficiency or for the site of action of Ca^{++}, nor does it concern itself with the activation of adenyl cyclase by secretagogues, or with the release-inducing effects of cAMP and theophylline. The effect of elevated $[K^+]$ can best be attributed to depolarization of the cell membranes, although it is possible that it could act indirectly since high $[K^+]$-induced increases in cAMP concentrations have been reported

Table 3. Effects of Cations on Pituitary Gonadotropin Release From the Incubated Rat Anterior Pituitary.

Hormone Released	Stimulation	Inhibition*	Normal
1. LH	60 mM K^+ (16,21,22)	0 mM Ca^{++} (16,22,23)	
		20 mM Mg^{++} (22)	0 mM Mg^{++} (22)**
2. FSH	50-60 mM K^+ (12,22)	0 mM K^+ (24)	
	0 mM Na^+ (22)	0 mM Ca^{++} (22,25)	
		20 mM Mg^{++} (22)	

*Inhibition of releasing factor and/or high $[K^+]$-induced release.
**Effect on high $[K^+]$ and releasing factor-induced release.

in non-pituitary tissues. Zor and his co-workers (27) have found, however, that 10-fold $[K^+]$ did not stimulate an increase in anterior pituitary cAMP levels in their experiments.

The relationship between adenyl cyclase - cAMP levels and $[Ca^{++}]$ may be quite complex, and recent reports would indicate a variable effect of Ca^{++} or its deprivation on adenyl cyclase activitiesin different tissues. It is known, however, that high $[K^+]$- or epinephrine-provoked increases in cAMP levels in the parotid gland, and hypothalamic- (20) or stalk-medium eminence-induced (27) increases in pituitary adenyl cyclase or cAMP levels are unaffected by the absence of Ca^{++} from the medium. The absence of Ca^{++}, however, is sufficient to prevent endogenous cAMP from promoting protein release, as well as to inhibit completely the effect of exogenous cAMP on FSH release (25). Thus, Ca^{++} is apparently not needed for cyclase function, and increased intracellular cAMP concentrations are not, of themselves, sufficient stimulus for release.

The exact function of Ca^{++} is unknown, and any suggestion offered should take into account the reported stoichiometry between release and $[Ca^{++}]$ at suboptimal concentrations of the latter. Table 4 lists a number of possibilities for the action of Ca^{++}. The bases for each of these suggestions, other than the last, are to be found elsewhere (3). The last is considered in the paragraph which follows.

The mode of action of cAMP is also clothed in mystery. I have suggested in Table 4 an effect of Ca^{++} on a protein kinase, and one may visualize a kinase which may be activated either by Ca^{++} or by Ca^{++} and cAMP. Kuo and Greengard have suggested that a wide variety of cAMP effects may be mediated by stimulation of protein kinases (28). Certainly if some stimuli for secretion

Table 4. Possible Modes of Action of Ca^{++}*

1. Promotion of the dissociation of a hormone-carrier protein complex.

2. Production of a conformational change in the macromolecules of the granule and/or plasma membranes, perhaps by bridging between neighboring negatively-charged groups in the membranes, resulting in a change in membrane reactivity.

3. Activation of a phospholipase, which by modifying membrane lipids alters membrane reactivity.

4. Promotion of the adhesion of the granule to the cell membrane, either by divalent bridging (see 2 above) or by enhancing the solvation of a component of the granule membrane in the lipid phase of the plasma membrane.

5. Alteration of the colloidal state of the cytosol, so as to promote granule movement.

6. Relief of the inhibition of an ATPase, thus promoting contraction of the postulated actomyosin-like microfilaments linking the granules to the cell membrane.

7. Activation of a protein kinase, which by phosphorylating a membrane protein either activates an enzyme or produces a conformational change in a structural protein. The net result of either is an altered membrane reactivity or an induced capability of membranes for fusion.

*The reader is referred to ref. 3 for a more extended discussion of most of these suggestions.

do not provoke an increase in adenyl cyclase activity and if cAMP does not stimulate release in the absence of Ca^{++}, some independent effect of Ca^{++} must be postulated which must be distal to the production of cAMP, and yet also involve available cAMP.

HORMONE SYNTHESIS

The methods employed to determine whether hypophysiotropic factors affect the synthesis of the pituitary hormones whose release they promote have been mentioned above. The method of demonstrating synthesis by an increase in the total amount of hormone in a system has been the one most extensively employed, but it has been criticized because too often the increments have been so small as to tax the precision of the bioassays used. Occasionally, as is reported below, large differences have been found, but then generally no proof has been offered which would eliminate activation of a prohormone or inhibition of an intracellular hydrolytic system as the cause of the increase. The more direct method of quantitating protein or glycoprotein synthesis, by measuring the incorporation of a radioactive amino acid or monosaccharide into the macromolecule, also has its limitations: conditions for protein synthesis in vitro must be optimal, the intracellular pools of the amino acid or monosaccharide must be unchanging, and adequate methods must be available for resolving the macromolecule from any rapidly labelled contaminants.

The evidence for stimulation of synthesis by the gonadotropin releasing factors is given below.

1. In 13 of 17 female rats bearing pituitary autografts beneath the kidney capsule for 5 to 96 days prior to continuous perfusion of the graft with hypothalamic extract for an additional 6 to 38 days, the presence of PAS-positive cells was noted in the grafts. Eleven of the 13 rats were also found to have large follicles in their ovaries, and in 9 of these 11 vaginal estrus occurred durring the infusion period (29). Since such grafts are inactive and probably contained little hormone at the onset of the infusion, synthesis of sufficient quantities of hormones to produce the observed effects must be assumed.

2. When normal female rat anterior pituitary is maintained in organ culture, the addition of hypothalamic extract produces an increase of the ovarian ascorbic acid depleting activity of the culture and an increase in the uptake of tritiated leucine by the PAS-positive cells of the pituitary (30).

3. Incubation of pituitaries derived from castrated, estradiol-progesterone treated rats for two hours with an LRF preparation, led to a sometimes significant increase in the total LH of the system (23,31).

4. In preliminary studies, an increase in total immunoassayable LH has been found only after incubation of rat pituitary halves with hypothalamic extract (32).

5. Organ culture of normal female rat pituitaries for a period of three days in the presence of highly purified preparations of LRF led to a mean increase of 20% in the total LH content of the system as determined by radioimmunoassay. The greatest increases, 34% and 67%,were produced by the highest concentrations of LRF (33).

All of the above evidence supports a stimulatory role of releasing factors on LH synthesis.

6. However, the incorporation of radioactive leucine or glucosamine into LH was not increased above control values during 4-hour incubations of pituitaries from ovariectomized rats, some of which were pretreated with estradiol-progesterone, or during 6-or 24-hour incubations of pituitaries from normal rats, or during 6-hour incubations of pituitaries from testosterone-treated rats, all in the presence of hypothalamic or stalk-median eminence extracts or crude LRF (6,34).

It should be noted that investigators using both total hormone and radioactive amino acid incorporation methods are in agreement that high $[K^+]$ does not stimulate the rate of LH synthesis (16,23,35), although it has been claimed that by the criterion of the former method FSH synthesis is increased (12).

The data on FSH are far more varied and interesting.

7. In 2 or 4 hour incubations, with a crude FSH-RF, of pituitaries from normal male rats or ovariectomized rats pretreated with estradiol-progesterone, the total amount of FSH in the system increased by 16 to 40% (9,12,25). The increase in the total FSH activity was found to be Ca^{++}-dependent (25), whereas others had previously claimed that the incorporation of radioactive leucine into LH was Ca^{++}-independent (16). Rather interestingly the authors (25) state "that synthesis of FSH or activation of a precursor of FSH may take place in the presence of FRF", although in an earlier publication (12) they had stated that since FRF had no effect on homogenates it could not be activating a precursor.

8. Under conditions identical with those given in 5 above, the presence of an LRF stimulated a mean increase in total immunoassayable FSH of 106% (33).

9. Rat stalk-median eminence extract injected intrajugularly into intact mature male rats 45 minutes after an initial dose of the extract, at a time when depletion of pituitary FSH was maximum, stimulated the reaccumulation of pituitary FSH, so that within two hours the pituitary FSH content was more than 30% greater than the initial, pre-injection levels (36). Moreover, in mature male rats with median eminence lesions placed seven days earlier, in which the pituitary FSH concentration is about 65% of normal, injections of such extracts produce a 75% increase in pituitary FSH concentration 45 minutes later (37), and a log dose-response relationship for such "FSH-synthesizing factor" activity has been obtained (38). Corbin has stated that "the hypothalamus controls both the synthesis and release of FSH and whether or not synthesis or release of FSH occurs appears to depend on the initial level of FSH in the pituitary" (38).

Corbin's findings are especially interesting, particularly if the reported increases in pituitary FSH levels do indeed represent synthesis of the hormone, for the question of the control of protein synthesis by the hypothalamic factors has been particularly vexing. Although the bioassay evidence clearly indicates increases in total system hormone for many of the pituitary hormones when glands are incubated, or preferably cultured, in the presence of crude or purified releasing factors, incorporation studies have failed to support such claims, with a possible exception in the case of ACTH. Such a discrepancy could result from any of the previously mentioned shortcomings of the two methods of analysis.

If it is assumed that synthesis is indeed stimulated, then one may ask whether the effect is a primary one, or whether it is secondary to release. Although either release or synthesis can be uniquely inhibited (e.g., for LH by Ca^{++}-deprivation or by puromycin, respectively [16]), there is no clear-cut evidence available from studies on pituitary hormones to indicate whether an increase in the rate of synthesis may be tied to release. Corbin's findings suggest that it may not. From studies on insulin secretion in in vitro or perfused systems, there is evidence that substances such as ribose, xylitol, and tolbutamide may promote release without enhancing synthetic rates (39), so that there need not be any link between the two processes. Recently, Grand and Gross (40) have attempted to resolve the question by studying the effect of epinephrine, a secretagogue for amylase release from the parotid gland, on amylase synthesis. In slices of the gland, epinephrine produces more than a two-fold increase in the incorporation of radioactive amino acids into amylase during the period of active enzyme extrusion into the medium. Subsequently, the rate of protein synthesis declines as enzyme release returns to near its original rate, and if epinephrine is again added during this period, the rate of incorporation again doubles, but at this point there is no change in the rate of amylase secretion.

Samli and Geschwind(6) originally raised the possibility that the release process itself, as stimulated by a releasing factor, could lead to feedback mechanisms allowing the synthesis of additional pituitary hormone, a view also espoused by others (e.g., 23), and more recently I have suggested (2,3) that cAMP may serve to link release and synthesis. This could be accomplished if cAMP has a direct, independent effect on both processes; if activation of cell membrane-associated adenyl cyclase causes a Ca^{++}-dependent change in membrane activity, while the cAMP formed stimulates protein synthesis; or if cAMP in some fashion affects the cytostructure, the alteration of which then leads independently to both secretion and synthesis. Much of the evidence supporting a role of cAMP in selected protein biosynthesis, especially in microorganisms, has been reviewed (3). To that evidence we may add the following additional support derived from experiments in higher organisms: cAMP stimulates the protein synthetic capacity of thyroid polysomes and monosomes in vitro (41); cAMP and DBC induce tyrosine transaminase in explants of fetal rat liver maintained in organ culture, the induction process being inhibited by cycloheximide (42); and DBC stimulates the incorporation of amino acids into parotid amylase at the same time that it provokes release of the enzyme (40). Directly pertinent to our considerations is the report that when pituitaries are incubated for 4 hours in the presence of cAMP, the total FSH activity of the system increases by about 35% (23).

These considerations suggest as a working hypothesis that a secretagogue stimulates both processes by primarily activating cell membrane-associated adenyl cyclase. The hypothesis, in the form presented in the paragraph above, could account for both Corbin's and Grand and Gross' results if the following stipulations are accepted: when release is occurring from a pituitary in which the initial level of FSH is high, synthesis is taking place simultaneously, as the inhibitor studies would suggest; and in a cell (parotid or pituitary) from which most of the readily-releasable products have been discharged (e.g., amylase or FSH), neither cell membrane nor cytostructure alteration nor cAMP itself can promote much further release of product, but protein synthesis is still capable of being stimulated. The hypothesis, however, must allow for secretion to occur by more than a single process, in order to accomodate, for example, the finding that compounds such as ribose and tolbutamide can only stimulate insulin release and not its synthesis. Furthermore, it appears that at times the cAMP effects can be mimicked by high $[K^+]$, (e.g., the reported increases in FSH synthesis and release), although both the failure of high $[K^+]$ to promote increases in adenyl cyclase and cAMP levels in the pituitary, and the additive effect on release of high $[K^+]$ and LRF or FSH-RF, would suggest that elevated $[K^+]$ and the releasing factors are not operating through the same mechanism, i.e., activation of adenyl cyclase.

ACKNOWLEDGMENTS

The research from my laboratory which is reported in this review was supported by USPHS Research Grant HD-00394.

I am indebted to Drs. Alan Corbin, Marian Jutisz, S.M. McCann, Andrew V. Schally, and Wilfrid F. White for their kindness in making findings from their laboratories available to me prior to publication.

REFERENCES

1. White, W.F. In Workshop Conference on the Bioassay and Chemistry of the Hypophysiotropic Hormones of the Hypothalamus, ed. Meites, J., Williams and Wilkins, in press, 1970.
2. Geschwind, I.I. In Frontiers in Neuroendocrinology, 1969 eds. Ganong, W.F. and Martini, L., Oxford University Press p. 389, 1969.
3. Geschwind, I.I. In Workshop Conference on the Bioassay and Chemistry of the Hypophysiotropic Hormones of the Hypothalamus, ed. Meites, J., Williams and Wilkins, in press, 1970.
4. Amsterdam, A., Ohad, I., and Schramm, M., J.Cell Biol., 41: 753, 1969.
5. Jutisz, M., Berault, A., Novella, M.A., and Chapeville, F. C. R. Acad. Sci. (Paris), 263: 664, 1966.
6. Samli, M., and Geschwind, I.I. Endocrinology, 81: 835, 1967.
7. Crighton, D.B., Watanabe, S., Dhariwal, A.P.S., and McCann, S.M. Proc. Soc. Exp. Biol. Med., 128: 537, 1968.
8. Schally, A.V., Bowers, C.Y., Carter, W.H., Arimura, A., Redding, T.W., and Saito, M. Endocrinology, 85: 290, 1969.

9. Jutisz, M., and de la Llosa, M.P. Endocrinology 81: 1193, 1967.
10. Watanabe, S., Dhariwal, A.P., and McCann, S.M. Endocrinology, 82: 674, 1968.
11. Schally, A.W., Saito, T., Arimura, A., Sawano, S., Bowers, C.Y., White, W.F., and Cohen, A.I. Endocrinology, 81: 882 1967.
12. Jutisz, M., and de la Llosa, M.P. Bull. Soc. Chim. Biol., 50: 2521, 1968.
13. Kirshner, N., and Smith, W.J. Life Sci.,8: 799, 1969.
14. Rubin, R.P. J. Physiol., 202: 197, 1969.
15. Bauduin, H., Colin, M., and Dumont, J.E. Biochim. Biophys. Acta, 174: 722, 1969.
16. Samli, M., and Geschwind, I.I. Endocrinology, 82: 225, 1968.
17. Howell, S.L., Young, D.A., and Lacy, P.E. J. Cell Biol., 41: 167, 1969.
18. Jutisz, M., and de la Llosa, M.P. C. R. Acad. Sci. (Paris), 268: 1636, 1969.
19. Zor, U., Kaneko, T., Schneider, H.P.G., McCann, S.M., Lowe, I.P., Bloom, G., Borland, B., and field, J.B. Proc. Nat. Acad. Sci. USA, 63: 918, 1969.
20. Steiner, A.L., Peake, G.T., Utigar, R., and Kipnis, D. J. Clin. Invest., 48: 80a, 1969.
21. Vale, W., and Guillemin, R. Experientia,23: 855, 1967.
22. Wakabayashi, K., Kamberi, I.A., and McCann, S.M. Endocrinology, 85: 1046, 1969.
23. Jutisz, M., de la Llosa, M.P., Berault, A., and Kerdelhue, B. Proceedings of the "Colloque de Neuroendocrinologie" of the C.N.R.S. (Paris), in press.
24. Jutisz, M., and de la Llosa, M.P. Excerpta Medica International Congress Series, 157: 137, 1968.
25. Jutisz,M., and de la Llosa, M.P. Endocrinology, in press, 1970.
26. Banks, P., Biggins, R., Bishop, R., Christian, B., and Currie, N. J. Physiol., 200: 797, 1969.
27. Zor, U., Kaneko, T., Schneider, H.P.G., McCann, S.M., and Field, J.B. J. Clin. Invest., 48: 93a, 1969.
28. Kuo, J.F., and Greengard, P. J. Biol. Chem. 244: 3417, 1969.
29. Evans, J.S., and Nikitovich-Winer, M.B. Neuroendocrinology, 4: 83, 1969.
30. Kobayashi, T., Kobayashi, T., Kigawa, T., Mizuno, M., Amenomori, Y., and Watanabe, T. Endo. Japon.,13: 430, 1966.
31 Jutisz M., Berault, A., Novella-M.A., and Ribot, G. Acta Endocr. (Kobenhavn), 55: 481, 1967.
32. Midgley, A.R., Jr., Gay, V.L., Caligaris, L.C.S., Rebar, R.W., Monroe, S.E., and Niswender, G.D. In Gonadotropins 1968, ed. Rosemberg, E., Geron-X, Los Altos,Calif, p 307, 1968.
33. Mittler, J.C., Arimura, A., and Schally, A.V., personal communication.
34. Wakabayashi, K., and Seldin, D.W. Fed. Proc., 28: 831, 1969.

35. Wakabayashi, K. Personal communication from S.M. McCann.
36. Corbin, A., and Daniels, E.L. Experientia, 24: 1260, 1968.
37. Corbin, A. In Workshop Conference on the Bioassay and Chemistry of the Hypophysiotropic Hormones of the Hypothalamus, ed., Meites, J. Williams and Wilkins, in press, 1970.
38. Corbin, A., personal communication.
39. Taylor, K.W., presented at the Third International Congress of Endocrinology, Mexico City, 1968.
40. Grand, R.J., and Gross, P.R. J. Biol. Chem., 244: 5608, 1969.
41. Lissitzky, S., Mante, S., Attali, J.C., and Cartouzou, G. Biochem. Biophys. Res. Commun., 35: 437, 1969.
42. Wicks, W.D. Science, 160: 997, 1968.

DISCUSSION

MEANS: Dr. Geschwind, as you probably know, if cyclic AMP is going to do all the things that it does in all of these various target organs, somewhere along the line some specificity must be invoked. If increases in protein and nucleic acid synthesis occur there has to be some manner of control. Dr. Jensen has recently reported that calcium is very necessary for the stability of the estrogen receptor molecule. If we couple this with L. Garren's findings that in the adrenal gland there may be a protein that in fact specifically binds cyclic AMP, this could in fact impart a means of specificity. If this occurs, then this might also provide a reason why one cell type with two distinctly different hormones acting upon it could possibly exhibit differential effects if the receptor sites for cyclic AMP were either different, or if the receptor proteins for the cyclic AMP were different.

GESCHWIND: One is dealing with a release process and I have pointed out that a high potassium ion concentration also requires calcium ion in order to stimulate release. Thus, the consideration of receptors is important and one has to look for something much more basic. I have also pointed out that if cyclic AMP is already present, then calcium ion is also required in order to effect release. Everyone who has studied release processes from both endocrine or exocrine glands has always found the same thing; calcium is absolutely necessary for the release process.

HELLER: I would ask you to differentiate between pharmacological effects of hormones which can invoke feedback mechanisms and physiological effects which can be as simple as utilization of FSH and ICSH by the testis. I am sure I will be challenged by some of you on this, but please let us remember that two mechanisms may be involved.

SAVARD: I would like to speak on this matter of adenyl-cyclase. I believe that the concept of cyclic AMP with its apparently ubiquitous presence in so many cellular systems, is entirely acceptable, but only if one invokes morphologic considerations. This, I admit, might be considered heretical for a biochemist to express, but nevertheless it makes sense. Sutherland himself has suggested that the system of adenyl cyclase - 3'5'-AMP is a very primitive control systen, which may have developed very early in biochemical evolution. One of these may be the activation of phosphorylase; there may be others which are very basic to cellular metabolism. With this as a primitive control system, at the simple unicellular level, as more sophisticated systems evolved, their mechanism utilized this basic cellular system of adenyl cyclase. Consequently, we must introduce into our thinking the idea that perhaps each cell has its own adenyl cyclase which is activated by secondary, but more sophisticated control mechanisms. These latter have the so-called specificity properties, but in each case they may activate a particular cell's adenyl cyclase. The process then becomes strictly an intracellular one with the generated cyclic AMP exerting its stimulatory message to whatever particular process the cell is programmed for. The point I wish to make is that neither adenyl cyclase nor cyclic AMP should be considered as circulating or peripheral factors otherwise all endocrine specificities are lost. These agents must be viewed as strictly intracellular agents, waiting to be turned on by a specific extracellular factor (a hormone for instance) and serving to stimulate a process unique to the particular cell involved. In this way it makes sense, at least to me.

LIPSETT: Dr. Pastan at the National Cancer Institute recently has shown that in a soluble system derived from E. coli, cyclic AMP promotes the synthesis of inducible enzymes. In particular, with respect to β-galactosidase, he can localize this effect to the promoter gene of the lac operon. Thus here is a direct effect of cyclic AMP on transcription localized at a particular site. Even though it is in a bacterial system, it may be relevant to our considerations of cyclic AMP and the synthesis of enzymes necessary for steroid synthesis.

HYPOTHALAMIC CONTROL OF GONADOTROPIN SECRETION IN THE MALE

L. Martini

Department of Pharmacology, University of Milan, Italy

I. LOCALIZATION OF THE NUCLEI WHICH SYNTHESIZE THE GONADOTROPIN-RELEASING FACTORS.

Three groups of experiments have been performed in order to clarify which regions of the hypothalamus synthesize the releasing factors (RF) controlling the secretion of pituitary gonadotropins in the male rat.

A. Hypothalamic Lesions

The first technique used was that of placing separate electrolytic lesions in each of the hypothalamic areas which are believed to play some role in the control of gonadotropin secretion (1), and studying whether such lesions modify the concentrations of FSH-releasing factor (FSH-RF) and LH-releasing factor (LH-RF)[1] at the level of the median eminence (ME), i.e. of the region of the hypothalamus which is specifically responsible for the storage of hypophysiotropic principles, and for their delivery to the anterior pituitary through the portal circulation. It was assumed that a lesion placed exactly in an area in which a RF is produced would prevent its synthesis, and consequently reduce its accumulation in the ME.

1. When dealing with the male, the name of Interstitial Cell Stimulating Hormone-Releasing Factor (ICSH-RF) would probably be more appropriate; however, the abbreviation LH-RF) will be used throughout this paper, because it is the only one usually employed in the neuroendocrine literature.

Three independent areas of the brain were bilaterally lesioned; they will be referred to as: a) paraventricular area; b) suprachiasmatic area; and c) arcuate-ventromedial area. Five days following placement of the lesions the animals were killed and their ME were collected in order to evaluate their content in FSH-RF and in LH-RF. For the assays of these principles the "pituitary depletion methods" described by Fraschini et al. (2) and by Motta et al. (3) were used. Using this approach it has been possible to localize, within the hypothalamus of the male rat, a circumscribed region in which FSH-RF is synthesized; it has actually been shown that lesions in or around the paraventricular nuclei are the only ones which reduce the concentration of this RF at ME level (Fig. 1). The synthesis of LH-RF takes place apparently in two different regions, since the content of this RF in the ME is reduced when lesions are placed either in the suprachiasmatic area or in the arcuate-ventromedial nuclei (Fig. 1) (4,5).

B. Hypothalamic deafferentation

The second approach devised to study the localization of the nuclei synthesizing the RF, which control the secretion of gonadotropins in the male, was that of evaluating the concentrations of FSH-RF and of LH-RF in the hypothalamic islands of rats submitted to a complete hypothalamic deafferentation (6). This operation permits a total separation of the paraventricular region from the rest of the hypothalamus (Fig.2); consequently, if it is true that FSH-RF originates in the paraventricular area, the complete disappearance of FSH-RF from the island a few days after the operation would be expected. On the other hand, the suprachiasmatic and the arcuate-ventromedial regions are still included within the hypothalamic island; consequently, if LH-RF is really produced by these two zones, its concentrations in the island should not be reduced following the operation.

The content of FSH-RF and of LH-RF in the deafferented island of adult male rats was measured eight and fifteen days following the operation, using the techniques described by Fraschini et al. (2) and by Motta et al. (3). The results shown in Fig. 3 indicate that FSH-RF stores are significantly reduced in the hypothalamic island eight days after a complete deafferentation; FSH-RF disappears completely from the isolated hypothalamus fifteen days after the operation. Eight and fifteen days after deafferentation LH-RF is still present in the isolated island (Fig.4); surprisingly, the concentration of this RF in deafferented animals is even higher than usual (7,8).

These data confirm with a new technique that FSH-RF is synthesized in the paraventricular region and that LH-RF is probably manufactured in the suprachiasmatic and in the arcuate-ventromedial regions. The fact that the stores of LH-RF are increased following

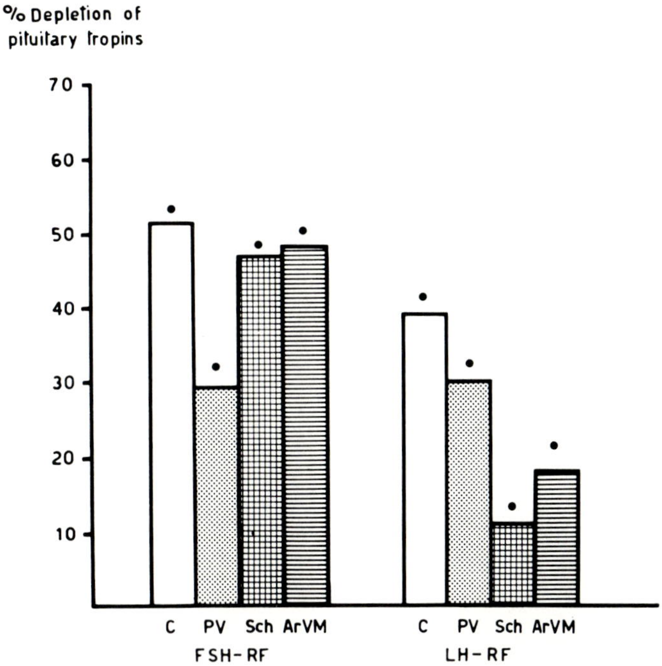

Fig. 1. Effect of lesions localized in the paraventricular (PV), suprachiasmatic (Sch) and arcuate-ventromedial (ArVM) areas on FSH-RF and LH-RF activity of the median eminence of male rats. Columns represent the depletion of pituitary tropins induced in normal male rats by the intracarotid injection of hypothalamic extracts prepared from non-lesioned controls (C) or from animals with the different hypothalamic lesions.

deafferentation suggests that, after the operation, all the LH-RF which is synthesized is accumulated in the island, because the extrahypothalamic neural stimuli necessary for its release are no longer transmitted to the hypothalamus (see below) (7,8).

C. Hypothalamic Implants of Inhibitors of Protein Synthesis

In the third group of experiments, the hypothesis that FSH-RF might be synthesized in the paraventricular nuclei was tested by implanting cycloheximide (Actidione), an inhibitor of protein synthesis, into the paraventricular region of adult, castrated, male rats, and by evaluating the effects of such implants on FSH-RF stores in the ME. Cycloheximide was implanted either unilaterally or bilaterally. When unilateral implants were performed, at the time of autopsy, ME tissue was collected in a way which permitted the separation of the half ME corresponding to the implanted side

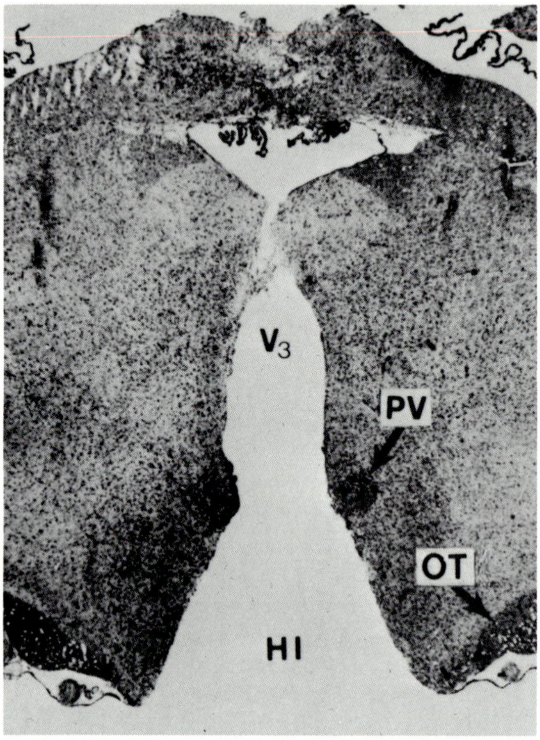

Fig. 2. Frontal section of the rat brain following total hypothalamic deafferentation and removal of the hypothalamic island. OT = Optic Tract; PV = Paraventricular Nuclei; V3 = Third Ventricle; HI = removed Hypothalamic Island.

from the half corresponding to the non-implanted one; the two halves of the ME were then tested separately for their content of FSH-RF and of LH-RF (2,3).

The data shown in Fig.5 indicate that, five days after unilateral implantation of cycloheximide, FSH-RF disappears only from the ipsilateral half of the ME; complete disappearance of FSH-RF from the ME is induced by bilateral implants. It may be concluded from these results that inhibition of protein synthesis in the cells of the paraventricular nuclei interfere with some biochemical process which is essential for the synthesis of FSH-RF in this region; these data, however, are not taken as indicating that FSH-RF itself is a protein or a polypeptide (9). It is also clear from the results that fibers originating in one paraventricular nucleus do not cross and carry FSH-RF only to the ipsilateral half of the ME.

Fig. 6 shows once more that the paraventricular region is not

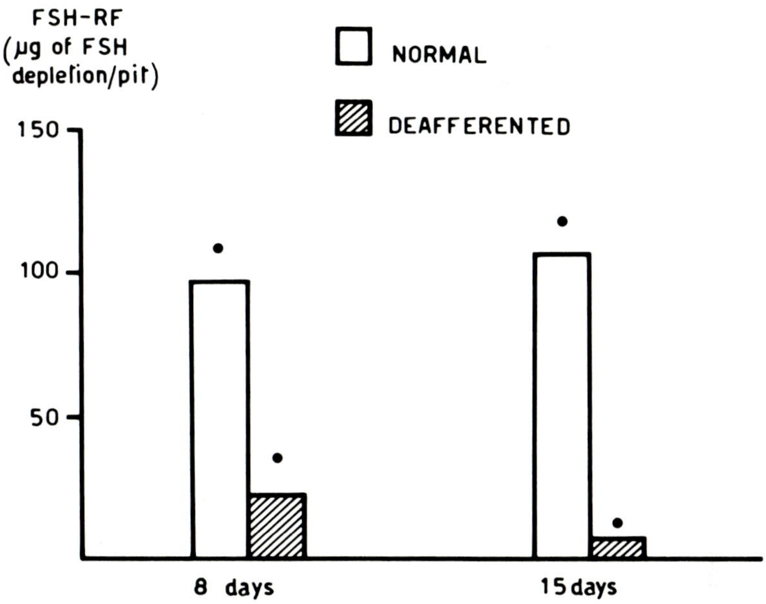

Fig. 3. Effect of hypothalamic deafferentation on the FSH-RF content of the hypothalamic island of adult male rats (eight and fifteen days after the operation). Columns represent the depletion of pituitary FSH induced in normal male rats by the intracarotid injection of hypothalamic extracts prepared from normal or from deafferented animals.

strictly involved in the synthesis of LH-RF. Animals implanted with cycloheximide either unilaterally or bilaterally in this region of the brain have normal amounts of LH-RF in the ME. These results, when considered in conjunction with the evidence previously described indicating that LH-RF is synthesized in the suprachiasmatic region, suggest that the effect of cycloheximide is very localized, and that no significant diffusion of the drug toward the basal hypothalamus takes place.

II. DATA SUGGESTING THE EXISTENCE OF A FOLLICLE STIMULATING HORMONE-SYNTHESIZING FACTOR

The three sets of results presented in the preceding sections of this paper agree in indicating that, in male rats, FSH-RF is synthesized in the area of the paraventricular nuclei. It is interesting that, both following paraventricular lesions and after hypothalamic deafferentation, the concentration of FSH in the anterior pituitary of the operated animals was perfectly normal, although

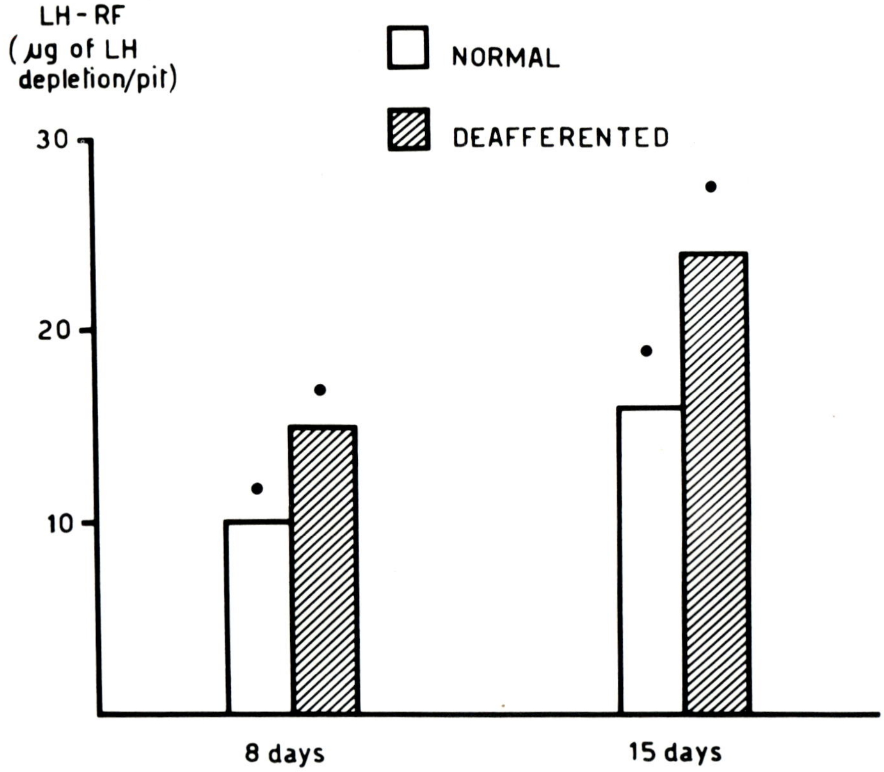

Fig. 4. Effect of hypothalamic deafferentation on the LH-RF content of the hypothalamic island of adult rats (eight and fifteen days after the operation). Columns represent the depletion of pituitary LH induced in normal male rats by the intracarotid injection of hypothalamic extracts prepared from normal or from deafferented animals.

the synthesis of FSH-RF had been considerably reduced. This result is surprising, since it is generally believed that RF control not only the release of anterior pituitary hormones, but also their synthesis (10). In accordance with this view, one whould expect the synthesis of a pituitary hormone to be interrupted when the corresponding RF is no longer available.

The presence of normal amounts of FSH in the anterior pituitary of animals in which the synthesis of FSH-RF had been experimentally suppressed, might be tentatively explained by suggesting that the hypothalamus controls FSH secretion through the production of two independent humoral factors: one devoted to the control of FSH release (FSH-RF), the other to the control of FSH synthesis (FSH - synthesizing factor or FSH-SF). It was believed that such a

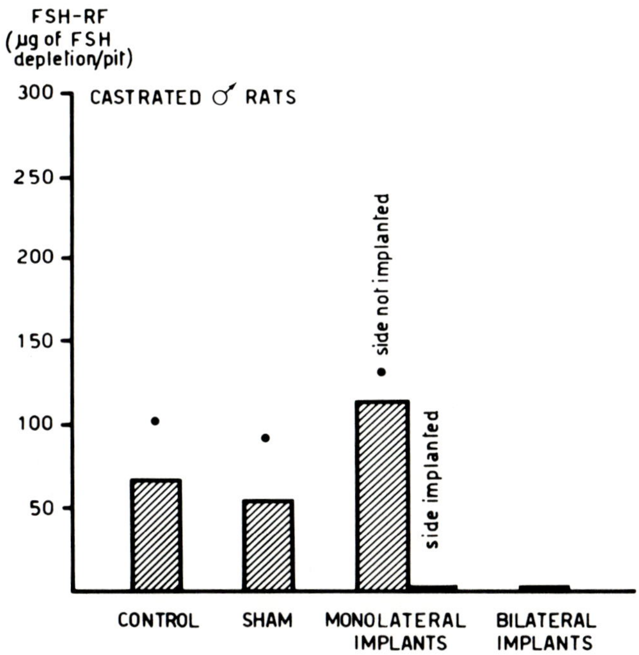

Fig. 5. Effect of implants of cycloheximide (Actidione) in the paraventricular region on the FSH-RF content of the median eminence of adult castrated male rats. See text for more details. Columns represent the depletion of pituitary FSH induced in normal male rats by the intracarotid injection of hypothalamic extracts prepared from controls or from implanted animals.

Control: unimplanted animals
Sham; animals implanted with empty cannulae
Monolateral implants: animals implanted with cycloheximide in one paraventricular nucleus
Bilateral implants: animals implanted with cycloheximide in both paraventricular nuclei.

hypothesis might be tested by evaluating whether hypothalamic extracts prepared from animals submitted to a complete hypothalamic deafferentation (and consequently devoid of any FSH-RF activity) might induce the synthesis of FSH in animals in which this had been interrupted by appropriate experimental manipulations. Corbin and Daniels (personal communication) have recently shown that ME lesions, performed in adult male rats, result, in one to two weeks, in a significant decrease in the amounts of FSH stored in the anterior pituitary. The decrease of FSH in the pituitary of lesioned animals has been interpreted as being due to the fact that hypophysiotropic principles endowed with synthesizing capacities cannot be

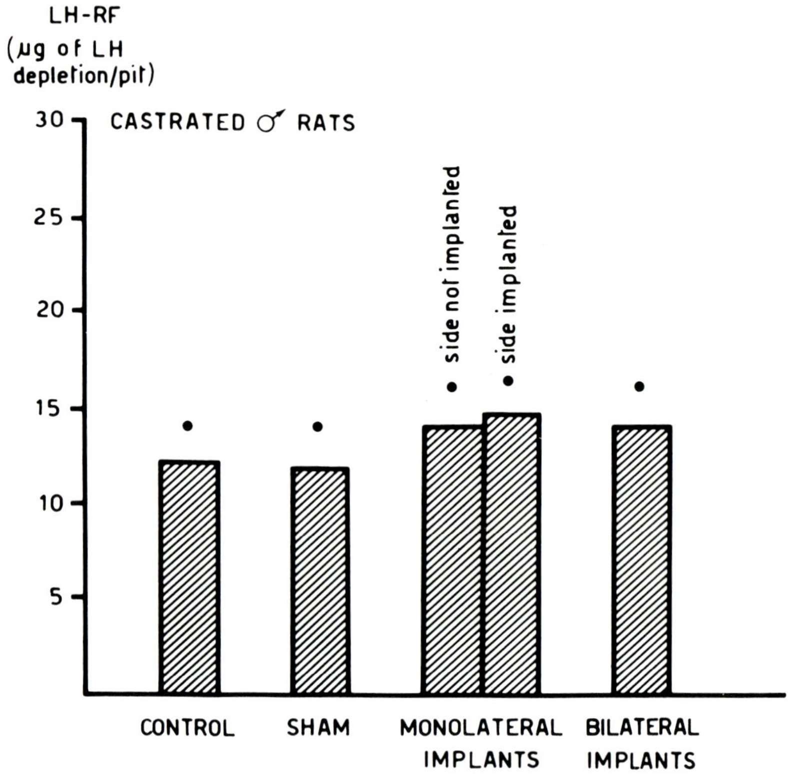

Fig. 6. Effect of implants of cycloheximide (Actidione) in the paraventricular region on the LH-RF content of the median eminence of adult castrated male rats. See text for more details. Columns represent the depletion of pituitary LH induced in normal male rats by the intracarotid injection of hypothalamic extracts prepared from controls or from implanted animals.

Control: unimplanted animals
Sham: animals implanted with empty cannulae
Monolateral implants: animals implanted with cycloheximide in one paraventricular nucleus.
Bilateral implants: animals implanted with cycloheximide in both paraventricular nuclei.

transported to the anterior pituitary. Daniels and Corbin (personal communication) have also shown that the intravenous injection of crude hypothalamic extracts prepared from the brain of normal rats induces a rapid and significant increase of FSH stores in ME-lesioned recipient animals. They have concluded that, under the conditions of their experiments, crude hypothalamic extracts are able to facilitate the resynthesis of FSH.

A similar approach has been recently used by Daniels, Motta and Martini (unpublished observations). These authors have confirmed that electrolytic lesions placed in the ME region of adult male rats are followed in 10 days by a significant decrease in pituitary FSH concentration (Table 1). As in the experiments of Daniels and Corbin, the intravenous injection of a hypothalamic extract prepared from the brain of normal animals induced, in 45 minutes, a significant increase in the amounts of FSH stored in the pituitary of ME-lesioned rats. In addition, Daniels, Motta and Martini have shown that the concentration of FSH in the pituitary of lesioned animals is also brought back to normal by the intravenous injection of a hypothalamic extract prepared from the brain of deafferented animals (Table 1) in spite of the fact that this hypothalamic extract does not contain any FSH-RF.

The results indicate that both normal hypothalamic extracts and hypothalamic extracts prepared from animals submitted to complete hypothalamic deafferentation contain a factor which is able to increase the concentration of FSH in the pituitary of ME-lesioned animals. There are two mechanisms through which this factor may operate: a) to facilitate the synthesis of new FSH; or b) to inhibit the release of stored FSH. The first possibility is the one favored by the authors, since it is not believed that, in ME-lesioned animals, release of FSH occurs so rapidly as to permit a significant reaccumulation of the hormone 45 minutes after blockade of the release process. In addition, no factors able to suppress FSH release have been described so far; inhibiting factors have been recognized to exist for the control of the secretion of prolactin (11), melanocyte stimulating hormone (12) and growth hormone (13).

The results obtained using the hypothalamic extract prepared from the deafferent animals suggest that the hypothetical FSH-SF is different and independent from FSH-RF; moreover, its site of origin is within the deafferented island and not in the paraventricular region.

III. MEDIATORS INFLUENCING THE NUCLEI WHICH SYNTHESIZE THE LUTEINIZING HORMONE-RELEASING FACTOR

It is a generally accepted concept that extrahypothalamic nervous structures (e.g., amygdala, cortex, hippocampus, midbrain) may influence the neurons which secrete the gonadotropin-releasing factors (1,6,14). The validity of this concept is proved once more by the observation, reported in a previous section of this paper, that LH-RF is accumulated in the deafferented hypothalamic island when all inputs from extrahypothalamic structures are eliminated.

Table 1. Effect of Median Eminence (ME) Lesions and of Intravenous Injections of Median Eminence Extracts (MEE) on Pituitary Concentrations of FSH in Adult Male Rats

Groups [a]	Intravenous Treatment	Pituitary FSH [b] (μg/ mg)	P
Normal (20)	Saline	42.54 ± 3.82 [c]	
ME-lesioned (25)	Saline	32.27 ± 3.38	< 0.05 Vs Normal
ME-lesioned (18)	2 MEE from Normal Rat	43.19 ± 3.10	< 0.05 Vs ME-lesioned, saline treated
ME-lesioned (18)	2 MEE from Deafferented Rat	45.68 ± 5.21	< 0.05 Vs. ME-lesioned, saline treated

a. Number of rats in parentheses; b. Microgram equivalents of NIH-FSH-S-5 per milligram wet weight of pituitary tissue; c. Values are means ± SE.

The chemical nature of the humoral mediator(s) involved in transferring the information from extrahypothalamic centers to the hypothalamic nuclei has not been fully clarified so far. A lot of data seem to suggest that traditional central nervous system mediators (e.g., epinephrine, norepinephrine, serotonin, dopamine, acetylcholine, etc.) may be involved in such a process (15,16,17,18).

The possibility that acetylcholine(Ach) might be the mediator involved in transmitting extrahypothalamic influences to the nuclei synthesizing LH-RF, has been tested recently using an in vitro procedure by Fiorindo and Martini (unpublished observations). They have shown that the anterior pituitary of normal adult male rats, when incubated alone, secretes very low amounts of LH. The release of LH from the incubated pituitaries is increased, but not significantly, by the addition of fragments of male hypothalamus; such fragments have been prepared in a way to include the ME and the arcuate-ventromedial region, i.e. one of the areas in which LH-RF is synthesized. Ach, added to incubation flasks containing only anterior pituitary tissue, does not increase LH output. The cholinergic mediator does increase LH secretion in flasks containing hypothalamic fragments together with anterior pituitary tissue; under these circumstances, the increase in LH release is proportional to the dose of Ach added to the medium. The data have been interpreted as indicating that Ach stimulates the release of LH-RF from the hypothalamic fragments; the LH-RF released under the influence of the drug enhances the secretion of LH from the incubated pituitary.

This interpretation is supported by the results of additional experiments performed by Fiorindo and Martini (unpublished observations) using drugs which either counteract or prolong Ach action. Atropine, a drug inhibiting the peripheral effects of Ach, has been shown to counteract in vitro the LH-releasing effect of Ach added to the medium containing anterior pituitary tissue and hypothalamic fragments. It is interesting that atropine also inhibits the small release of LH which is observed when hypothalamic tissue is added to anterior pituitaries in the absence of Ach; this result suggests that atropine may be able to block the effects on LH-RF release of endogenous Ach present in the incubated hypothalamic tissue. Prostigmine,a drug which inhibits cholinesterases, enhances the LH-releasing effect of Ach, when this mediator is added to media in which hypothalamic fragments are incubated together with anterior pituitary tissue. Prostigmine also increases the release of LH from anterior pituitaries incubated with hypothalamic fragments, but without exogenous Ach. This result may be explained by the fact that prostigmine enhances the activity of the endogenous Ach present in the hypothalamic tissue incubated.

In a similar set of experiments, Schneider and McCann (19) have found that the adrenergic mediator dopamine is able to release

LH in vitro when added to incubation media containing hypothalamic fragments and anterior pituitary tissue. They have suggested that dopamine might be the mediator liberating LH-RF. The possibility then exists that both cholinergic and adrenergic mechanisms participate in the control of the release of LH-RF from the neurons in which this factor is synthesized. The relative role of the two types of mediators remains to be ascertained.

IV. FEEDBACK CONTROL OF GONADOTROPIN SECRETION IN THE MALE

There are three different levels of feedback control of the activity of the hypothalamo-pituitary-gonadal axis of the male; a) a "long" feedback system, in which the inhibiting messages are provided by the hormonal steroids (mainly, but not exclusively, androgens) produced by the testes and possibly by the adrenals; b) a "short" feedback system, in which the inhibitory signals are represented by the gonadotropic hormones synthesized in the anterior pituitary gland; and c) an "ultrashort" feedback system, in which the releasing factors directly control their rate of production (20, 21).

A. "Long" Feedback System

The classic findings about the "long" feedback control of gonadotropin secretion in the male may be found in two reviews by Davidson (22,23) and in two articles by Martini and co-workers (5, 24). Consequently, only one aspect of the problem will be dealt with in detail in this paper: the type of androgenic hormone active on feedback receptors.

Recent evidence suggests that the potent androgenic steroid 17-betahydroxy-5-alpha-androstan-3-one (androstanolone, dihydrotestosterone, DHT) may be the active form of testosterone on androgen-sensitive target structures (see 25 for references). Conversion of testosterone into DHT has been reported to occur in the prostate , the seminal vesicles, the preputial glands and in other accessory organs of male reproduction (see 25 for references). If the formation of DHT is a general feature of testosterone action, one might expect this derivative to be formed also in the sites in which androgens exert their feedback effect on gonadotropin secretion. This hypothesis has been recently tested by Kniewald and Martini (unpublished observations). They have incubated in vitro labelled testosterone with slices of hypothalamus, pituitary gland, amygdala, cerebral cortex and prostates and identified the metabolites formed. All tissues were taken from adult male rats. The results indicate that testosterone is converted into DHT by all tissues examined; the prostates were the structures which effected such a conversion to the greatest extent; they were followed by the pituitary gland and by the hypothalamus; the cerebral cortex and the amygdala were also able to transform testosterone into DHT, but the rate of conversion was not as great as that found in the other tissues. Androstenedione (a metabolite of testosterone which is formed also in other androgen-sensitive target tissues) (26-28) was found together with DHT in all incubation media; traces of androstanediol and of androstenedione were also formed by some of the tissues.

These data, as well as the similar ones recently reported by Jaffe (29), suggest that the transformation of testosterone into DHT is probably necessary also for initiating androgen-induced feedback responses. They also indicate that the hypothalamus is not the only target organ of the feedback effect of testosterone, as it is generally assumed: (22,23); apparently, the anterior pituitary and other nervous structures (e.g., the amygdala, the cerebral cortex) must also be incorporated into androgen feedback circuits. That cerebral receptors for androgens are not exclusively localized in the hypothalamus is supported also by the study of the distribution of labelled androgens in vivo (27,28,30).

B. "Short" Feedback System

In an attempt to assess whether FSH might modify its own rate of secretion through a "short" feedback effect, Fraschini and coworkers (31,32) have studied the effects of the administration of exogenous FSH on the pituitary stores of FSH and on the hypothalamic content of FSH-RF in castrated adult male rats. Orchidectomized animals were used in order to avoid the possibility that the injected FSH might activate the gonads and operate through a "long" feedback effect. FSH was measured according to the assay of Steelman and Pohley (33) and FSH-RF using the "pituitary depletion method" described by Fraschini et al. (2). The data summarized in Fig. 7 indicate that treatment with exogenous FSH results in a significant drop of pituitary stores of FSH and of the hypothalamic content of FSH-RF. The data shown in the figure also suggest that the inhibitory signal provided by FSH is specific; it has been impossible to duplicate its effects by injecting ACTH and LH into the castrated animals.

The demonstration that an artificial increase in FSH in the general circulation reduced hypothalamic FSH-RF content suggested that the opposite phenomenon could be studied also, i.e., what happens to the secretion of FSH-RF when endogenous FSH is eliminated. Different groups of adult male rats were subjected to castration, hypophysectomy, or castration followed by hypophysectomy. Their hypothalamic stores of FSH-RF were then evaluated utilizing the in vivo procedure of Fraschini et al. (2). Three weeks following castration a significant increase in the amounts of FSH-RF stored in the hypothalamus was observed (Fig.8). One week following hypophysectomy a slight, but insignificant, increase of FSH-RF was detected. It is uncertain whether this small increase was due

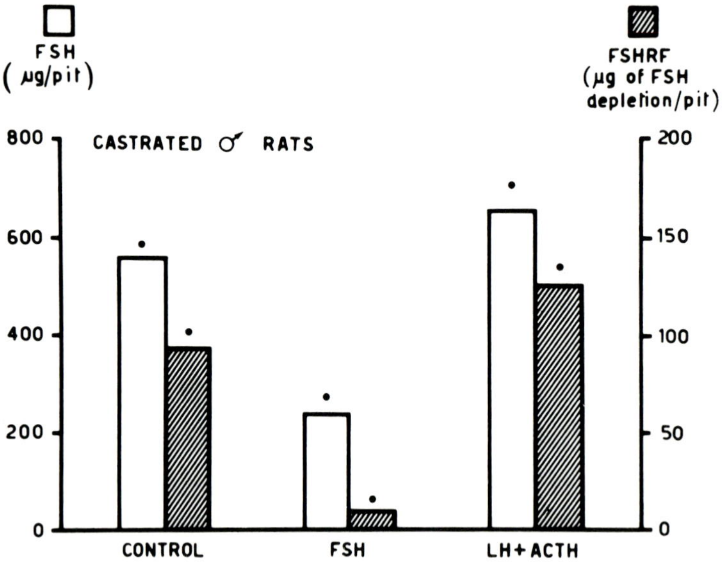

Fig. 7. Effect of systemic administration of FSH on pituitary FSH content and on hypothalamic FSH-RF stores of castrated male rats.

to the elimination of the "short" signal or to the reduction of testosterone secretion brought about by hypophysectomy, but the latter appears a likely explanation since all testosterone-dependent structures (prostates and seminal vesicles) were atrophied in this group of rats. In the animals subjected to the removal of the pituitary and the testes, hypothalamic FSH-RF stores reached a level well above that observed following the elimination of either gland alone (20,21). These data indicate that the effects of castration and of hypophysectomy are additive. It is also clear that in castrated animals FSH-RF stores do not reach the high levels found following castration plus hypophysectomy because of the "short" negative feedback signals provided by FSH. The fact that the elimination of the "short" feedback signal increases release as well as synthesis of FSH-RF is documented by the observation that, after hypophysectomy, FSH-RF appears in the peripheral plasma (34,35).

Additional information and data on the "short" feedback mechanism controlling LH secretion may be found in the chapter by Motta et al. (21).

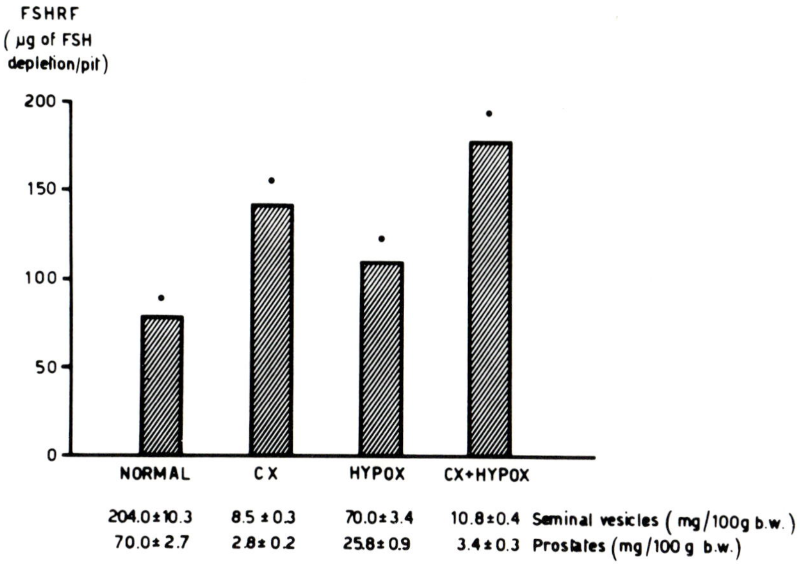

Fig. 8. Effect of castration (Cx), hypophysectomy (Hypox) and castration plus hypophysectomy (Cx + Hypox) on hypothalamic FSH-RF stores and on seminal vesicle and prostate weight of male rats.

C. "Ultra-short" Feedback System

It is clear from the data presented in previous sections of this paper that the concentration of FSH-RF in the hypothalamus can be modified by changes in the level of the hormones produced either in the peripheral target glands or in the anterior pituitary. Motta et al. (20,21) have recently explored the possibility that the synthesis, storage, and release of FSH-RF might also be influenced by changes in titer of this same principle in the general circulation. Two groups of male rats that had been castrated for three weeks and hypophysectomized for one week were used. One of these groups was injected subcutaneously with an extract of rat hypothalamus rich in FSH-RF (1 ME/rat per day, for five days); the other was treated in a similar way with saline solution. Animals were killed three hours after the last injection. Normal controls were also studied. The content of FSH-RF in the hypothalami of the different groups of animals was measured by the "pituitary depletion method" described by Fraschini et al. (2).

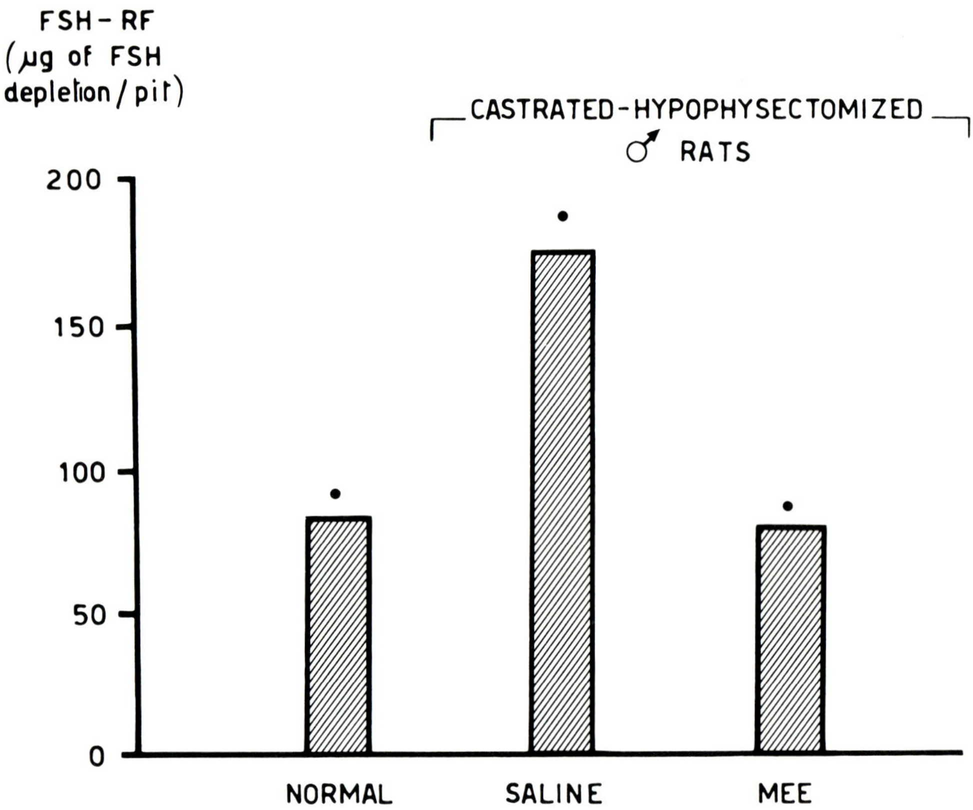

Fig. 9. Effect of treatment with a median eminence extract (MEE) rich in FSH-RF on hypothalamic FSH-RF stores in castrated-hypophysectomized male rats.

Fig. 9 shows that the treatment with the hypothalamic extract brings back to normal the elevated hypothalamic stores of FSH-RF typical of castrated hypophysectomized rats. This result is not due to contamination of the hypothalamic extract with FSH; the extract was assayed by the Steelman and Pohley procedure (33), and this hormone was not detected. It is difficult, of course, to establish whether this reduction of stores is due to inhibition of the synthesis of FSH-RF or to stimulation of its release. However, it appears that brain elements may exist which are sensitive to changing levels of releasing factors.

ACKNOWLEDGEMENT

The experimental work performed in the author's laboratory and here described has been supported by funds of the Department of Pharmacology of the University of Milan and by the following grants: 67-530 of the Ford Foundation, New York; 5-R01 AM 11783-01-02 of the

National Institutes of Health, Bethesda, Maryland. Gifts of FSH and LH were made by the National Institutes of Health, Bethesda, Maryland. All such support is gratefully acknowledged.

REFERENCES

1. Szentagothai, J., Flerko, B., Mess, B., and Halasz, B. Hypothalamic Control of the Anterior Pituitary, Akademiai Kiado, Budapest, 1968.
2. Fraschini, F., Motta, M., and Martini, L., In Methods in Drug Evaluation eds. Mantegazza, P. and Piccinini, F., North Holland Publishing Company, Amsterdam, p 424, 1966.
3. Motta, M., Piva, F., Fraschini, F., and Martini, L., In Chemistry of Hypophysiotropic Hormones of the Hypothalamus, ed. Meites, J., In press.
4. Mess, B., Fraschini, F., Motta, M., and Martini, L., In Hormonal Steroids, eds. Martini, L., Fraschini, F. and Motta, M., Excerpta Medica, Amsterdam, p. 1004, 1967.
5. Martini, L., Fraschini, F., and Motta, M., Recent Progr. Hormone Res., 24: 439, 1968.
6. Halasz, B., In Frontiers in Neuroendocrinology, 1969, eds. Ganong, W.F., and Martini, L., Oxford University Press, New York, p. 307, 1969.
7. Tima, L., Motta, M., and Martini, L., Program of the 51st Meeting of the Endocrine Society, p. 194, 1969.
8. Motta, M., Piva, F., Tima, L., Zanisi, M., and Martini, L, Mem. Soc. Endocrinology, 18: 407, 1970.
9. McCann, S.M., and Dhariwal, A.P.S., In Neuroendocrinology, eds. Martini, L., and Ganong, W.F., Vol. I, Academic Press, New York, p. 261, 1966.
10. Geschwind, I.I. In Frontiers in Neuroendocrinology, 1969, eds. Ganong, W.F., and Martini, L., Oxford University Press, New York, p 389, 1969.
11. Meites, J., In Neuroendocrinology, eds. Martini, L., and Ganong, W.F., Vol. I, Academic Press, New York, p. 669, 1969.
12. Kastin, A.J., and Schally, A.V., Gen. Comp. Endocr., 8: 344, 1967.
13. Krulich, L., Dhariwal, A.P.S., and McCann, S.M., Endocrinology, 83: 783, 1968.
14. Mess, B. and Martini, L., In Recent Advances in Endocrinology, ed. James, V.H.T., J. and A. Churchill, London, p. 1, 1968.
15. Kobayashi, H., and Matsui, T., In Frontiers in Neuroendocrinology, 1969, eds. Ganong, W.F., and Martini, L., Oxford University Press, New York, p. 3, 1969.
16. Fuxe, K., and Hokfelt, T., In Frontiers in Neuroendocrinology, 1969, eds. Ganong, W.F., and Martini, L., Oxford University Press, New York, p. 47, 1969.
17. Ganong, W.F., and Lorenzen, L. In Neuroendocrinology, eds. Martini, L., and Ganong, W.F., Vol. II, Academic Press, New York, p. 583, 1967.

18. Piva, F., Sterescu, N., Zanisi, M., and Martini, L., Bull Wld. Hlth. Org., 41: 275, 1969.
19. Schneider, H.P.G., and McCann, S.M., Endocrinology, 85: 121, 1969.
20. Motta, M., In Progress in Endocrinology, ed., Gual, C., Excerpta Medica, Amsterdam, p. 523, 1969.
21. Motta, M., Fraschini, F., and Martini, L., In Frontiers in Neuroendocrinology, 1969, eds. Ganong, W.F., and Martini, L., Oxford University Press, New York, p. 211, 1969.
22. Davidson, J.M., In Neuroendocrinology, eds. Martini, L., and Ganong, W.F., Vol. I, Academic Press, New York, p. 565, 1966.
23. Davidson, J.M., In Frontiers in Neuroendocrinology, 1969, eds. Ganong, W.F., and Martini, L., Oxford University Press, New York, p. 343, 1969.
24. Martini, L., Fraschini, F., and Motta, M., In Endocrinology and Human Behaviour, ed. Michael, R.P., Oxford University Press, London, p. 175, 1968.
25. Gloyna, R.E., and Wilson, J.D., J. Clin. Endocr., 29: 970, 1969.
26. Harding, B.W., and Samuels, L.T., Endocrinology, 70: 109, 1962.
27. Resko, J.A., Goy, R.W., and Phoenix, C.H., Endocrinology, 80: 490, 1967.
28. Whalen, R.E., Luttge, W.G., and Green, R. Endocrinology, 84: 217, 1969.
29. Jaffe, R.B., Steroids, 14: 483, 1969.
30. Pfaff, D.W., Experientia, 24: 958, 1968.
31. Fraschini, F., Motta, M., and Martini, L., Experientia, 24: 270, 1968.
32. Fraschini, F., In Progress in Endocrinology, ed. Gual, C., Excerpta Medica, Amsterdam, p. 637, 1969.
33. Steelman, S.L., and Pohley, F.M., Endocrinology, 53: 604, 1953.
34. Saito, T., Sawano, S., Arimura, A., and Schally, A.V., Endocrinology, 81: 1226, 1967.
35. Negro-Vilar, A., Dickerman, E., and Meites, J., Endocrinology, 82: 939, 1968.

DISCUSSION

LUNENFELD: Dr. Martini, you mentioned that progesterone exerts a positive feedback mechanism; could you elaborate on this assumption? Also, I seem to be at a loss about the present state of releasing factors. Do we have a releasing factor for FSH and a releasing factor for LH or not?

MARTINI: The "positive" feedback effect of progesterone is on LH and not on FSH. As for your second question, I still believe that there are two separate hypothalamic factors for the control of gonadotropic secretion: one controlling FSH, the other LH. I think that our data, which indicate that following a total hypothalamic deafferentation FSH-RF disappears while LH-RF is still present,

present good proof for the existence of two separate releasing factors.

GESCHWIND: It is a little difficult to reach a decision unless one personally works with both of these releasing factors. I mentioned one experiment from Dr. Schally's group in which they observed approximately a 100% increase in the total amount of FSH in the system upon culturing the pituitary gland. It so happened that the releasing factor used for this experiment was LRF and not FRF. They used one of Dr. Schally's purest preparations. W. White at Abbot, who has collaborated with Dr. Schally in this work, is also of the opinion that they are both one and the same substance. There is one very important experiment which was done about a year ago by Paul Nakane, who obtained from Dr. Midgley antibodies to FSH which did not cross react with LH, and antibodies to LH which did not cross react with FSH, and hooked peroxidase on to both of these. Dr. Nakane then attempted to localize both of these hormones in the anterior pituitary of the rat, and found that both labelled antibodies localized in the same cells. It is a little difficult to understand how you can get separate control of FSH granules and LH granules within the same cell with two different releasing factors.

JUTISZ: We did not purify LRF and FRF to the same extent as Dr. Schally did, but as we purified FRF the LRF activity steadily diminished. We never eliminated this activity completely, but we obtained an FRF preparation with a low LRF activity and an LRF preparation with very low FRF activity.

LIPSETT: Dr. Martini, I have never had any difficulty accepting your data on the short feedback and I am quite willing to accept your data on the ultra short feedback, but as a physiologist I have real difficulty in comprehending how such a system would possibly work.

MARTINI: It is our impression that the hypothalamus is able to realize and evaluate how much of each releasing factor is stored in the median eminence. We have indicated that unilateral implants with a blocker of protein synthesis, such as cycloheximide, performed in the paraventricular region of the hypothalamus, inhibit FSH-RF synthesis only on one side and make FSH-RF disappear from the ipsilateral side of the median eminence. I do not know whether you noticed that the non-implanted side contained twice the amount of FSH-RF which is found in normal animals. We think that this may be due to the fact that the paraventricular nuclei of the non-implanted side have got the indication that half of the median eminence was devoid of any FSH-RF.

E. STEINBERGER: Dr. Martini, in the experiments where the hypothalamus was separated, you showed a decrease in FSH-RF with normal levels of FSH in the pituitary and interpreted this finding by bringing in the possibility of a synthesizing factor. If FSH-RF was diminished, and the FSH release was impaired, could these findings be due to simple storage of FSH in the pituitary? I think that simultaneous determinations of pituitary and plasma levels of FSH and LH could have shed some light on this question. In experiments with castrated animals, you made an assumption that when an animal is castrated you have removed the feedback related to testosterone. Other experiments suggest different explanations for these findings.

MARTINI: I agree with you on the second question; actually our data indicate that also estrogen and progesterone may participate in the feedback control of gonadotropin secretion in the male rat. With regard to your first question, it is still difficult to provide an answer mainly because of the lack of a good FSH-radioimmunoassay to be used in the rat. It is however interesting to note that the weight of the testes of the animals whose hypothalamus had been completely deafferented for two weeks was perfectly normal. Apparently, even in the deafferented animal, there is enough leakage of FSH from the pituitary to maintain the testicular weight, if testicular weight is an indication of circulating FSH.

PURIFICATION AND CHEMISTRY OF GONADOTROPIN RELEASING FACTORS

Marian Jutisz

Laboratoire de Physiologie Cellulaire, College de France,

11, Place Marcelin Berthelot, Paris Ve, France.

INTRODUCTION

Historical Data

Although the humoral mechanism for the control of secretion of pituitary gonadotropins has been proposed for many years (1,2), the first attempts to demonstrate the presence of an LH (luteinizing hormone)-releasing factor (LRF) in hypothalamic extracts are relatively recent. It was actually Harris and Campbell et al. (3,4) and McCann et al. (5,6) who in 1960 independently demonstrated the presence of LRF in the acid extracts of cattle and rat hypothalamus. The existence in hypothalamic extracts of an LRF capable of stimulating release of LH has now been established in the following nine species: rat (5-8), cattle (4,9-11), sheep (8,11-14), pig (14), rabbit and dog (10,15), monkey (10), guinea pig (16,17) and man (18). Although LRF from some of these species has been prepared in a highly purified state, nobody, to our knowledge, has obtained pure LRF.

The presence of an FSH (follicle stimulating hormone) releasing factor (FRF) in rat hypothalamic extract was first demonstrated by Igarashi and McCann (19) in vivo and by Mittler and Meites (20) in vitro. Independently, Kuroshima et al. (21) demonstrated the presence of FRF in hypothalamic extracts of cattle and sheep. The existence of an FRF in hypothalamic extracts of pig (22) and man (18) have also been demonstrated. Highly purified preparations of FRF have been obtained only from some of these species.

A well documented review on the purification and chemistry of hypothalamic neurohormones regulating anterior pituitary function has recently been published by Schally et al. (23).

Nomenclature

The most widely used term for designating the hypothalamic principles is the term "releasing factors" (RF) proposed by Saffran et al. (24). Thus the principle acting on the secretion of luteinizing hormone is called LH-RF or LRF, that acting on the secretion of follicle-stimulating hormone, FSH-RF or FRF. Schally et al. (23) recently suggested designating the releasing factors by the term "releasing hormones", i.e., LRF by the abbreviation LH-RH or LRH and FRF by FSH-RH or FRH. In order to avoid confusion, we thought it preferable to keep the old nomenclature which is understood and accepted by a large number of scientific workers.

BIOLOGICAL TESTS

It is very important for purification work to have available a sensitive, specific and relatively simple biological test or assay for releasing factors.

LRF

1. In vivo. To assay LRF, Campbell et al. (4,10) and Nikitovitch-Winer (9) have used the test of ovulation obtained in the female rabbit or rat by direct intrapituitary infusion of an acidic extract of median eminence of cattle or rat. This same extract, when injected intravenously, was unable to produce ovulation. The cycle of the female rat, an animal with spontaneous ovulation, is blocked at the time of proestrus by the administration of pentobarbital (9). To assay LRF, the ovulation test has also been used in androgenized female rats (13,25) and in rats rendered anovulatory by hypothalamic lesion (26).

The most frequently employed test for routine assay of LRF was the ovarian ascorbic acid depletion (OAAD) test of Parlow (27). In this test (5,28), a stalk-median eminence extract (SME) is infused intravenously directly into immature female rats pretreated with pregnant mare serum-gonadotropin (PMS) and human chorionic gonadotropin (HCG) and the ovarian ascorbic acid depletion is taken as the response. To allow for the possible presence of LH-like activity in LRF preparations, the animals were hypophysectomized, treated with prolactin and used for assay one hr after hypophysectomy (29). It should be pointed out, however, that this assay has a low sensitivity for LRF (30), and that sufficient doses of vasopressin can deplete ovarian ascorbic acid (31).

A much more sensitive and specific test is the determination of the elevation of plasma LH levels in chronically ovariectomized, estrogen and progesterone-treated rats (32). The extracts are infused i.v., and the rats bled 10 minutes later. The plasma LH levels were determined by the OAAD-assay (27).

2. In vitro. Pituitaries from chronically ovariectomized, estrogen and progesterone-treated rats (32) were also used for demonstrating the action of LRF in vitro (11). The pituitaries were bisected and incubated for one or two hrs in a Krebs-Ringer bicarbonate-glucose medium. At the end of the incubation, the LH was assayed in the incubation medium using the OAAD test. It has been shown that a linear log-dose response curve was obtained (33).

FRF

1. In vivo. FRF or a crude stalk median eminence (SME) raise plasma FSH activity in chronically ovariectomized rats pretreated with estrogen and progesterone (19,29). FRF or a crude SME also deplete the pituitary FSH content in normal male rats (34,35), castrated male rats pretreated with testosterone (36), and in ovariectomized female rats pretreated with estrogen and progesterone (37). The Steelman-Pohley test (38) was used for the assay of FSH in the pituitary tissue.

2. In vitro. Mittler and Meites showed that crude rat SME stimulates FSH release from normal male rat pituitaries cultured for 9 days (20) or incubated in tissue culture medium for 6 hours (39). A linear log-dose response curve was obtained. Using incubation of pituitaries from chronically ovariectomized, estrogen and progesterone-treated rats in a Krebs-Ringer bicarbonate-glucose medium, a significant release of FSH under the influence of FRF or crude SME was also observed after a one hr incubation (21) or after a 2 hr incubation (40). Pituitaries from normal male rats may also be employed in the short time incubation method (41) and give a linear log-dose response curve.

PURIFICATION STUDIES

Purification of LRF

1. Ovine LRF. The first attempt to partially purify LRF, starting from ovine hypothalamus, was made in 1963 by Guillemin et al. (12). The method proposed consisted of the following steps: preparation of acetone-ether dried powder from frozen sheep hypothalamic tissue; extraction with 2 N acetic acid at 4°C; gel filtration on a Sephadex G-25 column in 0.1 M pyridine acetate buffer pH 5.0; and chromatography on a carboxymethylcellulose (CMC) column equilibrated with 0.01 M ammonium acetate buffer, pH 4.5. The LRF activity was eluted with a gradient to pH 7, 0.1M buffer. This method has since been used by several authors as a general procedure for the purification of all hypothalamic hormones. It was further slightly modified in our laboratory (42) and adapted for large batches of tissue. In order to completely eliminate inorganic salts, one step was added to the original method; the phenol extraction (43). An example of the new version of this method is

given below: frozen fragments of sheep hypothalamic tissue (Sorga, Paris) are lyophilized and the region of median eminence containing the pituitary stalk (SME) is cut off from the dry fragments by means of a stainless steel cutter. Tissues are ground in acetone with an Ultra-Turrax[1] homogenizer, defatted with acetone (50 ml, then 25 ml/g) and peroxide-free ether and extracted twice with 2N acetic acid at 4° C (5 ml/g for each extraction).

A lyophilized extract from 20,000 hypothalamic fragments (84 g) is extracted twice with 600 and 300 ml of cold 0.1 M pyridine acetate buffer, pH 5.0, and applied to a Sephadex G-25 column (19 x 105 cm) maintained in a cold room at 4° C. Fractions of 240 ml are collected every 20 min. Fig. 1 shows the chromatographic pattern and biological activities observed during gel filtration.

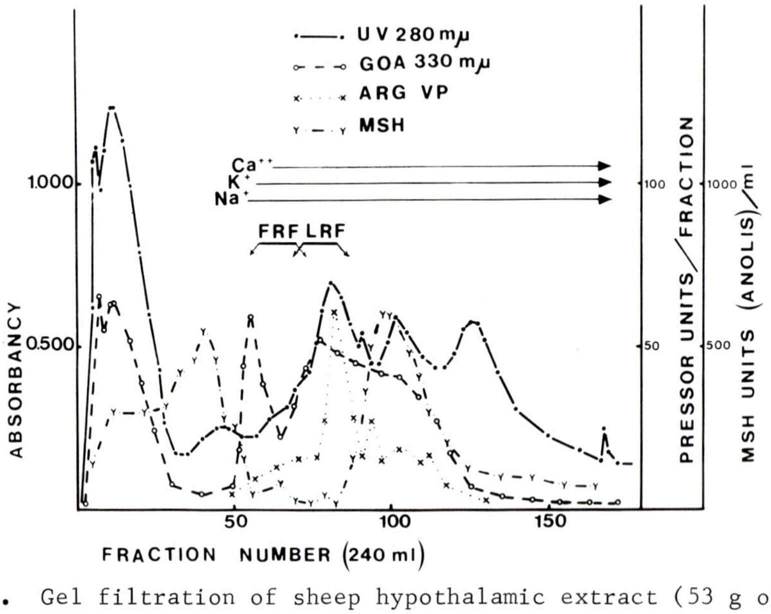

Fig. 1. Gel filtration of sheep hypothalamic extract (53 g of material corresponding to 20,000 SME) on a column of Sephadex G-25 (19 x 105 cm) in 0.1 M pyridine acetate buffer, pH 5.0. Fraction size, 240 ml; 300 μl aliquots taken for biuret colorimetry (Goa, 44). From Berault (42).

The concentration of different products in the fractions is determined by the measurement of absorbancy at 280 mμ and biuret colorimetry at 330 mμ (44). The first large peak (Fig. 1) corresponds to substances excluded from Sephadex G-25 and contains activities of the type of LH, TSH (thyroid stimulating hormone) and ACTH. LRF emerges in fractions 73 to 84. The FRF, melanocyte stimulating hormone (MSH) and vasopressin activities are also deter-

[1]Janke & Kunkel Kg., Staufen i. Br. (Germany).

mined. There is some overlapping of FRF and LRF activities. The concentrations of Na^+, K^+ and Ca^{++} in the fractions are measured using flame photometry. Starting from the fractions 55 to 60, these ions are present in all fractions. The LRF activity is determined using either the OAAD test or the incubation method as described above. The lyophilized LRF fraction (3.9 g) is desalted by phenol extraction. The fraction is dissolved in 80 ml water saturated with H_2S and this solution is extracted twice with 40 and 20 ml phenol saturated with water and H_2S. The phenol extracts containing LRF are washed 4 or 5 times with water and 80 ml of water together with 500 ml of ether saturated with H_2S are added. After equilibration the ether-phenol phase is washed five times with water, the aqueous phases are combined and extracted several times with ether to remove traces of phenol. The aqueous phases are heated under vacuum to remove ether and lyophilized. All the LRF activity is concentrated in this material (0.38 g) which is dissolved in 30 ml of 0.01 M ammonium acetate buffer, pH 4.5 and chromatographed on a CMC column (2.4 x 40 cm) equilibrated with the same buffer. After 22 fractions of 10 ml had been collected, a gradient to pH 7, 0.1 M buffer through a 1000 ml mixing flask is set up. Fig. 2 shows the results of chromatography on CMC.

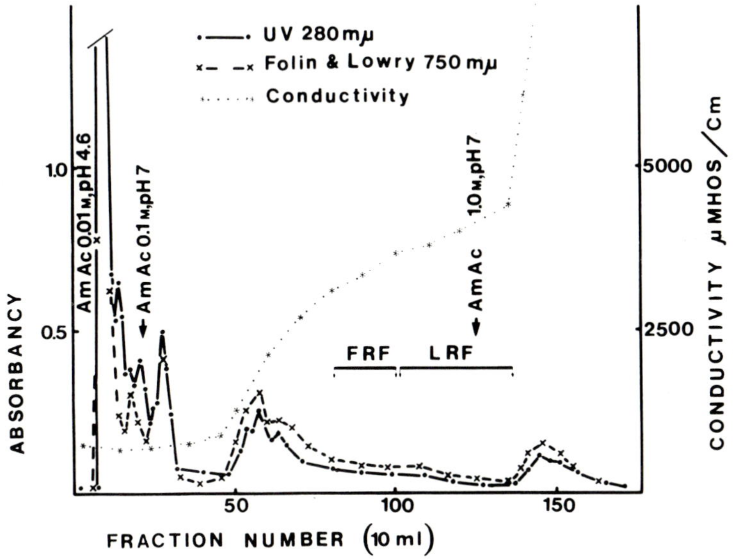

Fig. 2. Chromatography of FRF and LRF concentrates from Sephadex column and phenol extraction on CMC column (2.4 x 40 cm) equilibrated with 0.01 M ammonium acetate buffer, pH 4.5. Gradient to pH 7.0, 0.1 M buffer through 1000 ml mixing flask started at tube 22. Gradient to pH 7.0, 1.0 M buffer started at tube 125. Fraction size, 10 ml; 200 μl aliquots taken for Folin-Lowry colorimetry. From Berault (42).

The concentration of different products in the fractions is determined by the measurement of absorbancy at 280 mμ and Folin-Lowry colorimetry at 750 mμ. The conductivity of the fractions is also determined. LRF emerges in fractions 102 to 137 (Fig. 2), well separated from vasopressin (fractions 138 to 163). Some overlapping is observed between fractions containing LRF and FRF. After lyophilization of the fraction containing LRF, the yield is 15.5 mg of a dry product which is active in vivo at a dose of 3 to 6 μg on the elevation of plasma LH levels in ovariectomized estrogen and progesterone-treated rats. In vitro, a dose of 0.08 to 0.15 μg of the same product per mg or pituitary tissue is able to release a significant amount of LH from pituitaries of the same type of rats (see assay for LRF above).

A very similar method (but without phenol extraction) was used by Dhariwal et al. (45) for the purification of ovine LRF. Nikitovitch-Winer et al. (46) dialyzed a boiled acid extract of SME before fractionating the dialysate on a CMC column under conditions similar to those described above. Fawcett et al. (47) accomplished a partial purification of LRF by a procedure in five steps: Two cycles of gel filtration of a crude extract on Sephadex G-25 column; chromatography on DEAE-Sephadex A-25; gel filtration on Sephadex G-25 in ethanol - 0.2 N-acetic acid (1:5, v/v) medium; thin-layer chromatography on microcrystalline cellulose in a butanol-acetic acid-water solvent. Gel filtration in a partially organic medium allowed the recovery of two zones of activity separated by an inactive fraction. To prepare partially purified ovine LRF, Johnson (25) extracted the tissue with an acetate buffer at pH 4.6 and precipitated the activity with 4 x vol of acetone. Precipitation of the active material with acetone was repeated twice more. The final product was assayed using the OAAD-test and also the weaver finch assay of Witschi (48).

2. <u>Bovine LRF</u>. Schally et al. (49,50) purified bovine LRF using a similar method to that described above for ovine LRF: an extract of SME in 2 N acetic acid was heated to boiling point, chilled, and lyophilized. After reextraction with glacial acetic acid, the lyophilized extract was submitted to Sephadex gel filtration, phenol desalting, and chromatography on CMC. This material was then rechromatographed once more on an analytical column of CMC. A partial purification of bovine LRF was also obtained by Ramirez et al. (51) by extensive heat treatment of a crude acidic extract followed by gel filtration on a Sephadex G-25 column.

3. <u>Porcine LRF</u>. LRF with the highest specific activity and free from other contaminant hormones was prepared from pig SME extracts by Schally et al. (14,23); the hypothalamic fragments were extracted in batches of 25,000 to 35,000 as described above for bovine LRF. The concentrates made from these extracts were passed through a preparative column of Sephadex G-25 equilibrated with 1M acetic acid. The results of this chromatography are shown in Fig. 3.

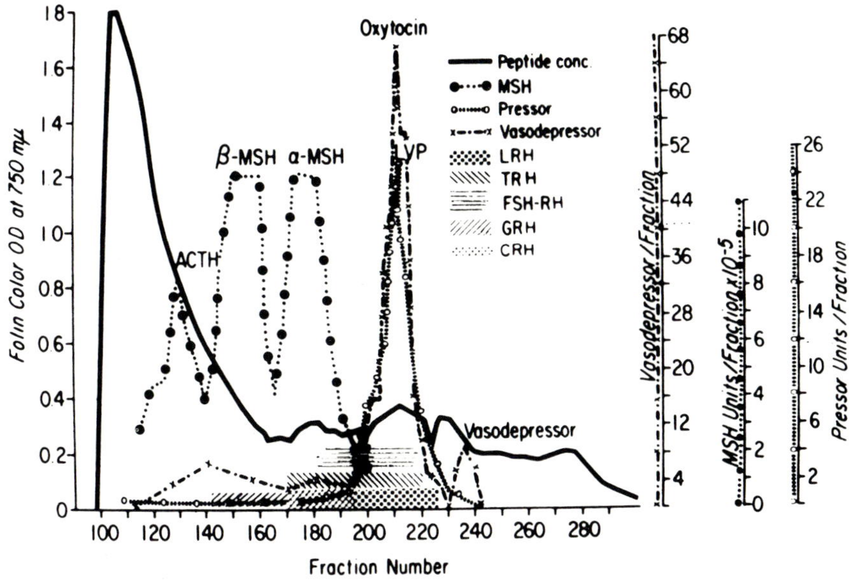

Fig. 3. Gel filtration of pig SME concentrates (10 g of material corresponding to about 3000 pig SME) on a column of Sephadex G-25 (7 x 170 cm) in 1.0 M acetic acid. Fraction sizes 25 ml; 50 μl aliquots taken for Folin-Lowry analysis. (From Schally et al. Recent Progress in Hormone Research, 24: 505, 1968.)

LRF activity emerged in fractions that also contained corticotropin releasing factor (CRF), thyrotropin releasing factor (TRF) and FRF activities. Zones containing these activities were combined and extracted together with phenol. Phenol desalted material was then submitted to CMC chromatography. This chromatography separated TRF and most of the vasopressin from CRF, LRF and FRF which emerged in the same zone together with α-MSH. Separation of CRF from a zone containing LRF activity and FRF activity was accomplished by a second chromatography on an analytical column of CMC. A complete separation of LRF from FRF was effected by preparative column electrophoresis illustrated in Fig. 4.

As shown in Fig. 4, FRF activity moved strongly towards the cathode and was well separated from the LRF zone. LRF thus prepared was active in vivo at a dose of 5 ng on the elevation of plasma LH level in ovariectomized, estrogen and progesterone-treated rats. In vitro, a dose of 20 ng/ pituitary was able to release a significant amount of LH (see LRF - 2 above). It was free of other known hypothalamic RF and of vasopressin.

4. LRF from other sources. Barry et al. (17) reported the partial purification of an LRF activity present in the lateral hypothalamus of guinea-pig. These authors used gel filtration on Sepha-

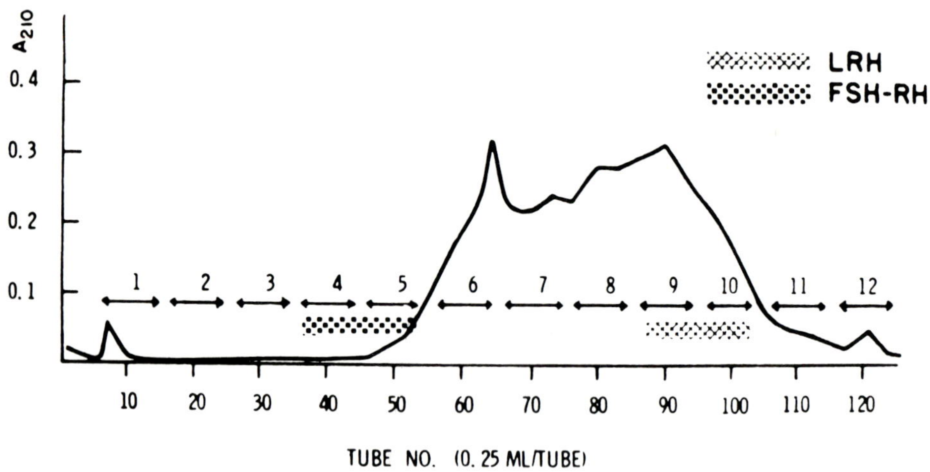

Fig. 4. Column electrophoresis of FRF (FSH-RH), LRF (LRH) concentrate from rechromatography on CMC. Elution pattern from vertical LKB apparatus No. 3340-c fitted with column 0.9 x 38 cm; supporting medium Sephadex G-25; fraction size, 0.25 ml/tube. A_{210} readings taken on fractions after removal of buffer by lyophilization. Starting material: 3.2 mg of solids. Conditions: 1000 V for 2.5 hr; cathode at bottom. Buffer was pH 6.5 pyridine acetate. (From Schally et at. Recent Progress in Hormone Research, 24: 543, 1968).

dex G-50 and a micro scale preparative electrophoresis (52) at pH 3.9. In this latter procedure, they isolated a small amount of a material that was active on the depletion of ovarian cholesterol in immature rats pretreated with PMS and HCG (53).

Starting from rat hypothalamic tissue Kobayashi et al. (54) partially purified LRF and separated it from FRF using gel filtration on a Sephadex G-25 column. LRF activity was assayed in an in vitro system in which rat anterior pituitaries were cultured by the organ culture method (55). The LH activity was estimated in the culture medium using the OAAD-test (27) and the FSH activity using the Steelman-Pohley method (38).

Purification of FRF

1. Ovine FRF. Partial purification of FRF has been accomplished in our laboratory (40,42) using the same method as that described above for ovine LRF. The following steps were followed; Extraction of SME with 2 N acetic acid; reextraction of lyophilized extract with glacial acetic acid; gel filtration on a Sephadex G-25 column; phenol extraction; chromatography on a CMC column. As shown in Fig. 1, the FRF activity emerges from Sephadex just before the LRF activity in fractions 59 to 71, but the two activities overlap to some extent. FRF is assayed using the in vitro method of incubation of pituitaries of either ovariectomized rats pretreated with

estrogen and progesterone, or normal male rats (see FRF - 2 above). During the chromatography on CMC, FRF emerges in fractions 82 to 102 and overlaps slightly with LRF (Fig. 2). Starting with 20,000 SME, the yield is 9.2 mg of FRF. This product is active in vitro at a dose of 5 ng per mg of pituitary tissue (41).

Dharival et al. (56) were the first to obtain a partial separation of ovine FRF from LRF on a Sephadex G-25 column. In another paper, Dhariwal et al. (57) reported on the chromatographic behavior of ovine FRF on CMC.

2. Bovine FRF. The same method was used for the purification of bovine FRF as for bovine LRF (50). FRF activity was estimated by measuring depletion of FSH from pituitaries of normal or testosterone-treated male rats, as well as elevation of plasma FSH activity in ovariectomized rats, pretreated with estrogen and progesterone (see FRF - 1 above). FRF activity was found to emerge from Sephadex before LRF and vasopressin and was found to be essentially free of LRF. The FRF zone from Sephadex was further purified by phenol extraction and chromatography on CMC. This step separated FRF from TRF. The FRF thus purified was able to deplete pituitary FSH content in vivo at doses of 10 to 47 μg.

3. Porcine FRF. Schally et al. (22,23) prepared highly purified porcine FRF essentially by the same steps as for porcine LRF. As shown in Fig. 3, FRF activity emerged from Sephadex in the same fractions as LRF, TRF and CRF, in contrast to bovine material. After extraction of the combined fractions with phenol, chromatography and rechromatography on a CMC column left FRF and LRF in the same fraction, completely separated from TRF and CRF. As shown in Fig. 4, a complete separation of FRF from LRF was achieved by preparative column electrophoresis. As in the case of bovine material FRF activity was estimated by the depletion of pituitary FSH content in rats. The highly purified fraction was found to be active at doses of the order of 10 ng. This product was free of LRF and other known hypothalamic RF.

4. FRF from other sources. Kobayashi et al. (54) prepared a partially purified rat FRF by gel filtration, as described above for rat LRF.

CHEMICAL PROPERTIES AND STABILITY

While this review was being written (December 1969), the exact chemical nature of LRF and FRF was still unknown. However, our knowledge in this field is progressing very rapidly and it is probable that in some months' time we should have more information on this subject. The generally accepted view that LRF and FRF are simple polypeptides has recently been questioned (58,59). In our opinion the question however still remains open. The story of the nature of TRF is a good example which shows how dangerous these kind of presumptions may be.

LRF

McCann (28) was the first to show that LRF activity was destroyed by incubation with trypsin, slightly reduced by pepsin, and that it was thermostable. In an early note from our laboratory (60), we reported that pepsin destroys and that trypsin greatly diminishes the LRF activity of ovine origin. The destruction of LRF activity (ovine) by proteolytic treatment with pepsin was also reported by Fawcett et al. (47). The stability of LRF to heat was generally accepted with the exception of Johnson (25) who found that heating to 100° C for 1 min inactivated LRF. Schally and Bowers (49) were the first to report an amino acid composition for their bovine LRF and stated that the purified material showed only one major ninhydrin-positive component on paper chromatography or electrophoresis. Similar results concerning ovine LRF were reported by Guillemin (61). The absence of cystine in bovine LRF has been demonstrated by Ramirez and McCann (62). All these results and also the position of LRF in the chromatographic pattern led several authors to the conclusion that LRF activity was associated with a basic polypeptide having a molecular weight of 1200 to 2000 (45,47, 49,60,61,63,64). Nikitovitch-Winer et al. (46) reported that their purified ovine LRF "is probably a small polypeptide which is dialyzable, heat stable, has little absorbancy at either 260 or 280 m μ, and does not give a positive reaction with ninhydrin after paper chromatography."

The polypeptidic nature of LRF has recently been questioned (23,58,59). Schally et al. (23) reported that pepsin does not inactivate highly purified LRF, and trypsin does so only at high enzyme/substrate ratios. They further reported that chymotrypsin inactivates LRF even at an enzyme/substrate ratio of 1/30. Overnight incubation at 38°C at pH 8 did not affect LRF activity, but a similar incubation at pH 2 slightly decreased it. They concluded that an apparent effect of chymotrypsin and trypsin can perhaps be accounted for by contamination with other enzymes or the ability of these enzymes to hydrolyze other bonds in addition to peptide linkage (ester, hydrazide, hydroxyamide, amide). This fact and also the observation that acid hydrolysis of highly purified porcine and bovine LRF revealed only trace amounts of amino acids (14,23) led Schally and Kastin (59) to the conclusion that LRF consisted of a non peptide, hydrosoluble molecule with a molecular weight of less than 1500 and with a basic isoelectric point.

FRF

Very little information is available on the nature of FRF. Several authors (21,56,57) reported that FRF is a small polypeptide with a molecular weight of 1200 to 2000. Further, Dhariwal et al.

(57) indicated that their purified FRF was a relatively small basic polypeptide (but less basic than LRF), heat stable, and that it was inactivated by tryptic digestion.

Recently White et al. (65) isolated five polyamines from porcine hypothalamus: histamine, putrescine, spermidine, spermine and lysine. They stated that taken together these substances account for most of the FSH-depleting activity in vivo of the crude extract. These and other results led Schally et al. (22,23) and White et al. (65) to consider that FRF is probably a polyamine derivative with a molecular weight of not more than 300. With de la Llosa (41) we checked the action of these polyamines in our in vitro system and we found that they were inactive on the release of FSH at doses of 0.05 to 1.25 μg per mg of pituitary tissue. This was confirmed recently by Mittler and Schally (23) who indicated that putrescine, cadaverine, spermine, spermidine and agmatine at doses of 2 to 10 μg per mg of pituitary tissue had no effect on release of FSH in vitro. They concluded that FRF is not one of these polyamines. Kamberi and McCann(66) reported that some biogenic amines enhanced the release of FSH in vitro, but only at high, nonphysiological doses. Thus the in vivo response stated by White et al. (65) may be indirect in nature and it seems evident from these results that it is not yet possible to assign FRF activity to a specific feature of the chemical structure.

SUMMARY

The most frequently employed tests for assay of LH-releasing factor (LRF) are, in vivo: The ovarian ascorbic acid depletion test of Parlow and the determination of the elevation of plasma LH levels in chronically ovariectomized, estrogen and progesterone-treated rats (EBP rats); in vitro: The incubation of pituitaries of EBP rats. FSH-releasing factor (FRF) is assayed in vivo by either determination of the elevation of plasma FSH levels in EBP rats or the determination of the depletion of the pituitary FSH content in different types of rats; in vitro by the incubation of pituitaries of normal male rats or EBP rats.

Highly purified preparations of LRF and FRF from three species have been obtained: sheep, cattle and pig, but they still seem heterogeneous. The most widely used method for purifing hypothalamic hormones consists of the following steps: Extraction of hypothalamic tissue with 2 N acetic acid; lyophilization and reextration with glacial acetic acid; lyophilization and gel filtration on Sephadex G-25; phenol extraction (desalting) and chromatography on CMC. The most highly purified preparations of LRF and FRF were obtained from porcine material.

The exact chemical nature of LRF and FRF is still unknown. The generally accepted view that these hormones are simple polypeptides has recently been questioned.

ACKNOWLEDGEMENT

This study was supported in part by research funds (R.C.P. no. 59) from the French National Research Council (C.N.R.S.).

REFERENCES

1. Harris, G.W., Neural control of the pituitary gland, Arnold, London, 1955.
2. Benoit, J. and Assenmacher, I., J. Physiol. (Paris), 47: 427, 1955.
3. Harris, G.W., in Villee, C.A., Control of Ovulation, Pergamon Press, New York, p. 56, 1961.
4. Campbell, H.J., Feuer, C., Garcia, G. and Harris, G.W., J. Physiol. (London), 157, 30p, 1961.
5. McCann, S.M., Taleisnik, S. and Friedman, H.M., Proc. Soc. Exp. Biol. Med., 104: 432, 1960.
6. McCann, S.M., and Taleisnik, S., Endocrinology, 68: 1071, 1961.
7. Piacsek, B.E. and Meites, J., Endocrinology, 79: 432, 1966.
8. Courrier, R., Guillemin, R., Jutisz, M., Sakiz, E. and Aschheim, P., C.R. Acad. Sci. (Paris), 253: 922, 1961.
9. Nikitovitch-Winer, M.B., Endocrinology, 70: 350, 1962.
10. Campbell, H.J., Feuer, G. and Harris, G.W., J. Physiol. (London), 170: 474, 1964.
11. Schally, A.V. and Bowers, C.Y., Endocrinology, 75: 312, 1964.
12. Guillemin, R., Jutisz, M. and Sakiz, E., C.R. Acad. Sci. (Paris), 256: 504, 1963.
13. Johnson, D.C., Endocrinology, 72: 832, 1963.
14. Schally, A.V., Bowers, C.Y., White, W.F. and Cohen, A.I., Endocrinology, 81: 77, 1967.
15. Endroczi, E. and Hilliard, J., Endocrinology, 77: 667, 1965.
16. Barry, J., Dautrevaux, M., Lefranc, G. and Fourlinnie, J.C., C.R. Acad. Sci. (Paris), 257: 4217, 1963.
17. Barry, J., Moschetto, Y. and Leonardelli, J., C.R. Acad. Sci. (Paris), 265: serie D, 1141, 1967.
18. Schally, A.V., Mueller, E.E., Arimura, A., Bowers, C.Y., Saito, T., Redding, T.W., Sawano, S. and Pizzolato, P., J. Clin. Endocr.,27: 755, 1967.
19. Igarashi, M. and McCann, S.M., Endocrinology, 74: 446, 1964.
20. Mittler, J.C. and Meites, J., Proc. Soc. Exp. Biol. Med., 117: 309, 1964.
21. Kuroshima, A. Ishida, Y., Bowers, C.Y. and Schally, A.V., Endocrinology, 76: 614, 1965.
22. Schally, A.V., Saito, T., Arimura, A., Sawano, S., Bowers, C.Y., White, W.F. and Cohen, A.I., Endocrinology, 81: 882, 1967.
23. Schally, A.V., Arimura, A., Bowers, C.Y., Kastin, A.J., Sawano, S. and Redding, T.W., Recent Progr. Hormone Res., 24: 497, 1968.
24. Saffran, M., Schally, A.V. and Benfey, B.G., Endocrinology, 57: 439, 1955.
25. Johnson, D.C., Experientia, 20: 311, 1964.

26. Schiavi, R., Jutisz, M., Sakiz, E. and Guillemin, R., Proc. Soc. Exp. Biol. Med., 114: 426, 1963.
27. Parlow, A.F., In Albert, A., Human Pituitary Gonadotropins, Thomas, C.C., Springfield, p. 300, 1961.
28. McCann, S.M., Amer. J. Physiol., 202: 395, 1962.
29. Guillemin, R. and Sakiz, E., Endocrinology, 72: 813, 1963.
30. Novella, M.-A., Alloiteau, J.-J. and Aschheim, P., C.R. Acad. Sci. (Paris), 259: 1553, 1964.
31. McCann, S.M. and Taleisnik, S., Amer. J. Physiol., 199: 847, 1960.
32. Ramirez, V.D. and McCann, S.M., Endocrinology, 73: 193, 1963.
33. Jutisz, M., Berault, A., Novella, M.-A and Ribot, G., Acta Endocr. (Kobenhavn), 55: 481, 1967.
34. David, M.A., Fraschini, F. and Martini, L., Experientia, 21: 483, 1965.
35. Corbin, A. and Story, J.C., Experientia, 22: 694, 1966.
36. Saito, T., Arimura, A., Mueller, E.E., Bowers, C.Y. and Schally, A.V., Endocrinology, 80: 313, 1967.
37. Kuroshima, A., Arimura, A., Saito, T., Ishida, Y., Bowers, C. Y. and Schally, A.V., Endocrinology, 78: 1105, 1966.
38. Steelman, S.L. and Pohley, F.M., Endocrinology, 53: 604, 1953.
39. Mittler, J.C. and Meites, J., Endocrinology, 78: 500, 1966.
40. Jutisz, M. and de la Llosa, M.P., Endocrinology, 81: 1193, 1967.
41. Jutisz, M. and de la Llosa, M.P., Bull. Soc. Chim. Biol., 50: 2521, 1968.
42. Berault, A., Thesis, University of Paris, 1969.
43. Schally, A.V., Bowers, C.Y. and Redding, T.W., Endocrinology, 78: 726, 1966.
44. Goa, J., Scand. J. Clin. Lab. Invest., 5: 218, 1953.
45. Dhariwal, A.P.S., Antunes-Rodriques, J. and McCann, S.M., Proc. Soc. Exp. Biol. Med., 118: 999, 1965.
46. Nikitovitch-Winer, M.B., Pribble, A.H. and Winer, A.D., Amer. J. Physiol., 206: 1286, 1965.
47. Fawcett, C.P., Reed, M., Charlton, H.M. and Harris, G.W., Biochem. J., 106: 229, 1968.
48. Witschi, E., Mem. Soc. Endocr., 4: 149, 1955.
49. Schally, A.V. and Bowers, C.Y., Endocrinology, 75: 608, 1964.
50. Schally, A.V., Saito, T., Arimura, A., Muller, E.E., Bowers, C.Y. and White, W.F., Endocrinology, 79: 1087, 1966.
51. Ramirez, V.D., Nallar, R. and McCann, S.M., Proc. Soc. Exp. Biol. Med., 115: 1072, 1964.
52. Hannig, K., Hoppe Seyle Z. Physiol. Chem., 338: 211, 1964.
53. Bell, E.T., Mukerji, A. and Loraine, J.A., J. Endocr., 28: 321, 1964.
54. Kobayashi, T., Kobayashi, T., Kigawa, T., Mizuno, M., Amenomori, Y., Watanabe, T. and Ichikawa, H., Endocrinol. Jap., 14: 101, 1967.
55. Kobayashi, T., Kobayashi, T., Kigawa, T., Mizuna, M., Amenomori, Y. and Watanabe, T., Endocrinol. Jap., 13: 430, 1966.

56. Dhariwal, A.P.S., Nallar, R., Batt, M. and McCann, S.M., Endocrinology, 76: 290, 1965.
57. Dhariwal, A.P.S., Watanabe, S., Antunes-Rodrigues, J. and McCann, S.M., Neuroendocrinology, 2: 294, 1967.
58. Guillemin, R., Ann. Rev. Physiol., 29: 313, 1967.
59. Schally, A.V. and Kastin, A.J., Triangle (Journal Sandoz des Sciences Medicales), 9: 19, 1969.
60. Jutisz, M., de la Llosa, P.. Sakiz, E., Yamazaki, E. and Guillemin, R., C.R. Soc. Biol. (Paris), 157: 235, 1963.
61. Guillemin, R., Proc. 23rd Intern. Congr. Physiol. Sci. Excerpta Medica I.C.S., 87: 284, 1965.
62. Ramirez, V.D. and McCann, S.M., Amer. J. Physiol., 207:441, 1964.
63. McCann, S.M., Antunes-Rodrigues, J. and Dhariwal, A.P.S., Proc. 23rd Intern. Congr. Physiol. Sci., Excerpta Medica I.C.S., 87: 292, 1965.
64. Jutisz, M., Europ. Rev. Endocrin. Suppl. 2, part 1, Pergamon Press, p. 47, 1966.
65. White, W.F., Cohen, A.I., Rippel, R.H., Story, J.C. and Schally, A.V., Endocrinology, 82: 742, 1968.
66. Kamberi, I.A. and McCann, S.M., Endocrinology, 85: 815, 1969.

FURTHER STUDIES ON MECHANISM OF ACTION OF LUTEINIZING HORMONE RELEASING FACTOR USING IN VIVO AND IN VITRO TECHNIQUES

Marian Jutisz, Bernard Kerdelhue and Annette Berault

Equipe de recherche du CNRS, Laboratoire de Physiologie Cellulaire, College de France, 11 Place Marcelin, Berthelot, Paris Ve, France.

Some attempts have recently been made to discover the mechanisms whereby hypothalamic luteinizing hormone releasing factor (LRF) stimulates the release of luteinizing hormone (LH) from the anterior pituitary and its subsequent biosynthesis (1-3).

We reinvestigated some of the reported results using a highly purified preparation of LRF and a new procedure of incubation of pituitary glands. The recent development in our laboratory of a radioimmunoassay for rat LH (4,5) has provided a sensitive and precise technique for these studies. Some of our preliminary results, obtained by in vivo and in vitro techniques, are reported in the present paper.

MATERIAL AND METHODS

The highly purified preparation of LRF was prepared by gel filtration of a crude extract of sheep hypothalamus on Sephadex G-25 followed by chromatography on carboxymethyl cellulose (6). Cyclic AMP was supplied by Boehringer A.G., Mannheim, Germany.

Rats used for this work were Wistar females (CF strain, CNRS, Gif-sur-Yvette, Yvelines, France) ovariectomized when 40 days old (140 g). Thirty to 40 days later, and three days before sacrifice, they were injected with 25 μg of estradiol benzoate and 12 mg of progesterone (EBP rats). This treatment with steroids was selected after an investigation of the influence of different doses of steriods on the plasma LH concentration in rats injected or not with LRF.

For in vivo studies, groups of three to five animals per treatment were anesthetized with ethylurethane (150 mg/100 g body wt; solution 300 mg/ml) and LRF solutions or normal saline injected into the external jugular vein. 500 µl of blood were withdrawn from the same vein 5 to 8 min, 14 to 15 min, and 22 to 28 min after injection. LH was assayed in serum using a radioimmunoassay previously described (4,5).

For in vitro experiments, hemipituitaries (4 to 5 per flask) were rinsed twice with 2 ml each time of Krebs-Ringer bicarbonate-glucose buffer (KRB) and "preincubated" for a period of 30 min in 2 ml of the same medium saturated with 93% O_2 /7% CO_2 to remove LH liberated from non-viable cells. After changing the medium, incubation proceeded for 4 hr in 2 ml of either normal or modified KRB. A high $[K^+]$ medium was prepared by increasing the concentration of K^+ from 5.9 to 59 mM and removing an equivalent amount of Na^+. In one case, cyclic AMP and LRF were added at the beginning of the incubation period in flasks containing hemipituitaries of each pair; the other hemipituitaries served as control. After a 2 hr period the media were replaced by fresh media of the same composition, and incubation proceeded for a further 2 hr period. In other experiments, incubation was started in normal or high $[K^+]$ KRB, in the presence or absence of cyclic AMP or theophylline. After 2 hr of incubation, and without changing the media, LRF or cyclic AMP were added to some flasks, media were gassed and incubation proceeded for a further 2 hr period. Ten µl of media were withdrawn at 30 to 60 min periods during the incubation, using Eppendorf pipettes, and were stored frozen until assayed. Results are expressed in terms of a highly purified rat LH laboratory reference preparation (preparation S15B; mean potency, 0.95 x NIH-LH-S1; see ref. 4). Following incubation groups of hemipituitaries were weighed to 0.05 mg.

RESULTS

Alteration of the Plasma LH Concentration After Injection of LRF.

Two doses of the LRF preparation were injected, 6 and 12 µg per rat. Fig. 1 shows that the concentrations of plasma LH increase rapidly during the first 5 to 8 min following injection to a value 2-3 times higher than that of the controls. Maximal levels of LH are reached in 14 to 15 min; the LH concentrations then decrease.

Kinetics of the Response of In Vitro Pituitaries to LRF, Cyclic AMP and High $[K^+]$

As shown in Fig 2, the response of pituitaries in vitro to LRF (4 µg/ml), cyclic AMP (15 mM), and high $[K^+]$ is very rapid but the amount of LH released after 2 hr of incubation is higher after stimulation with an optimal dose of LRF and with high $[K^+]$ than in the presence of an optimal dose of cyclic AMP. After a 2 hr incubation

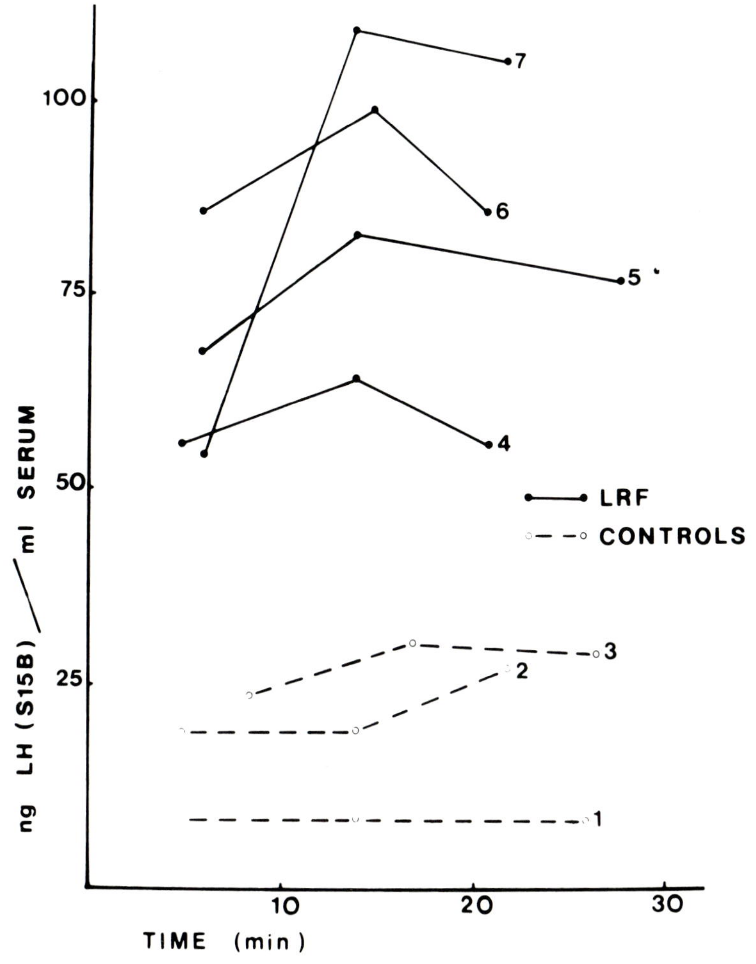

Fig. 1. Alteration of the plasma LH concentration in EBP rats after injection of LRF. At time 0, animals are injected into the external jugular vein with normal saline (1,2,3), 6 μg LRF (4,5), or 12 μg LRF (6,7). Assays of LH were performed using a radioimmunoassay method and results were expressed in terms of a laboratory reference preparation of rat LH (From: Kerdelhue et al. C. R. Acad. Sci. Ser. D., 270: 1010, 1970).

and changing the media, the release of LH was readily reinitiated under the same conditions as existed at the beginning of incubation, but the levels of LH were lower than during the first 2 hr. period.

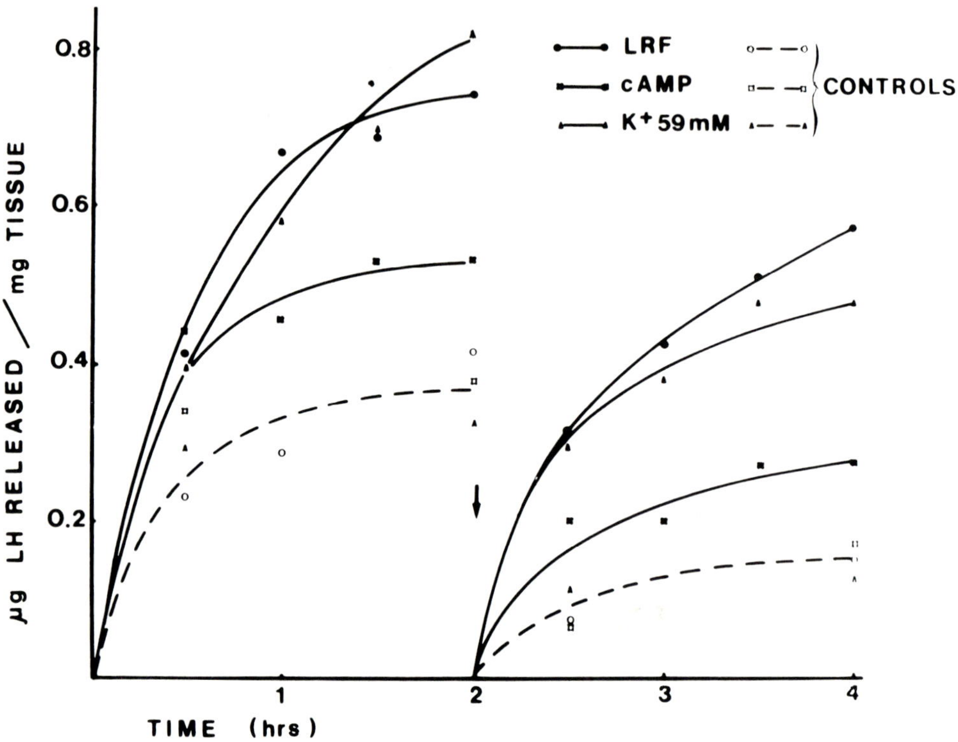

Fig. 2. Kinetics of the response to LRF, cyclic AMP (cAMP), and high [K^+] of pituitaries of EBP rats in vitro. Four groups of pairs of 4-5 hemipituitaries were incubated in 2 ml of either normal KRB (controls) or in KRB containing LRF (4 μg/ml), cyclic AMP (15 mM), or 59 mM K^+. One half of the pituitary served as a control for the other half. After a 2 hr incubation, media were replaced by fresh media of the same composition and incubation proceeded for a further 2 hr period. Assays were performed using a radioimmunoassay method and results were expressed in terms of a laboratory reference preparation of rat LH.

Potentiation of the Action of LRF by Theophylline

Two groups of pairs of hemipituitaries were incubated, one pair in each group in normal KRB, and another in KRB containing 1 mM of theophylline. As shown in Fig. 3, the addition of the same dose (4 μg/ml) of LRF to both groups provokes the release of LH, which is significantly greater in the medium containing theophylline. Under the same conditions, the addition of cyclic AMP (15 mM) instead of LRF, failed to alter significantly the release of LH, either in the presence, or in the absence of theophylline.

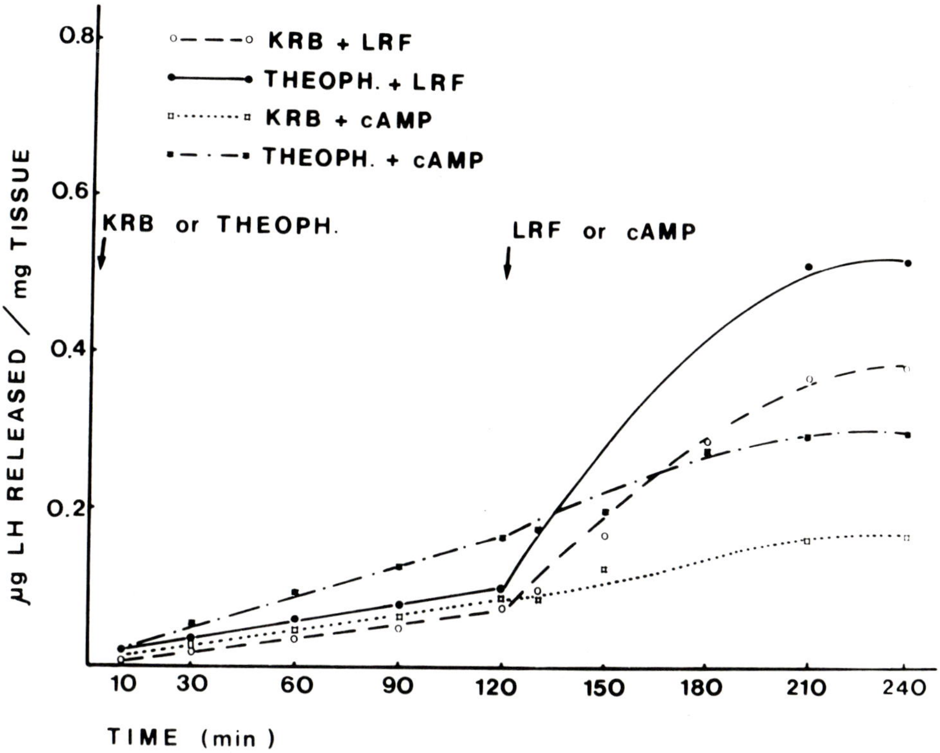

Fig. 3. Kinetics of the response to LRF and cyclic AMP (cAMP) of pituitaries of EBP rats incubated in the presence of theophylline. Two groups of pairs of 4-5 hemipituitaries were incubated, one pair in each group in a normal KRB, and another in KRB containing 1 mM of theophylline. After a 2 hr incubation, LRF (4 μg/ml) was added to one group of pairs and cyclic AMP (15mM) to the other group, and incubation proceeded for a further 2 hr period. Assays were performed using a radioimmunoassay method and results were expressed in terms of a laboratory reference preparation of rat LH.

Enhancement of the Effects of "Optimal" High [K+] by LRF on the Release of LH

One group of pairs of hemipituitaries was incubated separately for 2 hr in a high [K+] medium, then LRF (4 μg/ml) was added to one flask only and incubation continued for a further 2 hr period. Similarly another group of pairs of hemipituitaries was incubated in KRB containing 15 mM of cyclic AMP; after 2 hr incubation, LRF (4 μg/ml) was added to one flask, and the same amount of cyclic AMP as in the starting solution (15 mM) to the second flask. As shown in Fig. 4, when high $[K^+]$ and LRF were both present, the effects were greater than either alone produced. On the other hand, the results obtained with the second group confirmed those shown in Fig. 2, i.e., the amount of LH released with an optimal dose of LRF was higher than that released with an optimal dose of cyclic AMP. Fig. 4 shows also that the release of LH starts later in the presence of cyclic AMP than in the presence of LRF.

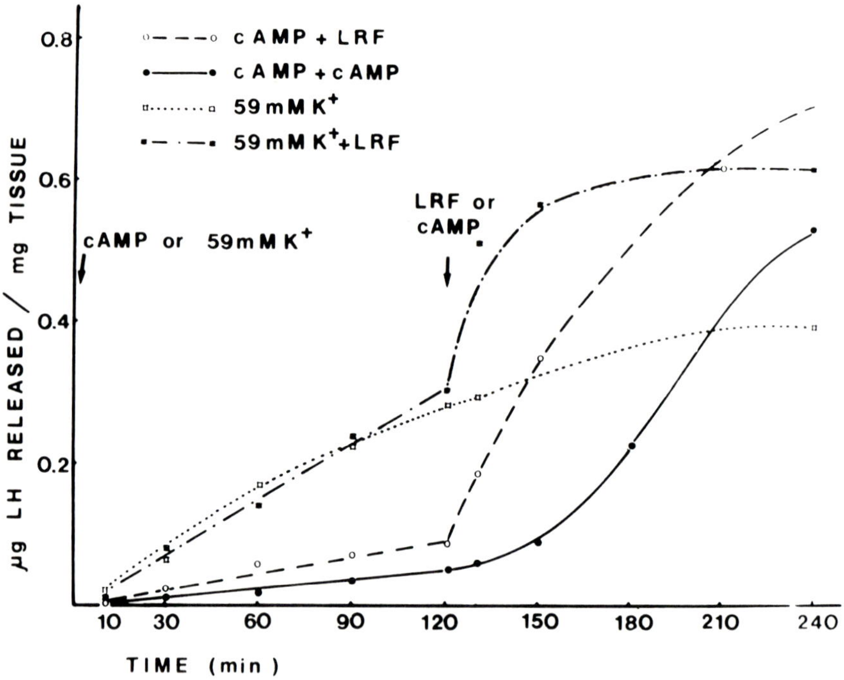

Fig. 4. Kinetics of the response to LRF and to a "double dose" of cyclic AMP (cAMP) of pituitaries of EBP rats incubated previously in the presence of cyclic AMP or in a high $[K^+]$ medium. Two groups of pairs of 4-5 hemipituitaries were incubated, one group in a normal KRB containing cyclic AMP (15 mM), and another in KRB containing 59 mM K^+. After 2 hr of incubation, in the first group, LRF (4 μg/ml) was added to one flask and cyclic AMP to the second flask; in the second group, LRF (4 μg/ml) was added only to one flask. Incubation proceeded for a further 2 hr period. Assays were performed using a radioimmunoassay method and results were expressed in terms of a laboratory reference preparation of rat LH.

DISCUSSION

Studies of the kinetics of the response of rats to LRF injected intravenously indicate that the response is rapid with maximal levels of LH being reached in 14 to 15 min. Similar results with a highly purified porcine LRF were obtained by Schally (maximal effect in 10 to 12 min, personal communication), and with a crude hypothalamic extract by Gay et al. (7).

Studies of the kinetics of the response of rat pituitary tissue to LRF, high $[K^+]$ medium and cyclic AMP indicate that the levels of LH released in 59 mM K^+ medium and in a normal KRB medium containing an optimal dose of LRF are very similar. The amount of LH released in the presence of cyclic AMP is much lower. Similar observations have been made in the case of FSH release as stimulated by FRF or by cyclic AMP (8). It is possible that penetration of cyclic AMP into the receptor cells is slower than is the action of LRF which may activate a cell membrane enzyme and therefore does not need to penetrate inside the cell (9). Another possibility is that cyclic AMP may be rapidly destroyed by phosphodiesterase (10). That the action of cyclic AMP on the release of LH is slower than the action of LRF is also shown in Fig. 4. Potentiation of the action of LRF by theophylline (Fig. 3) is good presumptive evidence of the participation of cyclic AMP. In the experiment shown in Fig. 3, the action of cyclic AMP was not potentiated by theophylline but it should be noted that this potentiation is often difficult to demonstrate as is the action of cyclic AMP itself. The reason for this difficulty is unknown.

The effects of "optimal" high $[K^+]$ are enhanced by LRF (Fig. 4) as has been already shown by Samli and Geschwind (2), and this may mean that high $[K^+]$ acts on the release of LH in a different way than does LRF. The release of neural hormones by a high $[K^+]$ was attributed by Douglas (11) to the depolarization of the specific cell membrane. Therefore, LRF may not act by the same mechanism.

REFERENCES

1. Samli, M.H. and Geschwind, I.I., Endocrinology, 81: 835, 1967.
2. Samli, M.H. and Geschwind, I.I., Endocrinology, 82: 225, 1968.
3. Jutisz, M., De La Llosa, M.P., Berault, A. and Kerdelhue, B., Proceedings of the Workshop Conference on the Integration of Endocrine and Non endocrine Mechanisms in the Hypothalamus, Eds. Martini, L. and Motta, M., Academic Press, New York, 1970 (in press).
4. Kerdelhue, B., Berault, A., Courte, C. and Jutisz, M., C.R. Acad. Sci., Ser. D, 269: 2413, 1969.
5. Kerdelhue, B., Berault, A., Ribot, G. and Jutisz, M., C.R. Acad. Sci., Ser. D, 270: 1010, 1970.
6. Jutisz, M, Berault, A., Novella, M.-A., and Ribot, G., Acta Endocr. (Kobenhavn), 55: 481, 1967.
7. Gay, V.L., Rebar, R.W. and Midgley, A.R. Jr., Proc. Soc. Exp. Biol. Med., 130: 1344, 1969.

8. Jutisz, M., and De La Llosa, M.P., C.R. Acad. Sci., Ser. D, 268: 1636, 1969.
9. Sutherland, E.W., Oye, I. and Butcher, R.W., Recent Progr. Hormone Res., 21: 623, 1965.
10. Robison, G.A., Butcher, R.W. and Sutherland, E.W., Ann. Rev. Biochem., 37: 149, 1968.
11. Douglas, W.W., Nature, (London) 197: 81, 1963.

CHAPTER IV

REGULATION OF TESTICULAR FUNCTION

SECTION 2: TESTICULAR-PITUITARY INTERRELATIONSHIP

INVESTIGATIONS INTO THE FEED-BACK MECHANISM BETWEEN SPERMATOGENESIS AND GONADOTROPIN LEVEL IN MAN

Svend G. Johnsen

Hormone Department, Statens Seruminstitut, Copenhagen, and the Male Hypogonadism Study Section, Medical Outpatients' Department, University Hospital of Copenhagen

It is a well established fact that there is a close relationship between spermatogenesis and gonadotropins. Selective damage of the germinal epithelium can easily be induced experimentally or found clinically and it has been shown by many authors that spermatogenetic failure is associated with castration changes in the hypophysis and increase in the gonadotropin level. The cause of spermatogenetic damage is unimportant. Hypophyseal changes have been shown to occur after anti-spermatogenetic compounds (1,2), cadmium(3), radiation (4), testicular ischemia (5), cryptorchidism (6, 7,8) and in various testicular disorders in man (9-14). When there is a failure of spermatogenesis, the gonadotropin rise primarily affects FSH (7,14,15), although LH also seems to be involved (16).

In the literature there have been two different theories on the cause of this gonadotropin increase. Nelson (17) and Heller et al. (11) believed that gonadotropins were used by the germinal epithelium, and if the germinal epithelium ceased to function the unused hormone was excreted. This explained the increased urinary gonadotropin excretion in cases of spermatogenetic failure. This "utilization hypothesis" therefore implies that FSH production is running at full speed whether or not gonads are present. Although still maintained by Heller (cf. Moore et al. (2)), the theory is incompatible with the fact that castration causes an increase of gonadotropins not only in the urine, but also in the hypophysis (18,19). It is also incompatible with the occurrence of castration changes in the hypophysis after spermatogenetic failure. Furthermore, no one has ever shown "utilization" of a hormone in a target organ.

Discarding the "utilization" theory, the only other possibility is that during spermatogenesis, a substance is produced which is capable of inhibiting FSH release from the hypophysis. According to this "inhibin" theory there is a true feed-back mechanism between spermatogenesis and the hypophysis: FSH stimulates spermatogenesis which in turn releases a substance depressing FSH.

Unfortunately, however, neither the site of production of the FSH inhibitor nor its chemical nature have been disclosed (cf. discussion) and this means that fundamental knowledge of the regulation of testicular function is still lacking.

This study is concerned with the identification of the stage of spermatogenesis which is involved in the testicular-hypophyseal feedback mechanism in man. In 284 patients with a variety of primary testicular disorders, the degree of spermatogenesis was determined from testicular biopsies by a new method (testicular biopsy score count) and correlated with gonadotropin analyses. The study involved a number of analyses which are described in detail elsewhere (20). This survey presents an outline of the general findings.

MATERIAL AND METHODS

Urinary hypophyseal gonadotropins(HG) were determined by the method of Johnsen (21,22). Results are expressed in mouse uterus units (MUU) per 24 hours. The MUU were compared with an HMG standard (1 ampoule of 2nd IRP-HMG = 133 MUU). At FSH/LH ratios found in clinical samples, the MUU expresses FSH + LH (23). In an analysis of a large series of normal men the log HG showed no deviation from a normal distribution and log HG is used throughout the study.

The evaluation of degree of spermatogenesis was performed using the testicular biopsy score count method (24). The full comprehension of the present paper requires familiarity with the principle of this method and the reader is referred to the cited paper as only a brief description follows. In this score count method, each tubular section in one testicular biopsy section is given a score from 10 to 1 according to the following (abbreviated) criteria: Score 10 = full spermatogenesis, normal epithelium, 9 = many spermatozoa, but disorganized epithelium, 8 = only few spermatozoa, 7 = no spermatozoa, but many spermatids, 6 = no spermatozoa and only few spermatids, 5 = no spermatozoa, no spermatids, but many spermatocytes, 4 = no spermatozoa, no spermatids and only few spermatocytes, 3 = spermatogonia are the only germ cells present, 2 = no germ cells, but Sertoli cells, 1 = no cells in tubular section. "Spermatozoa" are here defined as cells having achieved the small head form of the spermatozoon and correspond to Clermont's spermatid b_2, c, d_1 and d_2 (25).

In the testicular degeneration the tubules lose their cell content in a fixed sequence so that the more mature forms usually disappear before the next stage is seriously affected (cf. Johnsen (24)).

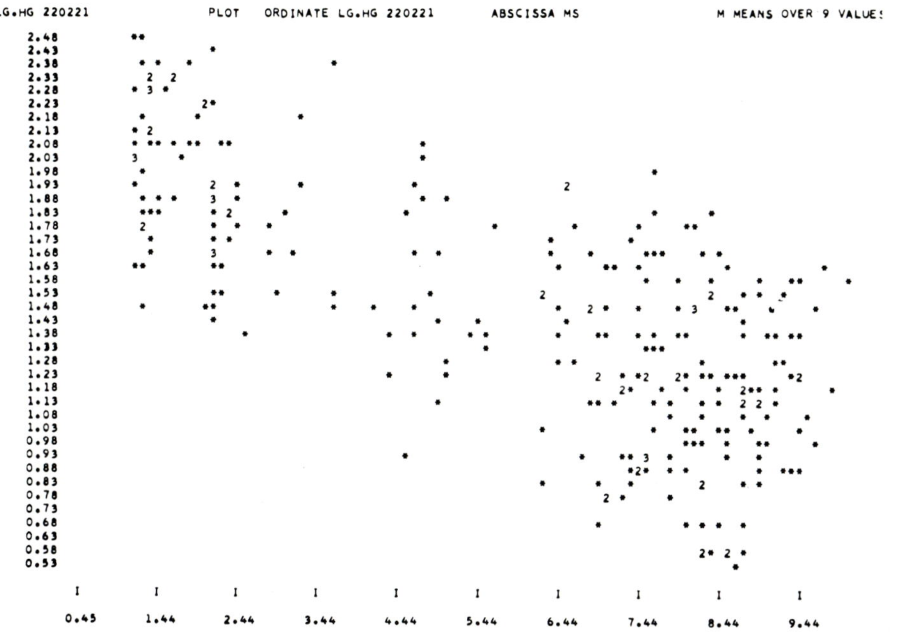

Fig. 1. Computer plot of the mean score of the testicular biopsy score count (abscissa) versus the log value of the excretion of hypophyseal gonadotropins in MUU per 24 hours (log HG) (ordinate). * = 1 value. M = over 9 values. 284 cases. (From: Johnsen, S.G., Acta Endocr.(Kobenhavn) in press).

The parameter in the present study is the cumulative percent (cum. %) of tubules scored at each step formed successively from step 10 to 2 (10 + 9, 10 + 9 + 8 etc). Thus, step 4 cum. % of 25 means that 25% of all tubules contained few spermatocytes, and that 75% did not show spermatocytes (these 75% might contain spermatogonia only, Sertoli cells only, or no cells at all). Cum. % 0 means absence of the cell recorded at the particular step and at all spermatogenetic stages above it (step 8 cum. % 0 = total absence of spermatozoa, step 6 cum. % = total absence of spermatids and higher stage, step 3 cum. % 0 = total absence of germ cells, etc.). A cum. % of 100 at a step means that all tubules contained at least the cell corresponding to this step.

In order to calculate a mean score (MS) the number of tubules recorded for each score is multiplied by that score and the sum of all 10 multiplications is divided by the total number of tubules. The mean number of tubules scored per biopsy was 113.

284 patients, all having primary testicular disorders, were used in the study. 98 had various degrees of oligospermia, 9 Sertoli-cell-only syndrome, 33 sequelae of testicular retention, 42 Kline-

felter's syndrome, 2 simple gynecomastia, 7 occlusion of the sperm tract, 73 varicocele (these were collected by Dr. P. Agger for a special study to be published elsewhere), 8 miscellaneous disorders and 12 were normal men. No evidence of impaired hypophyseal function was found in these groups.

RESULTS

Fig. 1 shows a plot of the mean score (MS) and log HG in the 284 patients. A very high correlation between the two was found. The correlation coefficient is 0.73 ($p < 0.001$) and the regression is given by: $\log HG = 2.125 - 0.113 \times MS$. The close relationship between spermatogenesis and gonadotropin output was thus confirmed.

It was thought that systematic plots and correlation between cumulative precentages (cum. %) and log HG at all score count steps in all 284 patients would be an effective tool in determining the stage of spermatogenesis involved in the feed-back mechanism. Theoretically, any stage could be involved and hypothetical curves for the correlations were drawn placing the determinative step at steps 8, 6, 4 and 3 corresponding to spermatozoa, spermatids, spermatocytes and spermatogonia. It was found that the determinative step would be the first step showing absence of low HG values at low cum. % (for example: if the presence of spermatocytes would determine the release of a gonadotropin inhibitor, then cases showing absence of spermatocytes (that is, low step 4 cum. %, cf. above) would show absence of low HG values. Cases with low HG values could, however, be present at low cum. % in higher steps because spermatocytes may be present in the absence of spermatozoa or spermatids. Therefore, taking the steps from above, step 4 would in this case be the first step showing the change). The determinative step would be the first showing a correlation between cum. % and log HG. The step above the determinative step would be the last step having low HG values at low cum. %, and the step below the determinative would be the first having some high HG values at high cum. % (high cum. % = cell scored fully present). If more than one spermatogenetic stage was involved, the HG at low cum. % should be expected to rise to a certain level at one step and further at another.

On this background, the systematic analysis at once revealed that the determinative step was step 8 (few or many spermatozoa present). Figs. 2, 3, 4 and 5 show the plots between log HG and cum. % from step 10 to step 7. Step 10 (Fig. 2) shows both high and low HG values at low cum. % and only low HG values at medium and higher cum. %. At step 9 (Fig. 3) there are less low HG values at low cum. %. When step 9 cum. % approaches zero the testis can at best contain tubules with few spermatozoa. Step 8 (Fig. 4) shows a great change. Low HG values at low cum. % have disappeared. When step 8 cum. % approaches zero spermatozoa are absent and it is seen that low HG values are absent also. At high cum. % at step 8 the HG values are, with a single exception, low. Step 7 (many spermatids present) is similar to step 8 at low cum. %, but a number of rather high HG values appear at high cum. %. Thus, whereas step 8 only had 1 log HG value > 1.64 at cum. % > 80, step 7 has 8 values and step 6, 10 values.

Table 1 shows the log HG values at low cum. % for all steps. It is seen that the gonadotropin level rises significantly from step 10 through step 9 to step 8. However, after step 8 no further rise is observed. When the cum. % is low at step 6 spermatids disappear, at step 4 spermatocytes disappear and at step 3 spermatogonia disappear, but the disappearance of these cells from the testis is associated with no further rise in gonadotropin level as seen when spermatozoa disappear.

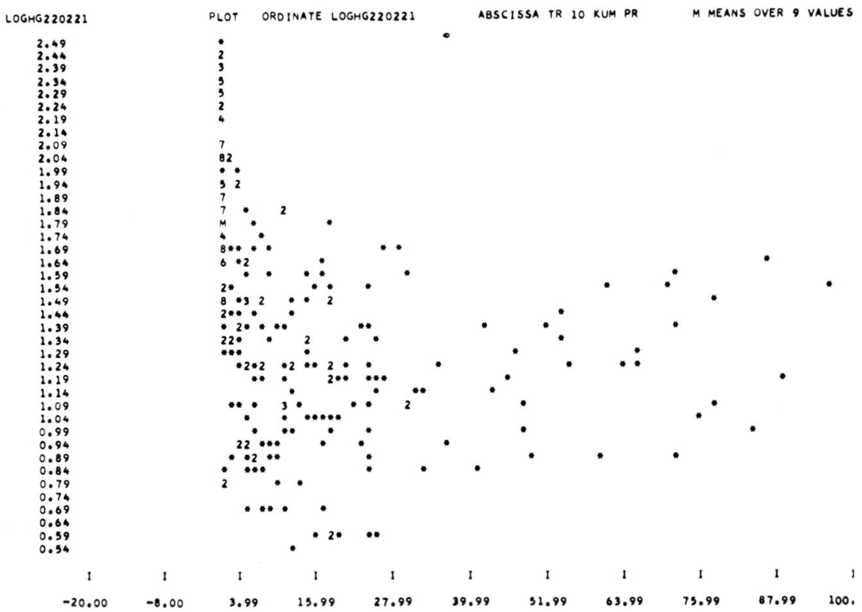

Fig. 2. Computer plot of the percent of tubules scored at step 10 of the testicular biopsy score count (abscissa) versus log HG. (From: Johnsen, S. G., Acta Endocr., (Kobenhavn) in press).

Correlation analyses between log HG and cum. % in the region 10-90 % showed no correlation at step 10 and step 9 ($p > 0.10$) but a high correlation at step 8 ($p < 0.001$). This correlation was

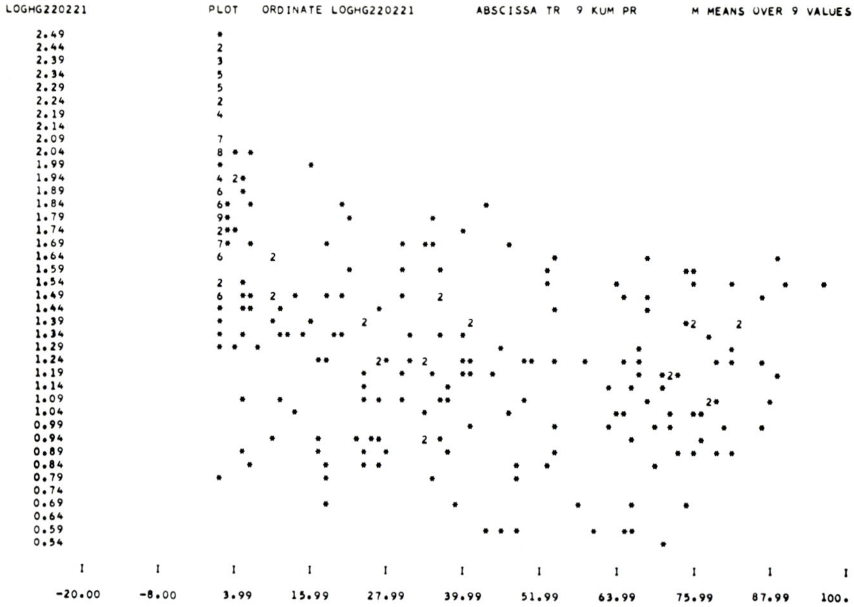

Fig. 3. Computer plot of the percent of tubules scored at step 10+9 (step 9 cumulative percent = 9 cum.%) (abscissa) versus log HG. (From: Johnsen, S. G., Acta Endocr., (Kobenhavn) in press).

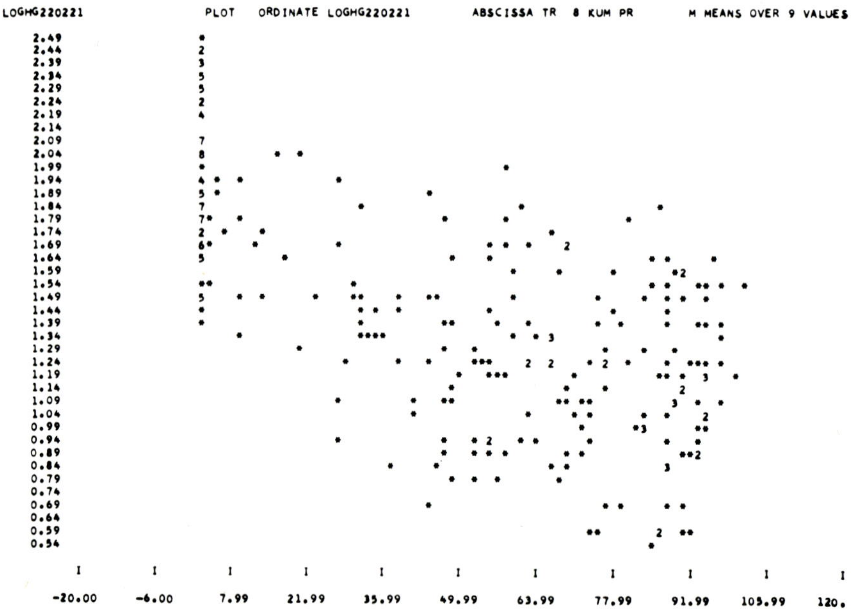

Fig. 4. Computer plot of step 8 cum. % versus log HG. (From: Johnsen, S.G., Acta Endocr ., (Kobenhavn) in press.)

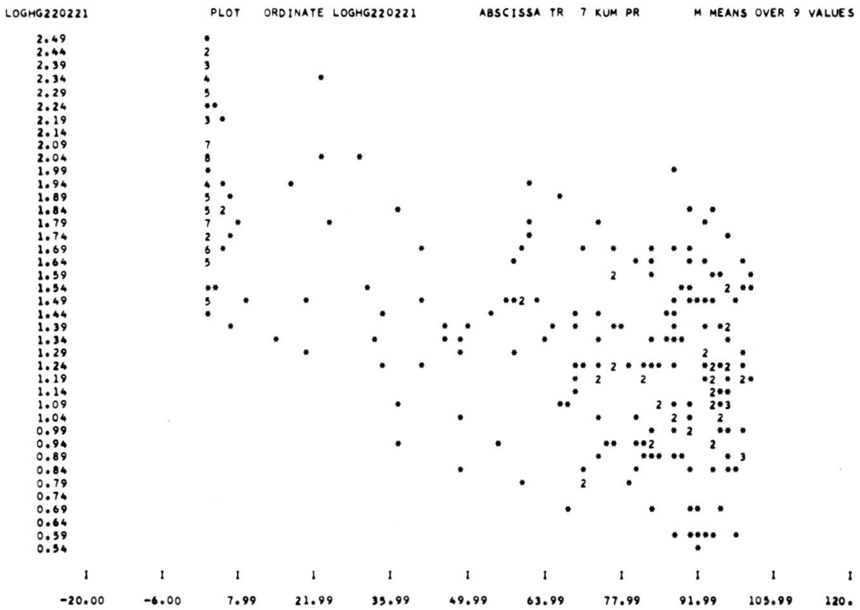

Fig. 5. Computer plot of step 7 cum. % versus log HG. (From: Johnsen, S.G., Acta Endocr., (Kobenhavn) in press).

Step	Number	Min.	Max.	Mean	s. d.	Mean: 95% fid. limits	p against preceding step
10	180	0.70	2.54	1.63	0.44	1.57 - 1.70	-
9	123	0.78	2.54	1.82	0.35	1.76 - 1.88	< 0.01
8	92	1.36	2.54	1.93	0.28	1.87 - 1.99	< 0.01
7	88	1.38	2.54	1.93	0.28	1.88 - 1.99	n. s.
6	85	1.38	2.54	1.94	0.28	1.88 - 2.00	n. s.
5	81	1.38	2.54	1.95	0.28	1.89 - 2.01	n. s.
4	78	1.45	2.54	1.96	0.27	1.90 - 2.02	n. s.
3	70	1.45	2.54	1.97	0.28	1.91 - 2.04	n. s.
2	11	1.62	2.46	2.02	0.25	1.87 - 2.17	n. s.

Table 1. Log values of excretion of hypophyseal gonadotropins when, at the steps of the testicular biopsy score count, the cumulative percent is 0 - 10 (= few or no cells, indicated by step number, present). n. s.: not significant. (From: Johnsen, S. G. Acta Endocrinologica, (Kobenhavn) in press).

Type of Biopsy	Elimination	No.	MEAN	s. d.	p against first group
No germ cells but Sertoli cells present	step 3 < 5 step 2 >90	22	1.80	0.24	-
No spermatozoa but spermatids present	step 8 < 5 step 6 >10	3	2.06	0.27	<0.10 >0.05
No spermatids but spermatocytes present	step 6 < 5 step 4 >90	3	1.66	0.18	<0.20 >0.15
No spermatocytes but spermatogonia present	step 4 < 5 step 3 >40	4	1.70	0.13	<0.25 >0.20
No germ cells No Sertoli cells	step 3 < 5 step 2 <10	11	2.02	0.25	<0.01

Table 2. Influence on log HG of spermatids in the absence of spermatozoa, spermatocytes in the absence of spermatids and higher stages, spermatogonia in the absence of spermatocytes and higher stages and Sertoli cells in the absence of germ cells. (From: Johnsen, S.G., Acta Endocrinologica, (Kobenhavn) in press).

maintained through all the following steps. All these showed a continuous shift of low HG values to the right. The correlation between log HG and cum. % took place at a still increasing HG level until at step 2 very high HG values were only found at cum. % lower than 100. However, depending on the number of tubules recorded at each step, these findings are more or less complicated by a mutual relationship between the cum. % at several steps and cannot be taken as evidence of a separate influence upon HG levels of steps below 8.

Screening procedures revealed that three patients possessed spermatids in the complete absence of spermatozoa, three had many spermatocytes in the complete absence of spermatids (complete meiotic arrest) and four had spermatogonia in the complete absence of spermatocytes. In Table 2 these 10 patients are compared with patients with only Sertoli cells and, as seen, no difference is found. This is a further indication that spermatids, spermatocytes and spermatogonia have no influence upon the HG level.

There was, however, a small but significant difference between patients possessing only Sertoli cells and patients having very few or no tubular cells (Table 2) and this indicated that Sertoli cells may have some influence upon the gonadotropin level although their depressing action is very small as compared with the effect of spermatozoa. It was here considered that the first group consists of cases of Sertoli-cell-only syndrome and the second of cases of Klinefelter's syndrome, and that the poor Leydig cell function described in the latter might be the explanation through an extra increase of LH. This possibility was, however, eliminated in a separate analysis where the group of 42 Klinefelter patients was compared with a group of 44 patients with severe hypospermatogenesis of non-chromosomal origin. In order to eliminate the influence of the germinal epithelium, the log HG was in all cases transformed to correspond to a mean score of 1 using the regression stated earlier (log HG transformed = log HG + 0.113 (MS - 1)). The XXY group thus had a mean value for log HG of 2.04 (s. d. 0.37) and the XY group 2.09 (s. d. 0.26). Thus, no separate extra-tubular influence upon HG was found in Klinefelter's syndrome and the demonstrated effect of Sertoli cells upon the HG level seems to be real.

The study has thus shown that the high correlation between spermatogenetic status and gonadotropin excretion is due to an effect of the spermatozoa (latest spermatids) in the testis. The last stage of spermatogenesis involving the maturation of the spermatozoa is the only spermatogenetic stage involved in the testicular-hypophyseal feed-back mechanism in man. Sertoli cells, either alone or accompanied by immature germ cells, seem to have a separate influence on the gonadotropin level. This is very small and only demonstrable when testes containing spermatozoa are excluded.

DISCUSSION

Possible Mechanism of the Inhibitory Action of the Spermatozoa

From a biological standpoint, the placement of the feed-back mechanism at the end of spermatogenesis is rational. The question remains how this end stage exerts the FSH inhibition.

Previously the author (12) put forward the hypothesis that the cytoplasm split off from the spermatozoa, as the residual body, which is rich in newly formed fat globules (26), contains a gonadotropin inhibitory substance. This theory places the feed-back at the spermatogenetic stage which we have shown here to be the effective one, but neither we, nor others, have published evidence to prove or disprove the theory.

Another possibility is that, by contact with the finished spermatozoon, a change is induced in the Sertoli cell so that this cell produces an FSH inhibitor. Brokelmann(27) found in the rat that, concurrently with spermatogenesis, structural changes indicating steroid secretion (cf. below) are induced in the Sertoli cell. Brokelmann showed that these changes occurred when the spermatozoa dived into the epithelium immediately prior to their escape. It is interesting that induction of Sertoli cell changes could be the first biological explanation of the meaning of the mysterious round trip journey of the nearly ripe spermatozoon down into the epithelium to the Sertoli cell nucleus.

The two theories are combined by Lacy (28-30) who showed that, in the rat, the residual bodies are phagocytosed by the Sertoli cells. He claimed that the residual bodies convey both information and material to the Sertoli cells which induce steroid production in them. Lofts (31) believes that the lipids found basally in Sertoli cells originate in the residual bodies. However, in our group, P. F. Larsen (unpublished observations) has, using electron microscopy studies in the human, been unable to find residual body remnants in the Sertoli cells.

Although the local effect of the spermatozoon is still open for speculation, the occurrence of changes in the Sertoli cell concurrently with spermatogenesis is well documented and suggests the possibility that the gonadotropin inhibitor is produced in this cell.

The Chemical Nature of the FSH Inhibitor

Androgens given in physiological doses suppress LH but not FSH (32-36). Gestagens have no physiological gonadotropin suppressing effect. It is, however, well documented that estrogens even at small doses suppress FSH (34-37). In fact estrogens are the only type of compound now known to be capable of suppressing FSH at a physiological dose level. This means that either spermatogenesis liberates estrogen, or an entirely new testicular hormone must exist. The second possibility appears very unlikely, and the key to the understanding of the regulation of the testis is therefore to look for estrogen production in the Sertoli cells.

Indications of Steroid Production in the Sertoli Cells

Brokelmann (27) found that the fine structure of the Sertoli cell "fits well into the cytoplasmic morphology of steroid producing cells." He found, concurrently with spermatogenesis, agranular endoplasmic reticulum, mitochondria with tubular christae and lipid droplets.

It has been found that Sertoli cells in higher animals do not possess a steroid 3β-ol-dehydrogenase (39-44) and thus presumably cannot perform a de novo steroid biosynthesis. However, they are known to possess certain steroid enzymes such as 3-, 16- and 17 - hydroxylases (45-47).

Christensen and Mason (45) found that in the tubules the complete biosynthesis from progesterone to testosterone can be carried out, and the presence of testosterone in the Sertoli cells was demonstrated immunologically by Woods and Domm (42).

Lacy et al. (48) claimed to have isolated estrone and estriol from the lipids which accumulate in rat Sertoli cells in large amounts when spermatogenesis is destroyed by irradiation, and according to Lofts (31) estrogens have been found in Sertoli cells of lower animals. Although further evidence is required, certain indications of estrogen production in the Sertoli cells exist and Sertoli cells definitely possess part of an androgen synthesis pathway.

It is a well-known fact that there is a considerable testicular estrogen production, and is believed that this estrogen is derived from the Leydig cells (49-52) because the estrogens increase when the testis is stimulated with HCG. If, however, the Sertoli cells can utilize a precursor from the Leydig cells for estrogen production, the argument favoring the Leydig cell origin of the estrogens is not valid. Another possibility is that Leydig cells can produce one estrogen and Sertoli cells another. In fact, estrogens comprise a whole family of compounds and the relative gonadotropin suppressive effect of them is practically unknown, particularly in man.

It would appear that important information can be derived from granulosa cells which are presumably homologous to the Sertoli cell (53). Ryan and Short (54) and Ryan and Petro (55) showed that isolated granulosa cells can convert progesterone or testosterone to estrogen, but a steroid 3 β-ol-dehydrogenase is lacking in the follicle (39). Falck (56) demonstrated that granulosa cells cannot perform de novo estrogen biosynthesis unless theca interna cells are present (presumably producing the necessary precursor for aromatization). If we believe that the two gonads have very much in common, this suggests that for estrogen production the granulosa cell homologue, the Sertoli cell, may be equally dependent upon precursors from its theca interna homologue, the Leydig cell.

In conclusion, it appears highly probably that the Sertoli cell is capable of producing the FSH inhibitor.

Suggestion for the Complete Arrangement

An interposition of the Sertoli cell between the spermatozoa and gonadotropin inhibition fits well with the findings in this study. A possible interpretation of the results is that the Sertoli cell alone (or the Sertoli cell with only immature spermatogenetic cells attached) has a small, basal level of gonadotropin inhibitor production which is enormously stimulated when maturation of spermatozoa takes place at the cell.

On the basis of the present state of knowledge, the complete arrangement for regulation of spermatogenesis could tentatively be described as follows:

The stimulator of spermatogenesis is FSH which penetrates the tubules (57). The FSH inhibitor is an estrogen produced by the Sertoli cells from a precursor from the Leydig cells. A certain Leydig cell stimulation with LH is therefore indirectly of importance. Left alone, the Sertoli cell has only a minimal production of FSH inhibitor. However, either by direct contact with the spermatozoon during its diving into the epithelium down to the Sertoli nucleus, or perhaps in some animals via information from the phagocytosed residual body, the secretory apparatus in the Sertoli cell is changed, and significant amounts of FSH inhibiting estrogen are released. The factor controlled by this arrangement will then be the number of spermatozoa produced per unit time.

It is interesting that a system involving the Leydig cell, the Sertoli cell, the spermatozoon (late spermatid) and perhaps the residual body, could offer a logical explanation for the development of the entire testicular structure.

ACKNOWLEDGEMENT

Supported by the Ford Foundation.

REFERENCES

1. Nissim, J.A., Lancet, 1: 304, 1957.
2. Moore, D.J., Roscoe, R.T., Matson, L.J. and Heller, C.G., Clin. Res. 10: 88, 1962.
3. Allanson, M. and Deanesly, R., J. Endocr., 24: 453, 1962.
4. Heller, C.G., Wootton, P., Rowley, M.J., Lalli, M.F. and Brusca, D.R., Proc. VIth Pan-Amer. Congr. Endocrinol. p 408, 1965.
5. Hinman, F., Jr. and Smith. G.I., J. Urol. (Baltimore) 83: 706, 1960.
6. Tornblom, N., Upsala Lak.-Foren. Forh. 48: 1, 1943.
7. Taira, A.M. and Tarkham, A.A., Acta Endocr. (Kobenhavn) 40: 175, 1962.
8. Morehead, J.R and Morgan, C.F., Fertil. Steril., 18: 530, 1967.
9. Klinefelter, H.F., Jr., Reifenstein, E.C., Jr. and Albright, F., J. Clin. Endocr., 2: 615, 1942.
10. McCullagh, E.P., Sirridge, W.T and McIntosh, H.W., J. Clin. Endocr., 10: 1533, 1950.
11. Heller, C.G., Paulsen, C.A., Mortimore, G.E., Junck, E. C. and Nelson, W. O., Ann. N. Y. Acad. Sci., 55: 685, 1952.
12. Johnsen, S.G.,Acta Endocr. (Kobenhavn) Suppl. 90: 99, 1964.
13. Johnsen, S.G.,Acta Endocr. (Kobenhavn) Suppl. 124: 17, 1967.
14. Paulsen, C.A., In Clinical Endocrinology, eds. Astwood, E. B. and Cassidy, C.E., Vol 2, Grune and Stratton, Inc. New York p 569, 1968.
15. Paulsen, C.A., In Gonadotropins 1968, Rosemberg, E. ed. Geron-X, Inc. Los Altos, Calif. p 163, 1968 .

16. Wide, L. and Kjessler, B., Acta Endocr. (Kobenhavn), 62: 299, 1969.
17. Nelson, W.O., Ciba Found. Colloq. Endocr • , 4: 271, 1952.
18. Bahn, R.C., Lorenz, N., Bennett, W.A. and Albert, A., Endocrinology, 53:455, 1953.
19. Davidson, J.M., Coutopoulos, A.N. and Ganong, W.F., Acta Endocr., (Kobenhavn), 34: 169, 1960.
20. Johnsen, S.G., (1970) to be published.
21. Johnsen, S.G., Acta Endocr. (Kobenhavn), 28: 69, 1958.
22. Johnsen, S.G., Acta Endocr. (Kobenhavn), 31: 209, 1959.
23. Rosemberg, E. and Joshi, S.R., In Gonadotropins 1968, Rosemberg, E. ed. Geron-X, Inc., Los Altos, Calif. p 91, 1968.
24. Johnsen, S. G., Hormones, 1, 1970, January issue.
25. Clermont, Y., Amer. J. Anat., 112: 35, 1963.
26. Kingsley Smith, B.V. and Lacy, D., Nature (London), 184: 249, 1959.
27. Brokelmann, J., Z. Zellforsch., 59: 820, 1963.
28. Lacy, D., J. Roy. Micr. Soc. 79: 209, 1960.
29. Lacy, D., Brit. Med. Bull., 18: 205, 1962.
30. Lacy, D., Endeavour, 26: 101, 1967.
31. Lofts, B., In Perspectives in Endocrinology, Barrington, E.J.W. and Barker Jorgensen, C., eds., Academic Press, London and New York, p 239, 1968.
32. Hellbaum, A.A. and Greep, R. O., Endocrinology 32: 33, 1943.
33. Davis, T.E., Lipsett, M.B. and Korenman, S.G., J. Clin. Endocr., 25: 476, 1965.
34. Kirschner, M.A., Lipsett, M.B., and Collins, D.R., J. Clin. Invest., 44:657, 1965.
35. Peterson, N.T., Midgley, A.R. and Jaffe, R.B., J. Clin. Endocr., 28: 1473, 1968.
36. Swerdloff, R.S. and Odell, W.D., In Gonadotropins 1968, Rosemberg, E., ed. Geron-X, Inc., Los Altos, Calif. p 155, 1968.
37. Biddulph, C., Meyer, R.K. and Gumbreck, L.G., Endocrinology, 26: 280, 1940.
38. Greep, R.O., In Sex and Internal Secretions, ed. Young, W.C., 3rd ed. Williams & Wilkins, Baltimore, p 240, 1961.
39. Wattenberg, L.W., J. Histochem. Cytochem. 6: 225, 1958.
40. Levy, H., Deane, H.W. and Rubin, B.L., Endocrinology,65: 932, 1959.
41. Jirasek, J.E. and Raboch, J., Fertil. Steril., 14: 237, 1963. 1963.
42. Woods, J.E. and Domm, L.V., Gen. Comp. Endocr., 7: 559, 1966.
43. Koudstaal, J., Frensdorf, E.L., Kremer, J., Mudde, J.M. and Hardonk, M.J., Acta Endocr. (Kobenhavn), 55: 415, 1967.
44. Sengoku, K., Bull. Tokyo Med. Dent. Univ., 14: 51, 1967.
45. Christensen, A.K. and Mason, N.R., Endocrinology, 76: 646, 1965.
46. Baillie, A.H. and Mack, W.S., J. Endocr., 35: 239, 1966.
47. Baillie, A.H., Calman, K.C., Ferguson, M.M. and Hart D. McK., J. Endocr., 34: 1, 1966.
48. Lacy, D., Lofts, B., Kinson, G., Hopkins, D. and Dott, H., Gen. Comp. Endocr., 5: 693, 1965.

49. Maddock, W.O. and Nelson, W.O., J. Clin. Endocr., 12: 985, 1952.
50. Plate, W.P., Ned. T. Verlosk. 63: 83, 1963.
51. Lipsett, M.B., Wilson, H., Kirschner, M.A., Korenman, S.G., Fishman, L.M., Sarfaty, G.A. and Bardin, C.W., Recent Progr. Hormone Res., 22: 245, 1966.
52. Fishman, L.M., Sarfaty, G.A., Wilson, H. and Lipsett, M.B., In Endocrinology of the Testis, Wolstenholme, G.E.V., ed., J. and A. Churchill Ltd., London, p 156, 1967.
53. Witschi, E. and Chang, C.Y., In Comparative Endocrinology, Gorbman, A. ed. John Wiley, New York and London, p 149, 1959.
54. Ryan, K.J. and Short, R.V., Endocrinology, 76: 108, 1965.
55. Ryan, K.J. and Petro, Z., J. Clin. Endocr., 26: 46, 1966.
56. Falck, B., Acta Physiol. Scand., Suppl. 47: 163, 1959.
57. Mancini, R. E., Castro, A. and Seiguer, A.C., J. Histochem. Cytochem., 15:516, 1967.

DISCUSSION

LUNENFELD: Dr. Johnsen, it is difficult for me to understand that a change in pituitary gonadotropin secretion will occur after the change in spermatogenesis.

JOHNSEN: I think that this question can be answered quite easily. If failure of spermatogenesis is induced experimentally, gonadotropin excretion rises.

PAULSEN: Dr. Lunenfeld, if you expose the testes of normal males to acute doses of irradiation, the germinal epithelium is damaged. Serum and urinary FSH levels increase from normal to pathologically elevated levels. When spermatogenesis recovers FSH levels return to normal.

CHRISTENSEN: This question of possible estrogen secretion by the Sertoli cells has been debated, of course, for many years. Some of the evidence comes from tumors, which are always a little suspect, but as I understand it, interstitial cell tumors are commonly masculinizing, Sertoli cell tumors are sometimes feminizing (in dogs) and seminomas of the germ cells usually produce no hormones. A number of years ago I developed a way of separating the interstitial tissue from the seminiferous tubules in the rat testis, and N. Mason and I tested the transformation of progesterone to androgens by these components in vitro (Christensen and Mason 1965). In parallel runs we incubated with androgens to see if they would be transformed into estrogens, and we obtained no activity in either the seminiferous tubules or the interstitial tissue. I understand that Lofts has taken this up and has claimed some activity, although it has only been published in abstract form. With regard to electron microscopy, it is true that Sertoli cells have smooth endoplasmic reticulum to an extent, but not nearly as well developed as in the interstitial cells.

It varies a good deal with the species. Jost Brokelmann studied the rat, and I am not aware that he saw any changes at the time when the sperm are descending in the trunks of Sertoli cell cytoplasm toward the basement membrane, which one would expect if your interpretation is correct. That would be good to examine with the electron microscope. The mitochondria in Sertoli cells are not unusual, and in fact are quite slender and not particularly characteristic of those seen in steroid secreting cells. But one should not be surprised about this if the cells lack the 3β-hydroxysteroid dehydrogenase. If this is so, then they probably also lack the 20, 22-lyase, and the mitochondria would not therefore be playing any direct role in steroid biosynthesis.

JOHNSEN: I think I quoted Brokelmann correctly in saying that he found these functional changes when the spermatozoa had dipped down in the epithelium. Dr. P. F. Larson in our group is continuing this kind of research in the human. It is unpublished yet, but Dr. Larsen thinks that he is able to demonstrate marked changes in the smooth endoplasmatic reticulum in the Sertoli cell at the particular stage of spermatogenesis when the spermatozoon performs its diving and not in the others. That means that when a Sertoli cell has the dipping down of its own spermatozoa, these changes are observed.

CHRISTENSEN: The clusters of spermatids dip twice toward the Sertoli cell nucleus in rats.

LIPSETT: I cannot eliminate the possibility of a second hormone but I question whether it is an estrogen. After all, in men, the quantities of estradiol and of estrone are the same as in post-menopausal women, and yet we know very well that the levels of FSH and LH are greatly different in these two groups. To account for the differences you either have to postulate an entirely different type of hormone or a different estrogen.

BURGOS: Dr. Johnsen, you mentioned that only those stages which have spermatozoa or late spermatids are significant in producing an inhibitory substance. If this is true, the Sertoli cell related to late spermatids must be different from the others. Have you any comments on this possibility?

JOHNSEN: Dr. Larsen in our group has found that the Sertoli cell having late spermatids attached is different, but I am not able to go further into this at this moment.

COUROT: Could you comment further on the relationship between Sertoli and Leydig cells? What is the evidence for that?

JOHNSEN: It was purely hypothetical. If we think that the Sertoli cell produces steroids, we must realize that it cannot proceed to bio novo synthesis of steroids. Therefore, one must find some precursors for it. The Leydig cell may provide precursors.

DICZFALUSY: I wonder whether it would be possible to use specific anti-testosterone and anti-estradiol sera for localizing intracellular steroids?

PAULSEN: Certain aspects of Dr. Johnsen's data have deficiencies. Dr. Johnsen is still using the mouse uterine weight assay which measures the net effect of FSH and LH. According to Dr. Diczfalusy and others this assay is more sensitive to changes in LH than FSH levels. More importantly, there are patients with oligospermia who do not show spermatids in their testicular biopsy and who have normal FSH levels. I would like to show some data that Drs. J. Leonard, R. Leach and I have accumulated which bear on this issue.

Although the precise feedback mechanism controlling FSH secretion is unknown, it has been postulated that FSH levels are reciprocally related to spermatogenic activity. This concept is based largely on observations (Nelson, W.O., Fertil. Steril., 1: 477, 1950, Howard, R.P., Sniffen, R.C., Simmons, F.A. and Albright, F., J. Clin. Endocr., 10: 121, 1950, Heller, C.G., Paulsen, C.A., Mortimore, G.E., Jungck, E.C. and Nelson, W.O., Ann. N.Y. Acad. Sci., 55: 685, 1952, and Johnsen, S.G., Acta Endocr. (Kobenhavn), Suppl. 90: 99, 1964) made prior to the availability of specific methods for measuring FSH. To re-examine this thesis, the following studies were performed. Serum FSH was measured by radioimmunoassay in 64 androgenically normal but oligospermic males; all had normal serum LH as determined by radioimmunoassay. To our surprise, the majority had FSH levels within the range observed in our control population, that is 54 patients exhibited serum FSH levels between 230-580 mμg LER 907/ml. In the 10 patients that demonstrated elevated FSH levels, the values ranged from 600-1400 μg LER 907/ml. Our control population consisted of 42 androgenically normal males with sperm counts >60 million/ml. Furthermore, no direct correlation between FSH levels and sperm counts existed in this oligospermic group. Johnsen (Johnsen, S.G., Acta Endocr. (Kobenhavn), Suppl. 90: 99, 1964) initially suggested that in man, the residual body which is split off from the spermatid is the regulator of gonadotropin production. Today he has proposed that the Sertoli cell is the source of an undefined FSH inhibitor, possibly an estrogen, and that the release of this inhibitor by the Sertoli cell is directly dependent on the late stages of spermatogenesis. Our studies do not support the thesis of a direct reciprocal relationship between spermatogenic activity and FSH secretion. To study this question, the quantitative histologic characteristics of testicular biopsy specimens were examined in twelve additional oligospermic males in whom FSH measurements and sperm counts were also available. These men were divided into two groups on the basis of their urinary FSH titers (Steelman-Pohley method): a) normal FSH (n= 7) 3.0 to 18.0 I.U./24 hours; b) elevated FSH (n = 5) 26.0 to 54.0 I.U./24 hours. The severity of the oligospermia in the two groups was comparable, i.e. mean of 11.1 million/ml vs. 13.3 million/ml. Germinal cell quantitation was performed in the following manner. The histologic section of an entire biopsy was photographed and those tubules which had been cut perpendicular to their long axis were identified and numbered. The individual germinal cells were counted in 10 such tubules per biopsy specimen. The cell counts were expressed as the mean cell count per tubule and the data for the two groups compared. There was no significant difference in the germinal cell counts between these two groups, and therefore no direct correlation between germinal cell populations and FSH levels. One of the patients with normal titers of FSH and less than 1 million/ml sperm count had virtually no (fewer than 6) spermatids in an entire testicular biopsy section. Therefore, we have to reject the concept that the germ cells per se directly control FSH secretion. We have to consider that there is an "independent station" which controls FSH secretion. This station may be the Sertoli cell or the Sertoli cell plus the limiting membranes. You may have a normal "station" with abnormal spermatogenesis or an abnormal "station" with abnormal spermatogenesis. The nature of the feedback signal from this independent station remains unknown.

JOHNSEN: I am of course very well aware that a total gonadotropin assay is not the right answer; but the cases presented were collected over a five year period. We are now pursuing the matter by specific FSH and LH determinations in the urine by bioassay. Dr. Christensen, can confirm that, in the poor testis lacking spermatozoa, he finds a rise in FSH excretion. So, I do not have an explanation of the difference in our findings.

Dr. Paulsen, in your patient completely lacking spermatids you did not observe an FSH rise. Was hypopituitarism the cause of the spermatogenic defect?

PAULSEN: It does not seem reasonable to me to postulate that all patients with oligospermia and normal FSH levels have hypopituitarism. Our patients had no evidence of a pituitary lesion.

MACLEOD: Dr. Paulsen, I have a slight quarrel with you about your definition of oligospermia. For example, if we do take a population of men at large, we find that the mean sperm count will be in the region of 95 million/ml. But it does not follow that levels below, even far below that are not able to produce conception with relative ease. So that if you start at the 40 million level as your definition of oligospermia, I think you may be a little bit far afield in terms of defining it. I fully agree, though, with what you have said: that there is probably no relationship between even severe oligospermia (that is, under the 10 million level) and gonadotropin levels.

PAULSEN: I would agree, Dr. MacLeod. For our studies we arbitrarily selected 40 million/ml as the cut-off point. However, if you select cases with sperm counts below 10 million/ml, no correlation with FSH levels exists.

THE ROLE OF FSH, ICSH, AND ENDOGENOUS TESTOSTERONE DURING TESTICULAR SUPPRESSION BY EXOGENOUS TESTOSTERONE IN NORMAL MEN

Carl G. Heller, Howard C. Morse, Mike Su, and Mavis J. Rowley

Division of Reproductive Physiology, Pacific Northwest Research Foundation, 1102 Columbia Street, Seattle, Washington 98104

Testosterone administered to normal men is know to depress spermatogenesis to azoospermia, as reflected in the ejaculate, and to depress Leydig cell morphology to the point that only mesenchymal cells and fibroblasts are identifiable. It is also know that urinary total gonadotropins are concomitantly depressed to the point that they are undetectable in 24 hour urine aliquots administered to single assay rats (1). It has been widely assumed, but not proved, that the depression of human testicular function by administering testosterone is secondary to pituitary suppression.

Three possible mechanisms of action of testosterone upon the testis were originally postulated in the following investigation: 1) that the depression is solely due to total pituitary gonadotropin suppression, 2) that the depression is solely due to a direct effect of testosterone upon the germinal epithelium and/or Leydig cells or 3) that the depression is due to a combination of direct testicular and indirect gonadotropin suppression.

To test which of these three postulates apply, the following protocol was planned. Testosterone enanthate (200 mg intramuscularly (I.M.) per week) was to be administered to normal men until the following three events occurred: azoospermia, Leydig cell disappearance and disappearance of gonadotropins in 24 hour urine aliquots. Then, while continuing the testosterone administration at the same level, human chorionic gonadotropin (HCG) was to be added for its interstitial cell-stimulating hormone (ICSH) effect (4000 International Units (I.U.) HCG I.M. per two days). If Leydig cell morphology could thus be restored to normal, as revealed by testicular biopsy examination, then a direct effect of testosterone upon

Leydig cell depression could be eliminated from further consideration. The suppression of Leydig cells by testosterone would then be attributed to the suppression of pituitary ICSH (if no restoration occurred the direct effect of testosterone on Leydig cells must still be considered). Assuming restoration of Leydig cell morphology, the plan was to add follicle-stimulating hormone (FSH) in the form of Pergonal in order to restore spermatogenesis, while continuing to administer the testosterone enanthate and continuing the HCG at the same levels for each. If spermatogenesis were now restored we could conclude that the inhibitory effect of testosterone upon the germinal elements was mediated by suppression of FSH.

To this end three healthy men, ages 37, 33 and 29 were chosen to serve as subjects. They were determined to be reproductively normal by hormonal studies, sperm concentration and examination of control testicular biopsy specimens. Testicular biopsies were obtained and prepared using the methods of Rowley and Heller (2).

Testosterone enanthate (Delatestryl, Squibb) was administered at the rate of 200 mg I.M. once weekly for eight to 12 months. Human chorionic gonadotropin (APL, Ayerst, 4000 I.U. I.M. every second day) was added beginning four months after the initiation of testosterone enanthate administration. The duration of HCG administration was four and one-half months. Testosterone enanthate was continued alone on two subjects after HCG was discontinued.

Seminal fluid specimens were collected once weekly and examined for sperm concentration, motility and volume. Concentration was measured using the hemocytometer method. Each subject was used as his own control. Sperm morphology was examined by Dr. John MacLeod of Cornell University Medical College.

Twelve-hour (overnight) urine samples were collected and pooled in 48 hour collections. Total gonadotropins and ICSH determinations were performed on aliquots of the urine pools. Urines were kept below 5°C until the extraction procedures were carried out. Urinary gonadotropins were extracted using the kaolin-acetone method of Albert (3). Total gonadotropin levels were determined by measuring the ovarian weights of immature rats and expressed as mgU/24 hours of a standard human urinary postmenopausal preparation (Pergonal P-22C). Urinary ICSH was determined biologically using the method of Greep et al. (4), measuring the increase in ventral prostate weight in hypophysectomized immature male rats. The values were expressed as mgU/24 hours of the standard preparation (Pergonal P-26E). Testicular biopsies were examined quantitatively using the germ cell/ Sertoli cell ratio method as developed by Heller et al. (5).

The administration of testosterone enanthate 200 mg I.M. weekly for four months resulted in barely detectable or absent total urinary gonadotropins, azoospermia as judged from ejaculated seminal fluid samples, disappearance of Leydig cells as judged by testicular biopsy examination and marked reduction in numbers of Sd, Sc, Sb and Sa spermatids, marked reduction in pachytene, zygotene and leptotene spermatocytes, slight reduction in preleptotene spermatocytes and type B spermatogonia, questionable reduction of type A pale spermatocytes and no apparent reduction in type A dark spermatocytes (Figs. 1-2)

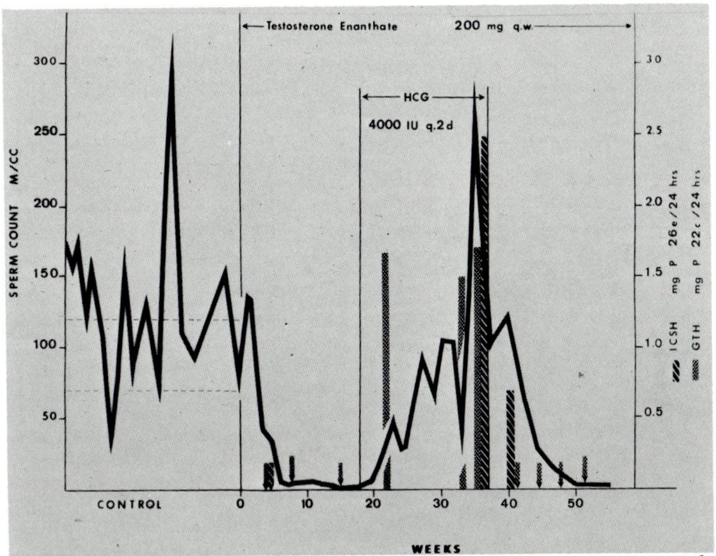

Fig. 1. Sperm count, total gonadotropin (gth) and ICSH values shown in a subject during control, testosterone and testosterone-HCG administration periods. Dashed lines across control period indicate range of normal gth and ICSH values. Bars with arrows pointing to bottom line indicate absent or barely detectable gth or ICSH.

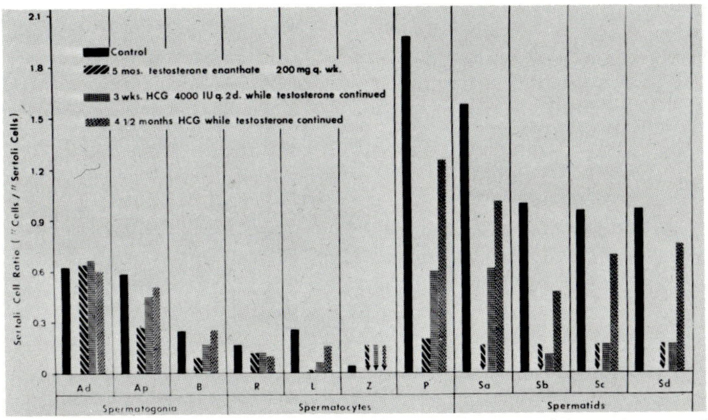

Fig. 2. Comparison of Sertoli cell ratios in biopsies taken during testosterone administration and twice during the additional administration of HCG. Control values for each cell type were determined from the average of the quantitation of 50 normal testicular biopsies. Arrows pointed to bottom line indiaate zero values.

Adding 4000 I.U. of HCG administered I.M. every second day brought about complete restoration of Leydig cell morphology in all five biopsies taken during HCG administration. Note should be made that two of these biopsies were taken as early as three weeks after the initiation of HCG administration.

Therefore, since testosterone caused Leydig cell disappearance and adding HCG caused restoration of Leydig cells to normal, we conclude that testosterone-caused Leydig cell depression is mediated by suppressing anterior pituitary ICSH secretion or release.

In the meanwhile, much to our surprise, the weekly seminal fluid examinations revealed an increase in sperm concentration by one month in one subject and by the second or third months in the other two. Between the third and the fourth month of HCG administration each subject had reached pre-testosterone treatment control levels (Fig. 1). Two reached the average of the control levels and one rose above the minimal control levels but did not rise as high as his pre-treatment average.

Quantitation of the elements of the germinal series in the two testicular biopsies obtained three weeks after the initiation of HCG revealed a partial restoration of leptotene and pachytene spermatocytes and significant but small increases in each of the four spermatid types. The second biopsy, obtained at four and one-half months following initiation of HCG, revealed complete restoration of each of the depressed germinal cells to pre-treatment levels in the two subjects whose sperm concentration had returned to average pre-treatment levels (Fig. 2). The third subject, whose sperm concentration had not reached the average of his pre-treatment levels, revealed definite but incomplete restoration of each of the germinal cells.

These results suggest that 1) testosterone does not exert a direct depressive effect upon either the germinal cells or the Leydig cells since both elements can be restored to normal by administering HCG, 2) administering HCG during testosterone administration restores spermatogenesis either by providing sufficient FSH to obtain this effect or because testosterone does not depress FSH secretion or release in normal male human subjects, and further 3) HCG stimulates enough Leydig cell androgen production to aid in the restoration of spermatogenesis in the presence of FSH.

As a consequence of the unexpected germinal cell response to HCG administration without the addition of FSH there was no reason to follow the original protocol. Thus no Pergonal was administered and the HCG was discontinued. In order to confirm the effect of testosterone upon the two testicular systems the testosterone was continued for an additional four months in the two subjects who had complete restoration of spermatogenesis.

The two subjects responded as before in that the weekly seminal fluid values decreased to azoospermia, and the gonadotropins dropped to levels barely detectable or absent. The Leydig cells disappeared and the germinal elements (except type A dark spermatogonia) again became depressed in the subject whose biopsy was available for examination. Parenthetically, observations on sperm morphology revealed a drop in normal forms during the initial testosterone enanthate administration and a return to normal during the administration of HCG.

As a general proposition, spermatogenesis appears to reach completion in most mammals under the influence of two different hormones, testosterone and FSH. First testosterone must be present in sufficient amounts to bring about maturation of the seminiferous tubules. The tubules may be considered a part of the rest of the genital system which is dependent upon testosterone for its maintenance and development, e.e., epididymis, was deferens, prostate, seminal vesicle, etc. In man, when such maturation of the seminiferous tubules is induced by testosterone, whether exogenous or endogenous, there is an accompanying differentiation of the previously undifferentiated Sertoli cells, spermatogonia and the occasional spermatocyte, but no noticeable progression of germinal cell maturation. This can be judged from administering HCG to true hypogonadotropic eunuchoids (6). After testosterone has provided basic testicular support, the second hormone, FSH, is able to initiate progressive and complete spermatogenesis. Follicle-stimulating hormone however is unable to influence human spermatogenesis when administered alone as HMG (Pergonal) (7).

With the above in mind we wished to explore the proposition that testosterone might differentially depress ICSH completely without concomitantly completely depressing FSH. The preferred way of testing this proposition would be, of course, to determine plasma FSH and ICSH levels. These determinations were not performed on the three subjects reported and must await a repetition of the experiment. As a substitute that could be performed with relative rapidity normal subjects were chosen for administration of a high potency and more rapidly acting androgen. Thus, testosterone propionate (Oreton, Schering) was administered I.M. at 100 mg levels daily for five days. Five control observations were recorded for plasma FSH and ICSH using modifications of Odell's radioimmunoassay methods (8,9). Daily observations were made during androgen administration and every two to three days for two weeks following cessation of androgen. ICSH disappeared entirely within 24 hours of the first injection and remained undetectable for the five day injection period (any value below 2.0 mU/ml is considered as zero or undetectable in our laboratory). In distinct contrast the plasma FSH values, determined simultaneously, remained unaltered during and following testosterone propionate administration. Thus under the specific circumstances of this experiment it must be concluded that testosterone can produce a dichotomous effect upon plasma FSH and ICSH levels (Table 1).

Table 1. Plasma Gonadotropin Before, During and After Testosterone Administration.

Date	SUBJECT PM 315 ICSH (mU/ml)*	SUBJECT PM 315 FSH (mU/ml)*	SUBJECT PM 214 ICSH (mU/ml)*	SUBJECT PM 214 FSH (mU/ml)*
Control				
3-9	5.66	8.07	4.43	7.03
4-11	3.13	7.47	3.98	7.30
4-12	6.00	7.03	4.23	7.30
4-14	5.25	7.20	3.58	6.75
10-11	4.40	7.75	3.45	6.50
Testosterone propionate 100 mg I.M. for five days				
10-12	1.90	7.65	1.43	6.40
10-13	1.70	7.17	2.08	6.75
10-14	1.63	7.25	2.05	6.50
10-15	1.73	6.63	2.03	6.18
10-16	1.75	6.50	1.68	6.60
Post-Testosterone				
10-20	8.25	7.20	5.23	6.45
10-23	7.38	8.25	6.90	6.68
10-27	5.03	8.03	3.70	6.73
10-30	5.15	7.53	3.93	6.85

* Standard:Human Pituitary Extract Reference Preparation LER 907

Swerdloff and Odell (10) administering 20 or 50 mg of fluoxymesterone daily for five days to five normal men and Franchimont (11) using a single injection of 50 mg testosterone propionate revealed a similar dichotomy in response, i.e., no change in FSH and undetectable ICSH (LH).

Neither Swerdloff and Odell's nor our experiments to date have been of sufficient duration to extrapolate the data to long-term effects. Bogdanove (12) has demonstrated a delayed effect of androgens on FSH release in rats.

The effect of androgen upon ICSH in the normal human male can be accepted as causing marked suppression. This is inferred from our observations of depression of total urinary gonadotropins, and suppression of urinary ICSH, in the one case, following testosterone enanthate administration. It is also inferred from the complete early plasma ICSH suppression following administration of fluoxymesterone and testosterone propionate. Thus there appears to be a strong likelihood that a dichotomy exists between ICSH and FSH suppression.

Assuming that FSH is not suppressed or only incompletely suppressed by administering 200 mg testosterone enanthate I.M. per week, we speculate that the restoration of spermatogenesis following the addition of HCG is due wholly or in part to the presence of plasma FSH of anterior pituitary origin.

Continuing with this assumption, each result of the testosterone enanthate plus HCG experiment is readily accounted for except one: the suppression of spermatogenesis by administering testosterone enanthate (or other androgens). The enigma that requires explanation is based upon the assumption that the presence of only two hormones, testosterone and FSH, is required for completion of spermatogenesis in man. In this experiment each hormone is assumed to be present; testosterone being administered exogenously and FSH not having been suppressed. The only immediately apparent interference with regulation of testicular function is the suppression of ICSH. This in turn stops the endogenous production of androgens, which in turn provides the explanation for the cessation of complete spermatogenesis. It is likely that the concentration of androgen provided by the Leydig cells, which are in such close approximation to the seminiferous tubules, is far higher than that provided to the germinal cells by an injection of 200 mg of testosterone enanthate given I.M. once weekly. Thus the effect of testosterone enanthate given I.M. is to lower the androgen levels available to the germinal epithelium, due to the inhibition of ICSH.

In applying this explanation, reference must be made to observations on the maintenance of spermatogenesis in the hypophysectomized rat by exogenously administered androgens (13-16). Woods and Simpson (17) found that spermatogenesis in hypophysectomized rats could be poorly maintained by ICSH alone but well maintained by ICSH plus FSH or testosterone propionate plus FSH. In these and many confirmatory observations the dosage administered and the concentration of plasma testosterone attained are far in excess of those possible for so much larger a mammal as man.

That the location of the Leydig cell so close to the germinal epithelium is an important factor in providing concentrated amounts of androgen is seen in man in the case of the "fertile eunuch" (18). Maintenance of spermatogenesis has been produced in hypophysectomized rats by Dvoskin (19) and in hypophysectomized rhesus monkeys by Smith (20) by intratesticular administration of testosterone in pellet form. Smith found tubules nearest the deposited androgen undergoing complete spermatogenesis and those more remote remaining in the degenerate state. Dvoskin reported that if the same amount of androgen was administered subcutaneously or intratesticularly the latter was far more effective in maintaining spermatogenesis.

We conclude that in normal men testosterone causes testicular Leydig cell and germinal cell depression without exerting a direct effect upon testicular activity, but does so indirectly by inhibiting production of ICSH. We postulate that FSH production is unaffected or only partially suppressed. Under these circumstances we assume that the inhibition of spermatogenesis is due to a decrease in the normally high androgen concentration at the germinal cell site due to the absence of ICSH effect upon Leydig cells.

ACKNOWLEDGEMENTS

We wish to thank Edward C. Reifenstein, Jr., M.D. of The Squibb Institute for supplying the Delatestryl, Jack Howard, M.D. of the Schering Corporation for the supply of Oreton and John Jewell, M.D. of Ayerst-McKenna for a supply of APL.

This investigation was supported by grants-in-aid from The Ford Foundation (680-0906), the Public Health Service (HD 00804) and the U.S. Atomic Energy Commission (AT (45-1)-1780).

REFERENCES

1. Heller, C.G. and Nelson, W.O., Recent Progr. Hormone Res., 3: 229, 1948.
2. Rowley, M.J. and Heller, C.G., Fertil. Steril., 17: 177, 1966.
3. Albert, A., Proc. Staff Meeting Mayo Clinic, 30: 552, 1955.
4. Greep, R.O., VanDyke, H.B. and Chow, B.F., Proc. Soc. Exp. Biol. Med., 46: 644, 1941.
5. Heller, C.G., Heller, G.V. and Rowley, M.J., In: Progress in Endocrinology, ed. Gual, C., Excerpta Medica Found., p. 1012, 1969.
6. Heller, C.G., Lalli, M.F. and Rowley, M.J., In: Pharmacology of Reproduction, Proc. 3rd Internat. Pharmacol. Meeting July 1966, Pergamon Press, Oxford and New York, 2: 61, 1968.
7. Paulsen, C.A., In: Gonadotropins, 1968, ed. Rosemberg, E., Geron-X Inc., Los Altos, Calif., p. 491, 1968.
8. Odell, W.D., Parlow, A.F., Cargille, C.M. and Ross, G.T., J. Clin. Invest., 47: 2551, 1968.
9. Odell, W.D., Ross, G.T., and Rayford, P.L., J. Clin. Invest., 46: 248, 1967.
10. Swerdloff, R.S. and Odell, W.D., In: Gonadotropins, 1968, ed. Rosemberg, E., Geron-X Inc., Los Altos, Calif., p 155, 1968.
11. Franchimont, P., Proc. Internat. Symp. on Protein and Polypeptide Hormones, ed. Margoulies, M., Excerpta Medica Found., Amsterdam, p. 99, 1968.
12. Bogdanove, E.M., Anat. Rec., 157: 117, 1967.
13. Walsh, E.L., Cuyler, W.K. and McCullagh, D.R., Amer. J. Physiol., 107: 508, 1934.

14. Nelson, W.O. and Gallagher, T.F., Science, 84: 230, 1936.
15. Cutuly, E., McCullagh, D.R., and Cutuly, E.C., Amer. J. Physiol. 119: 121, 1937.
16. Clermont, Y. and Harvey, S.C., In: Ciba Found Colloq. Endocr. 16: 173, 1967.
17. Woods, M.C. and Simpson, M.E., Endocrinology, 69: 91, 1961.
18. McCullagh, E.P., Beck, J.C. and Schaffenburg, C.A., J. Clin. Endocr., 13: 489, 1953.
19. Dvoskin, S., Anat. Rec., 99 : 329, 1947.
20. Smith, P.E., Yale J. Biol. Med., 17: 281, 1944.

DISCUSSION

ROSEMBERG: Dr. Heller, you indicated that testicular function was suppressed under testosterone administration; that is, the sperm count dropped. However, after subsequent addition of HCG, the sperm count increased. Hence, you postulated that HCG stimulated the Leydig cells to produce endogenous testosterone by virtue of the fact that testosterone may be near the germinal epithelium and then exerted a local effect. Do you have experimental proof for your statement? It seems to me that when exogenous testosterone is administered one is flooding the system.

HELLER: We do not have proof for our statement. The testosterone levels that we can conveniently produce in man by intramuscular injection are relatively low. In other words, the amount of testosterone theoretically reaching the germinal epithelium is much different in amount than what one can do, let us say in a hypophysectomized rat where one can maintain spermatogenesis by injecting testosterone. All the other evidence is rather indirect, as has been shown at this meeting. Dr. Steinberger showed a case with a testicular tumor in one testis in which the tubules that were near the testosterone-producing tumor continued to have normal spermatogenesis whereas on the other side no spermatogenesis was observed.

ROSEMBERG: Dr. Steinberger, what was the level of testosterone in this patient?

E. STEINBERGER: We are presently measuring the circulating hormone level, so I do not have the answer but I will be surprised if it is not extremely low.

ROSEMBERG: If this is so, it is difficult for me to visualize that the amount produced by the Leydig cells under HCG stimulation could overcome whatever is already there.

HELLER: The Leydig cells were morphologically altered by exogenous testosterone administration, suggesting lowered testosterone output.

But you ask me for proof; and I have no proof of this; it remains a logical assumption, but just an assumption.

SAVARD: There is a most important intra-testicular, as well as intra-ovarian, circulation of hormones produced within the gonad. I call your attention to the work of Lindner, some years ago in Dr. Mann's laboratories in Cambridge, who demonstrated the high testosterone content of the lymph of the testis. He found it many times greater than the peripheral testosterone concentrations, comparable and sometimes exceeding the concentrations of the spermatic venous blood. Lindner also suggested that this could perhaps explain the phenomenon of the syndrome of the fertile eunuch, who has sufficient local testosterone concentration to support spermatogenic function, yet not enough peripherally to masculinize him.

HUDSON: With the administration of fluoxymesterone, plasma levels of testosterone are suppressed. Continuing treatment with fluoxymesterone and administering HCG, peripheral plasma levels of testosterone are restored to normal. I really believe that Dr. Savard's comments are highly relevant: namely, what is the local concentration of testosterone around the tubules, and what is its significance on nurturing the germinal epithelium?

JOHNSEN: In Dr. Steinberger's case, there was only growth of the tubules and presence of a limited number of spermatocytes.

E. STEINBERGER: Dr. Johnsen, you are absolutely correct; as I clearly pointed out when discussing the photomicrographs, the spermatogenesis did not proceed beyond young spermatids. Dr. Heller's paper, together with data reported by Dr. Bergada on a case of Leydig cell hyperplasia showing localized areas of spermatogenesis and with our demonstration of spermatogenesis in a tumor-bearing testicle of a 6-year old boy, presents a good case for the critical role of testosterone in the process of initiation of spermatogenesis in the human testicle. Furthermore, we provided evidence that in the rat, FSH is necessary for the late stages of spermatid development. I think that demonstration of FSH by Dr. Heller in his experimental subject suggests that, in the human, FSH may also play an important role in maturation of the spermatids.

HELLER: Many years ago Carl Moore implanted crystals of testosterone. Wherever the crystals were, spermatogenesis was maintained; while peripheral to that, they were not.

PAULSEN: Dr. Heller, it occurs to me that something curious is going on which is not understandable. For example, when Maddock and Nelson administered HCG to normal adult men, oligospermia or azoospermia developed. Histologically, the seminiferous tubules became hyalinized and the Leydig cells became small and darkly stained.

They postulated that these changes were due to excessive steroid hormone production. Now suppose they had added testosterone to their HCG regimen. This would have further increased the intratesticular testosterone concentration. Thus the data of Maddock and Nelson appear to be in conflict with your experiment. Can you explain this?

HELLER: We have repeatedly confirmed the Maddock-Nelson work. And, for those of you who are not familiar with it, it consists simply of administering human chorionic gonadotropin long enough, in large enough amounts, resulting in azoospermia in normal men. During this time, not only are testosterone and the 17-KS steroids increased, but the hormone, in the urine at least, that increases the most is estrogen. I would postulate that human chorionic gonadotropin, under the circumstances of Maddock and Nelson's experiments and under the circumstances that we have given it, is causing failure of spermatogenesis because of the high concentration of estrogen.

PAULSEN: But you would still be getting the same equivalent amount of estrogen in the urine, Dr. Heller, with testosterone and HCG administration. Therefore, your explanation does not appear to be plausible. It still remains doubtful how you were able to restore spermatogenesis in your study. I would like to believe that it is the retention of normal endogenous FSH levels which was fundamental to the restoration of spermatogenesis in your study. But is it really fair, Dr. Heller, to compare your twenty-week administration of testosterone enanthate to the five-day administration of testosterone propionate?

HELLER: No it is not. Dr. Paulsen brings up the fact that we did not determine plasma ICSH and plasma FSH in the experiment with testosterone enanthate, which was a long-term experiment. This experiment is now under way.

DICZFALUSY: May I suggest another experiment. In the human female, those who tried to work on the mechanism of action of contraceptive steroids usually concluded that estrogen will inhibit FSH release and secretion, provided it is given for a long period of time. Dr. Heller, if you would give estrogen to your patients, you would see the following: 1) whether or not it was indeed the estrogen which, in combination with HCG, caused hyalinization, 2) whether or not you really need FSH from the pituitary and 3) whether you could replace FSH with HMG.

CHAPTER IV

REGULATION OF TESTICULAR FUNCTION

SECTION 3: GONADOTROPINS, PURIFICATION, AND MEASUREMENT

USE OF STANDARDS IN GONADOTROPIN ASSAYS

Eugenia Rosemberg

Medical Research Institute of Worcester, Inc.,

26 Queen Street, Worcester, Massachusetts

By definition a standard is "that which is set up and established by authority as a rule for a measure of quantity weight, extent, value or quality." Principles governing the appropriate use of standards in assays, whether the assays are biological, chemical, immunological or microbial, have been established for a long time.

The most important principle governing the use of standards in gonadotropin assays, is that a standard should be as alike the material tested as possible. This implies that the use of one hormone as a standard for another hormone represents a violation of the principle of similarity.

One of the major sources of confusion in the literature concerning both biologic and immunologic potency estimates of gonadotropic hormones has been the use of several standards. As an example, in the bioassay field, a disparity of some 12-fold in the assay of urinary LH was found when the assays were conducted by the ventral prostate weight method (VPW) and by the ovarian ascorbic acid depletion method (OAAD) (1). The discrepancy was understandable on the basis that it was attributable to the physical and chemical differences and possibly also to metabolic differences in the standard used (NIH-LH-SI, an ovine pituitary LH) and the material (urinary LH) tested (1-2). The discrepancy disappeared when a urinary standard was used for the assay of urinary LH. A similar observation was made testing an LH preparation obtained from human pituitary glands (R-469-2, kindly supplied by Drs. L.E. Reichert, Jr., and A. Wilhelmi), in both the VPW and OAAD methods using ovine NIH-LH-Sl as standard (3).

As shown in Table 1, another example of this discrepancy is

illustrated in the assay of ovine NIH-FSH-S1 and NIH-LH-S1 and the Second International Reference preparation of Human Menopausal Gonadotropin (2nd IRP) (WHO/BS/723) a gonadotropin preparation obtained from human urine.

TABLE 1

SPECIFIC ACTIVITY OF NIH-FSH-S1 AND NIH-LH-S1, IU 2nd IRP/mg

Assay System	No. of Assays	No. of Animals	Assay Characteristics		Weighted Mean Potency Ratio (95% CL)	
			bc	λ	NIH-FSH-S1 (IU/mg)	NIH-LH-S1 (IU/mg)
AR	10	245	239	0.14	26.5 (24.3-28.8)	
VPW	6	167	18.6	0.21		51.3 (43.9-59.9)
OAAD	21*	417	-26	0.30		588 (500-714)

*Lack of parallelism : 4 assays; Index of Discrimination $\frac{\text{OAAD}}{\text{VPW}} = 11.5$

The details of the assay methods used as performed in our laboratories have been described (1-4). (From: Rosemberg, E., In Gonadotropins 1968, ed. Rosemberg, E., Geron-X, Inc., Los Altos, Calif., p. 383, 1968.)

In the bioassay field, at least six reference preparations or standards were used to report values of gonadotropic activity in pituitary tissue and body fluids. These were HMG-20 A (5) obtained from the urine of menopausal and post-menopausal women; AMW (6) from the urine of normal males: the 1st International Reference Preparation for Human Menopausal Gonadotropin (1st IRP, WHO Tech., Rep. Series, P. 9, 1959); the ovine pituitary preparations NIH-FSH-S1 and NIH-LH-S1 (as well as subsequent batches), and the Second International Reference Preparation of Human Menopausal Gonadotropin (2nd IRP). Hence, one of the major sources of confusion concerning biologic potency estimates has been the use of various standards and therefore confusion arose concerning the conversion factors used to relate one standard to another.

1 mg. 1st IRP	∽	0.004 mg. NIH-FSH-S1	AR*	Rosemberg, E. et al. (J. Clin. Endocr. 24: 673, 1964)
1 mg. 1st IRP	∽	0.009 mg. NIH-LH-S1	VPW**	
1 mg. NIH-FSH-S1	∽	9.2 rat units	AR	Albert, A., Mayo Clinic Proc. 40: 216, 1965.
1 mg. NIH-LH-S1	∽	26.5 rat units	VPW	
1 mg. NIH-LH-S1	∽	166.0 rat units	OAAD†	
1 mg. 1st IRP	∽	0.14 IU 2nd IRP	AR	DRB/DF/82
1 mg. 1st IRP	∽	0.5 IU 2nd IRP	VPW	DRB/DF/82
1 mg. NIH-FSH-S1	∽	26.5 IU 2nd IRP	AR	Rosemberg, E. *In* Gonadotropins 1968, ed. Rosemberg, E., Geron-X, Inc., p.383, 1968.
1 mg. NIH-LH-S1	∽	51.3 IU 2nd IRP	VPW	
1 mg. NIH-LH-S1	∽	588.0 IU 2nd IRP	OAAD	

*AR: augmentation reaction assay (7); ** VPW: ventral prostate weight assay (1); † OAAD: ovarian ascorbic acid depletion assay (4). (From Rosemberg, E. *In* Gonadotropins 1968, ed. Rosemberg, E., Geron-X Inc., Los Altos, Calif., p. 387, 1968.)

It is well known that a protein molecule may lose functional or biologic activity without concomitant loss of immunologic activity. Hence, with the advent of immunological techniques for the measurement of gonadotropic activity in pituitary tissue and body fluids, the establishment of proper standards to be used in these systems is of paramount importance.

Ideally the test material and the standard should be identical at the molecular level. Hence, individual standards should be made available for each gonadotropic hormone of human or animal origin. However, the problem of setting up suitable standards for all forms of gonadotropins is a real dilemma. Moreover, antisera to individual hormones must be regarded as unique reagents. For example, although cross reactivity has been found between HCG and LH antisera, some antisera have been found to cross-react identically and others only partially. Moreover, some antisera to ovine LH have been shown to cross-react with human pituitary LH (HLH) (personal observations and personal communication from L.E. Reichert). Also, some antisera prepared against HFSH cannot recognize the difference between human FSH, LH, HCG or TSH.

In order to set up proper reagents to be used in immunoassays, it is obvious that it will be necessary to know the exact relationship between immunologically active and biologically active molecules; it would be also necessary to develop antisera specific to the hormone being measured. However, these conditions have not been met as yet. In the interim it was found necessary to make available antigens, antisera and a reference preparation for FSH and LH radioimmunoassays (RIA). Consequently, the Institute of Arthritis and Metabolic Diseases, NIH, through the National Pituitary Agency (NPA) made available the reagents for RIA of human pituitary follicle stimulating (HFSH) and luteinizing (HLH) hormones and a reference preparation designated as LER 907 derived from a human pituitary tissue extract which contains both FSH and LH activity.

The collaborative study conducted by the NPA (8) determined, by both bioassay and radioimmunoassay techniques, the FSH and LH content of four human pituitary tissue extracts differing widely in FSH/LH ratio and of three highly purified (immunochemical grade) preparations (one of HFSH and two preparations of HLH). The standard used was the 2nd IRP. However, the study was designed so that all preparations could be assayed in terms of any, such as the reference preparation LER 907, or all of the remaining preparations.

The NPA study confirmed that a tissue pituitary extract (LER 907) is satisfactory as a radioimmunoassay reference preparation for FSH and LH in pituitary tissue extracts. The study also showed that the use of the 2nd IRP (urinary) as a radioimmunoassay standard is associated with over estimation of the FSH and LH content of human pituitary tissue extracts. It has also been shown (9) that the use of a human pituitary tissue reference preparation is associated with radioimmunoassay under estimation of FSH and LH present in human urinary extracts. Moreover, it has been shown that the urinary 2nd IRP is a satisfactory standard for the radioimmunoassay of FSH and LH in urinary gonadotropic extracts, the index of discrimination (radioimmunoassay/bioassay) being close to unity (10). (A comprehensive review on the comparison of biologic and immunologic potency estimates of human luteinizing hormone and human follicle stimulating hormone has been published by R.J. Ryan (11)).

The availability of the NPA radioimmunoassay reagents (8) made possible the study of the LH biologic and immunologic activity of four human pituitary LH preparations and that of HCG. The standards used were the 2nd IRP and LER 907. The radioimmunoassay technique used was essentially that described by Odell et al. (12). For iodination, a purified human pituitary LH fraction DEAE-2-II, with an LH potency of 1,350 IU 2nd IRP/mg was used. The specific activity of the I^{131}-LH varied from 149 to 429 $\mu c/\mu g$.

BIOASSAY RESULTS

All bioassays were calculated by appropriate computer programs. For bioassay of LH activity, the OAAD method was employed; for the bioassay of FSH, the augmentation reaction assay (AR) was used. The concomitant standard and reference preparations tested with all bioassays were the 2nd IRP and LER 907, respectively.

Table 2 gives the bioassay results in terms of specific activity - i.e., International Units (IU) of FSH and LH activity per milligram of five preparations (including the reference material LER 907) and the specific activity by weight of the four pituitary preparations in terms of weight of the reference preparation LER 907. The FSH/LH ratios are also shown. The LH content of LER 907 was 54.2 IU/mg . One preparation, LER 856-1 exhibited an activity of 510 IU/mg. The other three preparations contained similar LH activity (IU/mg) which was about 2.5 times higher than that of LER 856-1. The four preparations differed in FSH/LH ratio by 74 to 185-fold from the reference preparation. However, the FSH/LH ratio of LER 856-1 differed by about 4-fold from the other three materials.

LH RADIOIMMUNOASSAY RESULTS

All preparations were tested at several dose levels. The concomitant standard and reference preparation used were the 2nd IRP and LER 907, respectively. All RIA assays were calculated by appropriate computer programs for parallel line assays. Table 3 presents the LH RIA assays and the comparison of bioassay and immunoassay results.

The RIA results are given in terms of specific activity by weight of the preparations in terms of weight of LER 907, and by specific activity in IU's of the 2nd IRP per milligram. One preparation, LER 856-1 differed in LH activity by about 5-fold from LER 907, and between 3.5 to 5.7-fold from the other three preparations. The LH activity of the last three preparations differed by about 20 to 30-fold from that of LER 907. The LH radioimmunoassay/bioassay (imm/Bio) ratio was close to unity when a pituitary preparation was used as reference material. However, the imm/Bio ratio varied from 3.2 to 6.9 when a urinary preparation (2nd IRP) was used as a concomitant standard.

These results confirm the observations recorded in the literature (8,13,14) in that bioassay and radioimmunoassay potency estimates obtained for pituitary preparations using a pituitary reference preparation are in agreement, and that bioassay potency estimates of pituitary preparations are lower than radioimmunoassay potency estimates when a urinary reference preparation is used.

Several factors might be responsible for the radioimmunoassay over estimation of LH content of the pituitary preparations when the 2nd IRP is used as the standard reference material. One is the possibility that a urinary preparation, such as the 2nd IRP, could have lost immunoreactive sites in the LH molecule as a result of metabolism attendant to its passage from pituitary to blood to urine, or

TABLE 2

BIOLOGIC CHARACTERISTICS OF HUMAN PITUITARY GONADOTROPIN PREPARATIONS

Preparations	OAAD Assay (LH)-Relative Potency (95% Confidence Limits)			AR† assay (FSH)	FSH/LH Ratio
	IU/2nd IRP/mg	IU LER 907/mg	mg LER 907/mg	IU/2nd IRP/mg	(2nd IRP std)
LER 907	54.2 (31.7 - 98.7)	-	-	20	0.37
LER 856-1	510 (320 - 830)	430 (280 - 660)	7.9 (6.7 - 8.7)	2.7	0.005
LER 1371	1,320 (760 - 2,290)	1,110 (640 - 1,910)	20.5 (19.3 - 20.6)	1.7	0.0013
LER 960	1,465 (630 - 3,460)	1,420 (740 - 2,770)	26.2 (23.0 - 28.0)	1.1	0.0008
DEAE-2-II ††	1,350 (560 - 3,250)	1,320 (680 - 2,550)	24.4 (21.5 - 24.8)	2.5	0.0019

†: Augmentation Reaction Assay; †† Prepared by Dr. Parlow for the NPA.

TABLE 3

LH RADIOIMMUNOASSAY BY HUMAN PITUITARY GONADOTROPIN PREPARATIONS

Preparations	Relative Potency (95% Confidence Limits) mg LER 907/mg	No. of Assays	IU 2nd IRP/mg	No. of Assays	IMM/BIO (OAAD) LER 907 std*	IMM/BIO (OAAD) 2nd IRP std**
LER 907	-		310 (320 - 340)	13		5.7
LER 856-1	5.5 (4.8 - 6.3)	9	1,633 (1,500 - 1,780)	8	0.70	3.2
LER 1371	18.9 (17.9 - 19.8)	6	6,235 (6,000 - 6,560)	6	0.92	4.7
LER 960	28.1 (27.2 - 29.1)	3	8,526 (8,230 - 8,800)	3	1.08	5.8
DEAE-2-II	29.7 (28.1 - 31.4)	7	9,349 (8,960 - 9,720)	7	1.22	6.9

*mg LER 907; **IU 2nd IRP.

from the extraction procedure used in the preparation of this standard. Another explanation has been introduced by Ryan (11) based on the hypothesis of the formation of hybrid molecules which could account for the immunologic deficiency of urinary LH. This hypothesis implies that a dissociated biologically inactive but immunologically recognizable form of LH, as well as the biologically active assiciated species of LH, is excreted in urine.

With the reservations pointed out by Albert (15) regarding the use of standards in the bioassay and radioimmunoassay of gonadotropins, it is hoped that an official body such as the World Health Organization (WHO) will undertake the preparation and distribution of suitable standards and reagents for radioimmunoassay. At present it seems very likely that the WHO will consider the distribution of the NPA reference preparation LER 907. If so, this material will become the WHO standard for FSH and LH radioimmunoassays and the values will probably be referred to in terms of the unitage assigned by the WHO to this preparation.

Finally, the use of one hormone as a standard for another hormone represents an unnecessary, confusing and potentially dangerous violation of the principle of similarity. Let us refer to the use of HCG International Standard (IS) for the bioassay and immunoassay of LH. While some LH bioassay systems, such as the OAAD, may fulfill the validity criteria for the bioassay, other biologic systems may not. Similarly, the use of HCG IS or commercial preparations of HCG of varying grades of biologically active purity as standard with or without the use of human pituitary LH preparations or the 2nd IRP as second standards in the LH radioimmunoassay system presumes complete cross-reactivity between LH and HCG.

Table 4 shows the biologic (OAAD assay) and radioimmunologic potency of a human pituitary LH preparation LER 856-1 (referred to in Tables 2 and 3) distributed by the NPA for clinical investigation, and that of HCG 2nd IS. The activity of LER 907 (shown in Tables 2 and 3) is included in this table.

The biopotency estimates of LER 856-1 and HCG 2nd IS were in good agreement both in terms of LER 907 and the 2nd IRP. The immunopotency estimates expressed in terms of LER 907 (for both preparations) agreed very closely with those obtained by bioassay using the same standard; the Immuno/Bio ratio being 0.70 and 1.3, respectively. However, the immunopotency estimates expressed in terms of the 2nd IRP were much greater than those obtained by bioassay; the Immuno/Bio ratio being 3.2 to 4.8, respectively. It is worth noting that the Immuno/Bio ratio of HCG is very similar to that observed with other HLH preparations (Table 3).

All assays fulfilled the necessary statistical criteria for validity. Specifically, all preparations (tested in the radioim-

TABLE 4

BIOLOGIC AND IMMUNOLOGIC POTENCY OF HLH-LER 856-1† AND HCG 2nd IS

Preparation	BIO Potency* in terms of		IMMUNO Potency in terms of		Ratio	
	LER 907	2nd IRP	LER 907	2nd IRP	IMM/BIO LER 907 std	IMM/BIO 2nd IRP std
LER 907	-	54.2 (IU/mg)	-	310 (IU/mg)	-	5.7
(HLH) LER 856-1	7.9 (mg/mg)	510 (IU/mg)	5.5 (mg/mg)	1633 (IU/mg)	0.70	3.2
HCG 2nd IS	10.8 (mg/mg)	592 (IU/mg)	14.0 (mg/mg)	2846 (IU/mg)	1.3	4.8

† Distributed by the NPA for clinical investigation; * OAAD assay.

munoassay at several dose levels) i.e., 2nd IRP, LER 907, LER 856-1, and HCG 2nd IS, elicited parallel dose-response curves. The presence of parallelism in the radioimmunoassay, although a valid criterion of assay, is not alone a sufficient criterion for judging identity of materials being tested in this case, human pituitary and urinary LH and HCG.

When adequate quantities of HFSH and HLH of sufficient chemical purity for use as immunologic reagents, appropriate specific antisera and suitable standards of acceptable and known stability will be made available by an official body, the present confusion in radioimmunoassay values for the levels of FSH and LH in man will disappear.

ACKNOWLEDGEMENTS

This work was supported by Grant AM-07564, USPHS, National Institutes of Health, Bethesda, Maryland.

We are indebted to the National Institute of Arthritis and Metabolic Diseases, NIH, and to the National Pituitary Agency for the generous supply of purified pituitary hormones and for the supply of immunologic reagents. We are also indebted to the Endocrinology Study Section, NIH, Bethesda, Maryland, for the supply of NIH-FSH-S1 and NIH-LH-S1 and to Dr. D. R. Bangham, Department of Biological Standards, Medical Research Council, Mill Hill, London for the gift of the 2nd IRP used in this study. The valuable technical assistance of George Bulat, Lawrence E. Fournier and Margaret M. Shea is gratefully acknowledged.

REFERENCES

1. Rosemberg, E., Solod, E.A. and Albert, A., J. Clin. Endocr., 24: 714, 1964.
2. Albert, A., Derner, I., Rosemberg, E. and Lewis, W.B., Endocrinology, 76: 139, 1965.
3. Albert, A., Hanten, C., Rosemberg, E. and Bulat, G., Endocrinology, 77: 588, 1965.
4. Rosemberg, E. and Engel, I., J. Clin. Endocr., 21: 1063, 1961.
5. Loraine, J. A. and Brown, J.V., J. Clin. Endocr., 16: 1180, 1956.
6. Albert, A., Proc. Staff Meet. Mayo Clinic., 31: 341, 1956.
7. Steelman, S.L. and Pohley, F.M., Endocrinology, 53: 604, 1953.
8. Albert, A., Rosemberg, E., Ross, G. T., Paulsen, C. A. and Ryan, R. J., J. Clin. Endocr., 28: 1214, 1968.
9. Faiman, C. and Ryan, R. J., Proc. Soc. Exp. Biol. Med., 125: 1130, 1967.
10. Faiman, C., Ryan, R.J. and Albert, A., J. Clin. Endocr., 28: 1076, 1968.
11. Ryan, R.J., In Immunoassay of Gonadotropins, ed. Diczfalusy, E., Bogtrykkeriet Forum, Publish., Copenhagen, Denmark, p 300, 1969.

12. Odell, W.D., Ross, G.T. and Rayford, P.L., J. Clin. Invest., 46: 248, 1967.
13. Albert, A., In Gonadotropins 1968, ed. Rosemberg, E., Geron-X Inc., Los Altos, Calif., p. 393, 1968.
14. Odell, W.D., Reichert, L.E. and Swerdloff, R.S., In Gonadotropins 1968, ed. Rosemberg,E., Geron-X Inc. Los Altos, Calif., p. 401, 1968.
15. Albert, A., J. Clin. Endocr., 28: 1683, 1968.

DISCUSSION

DONINI: I agree with Dr. Rosemberg that the use of appropriate standards in radioimmunoassays is extremely important. When we used a urinary standard, i.e., the second IRP-HMG, to determine the potencies of the different urinary preparations with different grades of purity and different FSH:LH ratios, we obtained a very good agreement between biopotency and the immunopotency. The ratio between the FSH and LH potencies as determined by bioassay and radioimmunoassay was close to unity. Our radioimmunoassay system for FSH and LH is a total urinary system. We use highly purified FSH and anti-urinary FSH sera; HCG for labelling, anti-HCG sera and the 2nd IRP-HMG as standards. We thus obtain very good agreement between biopotency and immunopotency.

ROSEMBERG: The reference preparation called LER 907 which is distributed by the NPA in the United States and abroad, is a mixture of human pituitary FSH and LH, and will probably be distributed by the WHO if the collaborative study will show that this material is suitable as a reference preparation. Hence, in the future, we may have this material labelled with a specific unitage assigned to it by the WHO. In the United States, we have used this material for some time and it is recommended to express results of radioimmunoassays in terms of weight of this reference preparation. However, in the future, if the WHO will decide on its distribution, things will be changed. I do hope and I am very hopeful that some continuity regarding unitage will prevail.

We have studied the biological and immunological LH activity of urinary gonadotropin preparations obtained from the urine of postmenopausal women, normal men and eunuchs.

These urinary extracts obtained from these three sources were kindly supplied by Dr. A. Albert, Mayo Clinic, Rochester, Minnesota. The urinary extracts were subjected to the purification steps described by Dr. Albert, in that fraction A, which represented the absorption of HPG on kaolin and subsequent dilution with ammonium, was further purified to fraction B, utilizing 10% ammonium acetate and 70% ethanol; from fraction B a more purified fraction, fraction C was obtained by removal of impurities by adsorption of fraction B with diethylaminoethylcellulose (DEAEC).

In our studies we only analyzed the LH activity of these preparations utilizing bioassay (BIO) and radioimmunoassay (RIA) systems. The bioassays used were the Ventral Prostate Weight (VPW) and Ovarian Ascorbic Acid Depletion (OAAD) assays. The purified human pituitary LH was used for labelling with I-131 and rabbit anti HCG serum was used as the first antibody. Goat anti-rabbit gamma globulin was used as the second antibody to separate free from bound labelled hormone.

Purified pituitary LH and anti HCG serum were kindly provided by the National Institute of Arthritis and Metabolic Diseases through the National Pituitary Agency and the goat anti-rabbit gamma globulin was kindly supplied by Dr. Alice Reiss, Ortho Research Foundation. The Second International Reference Preparation for Human Menopausal Gonadotropins (2nd IRP) was the reference standard. The relative potencies (RP) of fractions A, B, and C derived from the three urinary sources showed good agreement. Fraction A obtained from postmenopausal and eunuch urine showed good agreement between BIO and RIA values; this was not observed with fraction A from male urine. Fractions B and C obtained from these three sources showed higher activity in the RIA system as compared to that obtained with the use of BIO systems.

The mean purification corresponding to fractions A, B, and C, taking fraction A as 1 in the BIO system was similar to that originally published by Dr. Albert. The mean purification taking fraction A as 1 in the immunoassay system showed a similar trend, although, of a different magnitude than that obtained with bioassay. The $\frac{VPW}{OAAD}$ ratio was quite similar for the three fractions from PM, M and E urine; the IMM/BIO ratio increased with increased purification of these fractions.

It has been reported that the IMM/BIO activity of urinary fractions, specifically FSH fractions of urinary extracts, does not differ from unitage in a RIA system which utilizes purified urinary FSH for labelling and a rabbit anti-urinary FSH antiserum.

In this study, which refers to the IMM/BIO LH activity of urinary fractions, the RIA system involved the use of a human pituitary LH for labelling and anti HCG serum. It is possible that the use of this system may have resulted in the differences between IMM/BIO potency of the purified fractions. However, this study suggests that this immunoassay system could be utilized to check the degree of purification obtained when urinary fractions are subjected to various purification procedures.

DICZFALUSY: Chorionic gonadotropin preparations do possess FSH-like activity; this FSH-like activity can be removed, for instance, by Sephadex chromatography. However, there is another activity remaining which we could not remove thus far. If one immunizes rabbits with HCG preparations, one obtains very potent anti-FSH sera. This is due to a material that we call ANF, anti-gonadotropin neutralizing factor, and Dr. Petrusz and I have devised a bioassay for measuring it. The problem is that there are large quantities of biologically inactive, immunologically active materials in highly purified chorionic gonadotropin preparations, which will induce antibodies. These antibodies will neutralize FSH activity of pituitary as well as urinary preparations. Still, in most laboratories, including ours, such HCG preparations are used to obtain antisera which are later on considered to be specific to LH and HCG. By fractionation of chorionic gonadotropin on a Sephadex column one finds low molecular weight material which possesses little biological activity but which still contains a high amount of immunological activity. One obtains an entirely different ratio here than in a high molecular weight material. Therefore, I think that for the time being we should consider the distribution of different standards for bioassays and immunoassays.

ROSEMBERG: I would favor the preparation and distribution of several standards.

ROSS: In human chorionic gonadotropin there is good evidence that antigenic determinants exist that are similar to antigenic determinants in follicle stimulating hormone extracted from either human urine or human pituitary tissue. During purification of human chorionic gonadotropin, one removes substances with the apparent biologic activity of follicle stimulating hormone without completely removing substances with immunologic activity. This is not particularly surprising if one considers that both FSH and HCG are probably composed of subunits, all of which are required for biologic activity of either hormone, but which in biologically active material might still be capable of stimulating antibody formation. The important feature with respect to the nature of antibodies generated against these substances in my opinion relates to the differences in what the individual animal sees in the way of antigenic determinants, in the immunogen. I would like to ask Dr. Diczfalusy if all of the rabbits that are challenged with this particular preparation of chorionic gonadotropin make equally specific and equally potent antisera with respect to the capacity to neutralize the biologic activity of follicle stimulating hormone.

DICZFALUSY: One never obtains equally potent antisera when immunizing 30 rabbits. However, I would submit that in every rabbit we immunized thus far it was possible to detect measurable quantities of anti-FSH. I would say that with one exception we have not seen any rabbit serum thus far which contained less than 50 to 100 anti-

FSH units, and I wonder whether Dr. Lunenfeld would like to add further information to this point.

LUNENFELD: I wish to confirm Dr. Diczfalusy's statement. We have shown that all HCG preparations which we have utilized for immunization, also produced antibodies to FSH.

PREPARATIONS AND BIOLOGICAL CHARACTERISTICS OF HMG PREPARATIONS USED CLINICALLY

Piero Donini

Research Laboratories, Istituto Farmacologico

Serono, Rome, Italy

After the divergent and inconclusive effects obtained in treatment of female sterility with gonadotropin extracts obtained from animal pituitaries or from pregnant mare serum (PMS), our group, which was involved in the preparation of chorionic gonadotropin (HCG), started in 1949 to study the possibility of the preparation of human menopausal gonadotropin (HMG) suitable for treatment in humans. In the same year we published our first paper (1) on the preparation of HMG suitable for clinical investigation and Pergonal became available to physicians in Italy in 1950.

Following the same technique we also prepared Pergonal-23 which, in 1964, became the 2nd IRP HMG. Each ampoule of this reference preparation contains 5 mg of HMG, equivalent to 40 IU of FSH and 40 IU of LH.

Another possible source of human gonadotropins are human pituitaries obtained at autopsy. Although in some countries, e.g. U.S.A., England, and Sweden, collection banks for human pituitaries have been organized, this source does not permit the preparation of human gonadotropins on a large enough scale for general clinical use.

With respect to purification studies, Donini and Marchetti (2) reported the first attempt of chemical characterization of HMG in 1952.

The clinical effect of this HMG preparation in women with primary amenorrhea was reported by Borth et al. (3) and the results confirmed by Rosemberg et al. (4). Due to the relative low specific activity of the original preparations used in these clinical trials, further purification was attempted. Donini et al. (5) increased the relative potency of the HMG preparation so that the 75 IU of FSH and 75 IU of LH contained in one ampoule of Pergonal-500 (trade mark of purer HMG preparation) were equivalent to about 1-2 mg of HMG.

In diagram 1, reported by Lunenfeld (6), the extraction and purification procedure of our HMG preparation is illustrated. The extraction of gonadotropins from menopausal urine was done according to the method of Bradbury et al. (7) and the crude material obtained was then purified following the method of Albert et al. (8). This is based on the extraction of crude HMG with 10% ammonium acetate in 70% ethanol followed by absorption of the impurities on DEAE-C at pH 7. At this point of purification, we used Permutit column chromatography which, I believe, is the most important step for purification. With this step one can obtain an HMG preparation with a biological potency about 130-300 times higher than crude gonadotropic extract obtained by the first step or the kaolin-acetone precipitate.

It should be emphasized that by this single step of purification it was possible not only to increase the biological potency but to completely eliminate the phosphate salts contained in the buffer solution used for the step on DEAE-C.

By following the purification procedure described above, improved human menopausal gonadotropins could be prepared for therapeutic purposes; the LD_{50} in mice was very low, the specific FSH and LH potencies varied from batch to batch but the range was 40-90 IU per mg and the FSH:LH ratio was about 1:1. In some clinical trials the contents of 52 ampoules of Pergonal-500 were dissolved in 5 ml of saline and injected in one woman without relevant side-effects.

Initial clinical trials with Pergonal-500 were carried out and reported by Lunenfeld et al. (9,10). In one patient with primary amenorrhea, pregnancy with subsequent delivery of a normal infant was achieved.

It is well known that the gonadotropic extracts prepared from human pituitaries or menopausal urine contain two different hormones with different biological activities, i.e. follicle stimulating hormone (FSH), and luteinizing hormone (LH or ICSH). For a better understanding of the mechanism of these two gonadotropins, it was necessary to purify further and to separate these two biological activities. Due to the short time available for this presentation, I cannot present the details of studies carried out by several workers over the last ten years. But it would be of interest to examine the table previously published (11) which lists the biological potencies of urinary preparations obtained by different authors up to 1966 and expressed in terms of IU of the 2nd IRP-HMG.

Diagram 1. EXTRACTION AND PURIFICATION OF HUMAN MENOPAUSAL GONADOTROPINS.

Step 1: KAOLIN EXTRACTION

The kaolin is activated by washing with 1M-HCl, allowed to settle, the supernatant decanted and the kaolin subjected to repeated washings with water. Human Menopausal Urine adjusted to pH 4.5 with glacial AcH, then shaken with celite + 20% activated kaolin suspension.

Allowed to settle overnight at room temp.

sediment — supernatant discarded

centrifugation

supernatant discarded — precipitate washed twice with tap water adjusted to pH 4.5 with glacial AcH

elution twice with 1M-NH_4OH eluate (pH 11-11.3) adjusted to pH 8.5 with glacial acetic acid

Centrifugation

supernatant acidified to pH 5-5.5 with glacial acetic acid — precipitate discarded

2 volumes acetone added with stirring and left overnight

Precipitate washed with acetone, then with 95% EtOH, then with ether (HMG-K) — supernatant discarded

Step 2: CONDITIONING FOR DEAE-CELLULOSE TREATMENT

(HMG-K)

extracted twice by stirring with 70% EtOH + 10% ammonium acetate and filtered

ppt. discarded — clear extract

2 vols. of abs. EtOH + 10% ammonium acetate added allowed to settle overnight at 4-5° C, then ppt. centrifuged.

ppt. washed with 95% EtOH, then with ether and finally dried (HMG-PD) — supernatant discarded

Step 3: DEAE-CELLULOSE TREATMENT

The DEAE-cellulose is previously washed with 0.5 N-HCl, then with 0.5 N-NaOH and finally with 0.05 M-phosphate buffer (pH 7)

HMG-PD

dissolved in 0.05 M-phosphate buffer(pH 7) shaken with DEAE-cellulose, filtered through Buchner funnel, then ppt. washed twice with 0.05 M-phosphate buffer (pH 7).

filtrate acidified to pH 5.4 with glacial acetic acid then cooled to 4-5° C (HMG-D)

ppt. discarded

Step 4: CHROMATOGRAPHY ON PERMUTIT COLUMN

The permutit column is previously washed with 1M-NH_4OH, then with 1M-acetic acid, and finally equilibrated with 0.05 M-sod. acetate buffer (pH 5.4)

HMG-D

clear liquid poured into column in a cold room at 4-5° C

Column washed with 0.05 M acetate buffer (pH 5.4) until optical density of outflow is near 0 at 280 mμ

outflow discarded

elute adsorbed proteins with 40% EtOH + 10% ammonium acetate

discard outflow

add to eluate 95% EtOH (chilled at 2-4° C) with stirring, allow to settle overnight at 2-4° C, centrifuge ppt.

ppt. washed with abs. EtOH, then with ether and finally dried. (HMG-P)

supernatant discarded

(From: Excerpta Medica Proceedings of Second International Congress of Endocrinology, London, 1964. Excerpta Medica International Cong. Series, No. 83, p 814).

Later the urinary FSH and LH hormones were purified further. With respect to FSH, homogeneous preparations were obtained by Roos (12) and by our group (13,14). Both of us had the opportunity to make the physical chemical characterization and, in general, the findings obtained in the different laboratories agreed except for the sialic acid content which was much higher in our FSH preparation compared to that of Roos.

Diagram 2 depicts the different steps of purification which allowed us to prepare our purest and most active urinary follicle stimulating and luteinizing hormone preparations. In fact the FSH preparation contained 1255 IU-FSH as determined biologically according to the method of Steelman and Pohley, and only 3.2 IU-LH per mg as determined by radioimmunoassay according to the method of Donini et al. (16). Although the purest LH preparation was not homogeneous, as demonstrated by the different criteria commonly used for the physical-chemical characterization of proteins, it showed one of the highest biological and immunological activities reported, i.e. 982 IU and 1166 IU-LH, respectively. No FSH activity could be detected in this preparation at a dose level of 1260 µg.

These highly purified preparations of urinary FSH and LH were important not only to clarify the physical-chemical properties but also for other reasons. Other workers as well as our group have used these purified FSH preparations for labelling in radioimmunoassay systems and specificity studies of urinary anti FSH sera have also been carried out (17).

Furthermore, these same highly purified FSH preparations were used clinically by Mancini et al. who studied the effect of urinary FSH on the testes of hypophysectomized patients. The same group also studied the effects of highly purified LH and FSH and LH combinations at different ratios on the testis of the same patients. Their results will be reported elsewhere.

Bompiani and his group utilized the same highly purified FSH and LH preparations to study the effect of these hormones in the ovaries of one hypophysectomized patient. These results will also be published elsewhere.

With respect to the HMG preparations, which are used clinically in the therapy of female and male sterility, another point to be considered is their FSH:LH ratio. As reported herein, we can now prepare the HMG preparations with different FSH:LH ratios, but unfortunately we do not have good evidence as to which ratio can be considered the best in order to have the optimal effectiveness for induction of ovulation and pregnancy and to avoid hyperstimulation and multiple ovulation.

Diagram 2. PURIFICATION OF FOLLICLE-STIMULATING AND LUTEINIZING HORMONES FROM HUMAN MENOPAUSAL GONADOTROPIN. THE BIOLOGIC ACTIVITIES ARE EXPRESSED IN IU (2nd IRP-HMG)

HMG (Pergonal, 82.7 IU of FSH and 58.3 IU of LH per mg) 5.46 g

Batchwise separation of FSH and LH on DEAE-C

FSH fraction (2.88 g; 133 IU-FSH/mg) DEAE-C column chromatography

Eluted by borate phosphate buffer pH 8.0 +0.1 M NaCl (828 mg; 351 IU-FSH/mg) Gel filtration on Sephadex G-100

Other fractions with lower activity

Symmetric part of the 2nd protein peak (323.7 mg ; 692 IU-FSH/mg). Preparative disc electrophoresis

Other fractions with lower activity

Part of 2nd protein peak. Highly purified FSH 104.3 mg; 1255 IU-FSH/mg, 3.2 IU-LH/mg

Other fractions with lower activity

LH fraction (1.74 g; 86 IU-LH/mg) Batchwise chromatography on CMC-70

Eluted by 0.005 M phosphate buffer pH 6 + 0.5 NaCl (1.03 g; 102 IU-LH/mg) Gel filtration on Sephadex G-100

Impurities with lower activity

First part of ascending limb of elution curve (240 mg; 263 IU/mg) DEAE-Sephadex chromatography

Impurities with lower activity

Eluted by 0.002 M phosphate buffer pH 6.6 + 0.01 M NaCl (36.8 mg; 807 IU/mg) Gel filtration on Sephadex G-200

Impurities with lower activity

Symmetric and sharp part of the first peak. Highly purified LH 20.4 mg; 1166 IU/mg.

Fractions with lower activity

(From: Donini et al, In: Gonadotropins 1968, Rosemberg, E. ed., Los Altos, Calif. p 40, 1968).

Rosemberg and Nwe (18), Jones et al. (19), Taymor (20), and Bettendorf et al. (21) have studied this problem. In general we agree with Rosemberg's conclusion that, "Because the number of courses of medication is relatively small, investigation on the importance of FSH:LH ratios contained in HMG preparations used clinically should be continued." Nevertheless, it seems that if the FSH:LH ratio is too high, the effectiveness of the preparation is lower than when the FSH:LH ratio is about 1:1 with regard to the follicle ripening and estrogen excretion prior to ovulation. In other words, the total amount of FSH activity needed for follicular ripening is higher when the HMG preparation used has a high FSH:LH ratio (20). On the contrary, as reported by Rosemberg (18), "with preparations containing a higher proportion of LH activity relative to FSH, small increases in dosage were shown to cause an excessive pregnanediol excretion," and according to Bettendorf (21), "it is of interest that a higher incidence of ovarian enlargement was found in the group of patients who received the low FSH:LH ratio preparation than those patients who received a preparation having a high FSH:LH ratio."

In the last few years, our knowledge of the ovulatory mechanism in normal women is much better than in the past. We know that through the positive or negative feedback due to the action of ovarian steroids on the hypothalamus, the FSH and LH releasing factors regulate the release of follicle-stimulating and luteinizing hormones from the pituitary gland in such a way that these gonadotropins act in due time and in due amount on the ovaries. In the normal menstrual cycle, we also know the pattern of FSH and LH levels as determined in the urine or serum by bioassay or radioimmunoassay.

Up to now, as reported in several papers, induction of ovulation and pregnancy was tried in anovulatory women using HMG preparations having different FSH:LH ratios, i.e.: very high, 1:1, and very low. In these studies the same preparation and the same FSH:LH ratio were used during the entire course of a given treatment.

Another problem which should be kept in mind is that after stimulation of the follicle by HMG, to induce ovulation and to produce a functional corpus lutem, HCG has been injected instead of LH because LH was not available for extensive clinical trial. We know (22) that the disappearance rate from the blood is greater for LH than HCG. This finding could explain the ovarian hyperstimulation and the multiple pregnancy when HCG was injected. It is worth noticing that, according to the data obtained by radioimmunoassay, the ovulatory peak of LH is only about 24 hours long.

I believe that a new therapeutic approach with human gonadotropins could be tried in anovulatory women who are sterile due to a relative or absolute lack of pituitary gonadotropins. In the last two years several authors have reported that in the first part of the follicular phase of the menstrual cycle, most of the normal women studied showed in their serum and urine an FSH:LH ratio of about 2:1. Then in the second part of the follicular phase and before the ovulatory peak, the FSH:LH ratio was about 0.3:1. Later on in the cycle, the FSH:LH ratio is again about 1:1.

It would be worthwhile to evaluate the response to HMG preparations using different FSH:LH ratios during a course of treatment. It would also be worthwhile to use urinary or pituitary LH instead of HCG to induce the ovulation. One should keep in mind that the responsiveness to human gonadotropins varies from one patient to another and thus follicular stimulation should be carefully controlled by the rapid determination of estrogens by the method of Brown (23) or by other parameters like the fern test, karyopyknotic index, etc.

The same problems of FSH:LH ratio, dosage, and length of therapy, occur when male infertility has to be treated with human gonadotropins. Unfortunately, we do not have enough information on the physiology and the pathology of the human testis and I hope that this meeting will increase our knowledge on these problems.

In conclusion, using the methods of extraction and purification which have just been reported on, it is possible to have available a large amount of HMG with different grades of purity and with different FSH:LH ratios.

REFERENCES

1. Donini, P. and Montezemolo, R., Rass. Clin. Ter., 48: 143, 1949.
2. Donini, P. and Marchetti, E., Il Farmaco., 7: 418, 1952.
3. Borth, R., Lunenfeld, B., and Menzi, A., In Human Pituitary Gonadotropins. A Workshop Conference, ed. Albert, A., C. Thomas, Springfield, Ill., p 255, 1961.
4. Rosemberg, E., Coleman, J., Demany, M. and Garcia, C.R., J. Clin. Endocr., 23: 181, 1963.
5. Donini, P., Puzzuoli, D., and Montezemolo, R., Acta Endocr., (Kobenhavn), 45: 321, 1964.
6. Lunenfeld, B., Proc. 2nd Intern. Congress of Endocr. Publ. Excerpta Medica International Congress Series 83, p 814, 1964.
7. Bradbury, J.T., Brown, E.S., and Brown, W.E., Proc. Soc. Exp. Biol. Med., 71: 228, 1949.
8. Albert, A., Kobi, J., Leiferman, J., and Derner, J., J. Clin. Endocr., 21: 1, 1961.
9. Lunenfeld, B., Sulimovici, S., Rabau, E., and Eshkol, A., C.R. Soc. Franc. Gynecol. 35: 346, 1962.
10. Lunenfeld, B., Sulimovici, S., and Rabau, E., Proc. of Tel-Hashomer Hospital. 1: 25, 1962.
11. Donini, P., Puzzuoli, D., D'Alessio, I., Lunenfeld, B., Eshkol,

A., and Parlow, A.F., Acta Endocr. (Kobenhavn) 52: 169, 1966.
12. Roos, P., Acta Endocr. (Kobenhavn) 59: Suppl. 131, 5, 1968.
13. Donini, P., Puzzuoli, D., D'Alessio, I., Bergesi, G., and Donini, S. In Gonadotropins 1968, ed. Rosemberg, E., Geron-X, Los Altos, Calif., p. 37, 1968.
14. Donini, P., Puzzuoli, D., D'Alessio, I., Bergesi, G., and Donini, S., In Proceedings of meeting on 'Chemistry of Gonadotropins', Birmingham, 1969, in press.
15. Steelman, S.L. and Pohley, F. M., Endocrinology, 53: 640, 1953.
16. Donini, S., D'Alessio, I., and Donini, P., In Gonadotropins 1968, ed. Rosemberg, E., Geron-X, Los Altos, Calif., p. 263, 1968.
17. Donini, S. and Donini, P., In 1st Karolinska Symposium. Immunoassay of Gonadotropins, ed. Diczfalusy, E. Bogtrykkeriet Forum, Copenhagen, p. 57, 1968.
18. Rosemberg, E. and Nwe, T.T., Fertil. Steril. 19: 197, 1968.
19. Jones, G.S., De Moraes, R., Johanson, A.J., Ruiti, S. and Blizzard, R.M., Fertil. Steril., 20: 14, 1969.
20. Taymor , M.L. In Progress in Infertility, ed. Behrman, S.J. and Kistner, R.W., p. 393, 1968.
21. Bettendorf, G., Breckwoldt, M., and Neale, C., In Gonadotropins 1968, ed. Rosemberg, E., Geron-X, Los Altos, Calif., p. 453, 1968.
22. Yen, S.S.C., Llerena, O., Little, B., and Pearson, O.H., J. Clin. Endocr., 28: 1763, 1968.
23. Brown, J.B., MacLeod, S.C., Macnaughtan, C., Smith, M.A., and Smith, B., J. Endocr., 42:, 5, 1968.

DISCUSSION

JUTISZ: Dr. Donini, what physiochemical criteria did you use to show that your urinary FSH is a homogeneous protein? Can you also tell us about the contamination of this preparation with LH and other hormones? Finally, do you have any information about the amino acid and carbohydrate composition of this preparation, and is this the same as in human pituitary FSH? In other words, there is always a possibility of an alteration of the original molecule. I think that Mori showed some time ago that human pituitary FSH cross-reacts only partially with urinary FSH.

DONINI: The criteria used to demonstrate the homogeneity of our FSH preparation were the commonly used criteria, that is, 1) the pattern of sedimentation in the ultracentrifuge, where we observed only one peak; 2) disc electrophoresis on polyacrylamide gel. The disc electrophoresis pattern of the different fractions was as follows: in the less purified fraction (fraction A) many bands were seen; fraction B showed a smaller number of bands; with highly purified FSH only one band was observed. Also, with regard to the carbohydrate moiety we have demonstrated that urinary FSH is very similar to pituitary FSH. For example, we found that in our preparation one of the most important carbohydrate components, the sialic acid, was almost the same as that found in pituitary FSH; 8.4% of sialic acid was found in urinary preparations. About the same value was found by Dr. Reichert and by other investigators in pituitary FSH preparations. Some differences between urinary and pituitary FSH exists. The immunological behavior of some pituitary and urinary FSH preparations are different. We have demonstrated that our radioimmunoassay system with reagents of urinary origin is not suitable for radioimmunoassay of FSH in plasma. This means that at least some immunological differences exist between urinary and pituitary FSH. The activity of the highly purified FSH was determined biologically by the method of Steelman and Pohley. The LH contamination was determined by radioimmunoassay, because it was almost impossible, or difficult to waste so many milligrams of this preparation, to test its LH activity by biological methods. The FSH potency of this preparation was 1250 IU per mg and the LH contamination was 3.2 IU per mg. The differences between the amino acid composition of urinary and pituitary FSH are very small.

ROSEMBERG: Dr. Donini pointed out that in the preparation of HMG used clinically, the consideration of FSH:LH ratios is of importance. Dr. Diczfalusy, as well as ourselves, some years ago indicated that the FSH:LH ratio contained in HMG preparations was of importance in the treatment of female infertility. With the availability of purified material of urinary or pituitary origin it will be much easier to study this problem experimentally, mixing both hormones at a certain desired FSH:LH ratio. We have used purified HFSH and HLH at ratios similar to those described by Dr. Ross in his study of the blood levels of FSH and LH during the normal menstrual cycle. We have treated eight patients during 13 or 14 courses of medication. Most patients ovulated as judged by indirect indices of ovulation. Three of the patients became pregnant. There were no untoward effects. These were patients with intact pituitaries. We should test these combinations further in hypophysectomized patients. I think we are approaching the time when with the availability of purified materials,many of the previously unanswered questions will be clarified.

LUNENFELD: I would like to add that we now currently use urinary testosterone to monitor the amount of HCG to be given in addition to Pergonal in the treatment of males. We try to keep the testosterone at a desired level. I think this may be one of the ways to monitor treatment.

DONINI: Dr. Lunenfeld, how many international units of HCG or LH do you think are useful for the treatment of male infertility?

LUNENFELD: I do not think that we can make any general statement here. Before we start treating a patient we always evaluate Leydig cell function by dynamic tests. I was very impressed with Dr. Steinberger's presentation because it demonstrated that the testicular biopsy by itself might sometimes be misleading. We rely to a certain extent on urinary testosterone and estrogen as indicative of Leydig cell response to HCG. If, in a certain patient, there is very little or no response to HCG we treat this patient for 14 days with HCG alone and then re-estimate testosterone. If testosterone is increased, Pergonal therapy is initiated with the same amount of HCG which would keep the testosterone value at the desired level. This amount will vary from patient to patient.

PAULSEN: Dr. Lunenfeld, I assume you are referring to the treatment of patients with hypogonadotropic eunuchoidism.

PLASMA FSH AND LH MEASURED BY RADIOIMMUNOASSAY IN NORMAL AND PATHOLOGIC CONDITIONS IN MEN

Griff T. Ross

Endocrinology Branch, National Cancer Institute, National Institutes of Health, Bethesda, Maryland, 20014

Rational therapy of hypogonadal states in men depends in part upon determining whether the problem results from failure of the pituitary to secrete gonadotropins or from failure of the testes to respond. The use of double antibody radioimmunoassays for plasma follicle stimulating hormone (FSH) and luteinizing hormone (LH) in attempts to distinguish these pathophysiologic alternatives among patients seen on the clinical service of the Endocrinology Branch, National Cancer Institute will be reviewed here.

MATERIALS AND METHODS

1. Assays

Radioimmunoassays for FSH and LH activity in plasma were performed by methods which have been described in detail (1,2,3). All samples from an individual patient were assayed in the same assay. Not all samples from all subjects were included in a single assay, since this was not feasible for this study.

In both FSH and LH assays, dose response relationships of the Second International Reference Preparation of Human Menopausal Gonadotropin (IRP 2 HMG) have proved to be satisfactory for dose interpolation of concentrations of these hormones in samples of both plasma and urine. The immunoreactivity of 1 milli International Unit (mIU) of biological activity of this reference preparation is equivalent to that of 33 and 4 nanograms of the LER 907 reference preparation (Distributed by the National Pituitary Agency, USA) in these assays for FSH and LH respectively. In this discussion all concentrations will be expressed in milli International Units of IRP 2 HMG per milliliter (mIU/ml) of plasma.

The methods of Rodbard and associates (4) and of Weaver (5) were used for dose interpolation in most instances. Statistical quality control was maintained by the method of Rodbard et al. (6). In the assay of LH when 300 ml. plasma samples were used, a minimal detectable quantity was usually around 6 mIU per ml. Similarly, for FSH when 200 ml. plasma samples were used, the quantity was around 4 mIU per ml. In both assays potency estimates were less precise when concentrations were near either the upper or lower limits than when near the middle of the proportionate range of the dose response curve (6,7).

2. Clomiphene Tests

Clomiphene citrate was given in doses of 200 mg per day orally for six days. This regimen usually elicited significant increases in concentrations of immunoreactive FSH and LH when samples taken prior to and during administration of drug to normal men were compared (8-11). When coupled with simultaneous measurements of plasma testosterone concentrations, some evidence of Leydig cell response to LH was obtained (8,10).

3. Patients

Six eugonadal men, ages 19 to 57 years, served as controls. Eighteen men with hypogonadism were studied. Seven of these hypogonadal men had a syndrome characterized by retarded sexual and somatic development associated with skeletal anomalies and hyposmia, but with 46, XY karyotypes in cells cultured from peripheral blood (10). Seven of them were hypogonadal due to either neoplastic or idiopathic pituitary disease. The four anorchic patients included two who had been orchiectomized for treatment of carcinoma of the prostate and two with the "vanishing testis" syndrome (12).

RESULTS

Twenty-eight plasma samples taken on separate days, usually consecutively, from the six eugonadal men were assayed for FSH and LH. The mean, standard deviation of the mean and range of values obtained in each subject are summarized in Table 1. Plasma FSH concentrations varied from two to four-fold, within subjects between days. Values ranged from 4.7 to 27.3 mIU per ml when all determinations for all subjects were considered. Plasma LH values were somewhat less variable than plasma FSH values in this small series of samples although, on occasion, concentrations of LH in plasma samples randomly collected from other eugonadal men fell below the limits of detection in a given assay.

Means of FSH and LH concentrations in all specimens from the group of eugonadal men were compared with means of concentrations in randomly collected samples from the three groups of hypogonadal

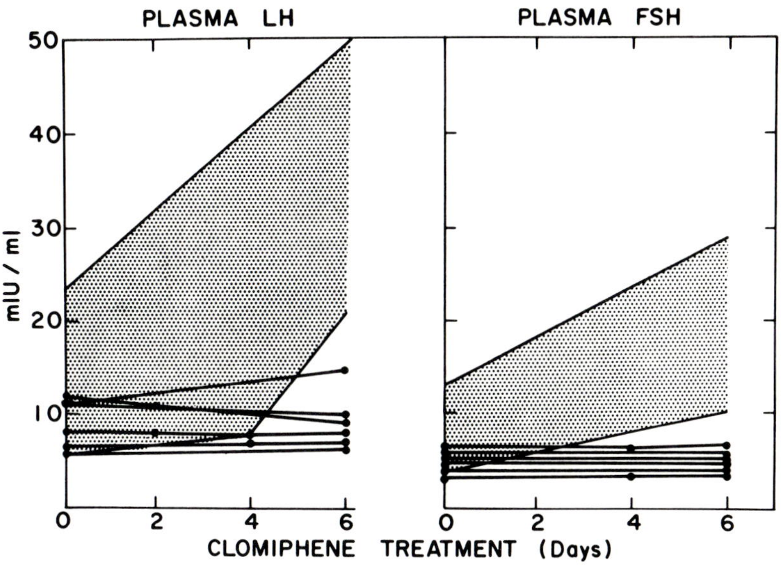

Fig. 1 Plasma FSH and LH concentrations prior to and during administration of Clomiphene to men with hypogonadism and hyposmia. Shaded areas depict range of responses in eugonadal men on the same regimen. (From: Bardin, C.W. et al., J. Clin. Invest., 48 2049, 1969.)

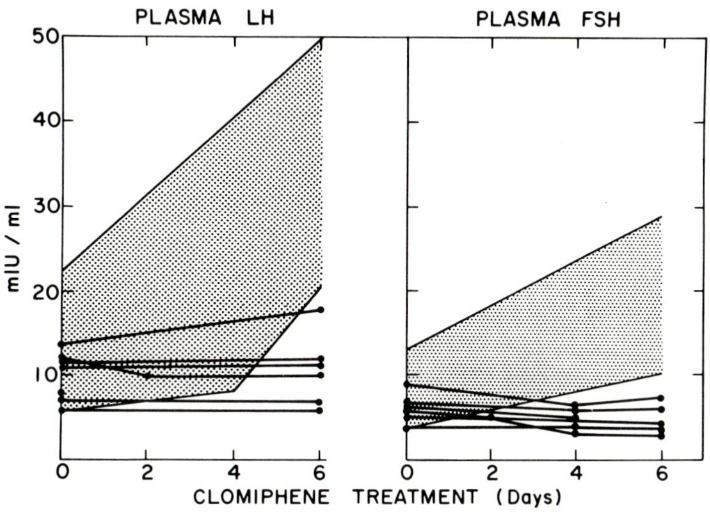

Fig. 2 Plasma FSH and LH concentrations prior to and during administration of Clomiphene to hypogonadal men with hypopituitarism. The shaded areas represent the range of values in eugonadal men on the same regimen. (From: Bardin, C.W. et al., J. Clin. Invest., 48: 2049, 1969.)

Subject	Number Samples	FSH*		LH*	
		Mean ± SD	Range	Mean ± SD	Range
A	4	6.9 ± 2.8	4.7 – 10.9	14.0 ± 4.0	11.1 – 19.9
B	5	16.7 ± 6.2	11.9 – 27.3	11.1 ± 1.0	10.4 – 12.8
C	5	9.9 ± 2.2	7.4 – 12.9	13.1 ± 3.0	9.9 – 17.6
D	4	10.0 ± 5.0	6.5 – 17.4	15.2 ± 2.1	12.5 – 17.5
E	5	15.3 ± 6.6	5.5 – 22.8	13 ± 1.3	11.7 – 14.5
F	5	12.3 ± 3.3	8.1 – 16.6	10.7 ± 1.3	9.5 – 12.9

* milli International Units per milliliter of plasma (radioimmunoassay, IRP 2 HMG)

Table 1 Mean, standard deviation and range of FSH and LH concentrations in plasma samples from six eugonadal men.

men. Results are shown in Table 2. Comparisons showed that mean concentrations for FSH and LH in each group of hypogonadal men were significantly different from mean concentrations for the group of eugonadal men. Thus, comparison of means of concentrations of FSH and LH in single random plasma samples distinguished the groups of hypogonadal men from the group of eugonadal men.

Therapeutic decisions must be made for individuals rather than for groups, however. Ranges of values in the six eugonadal men were compared with ranges of values in the three groups of hypogonadal men (Table 3). Concentrations in single samples discriminated between the six eugonadal men and the four anorchic hypogonadal men in every instance since the ranges of values obtained showed no overlap. In contrast, measurement of either FSH or LH or of both in single samples did not discriminate between individual eugonadal men and individual hypogonadal men, either hypopituitary or hyposmic. Thus, determinations of concentrations of FSH and LH in a single random plasma sample appeared to be of limited diagnostic value for any except anorchic subjects.

The possibility that assays of multiple specimens taken from a single subject might be diagnostic was considered. To test this possibility, values for LH were determined in four samples taken daily from two subjects with hypogonadism and hyposmia and the means calculated (Table 4). Tests for significance of differences were made using means for similar numbers of samples from the six individual eugonadal men(Table 1). Results were significant ($p < .05$) in only two of six contrasts for subject K, but in all six contrasts for subject L. Thus, means of determinations of plasma concentrations of LH in four daily specimens also failed to be diagnostic when hypogonadism resulted from failure of adequate pituitary gonadotropin secretion.

Group	Number Subjects	FSH*	LH*
Eugonadal men	6	12.1 ± 1.0	12.7 ± 0.5
Hypogonadal men			
A. Hypopituitary	7	5.7 ± 0.6†	9.4 ± 1.1†
B. Hyposmic	7	5.3 ± 0.5†	9.7 ± 1.2†
C. Anorchic	4	93.1 ± 6.6†	54.1 ± 3.6†

* milli International Units per milliliter plasma (radioimmuno-assay, IRP 2 HMG).

† $p < 0.05$ when compared with eugonadal controls.

Table 2 Mean and standard error of mean plasma FSH and LH concentrations in eugonadal and hypogonadal men.

Group	Number Subjects	FSH*	LH*
Eugonadal men	6	4.7 – 27	9.5 – 19.9
Hypogonadal men			
A. Hypopituitary	7	4 – 8	<6 – 14
B. Hyposmic	7	4 – 7	<6 – 14
C. Anorchic	4	66 – 120	37 – 86

* milli International Units per milliliter plasma (radioimmuno-assay, IRP 2 HMG)

Table 3 Range of FSH and LH concentrations in plasma samples from eugonadal and hypogonadal men.

Subject	Range	Mean	S.E.M.
K	8.8 – 11.2	10.0	0.5
L	6.4 – 8.0	6.8	0.4

Table 4 Range, mean, and standard error of the mean LH concentrations in four plasma samples from each of two hypogonadal men with hyposmia. Units are milli International Units per ml of plasma (radioimmunoassay, IRP 2 HMG).

When other tests had failed to be diagnostic, results of clomiphene tests were examined since plasma concentrations of FSH and LH always increased when eugonadal men were given clomiphene in doses of 200 mg per day for six days (8,9.10). Results of similar tests performed in the seven hypogonadal men with hypopituitarism and the seven hypogonadal men with hyposmia are shown in Figs. 1 and 2 respectively. Uniformly, these hypogonadal men failed to increase plasma FSH and LH concentrations in response to clomiphene, clearly discriminating them from eugonadal men.

DISCUSSION

The hypogonadal syndromes examined in this series are representative of the pathophysiologic varieties encountered by physicians in clinical practice. These include failure of gonadal function presumably due to either an intrinsic gonadal abnormality or to inadequate pituitary gonadotropin secretion, with a variety of nosologic entities in each group.

In this study, determination of concentrations of FSH and LH in a single randomly collected sample of plasma clearly discriminated men with normal gonadal function from men with hypogonadism secondary to gonadal failure per se. It is conceivable that in a larger group of anorchic men or in a larger group of normal men some might be found in whom concentrations of FSH and LH in random plasma samples would be identical. It seems likely, however, that in the majority of instances of hypogonadism due to gonadal failure, diagnostic information could be obtained from a single determination.

In contrast, the diagnosis of hypogonadism due to inadequate pituitary gonadotropin secretion was more complex. Hypogonadism associated with low levels of gonadotropin secretion in syndromes characterized by chronologically delayed spontaneous pubescence presented particularly difficult problems. It is noteworthy that in normal prepubertal males, as in hypogonadal males in this study, determination of FSH and LH activity in a single specimen of plasma occasionally failed to discriminate an individual prepubertal boy from a sexually mature normal male (5,13-17). Similarly, low but variable urinary total gonadotropin activity has been observed in concentrates of 24-hour urine collections in prepubertal boys (13). Thus, results of a single determination of either plasma or urinary gonadotropin activity may not permit definitive categorization of pituitary gonadotropin secretion among these patients.

Failure of measurements of plasma FSH and LH to provide diagnostically decisive results might be supposed to be due uniquely to reagents and methods of measurement used in this study. Since similar results have been obtained by others using different reagents, this explanation does not appear to be tenable (14,16,17).

The failure of measurement of FSH and LH in randomly collected plasma samples to be diagnostic is methodologic in part since it has been shown that both precision and specificity are less dependable when concentrations of gonadotropins are near the limits of detection by radioimmunoassay (6,7). When concentrations are low, it is frequently not possible to detect activity at sample volumes less than the maximum which can be tolerated without influencing specificity of measurements in some assay systems (18). Under these conditions, then, inability to demonstrate similarity in dose response relationships of unknown and reference preparation makes it impossible to employ this test for specificity.

When specificity of the assay is uncertain, discrepancies between results of these measurements and the degree of hypogonadism might be expected and, indeed, occur (13). Whether the discrepancies relate to substances which are antigenically active but biologically inactive gonadotropins cannot always be determined. It is tempting to speculate that differences between immunologic and biologic potency estimates shown for buffer solutions of a variety of pituitary extracts (19) may also exist for gonadotropins in plasma. Developments of methods for extraction and concentration of gonadotropins from plasma may permit systematic investigation of the antigenic and biologic properties of plasma gonadotropins. In addition, such techniques may serve to enhance both the precision and specificity of the determination, increasing the diagnostic value for the individual patient of either a single measurement or alternately of measurements of activity in a series of specimens.

In summary, then, when low plasma gonadotropin concentrations prevail, that is, when pituitary gonadotropin secretion is reduced, measurements of concentrations in four or five randomly collected plasma samples may not be completely reliable for diagnostic categorization. Under these circumstances, failure of concentrations of immunoreactive FSH and LH in plasma to rise in response to clomiphene is consistent with a diagnosis of hypogonadism secondary to inadequate pituitary gonadotropin secretion. Used in this manner, radioimmunoassays for plasma gonadotropins provide information diagnostically useful for evaluation of hypogonadism in men.

REFERENCES

1. Odell, W.D., Rayford, P.L. and Ross, G.T., J. Lab. Clin. Med., 70: 293, 1967.
2. Odell, W.D., Ross, G.T. and Rayford, P.L., J. Clin. Invest., 46: 248, 1967.
3. Cargille, C.M., Rodbard, D. and Ross, G.T., J. Clin. Endocr., 28: 1276, 1968.
4. Rodbard, D., Bridson, W.E. and Rayford, P.L., J. Lab. Clin. Med., 74: 770, 1969.
5. Weaver, C.K. and Cargille, C.M., unpublished observations.

6. Rodbard, D., Rayford, P.L., Cooper, J.L. and Ross, G.T., J. Clin. Endocr., 28: 1412, 1968.
7. Rodbard, D., Cooper, J.A., Proc. International Symposium on Radio Isotopes in Medicine: In vitro Studies. International Atomic Energy Agency, 1969.
8. Bardin, C.W., Ross, G.T., and Lipsett, M.D., J. Clin. Endocr., 27: 1558, 1967.
9. Cargille, C.M., Ross, G.T. and Bardin, C.W., Lancet, 2: 1298, 1968.
10. Bardin, C.W., Ross, G.T., Rifkind, A.B., Cargille, C.M. and Lipsett, M.B., J. Clin. Invest., 48: 2046, 1969.
11. Peterson, N.T., Midgley, A.R., and Jaffe, R.B., J. Clin. Endocr., 28: 1473, 1968.
12. Abeyaratne, M.R., Aherne, W.A. and Scott, J.E.S., Lancet, 2: 822, 1969.
13. Rifkind, A.B., Kulin, H.E. and Ross, G.T., J. Clin. Invest., 46: 1925, 1967.
14. Schalch, D.S., Parlow, A.F., Boon, R.C. and Reichlin, S., J. Clin. Invest., 47: 665, 1968.
15. Cargille, C.M., Rayford, P.L., and Howland, L.A.,Excerpta Medica Foundation: International Congress Series No. 157: 187, 1968.
16. Faiman, C. and Ryan, R., J. Clin. Endocr., 27: 444, 1967.
17. Saxena, B.B., Demura, H., Gandy, H.M. and Peterson, R.E., J. Clin. Endocr., 28: 519, 1968.
18. Burr, I.M., Brant, D.B., Sizonerho, P.C., Kaplan, S.L. and Grumbach, M.M., J. Clin. Endocr., 29: 948, 1969.
19. Albert, A., Rosemberg, E., Ross, G.T., and Paulsen, C.A. and Ryan, R.J., J. Clin. Endocr., 28: 1214, 1968

DISCUSSION

TROEN: I should like to report briefly on studies carried out by Dr. Howard Nankin and myself measuring serum gonadotropin levels in 11 men following bilateral orchiectomy for prostatic carcinoma. Six patients with normal preoperative FSH levels and five patients with elevated levels showed a steady increase in FSH during the days following surgery. The average increase each day was the same in both groups. In seven patients of this group with normal preoperative LH levels there was an early and marked increase in LH levels peaking on the second day and then falling to a lower but still elevated level. The different response of FSH and LH following orchiectomy suggests that release from gonadal inhibition (or metabolism of gonadotropin) yields a different pattern of synthesis and/or secretion of the two gonadotropins. This may be an inherent characteristic of the hypothalamic-pituitary axis or may reflect different inhibitory factors from the testis for each gonadotropin.

LUNENFELD: Dr. Ross, I was very interested in your clomiphene test. I think you have confirmed, once and for all, that this rules out clomiphene therapy for hypogonadotropic males.

ROSS: I have no experience in the use of clomiphene in the treatment of hypogonadotropic hypogonadism. However, I would suppose that clomiphene would be ineffective in instances of hypogonadotropic hypogonadism such as those we have studied in this series.

PAULSEN: Dr. Santen in our laboratory has studied the response to 30 days of clomiphene administration in patients with hypogonadotropic eunuchoidism. There was no LH rise.

ROSS: In our cases, there was clinical evidence of gonadal failure manifest in terms of low plasma concentrations of testosterone associated with loss of libido and potentia in these hypopituitary subjects. Some of them had failure of development of secondary sexual characteristics. The only patients in whom we had testicular biopsies were the seven subjects with hyposmia and hypogonadism. In a word, "immaturity" describes the nature of the testicular lesion. Functionally these individuals have what we call a "double defect", in that in addition to hypogonadotropism they fail to elevate plasma testosterone concentrations in response to administration of 4,000 IU of HCG per day for 5 days.

E. STEINBERGER: Dr. Ross, have you looked for a dose-response to clomiphene in individuals who did respond? Have you followed the gonadotropin levels in treated individuals after discontinuation of therapy? If so, for how long?

ROSS: In response to the first question, there is a dose response relationship, in that the mean values observed after 100 mg of clomiphene per day for six days are about half the mean values observed for 200 mg of clomiphene per day for six days. I cannot answer the second question since we have not systematically followed the plasma concentrations of FSH and LH serially after the discontinuation of clomiphene.

HUDSON: Dr. Lunenfeld asked about the treatment of hypogonadotropic males with clomiphene. We have observed two patients who have levels of between 110-200 ng/100 ml of testosterone when treated with clomiphene in doses of between 50 and 100 mg. per day. They had a further fall in the levels of their plasma testosterone. I have no explanation of this phenomenon.

ROSS: I am unable to explain this observation either. I would draw your attention to a paper by Kulin and his associates in Grumbach's laboratory in which effects of the administration of clomiphene on urinary FSH excretion by prepubertal males were reported. A decline in urinary excretion of follicle stimulating hormone associated with a decline in concentrations of testosterone in plasma was observed. The doses of clomiphene to which these prepubertal subjects were sensitive were of the order of magnitude of 1 mg or less per square meter of body surface, or less, per day. These patients differ from the classical patients with Kallman's syndrome in that these occurred sporadically, that is, not in family constellations in which the syndrome was recurrent. In addition, some of the signs and symptoms occurring in the classical syndrome were not seen in our patients. Our patients failed to detect odors at concentrations which differ by orders of magnitude from the concentrations at which any individual with normal sense of smell would be able to detect them and were thus classified as hyposmic rather than anosmic as in classical Kallman's syndrome. None of the nine subjects that we have had the opportunity to study up to now has had midline defects such as hare lip or cleft palate and only two were color blind. Our patients may have a syndrome which might be regarded as a subset of Kallman's syndrome.

CHAPTER IV

REGULATION OF TESTICULAR FUNCTION

SECTION 4: METABOLIC EFFECTS OF GONADOTROPINS

EARLY EFFECTS OF FSH UPON TESTICULAR METABOLISM

Anthony R. Means

Departments of Ob-Gyn and Physiology, Vanderbilt University School of Medicine, Nashville, Tennessee

Growth and maturation of the testis culminating in the onset of complete spermatogenesis are clearly some of the most profound physiological changes which occur during the postnatal development of the male. These events are regulated to a large degree by two peptide hormones elaborated in the anterior hypophysis, i.e. LH and FSH. However, the exact role of the pituitary gonadotropins in the initiation and maintenance of spermatogenesis is not clearly understood. The current concept, based primarily on morphological evidence, is that FSH maintains the germinal epithelium and LH facilitates the completion of spermatogenesis by stimulating the Leydig cells to produce testosterone (1).

It has been demonstrated that FSH, when given to immature or mature hypophysectomized rats, markedly increases the size of the testis but will not accelerate the appearance of mature sperm nor increase the secretory activity of the Leydig cells (2,3). Moreover, administration of FSH alone does not result in formation of germinal cells more advanced than spermatocytes (4,5). In addition, for final stages of spermatogenesis as well as for hypertrophy of the male accessory glands, an androgenic influence is needed (2,4, 5). This androgenic stimulation can be provided either indirectly by administration of LH or directly by testosterone (6). These studies, coupled with the demonstration by many investigators that LH stimulates testicular steroidogenesis (7,8), offers support to the suggestion that the primary function of LH is to direct the synthesis of testosterone which in turn is necessary for completion of the spermatogenic process. On the other hand the function of FSH remains uncertain.

There is a great lack of information concerning the biochemical effects of FSH in the mammalian testis. Furthermore, those studies which exist are primarily concerned with the long-term effects of FSH on testicular lipid metabolism. Gambal and Ackerman (9) have reported that following hypophysectomy the concentration of individual phospholipids in the testis changes, and administration of FSH helped to maintain the concentrations observed in untreated controls. FSH has also been shown to increase the incorporation of radioactive linoleic acid into lipid in testes from hypophysectomized rats (10).

Since LH was also shown to affect lipid metabolism (9,10) we undertook some studies to determine whether FSH stimulates phospholipid synthesis in the testis of hypophysectomized rats and if so whether the effect could be attributed to contamination with LH. It was demonstrated that FSH stimulated incorporation of various precursors into testicular phospholipids. Stimulation was demonstrated by incorporation of ^{32}P into a total phospholipid fraction as well as by incorporation of labelled choline and ethanolamine into total and individual phospholipids (1). Finally the stimulation was shown to be specific for FSH since treatment of this hormone with urea or with specific antibody to LH failed to destroy the stimulating activity.

Clearly the early effects of FSH upon testicular metabolism have been neglected. Since FSH increases testicular growth, effects upon protein and nucleic acid biosynthesis seem logical starting points in any attempt to study the mechanism of action of this gonadotropin. Therefore a series of studies were initiated in this laboratory designed to study the regulation of testicular protein biosynthesis following the administration of a single injection of FSH.

FSH was shown to enhance the testicular incorporation of various ^{14}C-labelled amino acids into acid-precipitable material within 30 minutes following a single injection to rats aged 20 days (12). This response to FSH was time-dependent (maximal stimulation was reached one hour after injection), was dose dependent within the range of 0.2 to 200 μg per rat, and was abolished by addition of puromycin in vitro or administration in vivo. Table 1 demonstrates this effect and also illustrates that stimulation of testicular protein biosynthesis by FSH was specific for that hormone and for other gonadotropins with FSH-like activity. It can be seen that PMS caused a significant stimulation at a dose of 100 I.U. whereas boiled FSH, LH, prolactin, TSH, HCG, or bovine serum albumin failed to exert any demonstrable increase in protein synthesis (12). Finally, treatment of the FSH preparation with neuraminidase, which inactivates this hormone, abolishes the stimulation, whereas the stimulating activity of FSH was unaltered under conditions where the LH contamination was destroyed by pretreatment with 6 M urea or 4 M guanidine-HCl.

Table 1. Specificity of the FSH-Mediated Stimulation of Testicular Protein Biosynthesis

Treatment	Specific Activity (dpm/mg protein)	P
Control	1620	
FSH	2829	.001
Boiled FSH	1602	NS
FSH + Neuraminidase	1631	NS
FSH + Urea	2861	.001
PMS	2209	.01
HCG	1802	NS
ICSH	1611	NS
Prolactin	1654	NS
TSH	1620	NS
Serum Albumin	1642	NS
Saline	1615	NS

All substances were injected intraperitoneally 1 hr prior to killing of animals. Amounts of substances injected were as follows: 20 µg each of FSH, boiled FSH, ICSH, prolactin, TSH, or bovine serum albumin; 150 I.U. HCG; 100 I.U. PMS. All compounds were dissolved in 0.2 ml of 0.9% aqueous saline. All rats were 20 days old and each served as its own control as follows: one testis was removed and 1 hr following injection of test compound the other testis was removed. Testis tissue was incubated at 37° for 30 minutes in Krebs-Ringer bicarbonate buffer containing 0.5 µC of lysine-^{14}C (0.1 mM). Values represent the mean from 6 animals (12). The hormone preparations used were ovine FSH (NIH-FSH-S3), ovine ICSH (NIH-LH-S9), ovine TSH (NIH-TSH-S2), bovine prolactin (NIH-P-B1), PMS (Ayerst Equinex) and HCG (Ayerst A.P.L.).

The stimulation of testicular protein synthesis by FSH was shown to be dependent upon the age of the animal, that is stimulation was observed in testes of rats aged 15-24 days, but not in testes of rats older than 25 days (13). On the other hand the testes of rats of any age will respond to FSH within 18 hours of hypophysectomy and will continue to respond for at least 25 days after operation. Glucose was also shown to stimulate testicular protein biosynthesis in an age-dependent fashion (14). However, sensitivity to glucose and to FSH were shown to occur at different ages (Table 2). Glucose did not increase protein synthesis in the testis before the age of 28 days and the stimulation observed in the adult gradually declined following hypophysectomy until no response was observed 25 days after operation.

Spermatids first appear between 26 and 28 days of age in the immature rat and disappear from the adult animal within 25 days of

Table 2. Effects of FSH or Glucose Upon Protein Biosynthesis in Testes of Intact or Hypophysectomized rats.

Intact Age (Days)	Specific Activity (dpm/ mg protein) Control	FSH	Glucose
15	900	1260	892
20	1605	2875	1640
24	1847	3368	1900
28	1954	2035	2262
30	1150	1203	1665
35	1222	1203	2005
40	1106	1112	2200
60	1210	1193	2492

Hypox Duration	Control	FSH	Glucose	FSH + Glucose
4 hr	900	884	1863	-
18 hr	920	1082	1850	-
3 days	842	1312	1706	-
5 days	530	922	980	-
15 days	277	452	398	536
25 days	235	408	230	420

Each animal served as its own control as previously described (13). FSH (50 μg/100 g body weight) was administered intraperitoneally 1 hr. before killing of animals. Glucose when present was added to the incubation at a final concentration of 9mM. Testis tissue (60-100 mg/flask) was incubated with 0.5 μC (0.1 mM) lysine-^{14}C for 30 min. at 37° as previously described (12). Numbers represent the mean value from 6 animals. The FSH preparation used was ovine NIH-FSH-S4.

hypophysectomy. Davis and Firlit (14) have reported autoradiographic studies on the incorporation of lysine-^{14}C into cells of the mature rat testis which indicate that the incorporation of the amino acid resulting from the addition of glucose to the medium occurs for the most part in spermatids. Our results would support this conclusion. On the other hand the effect of FSH is not related to the presence or absence of spermatids since the hormone stimulates protein biosynthesis in the young rat before these cells have appeared, fails to stimulate in the normal adult testis which contains spermatids, but increases protein synthesis within a few hours following hypophysectomy when spermatids are still present in large numbers. It is likely therefore that glucose and FSH exert their effects on different cell types within the testis.

The manner in which glucose stimulated testicular protein biosynthesis in the adult rat was then investigated. It was demonstrated that the effect of glucose was indirect, that is, through its ability to act as a source of energy and thus maintain testicular levels of ATP (15). Furthermore, the ATP produced from the oxidation of glucose was shown to serve at least a dual purpose; firstly in the transport of amino acids into the testicular cells, and secondly at some step(s) beyond the intracellular entry of amino acids (16). Finally, glucose had no effect upon cellular concentrations of ATP in the immature rat testis, which is in keeping with the inability of this substance to stimulate protein biosynthis.

Stimulation of testicular protein biosynthesis by FSH appears to be of a more direct nature. Two lines of evidence demonstrate that the stimulation cannot entirely be attributed to enhanced amino acid transport into testicular cells (12). In the first place FSH, under conditions where protein biosynthesis was stimulated, did not increase the cellular transport of the model compound, α-amino-isobutyric acid, which is transported in a manner similar to naturally occurring amino acids but is not metabolized or incorporated to any demonstrable degree. Secondly, the stimulation by FSH was not diminished by increasing the concentration of lysine in the incubation medium, i.e. further addition of substrate did not result in increased incorporation into protein. Likewise, FSH did not increase the activation of lysine-^{14}C into lysyl-transfer RNA.

Since FSH administration resulted in accelerated protein biosynthesis, but this gonadotropin did not increase the transport or activation of amino acids, we decided to investigate the effect of the hormone upon the activity of testicular polyribosomes. Therefore, polyribosomes were prepared from rat testis. Characterization of this preparation by sucrose gradient centrifugation, electron microscopy and analytical ultracentrifugation revealed a large predominance of ribonucleoprotein particles which contained more than two ribosomes (17). Furthermore, conditions were described for optimal incorporation of valine-^{14}C into peptide by a cell-free system. This ribonucleoprotein preparation was then used to investigate the mechanism by which FSH stimulates testicular protein biosynthesis.

When testes from rats which had received a single injection of FSH one hour before killing were incubated with valine-^{14}C before polyribosomes were prepared, the specific activity of protein associated with all polysomal fractions was higher than in similar preparations from control animals (Fig. 1) (18). On the other hand, FSH neither demonstrably influenced the proportion of testicular ribosomes appearing as polyribosomes nor altered the relative proportion of various polyribosomal species. Incorporation of valine-^{14}C into protein by polyribosomes in vitro was increased by prior treatment of the animal with FSH in vivo. No effect of the hormone upon protein synthesis was demonstrable until 1 hour after administration (Table 3). The response reached a maximum at 2 hours and

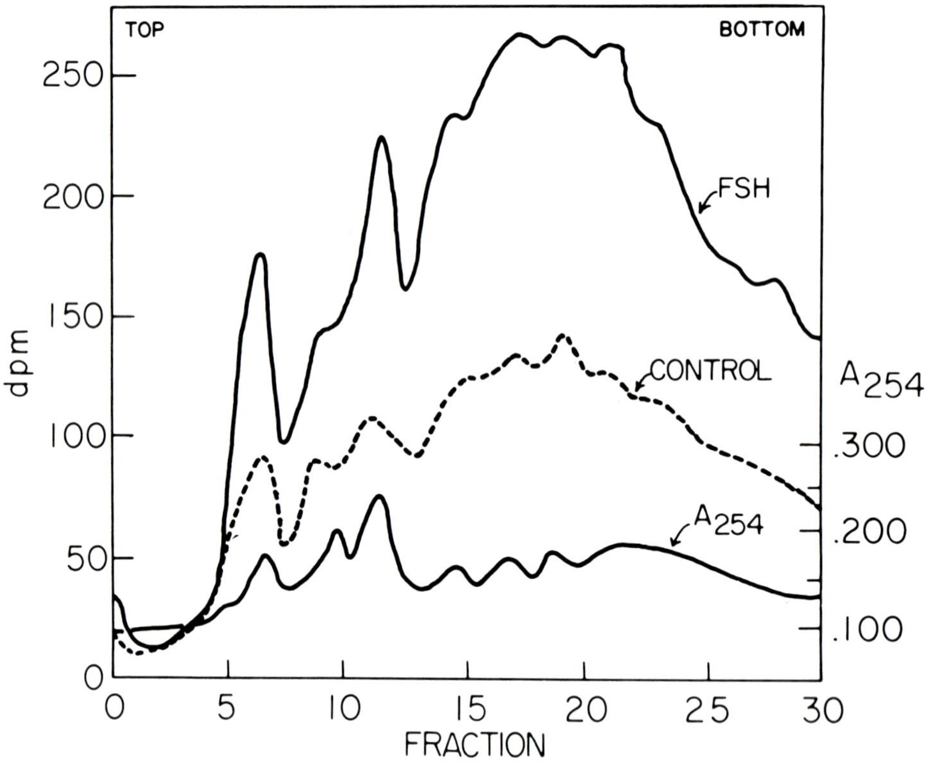

Fig. 1. Effect of FSH administered in vivo upon the radioactive labelling of testicular polyribosomes in vitro. FSH (200 μg/100 g body weight) was administered to hypophysectomized rats as a single intravenous injection 1 hr before killing. Testis tissue (2.5 g) was incubated with 10 μC of valine-^{14}C for 30 min at 37° and analyzed as previously described (18). The FSH preparation was ovine NIH-FSH-S6. (From: Means, et al. Biochemistry, 8: 4293, 1969).

Table 3. Influence of FSH upon Protein Biosynthesis by Testicular Polyribosomes in vitro as a Function of Time Following Intravenous Injection

Duration of FSH (minutes)	Specific Activity (pmoles val-^{14}C/mg ribosomal protein)
0	14.14
15	14.08
30	14.58
60	19.51
120	23.19
180	19.52
240	15.13
480	14.39

All animals were hypophysectomized at 150-160 g and used between 3 and 4 weeks postoperatively. FSH (200μ /100 g body weight) was injected intravenously at various times before sacrifice of animals. Polyribosomes (400μ /tube) were incubated in a cell-free system containing 1.0μC valine-^{14}C for 30 min. at 37°. The values represent the mean of determinations performed in triplicate and have been corrected for zero controls (17). The FSH preparation was ovine NIH-FSH-S6.

then began to decrease until by 8 hours no detectable difference was observed between incorporation activity by polyribosomes from control or FSH-treated animals. Moreover, it was demonstrated that the stimulation of peptide synthesis by FSH is independent of the source of enzymes necessary for amino acid activation (i.e. no difference was observed when pH 5 enzyme was from control or FSH-treated testis, or liver).

Injection of actinomycin D one hour before injection of FSH was shown to prevent the stimulation of protein biosynthesis by testicular polyribosomes in vitro without demonstrably decreasing the rate of synthesis by particles from control animals (18). Furthermore, although polyuridylic acid increased protein synthesis in vitro by polyribosomes from treated and from control animals, incorporation was equal with polyribosomes from these two sources in presence of excess poly U. It appears, therefore, that the capacity of polyribosomes to support peptide synthesis is the same whether these particles are isolated from hormone-treated or control animals. These observations suggested that FSH stimulates testicular protein synthesis by increasing the synthesis of RNA (possibly messenger RNA), although additional effects upon translation of mRNA cannot be excluded.

We then attempted to ascertain whether FSH increased testicular

Table 4. Effect of FSH upon Synthesis of Rapidly-Labelled Nuclear RNA and Uptake of Uridine-5-^{3}H in Testes of Rats Aged 20 Days

	Tissue Radioactivity				Specific Activity
Time After FSH (min)	Acid Soluble (dpm/mg DNAx10^{-3})	(%)	Acid Insoluble (dpm/mg DNA)	(%)	Nuclear RNA (dpm/mg)
0	100.6	98.9	1020	1.0	2500
15	109.0	96.9	1800	3.1	3680
30	107.0	96.5	2760	3.5	5100
45	103.0	97.0	2230	3.0	4060
60	106.0	97.4	2110	2.6	2600
120	105.0	98.0	1800	2.0	2220

FSH (50 μg/rat) was injected intravenously at various times before killing and all animals received 100 μC uridine-5-^{3}H intravenously 10 min prior to killing. Testes were homogenized and aliquots were taken for determinations of acid-soluble and acid-insoluble radioactivity as well as for DNA. Nuclei were isolated from the remainder of the homogenate and rapidly-labeled RNA was extracted. All of these methods have been described previously (19). Results represent the mean values of 6 experiments. Testes of 10 animals were pooled for each experiment. The FSH preparation was ovine NIH-FSH-S7.

RNA synthesis prior to the observed effect on protein biosynthesis. It can be seen from Table 4 that the specific activity of rapidly-labeled nuclear RNA was increased significantly within 15 minutes following a single injection of FSH. This response reached a maximum at 30 minutes and by one hour was declining rapidly toward control values. Moreover, simultaneous measurements of the acid soluble pool of uridine-5-^{3}H during these experiments showed that uptake of the nucleotide was unaltered by FSH. These changes in nuclear RNA synthesis clearly precede the enhancement of testicular polyribosomal incorporation activity first observed within one hour following FSH administration and argue for an early effect of the hormone upon genetic transcription.

The precise mechanism of action of FSH is still uncertain. Recent reports indicate that some effects of this gonadotropin may be mediated through a stimulation of adenyl cyclase (20,21). Regulation of protein synthesis may occur at two principal sites: at the level of transcription in the nucleus or in the cytoplasm at the level of translation. The early changes in rapidly-labeled nuclear RNA, the inhibitory action of actinomycin D and the time-course of events following FSH would suggest a very early action of this hormone at the nuclear level of protein synthesis. This then might result in new gene transcriptions and the subsequent de novo synthesis of protein molecules necessary for further growth and development of the seminiferous epithelium.

ACKNOWLEDGEMENT

The work presented herein was supported in part by Grant 66-16023 from the Australian Research Grants Committee (to P.F. Hall), Research Grant RA-5 from the Morrison Trust of San Antonio, Texas, and by U.S. Public Health Service Health Sciences Advancement Award 5-S04-FR06067 to Vanderbilt University. Thanks are extended to the Endocrine Study Section at NIH for gifts of peptide hormones used in these studies.

REFERENCES

1. Gemzell, C. and Roos, P., In The Pituitary Gland, eds. Harris, G.W., and Donovan, B.T., London, Butterworth Press Vol. 1, 492, 1966.
2. Greep, R.O., van Dyke, H.B. and Chow, B.F., Endocrinology, 30: 635, 1942.
3. Simpson, M.E., Li, C.H. and Evans, H.M., Endocrinology, 48: 370, 1951.
4. Lostroh, A.J., Acta Endocr. (Kobenhavn), 43: 592, 1963.
5. Lostroh, A.J., Johnson, R. and Jordan, C.W., Acta Endocr. (Kobenhavn), 44: 536, 1963.
6. Woods, M.C. and Simpson, M.E., Endocrinology, 69: 91, 1961.
7. Hall, P.F. and Eik-Nes, K.B., Biochim. Biophys. Acta, 63: 411, 1962.
8. Hall, P.F. and Young, D.G., Endocrinology, 82: 559, 1968.
9. Gambal, D. and Ackerman, R.J., Endocrinology, 80: 231, 1967.
10. Goswami, A. and Williams, W.L., Biochem. J., 105: 537, 1967.
11. Yokoe, Y., Means, A.R. and Hall, P.F., Biochim. Biophys. Acta, 187: 278, 1969.
12. Means, A.R. and Hall, P.F., Endocrinology, 81: 1151, 1967.
13. Means, A.R. and Hall, P.F., Endocrinology, 82: 597, 1968.
14. Davis, J.R. and Firlit, C.F., Amer. J. Physiol., 209: 425, 1965.
15. Means, A.R. and Hall, P.F., Endocrinology, 83: 86, 1968.
16. Means, A.R. and Hall, P.F., Endocrinology, 84: 285, 1969.
17. Means, A.R., Hall, P.F., Nicol, L.W., Sawyer, W.H. and Baker, C.A., Biochemistry, 8: 1488, 1969.
18. Means, A.R. and Hall, P.F., Biochemistry, 8: 4293, 1969.
19. Means, A.R. and Hamilton, T.H., Proc. Nat. Acad. Sci., U.S.A. 56: 686, 1966.
20. Murad, F., Strauch, B.S. and Vaughn, M., Biochim. Biophys. Acta, 177: 591, 1969.
21. Kuehl, F.A., Patanelli, D.J., Tarnoff, J. and Humes, J.L., Biol. Reprod. (in press).

DISCUSSION

SOLARI: Dr. Means' results agree with our unpublished results on the effect of FSH on rapidly labelled RNA in the rat testis. I would say from our data on the action of actinomycin on the adult rat testis that this action seems to be restricted to the spermatogonia and the Sertoli cells. Thus, it could be that the transient effect of FSH is also restricted to the Sertoli cells and the spermatogonia.

MEANS: One has to be very careful, I think, in interpreting data concerning actinomycin D. Firstly, actinomycin D is a very potent drug that has all sorts of systemic effects as well as affecting RNA systhesis. Secondly, it preferentially affects ribosomal RNA synthesis, that is to say even if one obtains an inhibition of RNA synthesis up to as much as 90 percent, messenger RNA synthesis (which may comprise only 2 to 3 percent of all the RNA synthesis in the cell) could continue merrily along its way. With regard to what cell types are targets for FSH, I purposely avoided that subject. We used rats aged 20 days and Dr. Clermont was kind enough to tell me that at least 50 percent of the cells present in the testis at that age are primary spermatocytes. I would find it difficult to imagine that these large increases in rapidly labelled nuclear RNA synthesis would be localized to one cell type unless this cell comprised a large proportion of the mass. I would rather suggest that we may unfortunately be looking at both specific and non-specific effects of this hormone. We are in the process now of isolating testicular DNA and separating on hydroxyapatite columns the unique sequences of the DNA from the repeating or the redundant sequences. When we hydridize our rapidly labelled nuclear RNA back against these two types of DNA sequences, I believe that this will obtain much more information about what is going on. If we find only increased competition in the redundant species this would indicate that we have a non-selective effect of FSH. Finally, in our hands this is a very transient effect and always when one has a transient effect one wonders about the reasons. This is particularly true in this case since we know that if one gives multiple doses of FSH to immature hypophysectomized rats one obtains an increase in testicular weight. Therefore, we probably have two things going on, but I would not be willing to make any comments at the present time about what cell types FSH is specifically affecting, except to rule out spermatids and spermatozoa.

LUNENFELD: We have found that Dr. Means' experiments on the effect of FSH or role of protein on nucleic acid synthesis in the testis give results extremely similar to ours on the effect of FSH on the mouse ovary. Furthermore, I was extremely interested in the effect of HCG. We found a similar effect of HCG on the ovary. We postulated that this might be due to an endogenous release of FSH and this was found to be true since when HCG was injected together with an antiserum to rat gonadotropin the effect of HCG was completely abolished.

CHRISTENSEN: I wonder if ordinary autoradiography at the light microscope level would not suffice to identify the cell type involved, since one administers soluble amino acids and can test for insoluble proteins. In the polyuridine experiments there was the implication that free ribosomes were being taken up into polysomes, and yet in your polysome profile, Dr. Means, you had an extremely small free ribosomal peak. Where did the ribosomes for that large an increase in protein synthesis come from?

MEANS: With regard to the autoradiography, I agree that this is a reasonable type of approach. We have some preliminary results that indicate very similar data to what Prof. Mancini has reported previously. We find radioactivity localized over the primary spermatocytes and there may be also an increase over the Sertoli cells. I feel obligated to stress that these studies are very preliminary in nature. With regard to the second question, you should realize that this is an absorbancy tracing and in these particular studies we are selectively isolating polyribosomes. Therefore, the monomer peak should be small. This is not to say, however, that all of the polyribosomes so isolated are active in protein biosynthesis, and in fact this is probably not the case. Secondly, we were applying only 10 A 254 NM of polyribosomes to each gradient since we were interested primarily in the optimal conditions for separation of the various species of polyribosomes which we had present in our preparation. Finally, it is well known that in any cell-free system as protein synthesis continues in vitro polyribosomes dissaggregate monomers and that the addition of an exogenous messenger will reestablish these ribosomes into functional polysomes. I tried not to make any particular conclusions from the data with Poly U except one simple point: if one believes the validity of such a study the data would indicate that the capacity of the ribosomes to synthesize protein is similar whether isolated from testes of control or FSH-treated rats.

OHNO: I wonder if cyclic AMP is mediating the generalized stimulation which you observed after FSH?

MEANS: Two recent reports by Murand and Kuehl bear directly on this subject. FSH was demonstrated by these two groups of workers to enhance production of cyclic AMP when added to a whole tissue preparation from the testis. This response was also very age-dependent as we have demonstrated for protein biosynthesis, with maximal activity occurring at 20 days of age. FSH added in vitro will actually cause a stimulation of adenyl cyclase activity. We have injected dibutyryl cyclic AMP directly under the tunica and indeed find an increase in protein synthesis with similar kinetics to the effect of FSH. We find that when we analyze the peptides synthesized by polyribosomes in vitro as we showed for the FSH they are again similar. However, at this point, we have one discrepancy that I have no explanation for at present. That is, that under no conditions does dibutyryl cyclic AMP plus or minus methyl xanthine derivatives exert any effect on rapidly labelled nuclear RNA synthesis. The mechanism of action of most trophic hormones is probably mediated by some sort of intercellular second messenger. Cyclic AMP is most definitely a likely candidate.

ROSEMBERG: Dr. Means, would you please indicate the dose of FSH used in the experiments presented tonight? Is this one of the NIH ovine materials?

MEANS: The most common dose given was about 200 micrograms per rat. All of the preparations used were NIH ovine preparations. In each case, the LH contaminating activity was removed.

A. STEINBERGER: Dr. Means, are you certain that nothing happens in the Leydig cells? Was there any particular reason for using ovine NIH-FSH which has some LH activity?

MEANS: We did get rid of the LH contaminating activity. I still cannot really say whether there is any effect on the Leydig cells or not. I think some information from several workers, one of whom is Dr. Hall, I believe, is important in this regard. They have isolated interstitial cells and seminiferous tubules, and looked at the effect of LH and FSH on steroidogenesis. They find that FSH has no effect on production of testosterone by isolated Leydig cells.

CHRISTENSEN: Even if the interstitial cells were carrying on protein synthesis, I doubt that it would show in your results, because the interstitial cells in rats only constitute about 1.5% of the testis volume.

PAULSEN: I think it is important to consider what effect testosterone might have in stimulating protein synthesis in the seminiferous tubules. Also in that regard, did you indicate that ICSH had an effect on protein synthesis?

MEANS: We have tried testosterone, in fact we have tried a number of naturally occurring steroids, none of which exert any demonstrable effect on the parameter measured. LH (ICSH) showed no effect. PMS and HCG did have some effect; but both of these substances have follicle stimulating activity.

MANCINI: Dr. Means, in order to localize the site of action of FSH, did you consider it useful to try to separate the seminiferous tubules from the interstitial tissue? Would you consider the effect of FSH a direct one or could it be mediated by some changes in the blood flow, which in turn by extravascular diffusion may offer to the seminiferous tubules an increased amount of nutrients?

MEANS: Blood flow has of course been shown by many people to be very important. Larry Ewing's very elegant studies with the perfused testis have indicated this point. I think that this is certainly a possibility, and would not rule it out. One of the problems readily apparent from our studies is that all of these data were obtained in vivo; that is to say the hormone was administered exogenously.

RADIOAUTOGRAPHIC STUDIES OF PROTEIN SYNTHESIS IN CELLS OF THE SEMINIFEROUS EPITHELIUM

Joseph R. Davis and Casimir F. Firlit[1]

Department of Pharmacology and Therapeutics,
Loyola University Stritch School of Medicine,
Maywood, Illinois, U.S.A.

Because of the complex histological pattern of the spermatogenic cycle, it has been exceedingly difficult to ascertain the specific metabolic functions of the various cell types involved in mammalian spermatogenesis. In addition, very little is known about the metabolism of cells undergoing meiotic division and of the biochemical events associated with the transition from somatic mitosis to meiosis. However, the continuous nature of the spermatogenic cycle which begins with a stem cell spermatogonium and ends with the mature spermatid seems to be uniquely suited for a comparative study of the three main phases of growth, namely mitotic division, meiotic division and morphogenic differentiation. It would appear that this aspect of testicular biochemistry is of extreme importance since not only is meiosis the mechanism by which the diploid number of chromosomes is reduced to the haploid number of chromosomes found in the gametes, but the recombination of chromosomal segments during the crossing-over phase of meiosis provides for constant changing of the cell's genotype.

For these reasons, our laboratory has initiated a series of experiments which have been designed to investigate protein biosynthesis as it occurs in the various cells of the germinal epithelium of the testis. Since it is not possible at the present time to physically separate and isolate the individual cells of the testicular germinal epithelium, we have utilized two experimental approaches designed to determine which of the several cell types of the seminiferous germinal epithelium of the testis were particularly susceptible to our previously reported effects of temperature (1), cryptorchidism (2) and glucose (3) on testicular protein biosynthesis. The

[1]Predoctoral Trainee, U.S. Public Health Service.

first approach involves the measurement of the incorporation of ^{14}C-lysine into acid-precipitable protein of various preparations of testes consisting primarily of only a very few cell types. The second and more specific approach involves the radioautographic determination of the incorporation of tritiated lysine into each of the successive cells of the cycle of the seminiferous germinal epithelium.

PROTEIN SYNTHESIS IN THE CRYPTORCHID RAT TESTIS

Cryptorchidism can easily be induced in the rat by gently forcing the testis into the abdominal cavity and anchoring it to the lateral abdominal wall. The contralateral testis of the same animal can then be allowed to remain in the scrotal sac to serve as a control. The predominant histological feature of the cryptorchid testis appears to be the total absence of spermatids (4). On the other hand, the immature testis of the rat appears to consist largely of primary spermatocytes (5).

Fig. 1 presents the in vitro incorporation of L-lysine-U-^{14}C into acid-precipitable protein of slices of immature, mature and cryptorchid rat testes. The normal descent with age of the immature abdominal testis into the scrotal sac was accompanied by a remarkable decrease in testicular protein labelling. In addition, protein labelling of the cryptorchid testis was observed to increase markedly following abdominal transplantation from the scrotal sac. It seemed quite surprising to us that a tissue such as the cryptorchid testis which was rapidly regressing in size should display an increased synthesis of protein. The question arose as to whether this increased protein labelling of the cryptorchid testis, on the one hand, was a reflection of an unmasking of the spermatogonia, primary spermatocytes and Sertoli cells resulting from the disappearance of the spermatids or, on the other hand, represented a true temperature-induced change in the protein-synthesizing capacity of these remaining testicular cell types.

Fig. 2 shows photomicrographs of the three types of seminiferous tubules which occurred in approximately equal numbers in the cryptorchid rat testis 30 days after abdominal transplantation. Only four cell types were found in the germinal epithelium of these tubules, namely "crust" spermatogonia, pachytene primary spermatocytes, normal-appearing Sertoli cells and atrophic-appearing Sertoli cells, accounting for 31, 3, 28 and 38 percent, respectively, of the total cells remaining in the seminiferous germinal epithelium of the cryptorchid rat testis.

Fig. 3 presents the radioautographic incorporation of tritiated lysine into each of the remaining cells of the cryptorchid rat testis 30 days after abdominal transplantation of the testis. Slices of testes were incubated at 37.5^{o}C in a Warburg apparatus with 100

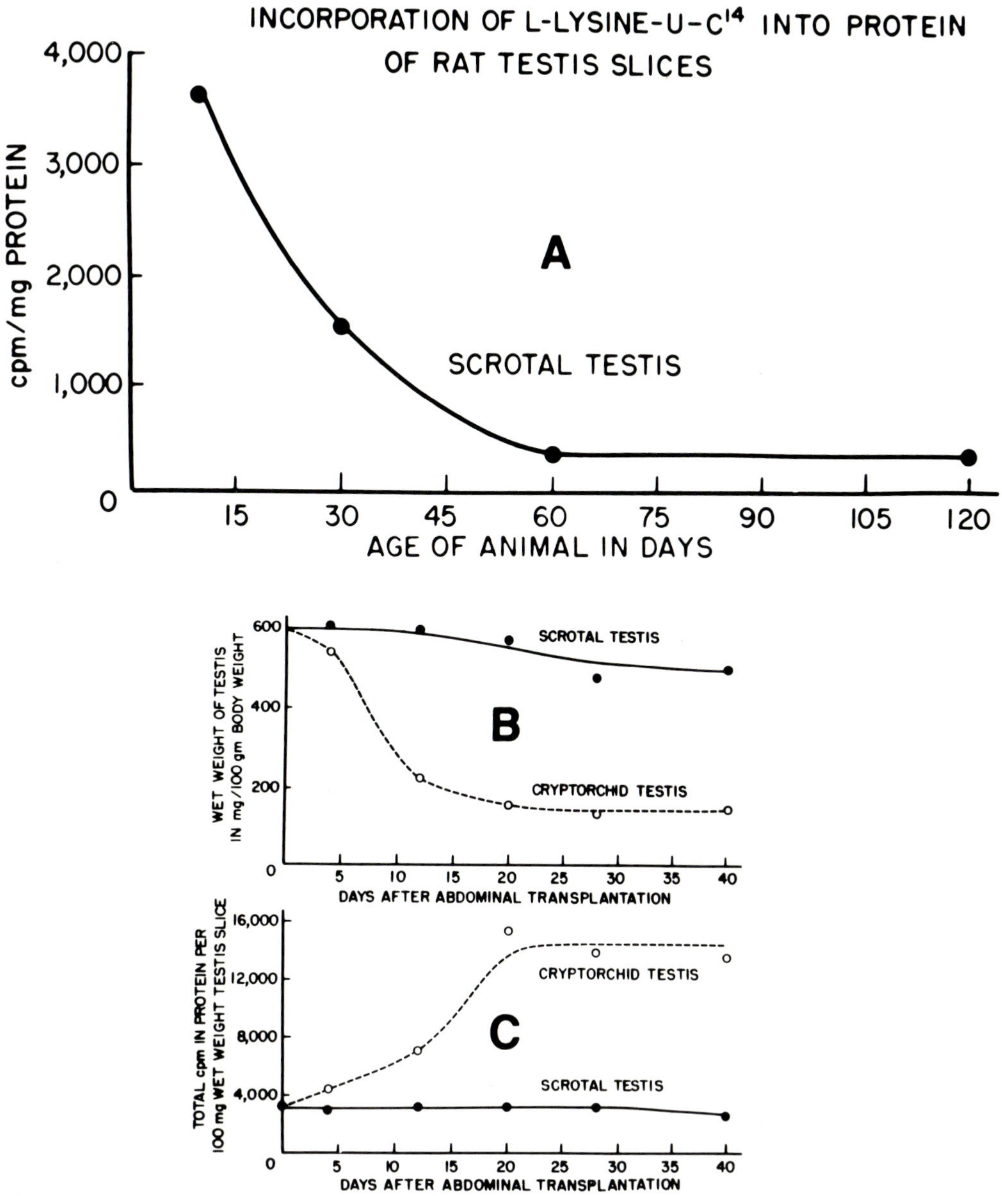

Fig. 1. Incorporation of L-lysine-U^{14}C into protein of rat testis slices. A. Effect of age of animal on protein labelling of normal testis. B. Effect of abdominal transplantation on testicular weights of experimentally-induced unilateral cryptorchid rats which were 60 days old at the time of surgery. C. Corresponding testicular protein labelling of experimentally-induced unilateral cryptorchid rats which were 60 days old at the time of surgery.

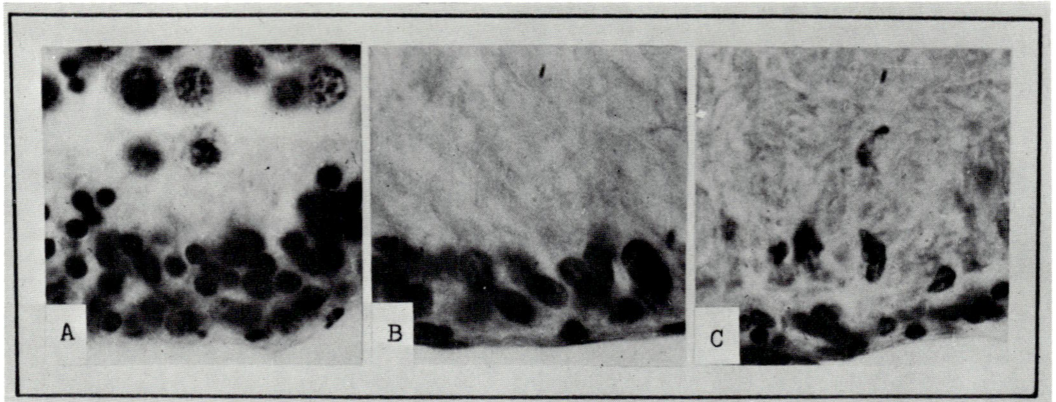

PERCENTAGE DISTRIBUTION OF CELL POPULATION IN SEMINIFEROUS TUBULES OF THE CRYPTORCHID RAT TESTIS 30 DAYS AFTER ABDOMINAL TRANSPLANTATION

Cells	*Type A tubule*	*Type B tubule*	*Type C tubule*
'Crust' spermatogonia	55·0±0·8	43·0±2·7	3·6±0·3
Pachytene 1° spermatocytes	8·6±1·1	0	0
Normal Sertoli cells	36·4±1·4	57·0±3·0	0
Atrophic Sertoli cells	0	0	96·4±0·3

The number of cells were determined in approximately twenty-five seminiferous tubules of each type for each of the four animals used.

All figures are percentages of total tubule cells ± standard error.

Fig. 2. Percentage distribution of the remaining cells of the seminiferous tubules of the cryptorchid rat testis 30 days after abdominal transplantation. The animals were 60 days of age at the time of surgery. (From: Davis, J.R. et al. J. Reprod. Fertil., 11: 125-131, 1966.)

μc of tritiated lysine in Krebs-Ringer bicarbonate buffer for 1 hour under aerobic conditions (6). At the end of the incubation period, the flask contents were poured through a 90-mesh stainless steel sieve in order to collect the testicular slices. The tissue held back by the sieve was then washed three times with cold Krebs-Ringer bicarbonate buffer containing 0.1% non-radioactive lysine and gently placed in cold Carnoy's solution by means of forceps. Following fixation overnight, the tissue was dehydrated, cleared, embedded in paraffin and sectioned at 5 μ. The sections were freed from paraffin, dipped in molten Kodak nuclear track emulsion type NTB3 and stored in the dark for 2 days. The exposed slides were developed, stained in hematoxylin solution and examined. Alternate sections which were not dipped with nuclear emulsion were stained with either hematoxylin alone or the periodic acid-Schiff reagent as outlined by Leblond and Clermont (7). Grain counting was performed under oil immersion using a Whipple micrometer eyepiece grid. Grains were counted within four squares in the Whipple micrometer and recorded as grains per 200 μ^2. A very dense radioautographic labelling pattern was observed over both the spermatogonia and the Sertoli cell cytoplasm in Type A tubules of the cryptorchid rat testis. The labelling of the Sertoli cell cytoplasm in Type B tubules of the cryptorchid rat testis was found to be quite similar to the labelling over the Sertoli cell cytoplasm present in Type A tubules. However, in contrast, the atrophic-appearing Sertoli cells found in Type C tubules of the cryptorchid rat testis were characterized by a marked decrease in the uptake of tritiated lysine into cellular protein. In comparison to the scrotal testis, the experimental induction of cryptorchidism was found to produce an approximate four-fold increase in protein labelling of both "crust" spermatogonia and pachytene primary spermatocytes. The induction of cryptorchidism was also found to result in a forty-fold increase in protein labelling from tritiated lysine in the normal-appearing Sertoli cells of both Type A and Type B cryptorchid tubules. It would therefore appear that the overall increase in labelling of acid-precipitable protein of slices of the cryptorchid rat testis is due not only to an unmasking of the remaining cell types with an inherent higher capacity for protein synthesis but is also due to a temperature-induced stimulation of protein synthesis occurring in these same testicular cell types, namely the "crust" spermatogonia, pachytene primary spermatocytes and the Sertoli cells.

EFFECT OF GLUCOSE ON RAT TESTICULAR PROTEIN SYNTHESIS

Although glucose has long been shown to maintain not only the oxygen uptake (8-12) but also the morphological integrity of adult testicular tissue (13), few studies have been carried out on the effect of this important substrate on testicular protein biosynthesis. Our laboratory has reported that the addition of 0.009 M glucose is capable of increasing the aerobic incorporation of radio-

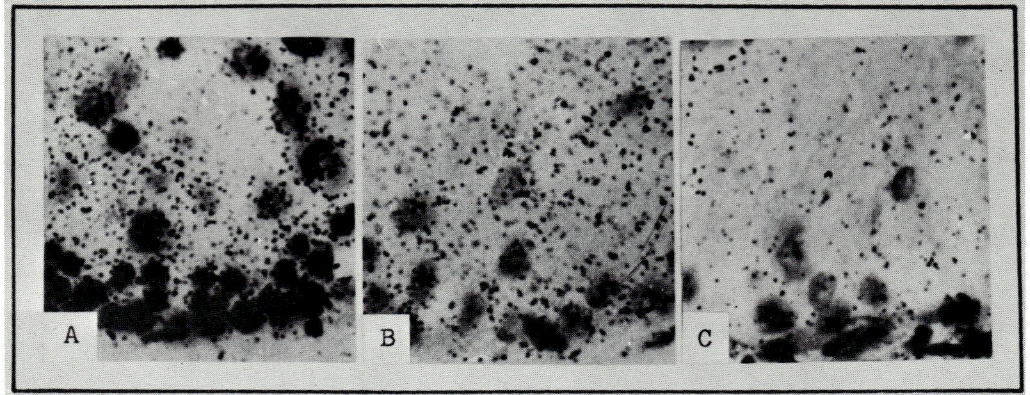

RADIO-AUTOGRAPHIC INCORPORATION OF L-LYSINE-^{3}H INTO CELLS OF THE GERMINAL EPITHELIUM OF THE CRYPTORCHID RAT TESTIS 30 DAYS AFTER ABDOMINAL TRANSPLANTATION

Cells	*Scrotal testis*	*Cryptorchid testis*		
		Type A tubule	*Type B tubule*	*Type C tubule*
'Crust' spermatogonia	19·3 ± 0·7	67·1 ± 1·0	66·2 ± 1·8	6·7 ± 0·3
Pachytene 1° spermatocytes	7·0 ± 0·7	27·5 ± 0·7	–	–
Normal Sertoli cells	1·6 ± 1·6	67·0 ± 0·6	61·5 ± 1·1	–
Atrophic Sertoli cells	–	–	–	19·1 ± 2·4

Grains/200 μ^2 were determined over each of the designated cell types in approximately 100 microscopic fields for each of the four animals used.

The data are presented as grains/200 μ^2 above background ± standard error.

Fig. 3. Radioautographic incorporation of tritiated lysine into cells of the germinal epithelium of slices of the cryptorchid rat testis 30 days after abdominal transplantation. The animals were 60 days of age at the time of surgery. (Davis, J. R. et al. J. Reprod. Fertil. 11: 125-131, 1966).

active lysine into acid-precipitable protein of slices of adult rat testes by 600 percent (3). In marked contrast, the addition of 0.009 M glucose was found to increase protein labelling of the head of the epididymis by 150 percent while causing no change to only a 50 percent enhancement of protein labelling in slices of jejunal mucosa, spleen, thymus, submaxillary gland, pancreas, tail of epididymis, kidney, brain, diaphragm, heart, lung, seminal vesicle, normal liver, regenerating liver, Walker 256 carcinosarcoma, Jensen sarcoma and Morris hepatoma 5123. It therefore appeared that with respect to a total of 15 different normal tissues of the adult male rat, as well as 3 varieties of transplantable rat tumors and a rapidly-growing non-malignant tissue such as the regenerating rat liver, glucose exerted a unique and characteristic stimulation of testicular protein biosynthesis.

Fig. 4A indicates the effect of exogenous glucose on the in vitro incorporation of L-lysine-U-^{14}C into acid-precipitable protein of slices of four different testicular preparations, each having its own individual histological structure. Whereas the absolute levels of protein labelling of the immature testis, the cryptorchid testis and the interstitial-cell testicular tumor were all higher than the adult scrotal testis, these tissues, which in no instance contained any spermatids, displayed essentially no effect of glucose on protein labelling as compared to the scrotal testis. In view of the fact that only the adult scrotal testis contained spermatids, these data pointed to the possibility that the spermatids were the most sensitive cell type of the seminiferous germinal epithelium with regard to glucose regulation of testicular protein synthesis. As suggested by Means and Hall, this remarkable stimulation of spermatid protein biosynthesis may be due at least partially to the maintenance of testicular ATP levels by glucose (14). Additional evidence that the spermatids are highly sensitive to glucose with regard to regulation of protein synthesis is presented in Fig. 4B. A marked increase in the stimulatory effect of glucose on protein labelling of slices of the normal rat testis was observed with an increase in the age of the animal from 20 to 50 days, corresponding to the appearance of the spermatids in the developing seminiferous tubular epithelium.

In order to investigate this possibility further, as well as to compare protein labelling in mitotic versus meiotic cell division, in vitro radioautographic studies were initiated on the effect of exogenous glucose on protein labelling from tritiated lysine in each of the successive cells of the cycle of the seminiferour epithelium of the rat. The fourteen stages of the cycle of the seminiferous epithelium in the rat have been classified according to the description of Leblond and Clermont (7). Slices of normal scrotal testes of the adult rat were incubated in Krebs-Ringer bicarbonate buffer under aerobic conditions with 100 μc of tritiated lysine in the presence and absence of 0.009 M glucose. It was found that the seminiferous epithelium of the rat testis retained its morphological integrity in the Warburg apparatus while shaking at a rate of 140 oscillations/minute. At the end of the 1 hour incubation period at 37.5°C, the tissues were sectioned and dipped in molten Kodak nuclear track emulsion. Exposure was carried out for four days, after which the slides were developed and stained in hematoxylin solution. Grains were counted within four squares in the Whipple micrometer and recorded as grains/200μ^2. A total of four cells occupied an area of 200μ^2 for each of the successive cell types of the seminiferous germinal epithelium with the exception of the larger pachytene primary spermatocytes of which a total of only two cells were observed to occupy an area of 200μ^2.

Fig. 5 demonstrates representative radioautographs of sections taken from slices of rat testes incubated with tritiated lysine in the presence and absence of exogenous glucose. A marked stimulation of protein labelling upon the addition of exogenous glucose was observed in the grain distribution over the pachytene primary spermatocytes present in stage VII. Glucose was also found to cause a great increase in the number of grains appearing over the area of the spermatids.

Fig. 6 presents a plot of the average grain count per 200μ^2 above background over each of the successive cells of the cycle of the seminiferous germinal epithelium of the rat testis one hour after incubation with tritiated lysine both in the presence and absence of exogenous glucose. In the control system, the cells which were found to incorporate the greatest amounts of lysine into protein were the early primary spermatocytes. In fact, immediately after the division of type B spermatogonia into the resting primary spermatocytes, there was a marked increase in the degree of labelling over these cells. In the glucose-supplemented system, a marked increase in the overall degree of protein labelling from tritiated lysine was observed in all the cells of the spermatogenic cycle, with the greatest grain count occurring over the pachytene primary spermatocytes. During the two meiotic cell divisions, shown over the secondary spermatocytes, a sharp decrease in the grain count was observed. Whereas few grains were seen over the spermatids in the control system, the addition of exogenous glucose was found to produce a marked increase in the number of grains appearing over the spermatids. These data indicate that of the various cell types found in the seminiferous germinal epithelium of the rat, the primary spermatocytes demonstrate the highest degree of protein labelling from radioactive lysine. On the other hand, protein labelling of the spermatids appears to have a great sensitivity to the addition of glucose. The data also suggest that glucose is capable of exerting a pronounced stimulation of protein labelling in the primary spermatocytes whose nuclei are at pachynema and whose chromosomes are undergoing crossing-over. The possibility therefore ex-

A

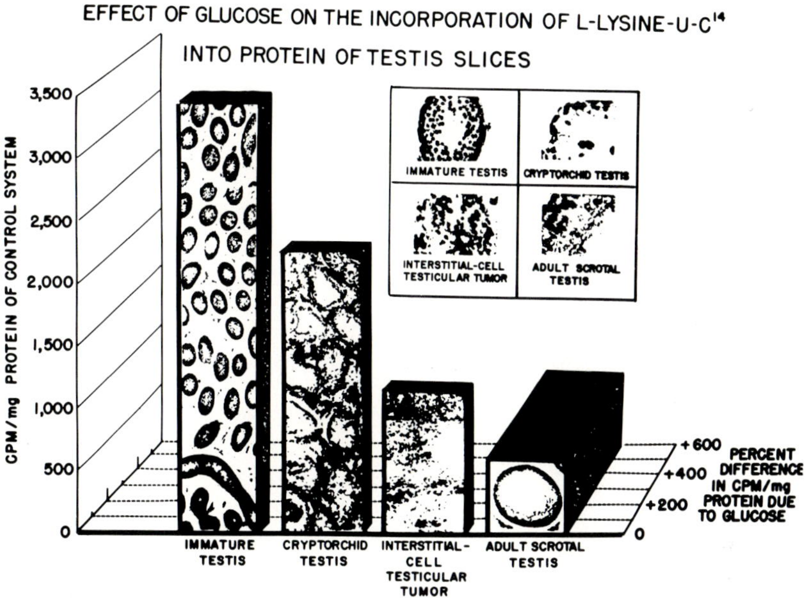

B

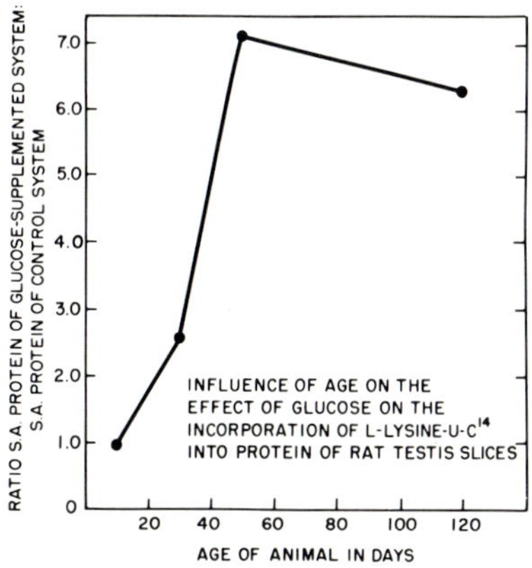

Fig. 4. Effect of glucose on the incorporation of L-lysine-U-^{14}C into protein of testis slices. A. Slices of four different testicular preparations, each with their own characteristic histological structure, were incubated in the presence and absence of 0.009 M glucose for 1 hour at 37.5^{o}C. Height of each bar represents the control specific activity (cpm/mg dry protein) while the depth of each bar represents percent stimulation of protein labelling by glucose. B. Influence of age on the effect of 0.009 M glucose on protein labelling of slices of the normal rat testis.

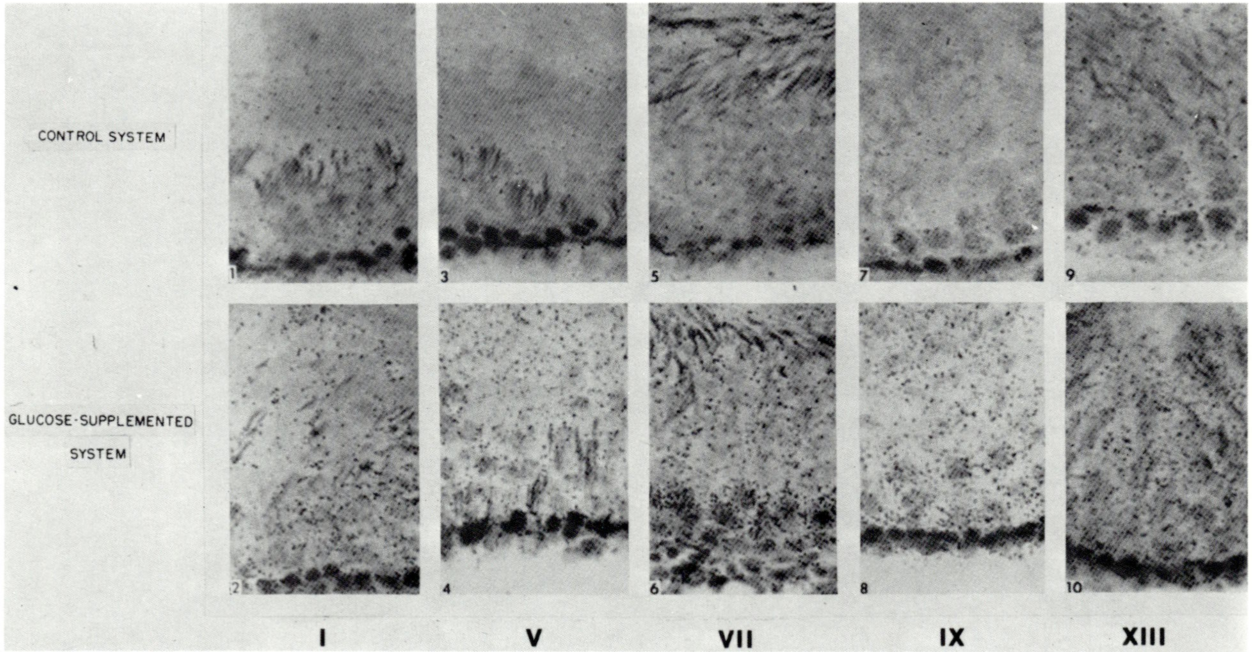

Fig. 5. Radioautographs of sections taken from slices of rat testes incubated for 1 hour with tritiated lysine in the presence and absence of 0.009 M glucose. 1 and 2 represent stage I; 3 and 4, stage V; 5 and 6, stage VII; 7 and 8, stage IX; 9 and 10, stage XIII. Sections were cut at 5 μ and stained with hematoxylin. Magnification approximately x 1,000. (From: Davis, J. R. et al. Amer. J. Physiol., 209: 425-432, 1965).

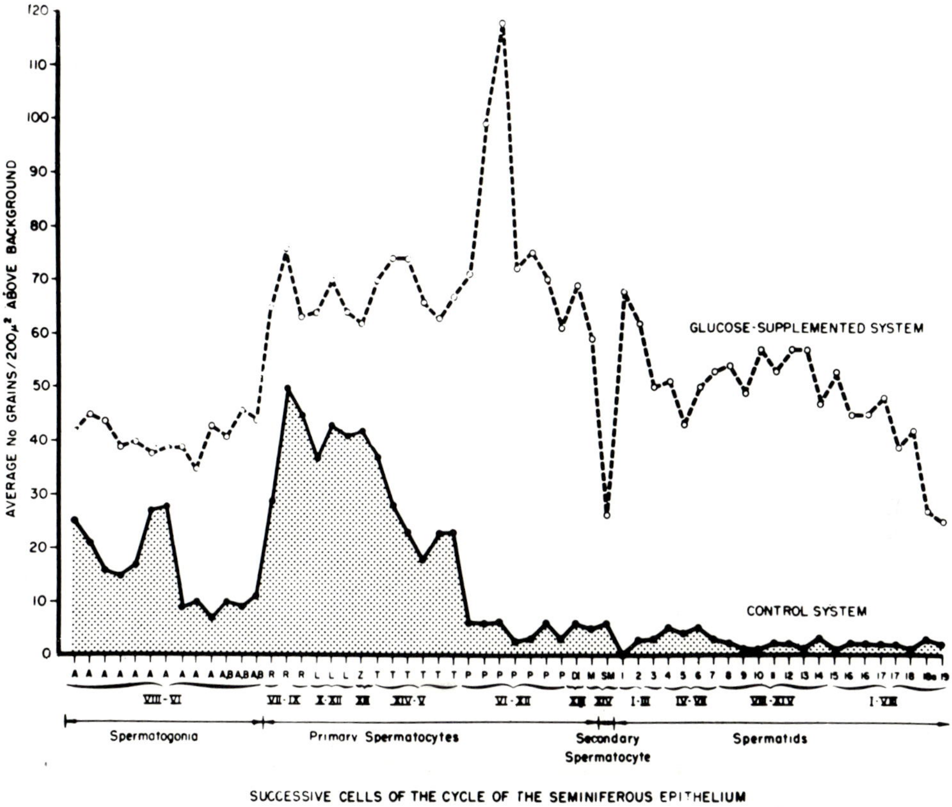

Fig. 6. Effect of glucose on the incorporation of tritiated lysine into protein of the successive cells of the seminiferous epithelium of the rat testis. Each point on the curves represents the average from 4 individual experiments, comprising 20 microscopic fields from each animal or a total of 80 determinations for each of the designated cells of the cycle of the seminiferous epithelium. Representative standard errors for cells in the control system averaged ± 3 grains/$200\mu^2$ above background; that for cells in the glucose-supplemented system averaged ± 7 grains/$200\mu^2$. I-XIV refer to stages of the cycle of the seminiferous epithelium of the rat according to the description of Leblond and Clermont (7). Numbers 1-19 refer to spermatids at various steps of spermiogenesis. (From: Davis, J.R. et al., Amer. J. Physiol., 209: 425-432, 1965).

ists that glucose may be involved in the mechanisms of recombination of chromosomal segments during meiosis, thereby playing an important role in the constantly changing patterns of the genome. In addition, the data also suggest that the transition from mitosis to the first meiotic prophase is associated with a marked increase in protein labelling from lysine.

EFFECT OF GLUCOSE ON HUMAN TESTICULAR PROTEIN SYNTHESIS

The question then arose as to whether the presently-described pattern of protein labelling of the various successive cells of the seminiferous germinal epithelium of the rat would be similar in slices of the human testis incubated with tritiated lysine. The problems of comparing experimental animal data with human data are well known and the difficulties involved in performing dynamic biochemical studies on viable human testicular slices provide no exception. We were fortunate to obtain large segments of normal testes of two males aged 65 and 70 years which were removed as a therapeutic measure for prostatic carcinoma. Incubation of human testicular slices with tritiated lysine was begun within 30 minutes of removal of the testis at surgery. At no time prior to the beginning of the incubation period was the temperature of the removed testis allowed to rise above $4^{o}C$. Slices of the human testis, weighing approximately 250 mg, were therefore incubated for one hour under aerobic conditions with 100 μc of tritiated lysine both in the presence and absence of 0.009 M glucose in a manner identical to that for the rat. At the end of the incubation period, slices of the human testis were sectioned, dipped in molten Kodak nuclear track emulsion and exposure carried out for five days. The slides were then developed, stained in hematoxylin solution and the six stages of the cycle of the seminiferous epithelium of the human testis identified as described by Clermont (15).

Fig. 7 demonstrates representative radioautographs of sections taken from slices of human testes incubated with tritiated lysine in the presence and absence of exogenous glucose. A definite enhancement of protein labelling was observed over the spermatogonia, primary spermatocytes and spermatids.

Fig. 8 presents a plot of the average grain count per $200\mu^2$ above background over each of the successive cells of the cycle of the seminiferous germinal epithelium of the human testis one hour after incubation with tritiated lysine both in the presence and absence of exogenous glucose. The pattern of protein labelling over each of the cell associations of the human seminiferous germinal epithelium is remarkably similar to that just described for the rat. Not only do the primary spermatocytes most actively incorporate lysine into protein, but there is also a rapid increase in protein

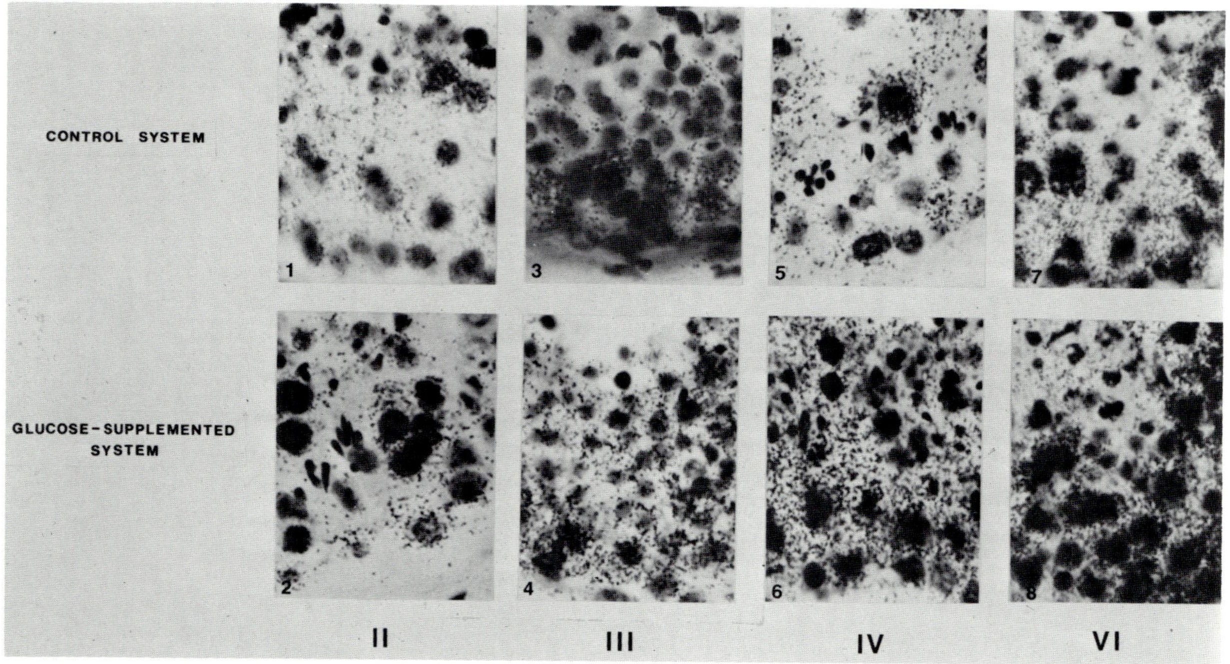

Fig. 7. Radioautographs of sections taken from slices of human testes incubated for 1 hour with tritiated lysine in the presence and absence of 0.009 M glucose. 1 and 2 represent stage II; 3 and 4, stage III; 5 and 6, stage IV; 7 and 8, stage VI. Sections were cut at 5 μ and stained with hematoxylin. Magnification approximately x 1000.

labelling following division of the spermatogonia into primary spermatocytes. A sharp decrease in protein labelling again occurred over the secondary spermatocytes in metaphase which was even more pronounced than that previously found in the rat. It is of interest to note that the meiotic divisions occurring during the development of Trillium anther have been reported to be associated with a fall in protein sulfhydryl groups (16). The only difference in the pattern of protein labelling in the successive cells of the seminiferous epithelium of the human testis as compared to the rat testis appears to involve the degree of stimulation that glucose exerts over the pachytene primary spermatocytes. The greater enhancement of protein labelling by glucose in the pachytene primary spermatocytes occurring in the rat seems to be due to the presence of lower control values of these cells in the rat. One possible explanation may be that in the absence of adequate levels of glucose, the earlier resting and leptotene primary spermatocytes have a higher capacity for protein synthesis than the later pachytene primary spermatocytes in younger animals as opposed to older animals. Experiments involving the influence of age on the effect of glucose on the radioautographic incorporation of tritiated lysine into the successive cells of the cycle of the seminiferous epithelium of both the rat and the human testis are now in progress in our laboratory.

The present studies have demonstrated characteristic quantitative radioautographic patterns of protein labelling in the various successive cells of the seminiferous germinal epithelium of both the rat and human. Although similar quantitative patterns for nucleic acid labelling are presently lacking for these two species, Monesi (17,18) has investigated the radioautographic incorporation of nucleic acid precursors in the mouse testis. DNA was found to be synthesized during the resting stage of the primary spermatocytes with RNA synthesis reaching a peak in middle pachytene, declining during late pachytene and then ceasing completely during metaphase and anaphase I and II. These observations on nucleic acid labelling in the mouse testis seem to be consistent with our findings for protein labelling in the various successive cells of the seminiferous germinal epithelium of both the rat and human testis. Any differences in protein biosynthesis of those cells of the spermatogenic cycle responsible for cell proliferation and renewal as compared to the more mature spermatids may have importance not only in investigations dealing with regulation of male fertility but also in investigations dealing with potential side-effects of drugs that may cause genetic damage with resulting congenital malformations. It is our opinion that the presently-described radioautographic patterns of protein labelling over each of the successive cells of the seminiferous germinal epithelium may provide an extremely practical initial screening procedure for the detection of any such possible side-effects of drugs on spermatogenesis. Drugs which are commonly administered to the male prior to the breeding performance may alter the radioautographic pattern of protein labelling over the successive cells of the spermatogenic cycle in a more sensitive manner

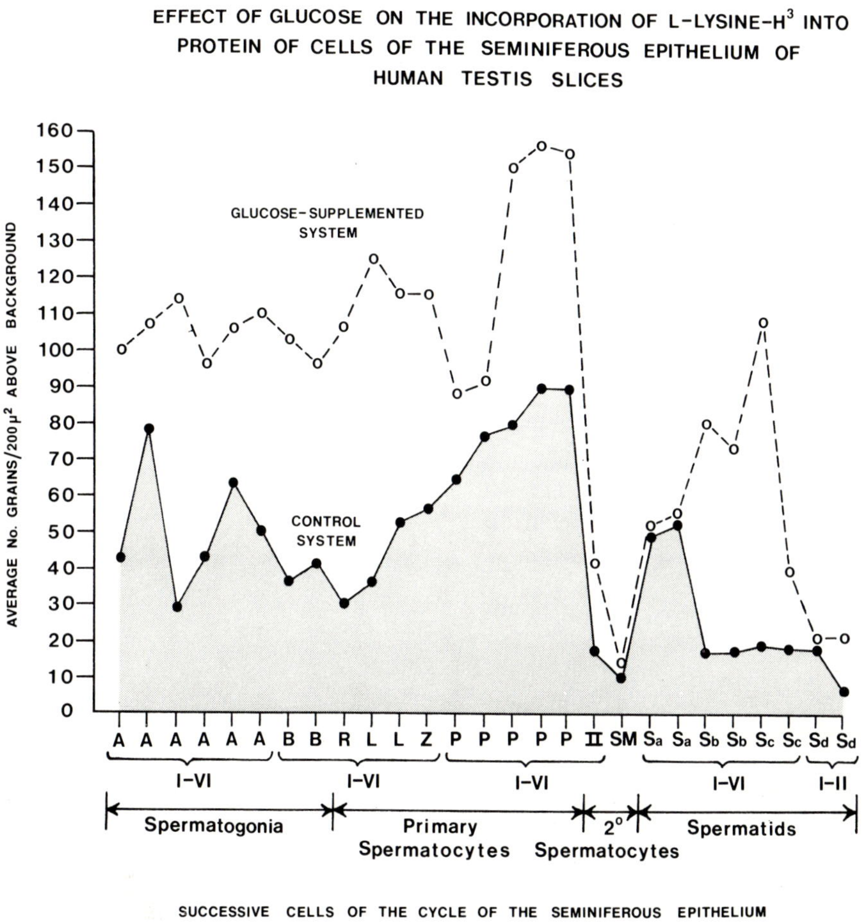

Fig. 8. Effect of glucose on the incorporation of tritiated lysine into protein of the successive cells of the cycle of the seminiferous epithelium of the human testis. Each point on the curves represents the average from 2 individual experiments, comprising 10 microscopic fields from each human testis or a total of 40 determinations for each of the designated cells of the cycle of the seminiferous epithelium. I-VI refer to stages of the cycle of the seminiferous epithelium of the human according to the description of Clermont (15). Sa-Sd refer to spermatids at various steps of spermiogenesis.

than a usual histological examination of the testis. Any drugs that are found to influence initially the radioautographic pattern of protein labelling of the successive cells of the seminiferous epithelium could then be studied further employing the more laborious technique of mating experiments with subsequent examination of offspring.

ACKNOWLEDGEMENT

This investigation was supported by U.S. Public Health Service Research Grant HD-01573 from the National Institute of Child Health and Human Development.

REFERENCES

1. Davis, J.R., Firlit, C.F. and Hollinger, M.A., Amer. J. Physiol., 204: 696, 1963.
2. Davis, J.R., Morris, R.N. and Hollinger, M.A., Amer. J. Physiol., 207: 50, 1964.
3. Davis, J.R. and Morris, R.N., Amer. J. Physiol., 205: 833, 1963.
4. Steinberger, E. and Nelson, W.O., Endocrinology, 56: 429, 1955.
5. Davis, J.R. and Firlit, C.F., Fertil. Steril., 17: 187, 1966.
6. Firlit, C.F. and Davis, J.R., J. Reprod. Fertil., 11: 125, 1966.
7. Leblond, C.P. and Clermont, Y., Amer. J. Anat., 90: 167, 1952.
8. Schuler, W., Helv. Chim. Acta, 27: 1796, 1944.
9. Tepperman, J., Tepperman, H.M. and Dick, H.J., Endocrinology, 45: 491, 1949.
10. Paul, H.E., Paul, M.F., Kopko, F., Bender, R.C., and Everett, G., Endocrinology, 53: 585, 1953.
11. Steinberger, E. and Wagner, C., Endocrinology, 69: 305, 1961.
12. Ewing, L.L., Baird, E.R. and VanDemark, N.L., Comp. Biochem. Physiol., 17: 455, 1966.
13. Mancine, R.E., Penhos, J.C., Izquierdo, I.A. and Heinrich, J.J., Proc. Soc. Exp. Biol. Med., 104: 699, 1960.
14. Means, A.R. and Hall, P.F., Endocrinology, 83: 86, 1968.
15. Clermont, Y., Amer. J. Anat., 112: 35, 1963.
16. Stern, H., J. Biophys. Biochem. Cytol., 4: 157, 1958.
17. Monesi, V., J. Cell Biol. 14: 1, 1962.
18. Monesi, V., Exp. Cell Res. 39: 197, 1965.

DISCUSSION

BURGOS: In guinea pig testes, we have found by electron microscopy that from the spermatogonia B to the primary spermatocyte in the pachytene stage, there is a remarkable synthesis of cytoplasmic membranes at the same stage at which the peak of maximal protein labelling occurs. The membranes start to appear at the leptotene stage and reach their greatest development at the end of the pachytene stage.

CHRISTENSEN: Dr. Davis, I might suggest that you use perfusion to administer the labelled amino acid to testes that have been removed from human beings. I think you might obtain a more uniform administration. On that first autoradiogram that you showed, it looked to me as if the grains were evenly distributed over the nuclei and over the cytoplasm. I wonder whether you are claiming nuclear protein synthesis?

DAVIS: With regard to your first comment, we have previously shown that the in vitro testicular slice technique for radioactive tracer experiments allows for a uniform penetration of the isotope throughout the entire seminiferous germinal epithelium. With regard to your second comment, we have expressed our results as grains per $200\mu^2$ over the entire cell inasmuch as it was not possible to rule out any cytoplasmic grains that might appear over areas of the nucleus in 5μ sections.

CHRISTENSEN: In the autoradiograph you showed, many of the grains were over the nuclei.

DAVIS: We are certainly keeping the possibility of a selective glucose-stimulated nuclear protein synthesis in the seminiferous germinal epithelium in mind and are presently designing experiments to investigate this point.

MEANS: I have one comment to add to what Dr. Christensen said about perfusion. We must realize that pool sizes are neglected in tissue slices because we have many cut surfaces of cells. A perfusion might be a very interesting approach to use if one is really trying to categorize and look at the clinical type of phenomenology that Dr. Davis was talking about.

JOST: I should like to ask Dr. Davis if the influence of glucose on the synthesis of protein is insulin-dependent, and what happens in diabetic patients?

DAVIS: We are certainly planning to study the possible influence of insulin on the radioautographic incorporation of tritiated lysine into the successive cells of the seminiferous germinal epithelium, employing our in vitro testicular slice technique, both in the presence and absence of exogenous glucose. Dr. Mancini has indicated that hypoglycemia will produce testicular atrophy and a number of investigators have reported that male diabetics can have reduced sperm counts. In addition, alloxan-diabetic rats have been shown to have testicular atrophy. Until we determine whether the testis is dependent upon insulin for glucose transport, all I would like to state at the present time is that it is apparent that the intracellular content of glucose is a most important regulator of protein synthesis occurring in the seminiferous germinal epithelium. We are currently quite interested in whether one possible explanation for any damaging effects of diabetes on the testicular germinal epithelium may involve the extremely sensitive regulation of testicular protein synthesis by glucose.

MACLEOD: I would like to amend the statement made by Dr. Davis that diabetics are infertile. We have found the contrary to be true. We have not found any higher incidence of infertility amongst diabetics than we have in any other population. It is true that diabetics may become impotent, but that is quite another matter.

DAVIS: All I can say is that I have read several papers expressing both viewpoints. I would like to suggest that the possibility of male infertility in diabetics be more extensively studied in non-treated cases but of course this would be extremely difficult to do. In answer to Dr. MacLeod's comment, there have been experiments performed in alloxan diabetic rats; and these have demonstrated destruction of the seminiferous germinal epithelium.

STUDIES OF SPERMATOGENESIS AND STEROID METABOLISM IN CULTURES OF HUMAN TESTICULAR TISSUE

A. Steinberger, M. Ficher and E. Steinberger

Division of Endocrinology and Reproduction Research Laboratories, Albert Einstein Medical Center, Philadelphia, Pa. 19141

INTRODUCTION

Study of the physiology of any organ in vivo is complicated by numerous interactions taking place within a living organism, and attempts to identify factors controlling testicular functions have been faced with a similar problem. Thus, while it has been established that pituitary gonadotropins play an integral part in the control of testicular physiology, the specific role of follicle stimulating hormone (FSH) or luteinizing hormone (LH), as well as the role of other factors in the spermatogenic and steroidogenic functions of the testis have not been clearly defined.

We have sought to alleviate some shortcomings of the in vivo systems by utilizing an in vitro culture method, which permits a more rigid control of the environmental conditions and offers an experimental model for the study of direct effects of various factors on testicular physiology. A culture method would seem particularly useful for the investigation of human testicular functions, since besides simplifying the experimental model from a biological viewpoint, it also alleviates many moral and legal problems connected with human experimentation in vivo. In view of the fact that relatively small amounts of tissue are needed to set up a culture, multiple cultures can be initiated from an average size testicular biopsy.

This communication summarizes our observations on the maintenance and differentiation of human testes grown as organ culture under several in vitro conditions, as well as the capacity of the cultured tissues to metabolize progesterone. Formation of steroid hormones from acetate by fetal human testes grown as organ culture was reported recently (1).

MATERIALS AND METHODS

a. Source of Tissue. Testicular tissues were obtained from adult individuals undergoing diagnostic biopsy or therapeutic orchiectomy. In one instance, testes from a 2-day old male were obtained at autopsy two hours following accidental death. Only testes with complete spermatogenesis and ability to metabolize progesterone to testosterone were utilized for these studies.

b. Culture Method. The method for organ culture of human testes was similar to that used in our laboratory previously for culture of testes from other mammalian species (2). Briefly, small tissue fragments (1 mm^3) were grown on top of a millipore filter (0.45 μ pore size) supported by a stainless steel wire grid at the liquid-gas interphase. The culture medium was maintained at pH 6.9-7.1 and was replenished every 3 to 4 days. Penicillin (100 IU), streptomycin (100 μg) and fungizone (5 μg) per ml of culture medium were used to minimize the incidence of microbial contamination. The various culture medium supplements, incubation temperatures and gas phases used in an attempt to define optimal conditions for cultivation of human testes will be discussed in the Results section.

c. Histologic Evaluation. Fresh testicular tissue and tissues cultured for various time intervals were fixed in Cleland's or Bouin's fixative and processed by standard histologic methods. Four micron sections were stained with periodic acid-Schiff followed by hematoxylin (PAS-H). The histologic appearance of the cultured tissues was evaluated microscopically, using the following criteria: 1) Maintenance of the overall tubular structure and the viability of supporting cells. 2) Duration of the survival of specific cell types in the germinal epithelium. 3) Degree of differentiation of the germinal cells in vitro.

d. Radioautography. Tritiated thymidine (specific activity 6.7 Ci/mmole) was added aseptically to the culture medium in a final concentration of 1 μCi/ml. After 40 minutes the ^{3}H-thymidine containing medium was replaced by "cold" medium. At various time intervals following the pulse, several tissue fragments were fixed in Bouin's fixative and processed by routine histologic methods.. Four micron thick sections were stained with PAS and coated with liquid Kodak NTB-2 emulsion. After 2 or 3 weeks of exposure in the dark at 4 ^{o}C, the emulsion was developed and the sections stained with hematoxylin. This procedure yielded better preparations than sections stained with PAS-H, either before or after development of the emulsion. The location of grains over cell nuclei was determined using a high magnification objective. A nucleus was considered labelled when the density of grains over the nucleus was more than two standard deviations above that of the background.

e. Incubation with ^{3}H-progesterone. The incubation procedure was similar to that described previously (3). Twenty to 80 mg. wet weight of fresh or cultured testicular tissue was minced in a small flask containing 1.5 ml of incubation medium and the substrate ^{3}H-progesterone (20 x 10^6 dpm, 3 mμmole). The incubation was carried out in a Dubnoff shaker for 3 hours at 37°, in an atmosphere of 95% air and 5% CO_2. After the incubation, ^{14}C-labelled tracers (40,000 dpm of each) dissolved in 10% ethanol in benzene were added to the incubate in order to correct for losses in subsequent manipulations. At this point, 10 ml of ethyl acetate was also added and the material was stored at -20° until further processing. The incubation medium (1.5 ml/flask) had the following composition:

1 ml Hank's balanced salt solution
125 μl 1.3% $NaHCO_3$
175 μl NADP,Na solution (3.257 μmole/ml)
175 μl G-6-P,Na_2 solution (36.17 μmole/ml)
25 μl ethanol

f. Extraction Procedure. Following repeated extractions with ethyl acetate and methanol-hexane partition, the material was extracted with chloroform. Appropriate cold carriers (50 μg of each) were added to the dry residue obtained from the chloroform extract.

g. Purification and Identification of Steroids. For the initial separation of steroids,aBush A chromatograph system (heptane, methanol, water - 100:80:20) was utilized, and the radioactive peaks were related to known steroid standards; the Δ^4-3-ketosteroids were located on the paper strips as dark zones under short-wave ultraviolet illumination. The materials from the radioactive peaks of the initial chromatogram were eluted and rechromatographed in a Bush 3 system (heptane, benzene, methanol, water - 66:34:80:20). Further identification of the steroids was accomplished by derivative formation and by the technique of isotopic dilution and recrystallization to constant specific activity or constant ratio $^{3}H/^{14}C$.

h. Measurement of Radioactivity. Paper chromatograms were scanned in a Packard model 7200 radiochromatogram scanner. Eluates from paper chromatograms were dried, dissolved in 10 ml of scintillation solution (0.4 percent w/v of 2,5-bis-[2'(5'-tert-butylbenzoxazolyl)] -thiophene in toluene) and counted in a Packard liquid scintillation spectrometer, model 3003, set for simultaneous counts of ^{3}H and ^{14}C. Further details on counting efficiencies and purification of chemicals used in these procedures were described previously (3). Calculation of percent conversion from progesterone was based on the following formula:

$$\frac{^{3}H \text{ dpm in last crystals X dpm of } ^{14}C \text{ steroid added X 100}}{^{14}C \text{ dpm in last crystals X dpm } ^{3}H \text{ progesterone in incubation medium}}$$

RESULTS

A. Maintenance of Human Testes in Organ Culture

1) The effect of basic culture conditions

Prior to initiating studies on the effect of hormones or other specific factors on mammalian testes cultured in vitro, basic environmental conditions had to be defined which would best support the over-all tissue viability for prolonged periods of time. Initial studies on the effect of several culture conditions were carried out, using organ cultures of rat testes (4,5,6). Conditions found to be optimal for maintaining rat testes in vitro were later utilized for culture of testes from several other mammalian species (2). In an attempt to define optimal conditions for cultivation of human testes in vitro, the effects of incubation temperature, oxygen tension and medium composition were re-investigated, using human testes.

a. Effect of incubation temperature: Multiple cultures of adult human testes were grown at 31°, 33° or 35° for varying periods of time. Microscopic examination of stained histologic sections revealed that with all other conditions kept uniform, best overall survival of germinal elements and differentiation of spermatogonia to late pachytene spermatocytes occurred in cultures grown at 31°. At temperatures of 33° or 35°, the results were much more variable and extensive degeneration of germ cells was often observed in cultures grown at 35°. The incubation temperature of 31° was, therefore, considered to be optimal for cultivation of human testes.

b. Effect of oxygen tension: To test the effect of higher oxygen tension, cultures were incubated in a gas atmosphere composed of 5% CO_2 and 95% air, or 5% CO_2 and 95% oxygen. The presence of 5% CO_2 in the gas phase was essential for the maintenance of pH (6.9-7.1). The increased oxygen tension was found to be damaging to the overall survival of testicular tissue and the survival of germ cells in particular.

c. Effect of culture medium composition: Several commercially available media were tested for their efficiency in supporting the viability of human testes in organ culture. Minimum Essential Medium (7) supplemented with 1 mM of Na pyruvate and 0.1 mM of each of the amino acids alanine, asparagine, aspartic acid, glutamic acid, glycine, proline and serine, appeared consistently somewhat superior to other media tested and was, therefore, adapted for routine use. In most cases, the medium was also supplemented with 10% calf serum, since it appeared beneficial for maintenance of the tissues for periods longer than four weeks. Until the fourth week of cultivation, no difference was observed in the morphological appearance of tissues grown in chemically defined media or media supplemented with serum. The calf serum was consistently superior to homologous serum. Additional supplements tested for enhancing effect on either maintenance or differentiation of the germinal cells in culture will be discussed below.

2) Sexually Mature Testes

A microscopic cross-section of a seminiferous tubule from a sexually mature human testis is shown in Fig. 1. Several cell associations (stages of spermatogenesis) are present within a single tubular cross-section, which is characteristic for the human testis (8). In organ cultures grown under optimal conditions, spermatids were present for approximately seven days of cultivation (Fig. 2), and spermatocytes for approximately three weeks of cultivation (Fig. 3). The basic tubular architecture was maintained and the Sertoli cells and spermatogonia remained viable for at least seven weeks (Fig. 4). Mitotic activity diminished gradually with time of cultivation, but was still evident after seven weeks (Fig. 4). The pale type A spermatogonia (Ap) survived in culture for longer periods than the dark type A (Ad) spermatogonia. This results in an increased ratio of Ap:Ad, which is close to 1.0 in normal tissues, and may become as high as 4.6 after several weeks of cultivation(9).

3) Differentiation of premiotic germ cells in vitro

The presence of spermatocytes in cultures for periods up to four weeks raised the question whether these cells were formed by in vitro differentiation of less mature germ cells or represented cells which were present in the tissues prior to cultivation. This question was resolved by using radioautography techniques following pulse-labelling of cell nuclei with ^{3}H-thymidine.

It has been shown (10) that one hour following injection of ^{3}H-thymidine into human testes in vivo, the most advanced germ cells which incorporate the precursor into nuclear DNA are the early leptotene or pre-leptotene spermatocytes. It was, therefore, possible to follow the development of these cells into more mature forms by obtaining testicular biopsies at time intervals and examining them following radioautography.

We utilized a similar approach to determine the fate of pre-leptotene spermatocytes in culture. The initial labelling was accomplished in vitro by growing the cultures for the first 40 minutes in medium containing ^{3}H-thymidine. At various time intervals following the pulse, several tissue fragments were fixed and processed for radioautography. After 40 minutes exposure to ^{3}H-thymidine, the most advanced germ cells that were labelled were pre-leptotene spermatocytes. After seven days of cultivation, the label was associated with leptotene or zygotene spermatocytes, and after two to

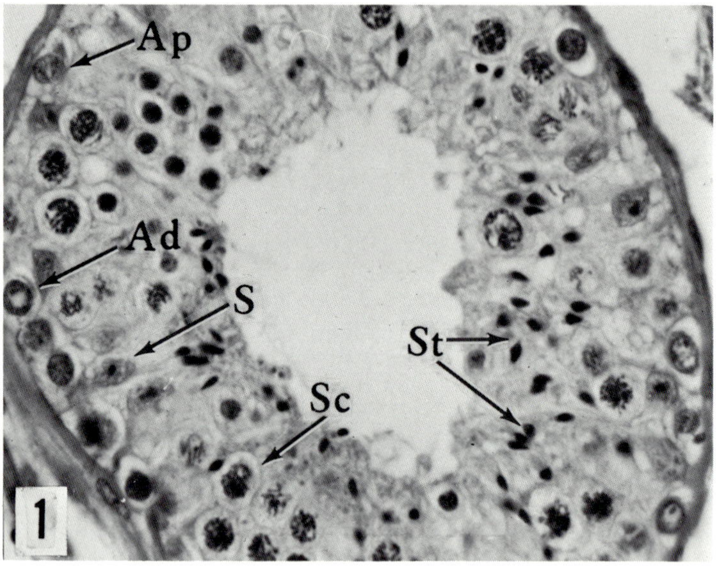

Fig. 1. Cross-section of a seminiferous tubule from a sexually mature human testis. The germ cells are present in several specific associations (stages of spermatogenesis) Ap-pale type A spermatogonia. Ad-dark type A spermatogonia. Sc-spermatocytes. St-spermatids. S-Sertoli cells. Magn. X 480.

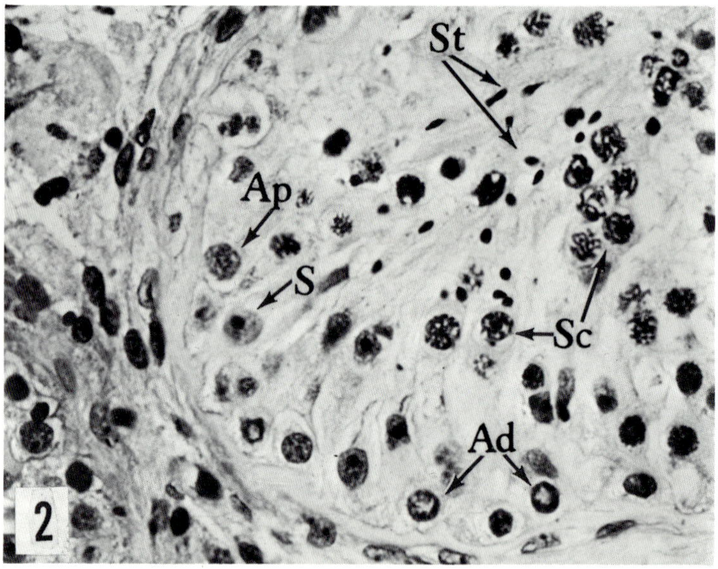

Fig. 2. Microscopic appearance of a sexually mature human testis after 7 days of cultivation. Magn. X 480.

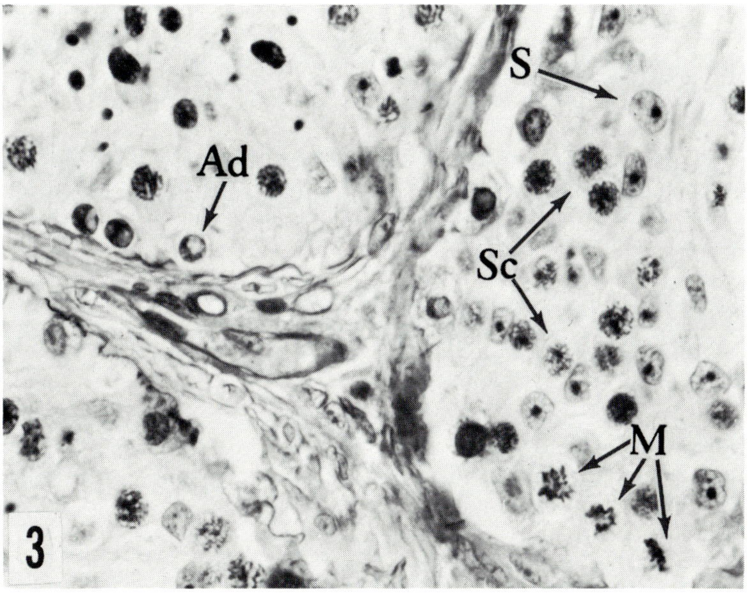

Fig. 3. Microscopic appearance of a sexually mature testis after 21 days of cultivation. Note presence of mitotic figures (M) and absence of spermatids. Magn. X 480.

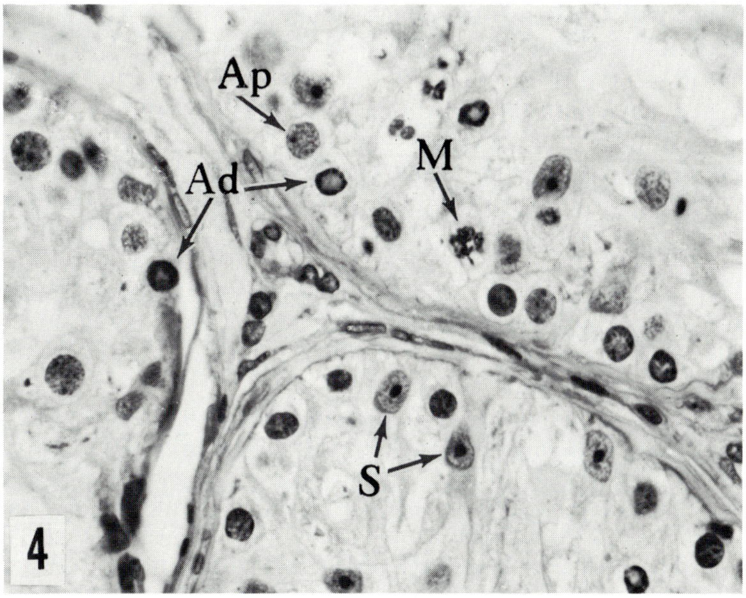

Fig. 4. Microscopic appearance of a sexually mature testis after 48 days of cultivation. The only germ cells remaining are spermatogonia. Magn. X 480.

three weeks of cultivation, with spermatocytes in the late pachytene stage of miosis. Differentiation of germ cells was observed only when either vitamins A (12 u), C (50 μg) and E (60 μg) per ml, or 4 mM of glutamine were present in the culture medium. Addition of various concentrations of testosterone or gonadotropic hormones (HCG, NIH-LH-B5, HIH-FSH-S-1, PMS) to the culture medium did not result in improved maintenance or stimulation of differentiation of the germ cells. In fact, high concentrations of the gonadotropins appeared toxic and produced pronounced vacuolation of Sertoli cell cytoplasm and scattered non-specific necrosis.

These results show unequivocally that in human testes differentiation of pre-leptotene spermatocytes through the leptotene, zygotene and pachytene stages of the miotic prophase takes place under appropriate culture conditions in the absence of gonadotropic hormones. Under no culture conditions tested could we maintain the entire spermatogenic process or show progression of differentiation beyond the late pachytene stage of spermatocytes. These findings are in agreement with our earlier observations on organ cultures of several other mammalian species (2).

4) <u>Sexually immature testes</u> (2-day old male)

The histologic appearance of normal testes from a 2-day old male, and of similar tissue following 28 days of growth in organ culture, are shown in Figs. 5 and 6, respectively. The cultures were grown at 31°C in an atmosphere of 5% CO_2 and 95% air, in a medium containing a 4 mM concentration of glutamine. It is apparent that the tubular structure, the supporting cells and the germinal cells were well maintained under these culture conditions, with some evidence of morphologic differentiation. The lumen of the tubules became somewhat larger and the number of germ cells increased. Since the human testes do not become sexually mature for about 13 years, we obviously did not expect to observe drastic differentiation in vitro in a matter of weeks.

B. Metabolism of Progesterone in Fresh and Cultured Human Testes

Although the qualitative results obtained in three separate experiments, using tissue from three different adult individuals, were similar, there were considerable quantitative differences in the amounts of converted progesterone and the amounts of the resulting metabolites. For this reason, the results obtained in each experiment (Exp. A,B,C) are shown in Tables 1-4. Tracings of the radioscans from the first chromatograms (Bush A system) obtained from fresh tissue and tissue cultured for seven days (Exp. A) are shown in Figs. 7 and 8, respectively. Both radioscans showed a major radioactive peak of highly polar material at the origin and four additional peaks of radioactivity with chromatographic mobilities corresponding to the following steroid standards: Testosterone

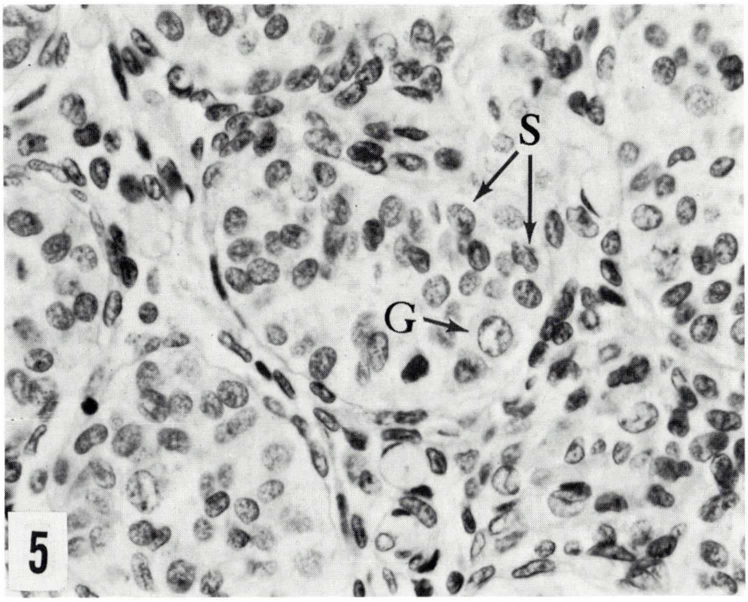

Fig. 5. Section of testis from a 2-day old human male. The seminiferous tubules contain only Sertoli cells (S) and undifferentiated germ cells (G). Magn. X 480.

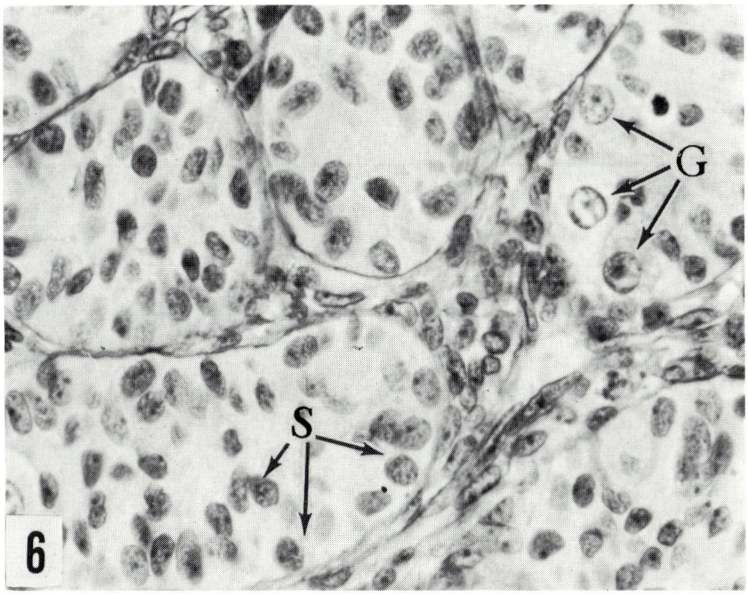

Fig. 6. Microscopic appearance of testis from 2-day old human male after 28 days of cultivation. The seminiferous tubules appear more differentiated. Magn. X 480.

TABLE 1. ISOTOPIC DILUTION AND RECRYSTALLIZATION OF TESTOSTERONE ACETATE TO CONSTANT $^{3}H/^{14}C$ RATIO

		Days in Culture							
		Exp. A			Exp. B		Exp. C		
FRACTION		0	7	14	0	14	0	3	31
Crystallization #1 methanol/water	xls [a]	24[c]	3.7[c]	3.0[c]	9.3[c]	0.503[c]	41[c]	3.9[c]	.580
	ML[b]	27	7.4[c]	6.1	4.0	0.413	15	1.6	2.426
Crystallization #2 methanol/water	xls	23[c]	3.7[c]	2.9[c]	9.0[c]	0.445[c]	41[c]	3.9[c]	0.510[c]
	ML	24[c]	4.8	3.2[c]	8.5	0.603	26	3.4	1.660
Crystallization #3 methanol/water	xls	24[c]	3.8[c]	2.9[c]	9.2[c]	0.505[c]	43[c]	3.7[c]	0.540[c]
	ML	24[c]	3.7[c]	3.0[c]	9.7[c]	0.539[c]	39[c]	5.2	0.790
MEAN ± S.E.		23.80 ±0.20	3.73 ±0.03	3.00 ±0.06	9.30 ±0.15	0.516 ±0.012	41 ±0.8	3.8 ±0.07	.525 ±0.015

a - crystals
b - mother liquor
c - $^{3}H/^{14}C$ ratios used for calculation of the mean ± S.E.

TABLE 2. ISOTOPIC DILUTION AND RECRYSTALLIZATION OF 17α-HYDROXYPROGESTERONE TO CONSTANT $^{3}H/^{14}C$ RATIO

		Days in culture							
		Exp. A			Exp. B		Exp. C		
FRACTION		0	7	14	0	14	0	3	31
Crystallization #1 methanol/water	xls[a]	110[c]	33[c]	23[c]	165[c]	20[c]	48[c]	7.4[c]	56[c]
	ML[b]	79	44	27	158	18[c]	44[c]	13.3	45
Crystallization #2 methanol/water	xls	110[c]	33[c]	21[c]	172[c]	20[c]	47[c]	7.4[c]	52[c]
	ML	103[c]	33[c]	23[c]	172[c]	20[c]	45[c]	8.2[c]	56[c]
Crystallization #3 methanol/water	xls	106[c]	32c	24[c]	174[c]	20[c]	47[c]	8.4[c]	55[c]
	ML	106[c]	34c	22[c]	167[c]	19[c]	47[c]	7.4[c]	57[c]
MEAN ± S.E.		107.00 ±1.30	33.00 ±0.32	22.60 ±0.51	170.00 ±1.70	19.50 ±0.34	46.30 ±0.60	7.8 ±0.22	55.60 ±0.88

a - crystals
b - mother liquor
c - $^{3}H/^{14}C$ ratios used for calculation of the mean ± S.E.

TABLE 3. ISOTOPIC DILUTION AND RECRYSTALLIZATION OF 20α-DIHYDROPROGESTERONE TO CONSTANT SPECIFIC ACTIVITY (dpm/μMole)

		Days in Culture							
		Exp. A			Exp. B		Exp. C		
FRACTION		0	7	14	0	14	0	3	31
Crystallization #1	xls[a]	443[c]	1,139[c]	1,076[c]	380[c]	95	320[c]	-d	1,430[c]
methanol/water	ML[b]	601	2,184	1,392	475	76[c]	1,520	-	1,980
Crystallization #2	xls	443[c]	1,139[c]	1,044[c]	380[c]	70[c]	310[c]	-	1,540
methanol/water	ML	475[c]	1,266	1,044[c]	443	79[c]	320[c]	-	1,460[c]
Crystallization #3	xls	443[c]	1,155[c]	886	348[c]	70[c]	310[c]	-	1,310[c]
methanol/water	ML	443[c]	1.202[c]	1,170	380[c]	57	320[c]	-	1,490[c]
MEAN ± S.E.		449 ±6.4	1,159 ±15.0	1,055 ±10.7	372 ±8.0	73.8 ±2.3	316 ±2.5	- -	1,422 ±40

a - crystals
b - mother liquor
c - specific activities used for calculation of the mean ± S.E.
d - not done

TABLE 4. PERCENT CONVERSION OF PROGESTERONE TO KNOWN METABOLITES

	Days in Culture							
	Exp. A			Exp. B		Exp. C		
METABOLITES	0	7	14	0	14	0	3	31
Progesterone[a] (unconverted substrate)	13	68	61	29	84	7	64	72
Testosterone[b]	4.5	0.7	0.5	2.5	0.14	10	0.9	0.14
17α-hydroxyprogesterone[b]	17	5	4	38	4.5	9	1.6	12
20α-dihydroprogesterone[a]	7	6	10	5	3	3	6	6
Androstenedione[a]	3	2	2	1	0.4	2	1	0.5

a - calculated on basis of recovered radioactivity in the first chromatogram (Bush A)

b - calculated on basis of recrystallization to constant $^{3}H/^{14}C$ ratio

and 17α-hydroxyprogesterone, 20α-dihydroprogesterone, androstenedione and progesterone.

It is evident that following seven days of cultivation, the amount of unconverted progesterone increased considerably, while the amount of radioactivity in the area corresponding to testosterone and 17α-hydroxyprogesterone showed a three-fold decrease. The peaks in the zones of 20α-dihydroprogesterone and androstenedione showed no significant change. The radioscans obtained from the cultured tissues also showed an additional peak of radioactivity in the area of less polar material than progesterone. This material has not been identified. The change observed in the first chromatogram after seven days of cultivation were slightly emphasized with additional time of cultivation.

The material from the radioactive peak corresponding in mobility to testosterone and 17α-hydroxyprogesterone was eluted and rechromatographed in a Bush 3 system following acetylation Two peaks of radioactivity were formed; one with an Rf value similar to that of 17α-hydroxyprogesterone, and another peak with the Rf value of testosterone acetate. Final identification of the materials in these two peaks was obtained by isotopic dilution and recrystallization to constant $^{3}H/14C$ ratio (Tables 1 and 2).

The materials migrating in the first chromatogram, like androstenedione and 20α-dihydroprogesterone standards, respectively, yielded single peaks upon rechromatography in the Bush 3 system. The chemical purity of 20α-dihydroprogesterone was further asserted by recrystallization to constant specific activity (Table 3).

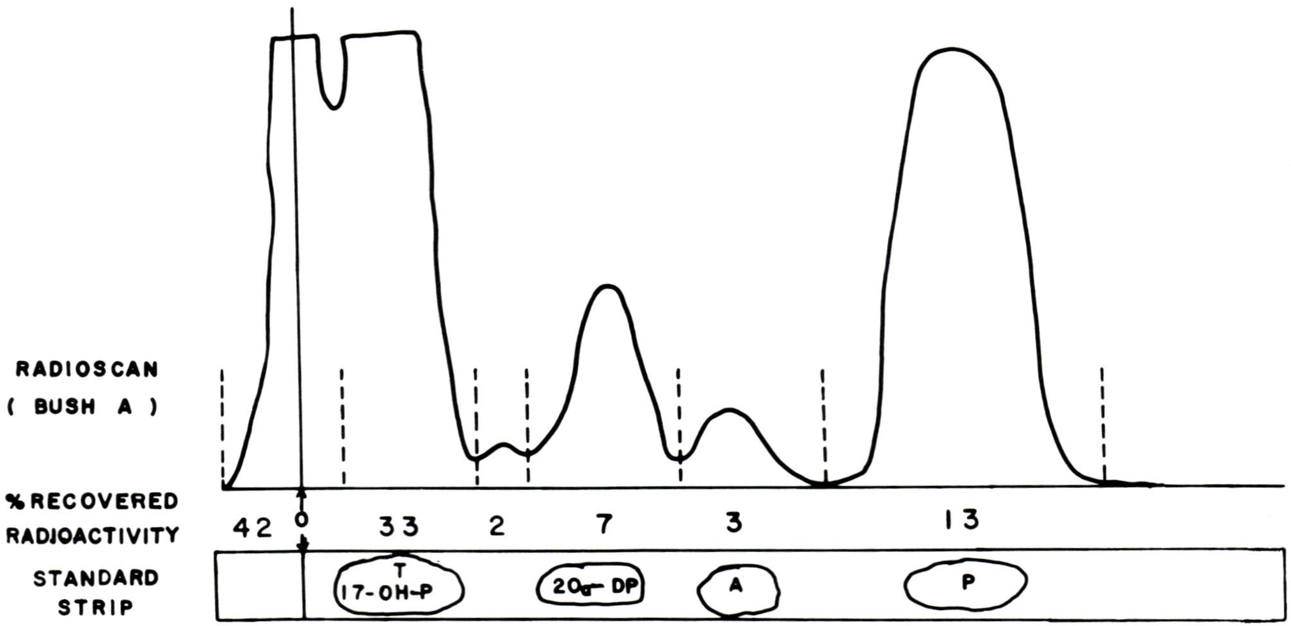

Fig. 7. Radioscan of the first chromatogram (Bush A obtained from incubate of fresh testicular tissue (adult human) with ^{3}H-progesterone in Exp. A.

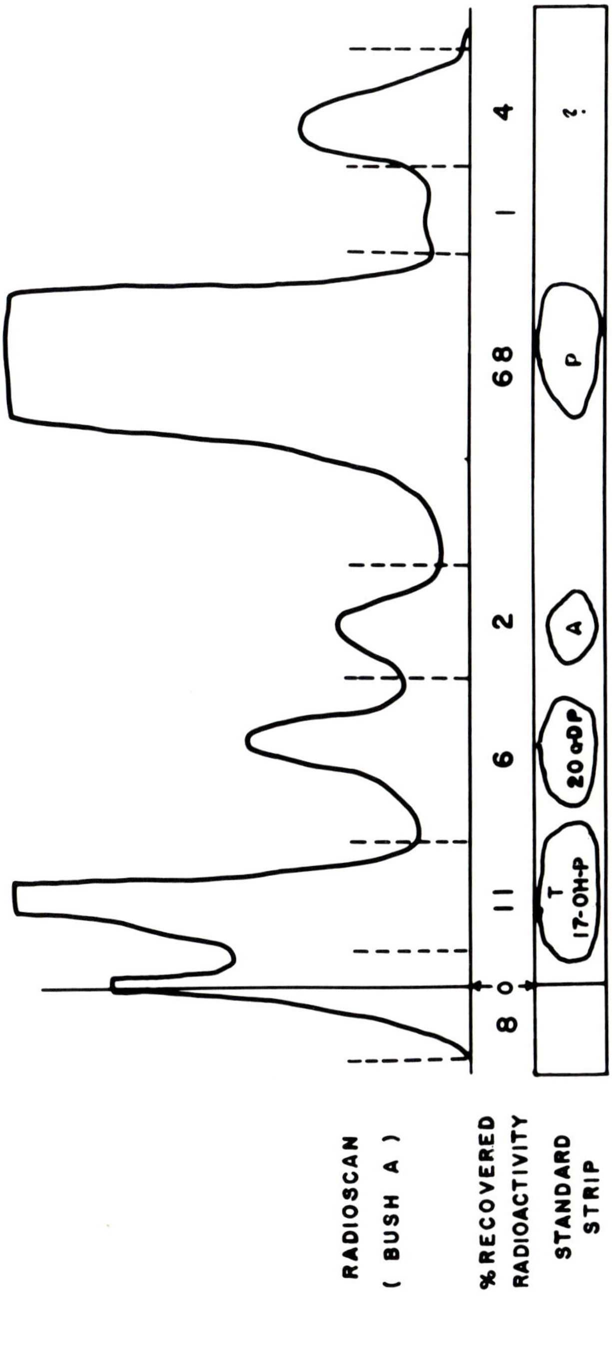

Fig. 8. Radioscan of the first chromatogram (Bush A) obtained from incubate of similar tissue with ^{3}H-progesterone after 7 days of cultivation in Exp. A.

The percent conversion of progesterone to several known metabolites obtained in all three experiments and the percentages of radioactivity associated with unconverted substrate are summarized in Table 4. The percent conversion of progesterone to testosterone and 17α-hydroxyprogesterone, respectively, are based on the results of recrystallizations to constant $^{3}H/^{14}C$ ratio using ^{14}C labelled carriers. The percent conversion of progesterone to 20α-dihydroprogesterone and to androstenedione was calculated on the basis of recovered radioactivity in the first chromatograms, since repeated chromatographies and recrystallizations to constant specific activities did not reveal any impurities. It is evident that the amount of progesterone converted to testosterone drops significantly within the first three days of cultivation, with a further small drop occurring upon additional culture period. The capacity of testicular tissue maintained in organ culture to convert progesterone to 17α-hydroxyprogesterone also appears to diminish, although not as drastically as the conversion of progesterone to testosterone. In one experiment (exp. C), the percent conversion of progesterone to 17α-hydroxyprogesterone diminished after three days of cultivation, but after 31 days of cultivation it was somewhat higher than in fresh tissue (Table 4).

DISCUSSION

While in vitro conditions, which would successfully maintain the entire spermatogenic process in the mammalian testes, have not been defined, some progress has been made in that direction. In organ culture of human testes, the overall tubular structure and viability of Sertoli cells and spermatogonia were maintained for at least seven weeks. The spermatids and spermatocytes survived for approximately seven days and 28 days, respectively. It was shown with the aid of radioautography that resting primary spermatocytes differentiate through the leptotene, zygotene and pachytene stages of the miotic prophase, in the absence of gonadotropins or testosterone, providing the culture medium contains vitamins A, C and E or a 4 mM concentration of glutamine. Addition of the hormones had no effect on either maintenance or differentiation of human testes in vitro. These results are generally similar to the results obtained with cultures of testes from several other mammalian species (2).

However, a unique characteristic of human testes is the retention of morphologic integrity of type A spermatogonia throughout the entire culture period, while in testes from other mammalian species the type A spermatogonia, after several days of cultivation, are replaced by primitive type A spermatogonia (11). The Ap spermatogonia survive in vitro for longer periods of time than the Ad spermatogonia, causing the Ap:Ad ratio to increase 3 to 5 fold within several weeks of cultivation. The significance of these observations is not clear.

The steroid studies indicate that the capacity of human testicular tissue to convert progesterone to 17α-hydroxyprogesterone and testosterone diminishes drastically within the first three days of cultivation, with only a slight further decrease occurring upon additional cultivation time. 20α-dihydroprogesterone and androstenedione were formed from progesterone by the cultured tissues, as well as by the fresh tissues. Since the major change in the pattern of progesterone metabolism occurs in culture rather rapidly, it could be due to the sudden removal of gonadotropic stimulation rather than a gradual loss of tissue viability. If the latter were the case, one would expect the changes to be more directly related to the time of cultivation. The decrease in the activity of 17α-hydroxylase, and particularly the decrease of 17-20 lyase activity could very well be a reflection of lack of gonadotropins, since diminution of the activity of these two enzymes was found in testicular tissue of human males with suppressed pituitary function (12).

Major metabolites, including testosterone, formed from progesterone in incubates of fresh tissue, were also formed by tissues cultured for up to 31 days. This would imply that all the necessary enzymes in the progesterone to testosterone metabolic pathway must have been functional under the culture conditions employed. Whether the quantitative relationships of progesterone metabolism can be affected by adding gonadotropic hormones to the cultures is presently being investigated.

Formation of a number of steroids, including testosterone from ^{14}C-acetate, was recently demonstrated in organ culture of human fetal testis (1). It is interesting that the amounts of testosterone and androstenedione formed by these cultures were also very small and were not significantly affected by addition of HCG to the culture medium.

It appears that organ culture may be a useful experimental model for the study of steroid biosynthesis and metabolism in testes exposed to various environmental conditions.

ACKNOWLEDGEMENTS

This study was supported, in part, by U.S. Public Health Service Grant No. HD 00399 and by a grant from the Ford Foundation. The excellent technical assistance of A. Gdowik, O. Luckyj, R. Ham and I. Haltrecht is gratefully acknowledged.

The following trivial names and abbreviations are used in this paper:

Androstenedione (A)	Δ^4-Androstene-3,17-dione
17α-Hydroxyprogesterone (17-OH-P)	Δ^4-Pregnene-17α-ol-3,20-dione
20α-Dihydroprogesterone (20α-DP)	Δ^4-Pregnene-20α-ol-3-one

Progesterone (P)	Δ^4-Pregnene-3,20-dione
Testosterone (T)	Δ^4-Androstene-17 β-ol-3-one
NADP,Na	Nicotinamide adenine dinucleotide phosphate, sodium salt
G-6-P, Na_2	Glucose-6-phosphate, sodium salt

REFERENCES

1. Rice, B.F., Johanson, C.A. and Sternberg, W.H., Steroids, 7: 1, 1966.
2. Steinberger, A. and Steinberger, E., J. Reprod. Fertil. Suppl., 2, 117: 1967.
3. Steinberger, E. and Ficher, M., Steroids, 11: 3, 1968.
4. Steinberger, A., Steinberger, E. and Perloff, W.H., Exp. Cell Res., 36: 19, 1964.
5. Steinberger, E., Steinberger, A. and Perloff, W.H., Endocrinology, 74: 5, 1964.
6. Steinberger, A. and Steinberger, E., Exp. Cell Res., 44: 429, 1966.
7. Eagle, H., Science, 130: 432, 1959.
8. Clermont, Y., Fertil. Steril., 17: 6, 1966.
9. Chowdhury, A.K., Steinberger, A. and Steinberger, E., Unpublished data.
10. Heller, C.G., Matson, L.J., Moore, D.J. and Clermont, Y., Procedures International Symposium on Effects of Ionizing Radiation in the Reproductive System, Pergamon Press, New York, 1963.
11. Steinberger, E., Steinberger, A. and Perloff, W.H., Anat. Rec., 148: 581, 1964.
12. Tamaoki, B. and Shikita, M., Steroid Dynamics, eds. Pincus, G., Nakao, T. and Tait, J.F., Academic Press, p. 493, 1966.

DISCUSSION

DICZFALUSY: Dr. Steinberger, do you have any information on the chemical nature of the metabolite which was less polar than progesterone? Could this possibly be a protein-bound form of progesterone? Have you done or do you intend to repeat your beautiful incubations with acetate instead of progesterone? The reason for asking this question is that in fetal perfusions using progesterone we found extremely limited incorporation of progesterone into testicular tissue. Using acetate we found that we could isolate as much as 10 to 15% of the total testicular radioactive material as cholesterol. Furthermore, when cholesterol and acetate were used together it was found that some 100 times more acetate was incorporated into the esterified cholesterol fraction than into unesterified cholesterol. A similar relationship was found in the fetal adrenals where much more acetate was incorporated into different conjugated steroids than into unconjugated forms. What I would like to find out is whether this is a particular situation in the fetal glands or does it also apply to the adult glands?

A. STEINBERGER: We have not identified the material, which is less polar than progesterone. The answer to the second question is that we are indeed planning to use acetate as a precursor in our incubations to test de novo synthesis of testosterone. The progesterone was used as a preliminary experiment. In this connection I would also like to quote a paper by Rice et al. (Steroids, 7: 79, 1966) who showed that acetate incubated with organ cultures of human fetal testis was incorporated into several steroids and I believe among others into testosterone and 17-hydroxyprogesterone.

MACLEOD: Dr. Steinberger mentioned that above the oxygen tension of air they did not obtain good culture development. I wonder if Dr. Steinberger would tell us under what experimental conditions this was found. Has the catalase activity of the various generations of germinal epithelium ever been measured? This question pertains to the observation we made about 25 years ago, namely that mature human spermatozoa are extremely sensitive to high oxygen tensions, and indeed extremely sensitive to any oxidations produced in their presence.

A. STEINBERGER: We found that in cultures grown by the usual method but under high oxygen tension (5% carbon dioxide and 95% oxygen) the germinal cells survive for a much shorter period of time, and do not show the progressive differentiation in the presence of glutamine or vitamins A, E and C. These observations are similar to our previous findings with cultures of mammalian testis of other species. Whether certain germ cells are specifically more affected by the oxygen I am not able to say, but the overall survival of the germ cells was impaired in higher oxygen tensions, and this is why we prefer using a gas phase composed of 95% air and 5% carbon dioxide. The carbon dioxide, incidentally, is necessary for the proper buffering capacity of the bicarbonate system used in the culture medium.

FORD: I understood Dr. Steinberger to say that in her organ cultures the spermatocytes developed up as far as the late pachytene stage. What total span of spermatocyte development would be covered? Would it be from zygotene to late pachytene or leptotene through to late pachytene?

A. STEINBERGER: The radioautography experiment showed definitely development of preleptotene spermatocytes into late pachytene spermatocytes. Possibly some spermatogonia also proceed into the late pachytene stage, but in this experimental design, this would be more difficult to assess since we were primarily following the most advanced labelled cells.

TROEN: I should like to report on some findings obtained by Dr. Takumi Yanaihara and myself in an organ culture study of steroid biosynthesis in testicular tissue of infertile males. Tissue obtained at diagnostic testicular biopsy from nine patients with oligospermia was studied in 24 to 48 hour organ cultures, using 3.8 to 6 mg and in one instance, 20 mg of tissue. Tritium and C^{14} labelled precursors were used in varying combinations and the metabolites identified and isotopic ratios determined. Δ^5-androstenediol and testosterone, and to a smaller extent, Δ^4-androstenedione were identified from precursor dihydroepiandrosterone. With mixed precursors, Δ^5-androstenediol and Δ^4-androstenedione there was greater conversion to testosterone from Δ^4-androstenedione. From mixed precursors, C^{14}-17-hydroxyprogesterone with tritiated 17-hydroxypregnenolone or C^{14}-pregnenolone with tritiated DHA or C^{14}-pregnenolone with tritiated 17-hydroxypregnenolone, there was a consistently greater tritium/C^{14} ratio in testosterone than in Δ^4-androstenedione. The radioactive intermediates in both Δ^4 and Δ^5 pathways were identified. It appears that DHA and 17-hydroxypregnenolone favor the Δ^5 pathway to testosterone more readily than does pregnenolone. Dr. Tominaga and I conducted experiments with adult human testis tissue in organ cultures for four days under hyperbaric oxygen, and have found that mitosis persists in the germinal epithelium and steroid biosynthesis continues or is even increased.

MANN: Among the interesting findings on which you reported, Dr. Steinberger, is the observation that organ cultures can maintain steroidogenesis during prolonged incubation periods, and as you quite rightly pointed out, that must mean that all the enzymes required for steroidogenesis have been preserved intact. However, you appear to be somewhat worried about the decreasing rates of steroidogenesis, particularly the rate of testosterone formation. I wonder if you are giving the best possible chance to all the enzymes to act under optimal conditions. Perhaps one might look into the possibility that, although the enzymes are peeserved excellently, the co-enzymes which they normally require have disappeared. I mean, for example, the diphosphopyridine nucleotide and the triphosphopyridine nucleotide. Would it not be worthwhile to look into the possibility that these co-enzymes are in fact, decreasing during incubation and, if so, one might perhaps add them to the organ cultures.

CHANDLEY: Dr. Steinberger, in your labelling studies, have you found any incorporation of tritiated thymidine during the leptotene/zygotene stage of meiosis? This has been claimed by Lima de Faria in human spermatocytes. This would mean looking at cells within one hour or half an hour of labelling, and seeing if there was any incorporation at this stage, in addition to the incorporation that is occurring at the premeiotic interphase or preleptotene stage.

A. STEINBERGER: We have not observed labelled leptotene or zygotene spermatocytes in sections of human testes following a short 40 minute pulse with ^{3}-H thymidine. The label was limited to the preleptotene stages. Similar results were obtained with other mammalian species as well.

CHAPTER IV

REGULATION OF TESTICULAR FUNCTION

SECTION 5: INFLUENCE OF GONADOTROPINS ON TESTICULAR FUNCTION

EFFECT OF GONADOTROPINS ON THE SEMINIFEROUS TUBULES OF THE IMMATURE TESTIS

M. Courot

I.N.R.A. - Station de Physiologie de la Reproduction,
37 - Nouzilly, France

INTRODUCTION

It is important first to define the "immature testis", at least with respect to the spermatogenetic function of the organ. We know that an "adult" or "mature" testis is that in which complete spermatogenesis occurs, with a satisfactory yield (although this may be related to the time of year or to the environment in which individuals are placed). This brings to light the characteristics of the immature testis; namely, a non-existent or incomplete spermatogenesis or a spermatogenesis not yet having attained normal cell yield. Thus there are several types of immature testes, depending on the degree of their spermatogenetic activity. A terminology has just been proposed (1) in which the following terms are used to describe the immature testis:

Impuberal testis type: the sex cords, future seminiferous tubules do not yet have a lumen and have no spermatogenetic activity. The germ cells present are gonocytes or stem spermatogonia; they divide by mitosis, but do not differentiate into primary spermatocytes. The somatic cells are Sertoli cell precursors, the supporting cells.

Prepuberal testis type: The germ cells evolve and different stages leading to the formation of the first spermatozoa may be observed as the Sertoli cells differentiate from the supporting cells. Puberty terminates this phase, i.e., the first spermatozoa are produced, but the testis is not yet mature because the cellular yield of the spermatogenetic process is very low.

Postpuberal testis type: during this stage, the cellular yield of the spermatogenetic processes increases, and the quantity of spermatozoa produced increases to become progressively comparable to that of the adult.

All of these stages constitute the immature phase of the testis, and we shall study the effect of gonadotropins on the immature seminiferous tubules thus defined. Since the literature available for the human generally concerns pathological cases in which organ receptivity may be changed, we shall also use the experimental results obtained on mammals for our analysis and then compare them to each other.

HYPOPHYSECTOMY

It is known that all stages of testis development, even the earliest ones, are regulated by the pituitary gland. After hypophysectomy, the weight of the testis in operated animals decreases in the impuberal (monkey (2); lamb (3)), prepuberal and postpuberal phases (rat (4)). Likewise, early pituitary imbalance of accidental or pathological origin prevents, or retards, testis development and onset of spermatogenesis in man (5-11). These effects concern both the germinal and endocrine testis functions, but we shall only discuss the former here. Hypophysectomy always involves a decrease in seminiferous tubule diameter, but its effect on the tubule cell population depends on the period in which it is performed.

In the impuberal period (Table 1) in the lamb, hypophysectomy mainly affects the somatic cells (supporting cells) which are the precursors of the Sertoli cells. Their number rapidly decreases (from day 5 onwards) and then remains relatively constant, the cell appearance remaining that of undifferentiated cells. On the other hand, germ cells seem less sensitive to pituitary endocrine regulation. Their number is unmodified by hypophysectomy, and it even continues to increase after the pituitary has been removed (Table 1), although less rapidly than in normal animals. However, the evolution of these cells is affected because they do not differentiate into primary spermatocytes (3). It is not possible to perform the equivalent experiment in man, but several pathological cases have been described. When the surgical operation is done at a young age, it prevents germ cell differentiation and spermatogenesis will not be established (11).

In the prepuberal period (Table 4); the number of Sertoli cells decreases in the rat testis following hypophysectomy. The somatic cells in the tubules are thus also under pituitary control, as they could be in the adult (8,12-14). The development of germ cells is greatly affected, the elongated spermatids disappear, the young spermatids quantitatively considerably decrease and in most instances are said to disappear. The number of primary spermatocytes also diminishes (only 12% of leptotene spermatocytes are formed in the

Table 1. Effect of Hypophysectomy on the Cellular Content of the Sex Cords in the Impuberal Lamb Testis.

	Initial	Delay After Surgery (days)				
	Control	3	6	15	30	250
No. of Animals	19	7	15	22	9	5
Testis Weight (g)	3.4+ (0.13)	2.9 (0.40)	2.3 (0.15)	1.9 (0.13)	1.9 (0.14)	2.1 (0.30)
Supporting Cells/ testis x 10^6	2540 (134)	2550 (333)	1930 (170)	1680 (147)	1540 (130)	1600 (252)
Spermatogonial Cells/ testis x 10^6	37 (35)	49 (72)	48 (3.3)	53 (6.0)	55 (5.0)	76 (18.0)

+ m ($\pm$ s_m) - 6 days and more after surgery, experimental data and initial control are significantly different ($P \leqslant 0.05$)

rat 48 days after hypophysectomy performed at 27 days). Nothing precise has been published on stem spermatogonia in the impuberal testis, but it may be that their number decreases as observed in the adult (13,15). This point should be carefully studied in the light of recent studies on stem spermatogonia (16) to determine if the renewing stem cells, A_1, and the reserve stem cells, A_0, are equally affected. Could there not be reserve stem cells not destroyed by hypophysectomy as is the case for the germ cells of the impuberal testis, the only affected cells being the renewing stem cells?

GONADOTROPIC SUPPLEMENTATION IN THE IMPUBERAL MALE

To our knowledge, only the monkey (2) and the lamb (3) have been the objects of analytical experiments on endocrine control of the impuberal testis, but since in the work on the monkey only slightly purified products were used, we will not present these results. In man, cases of impuberal testis have been studied in boys showing genital infantilism (5-10), treated after cranial surgery (11,17) or treated for unilateral cryptorchidism (11). In the last case, we shall limit the discussion to the normal testis.

In the lamb, spermatogenesis commences several months after birth thus leaving time for experimentation on a testis not yet presenting any spermatogenetic activity; a situation which does not exist in laboratory animals such as the rat or the mouse. Using hypophysectomized lambs, supplemented immediately after the surgical operation twice a day for 5 to 60 days,we have shown that ovine acetonic anterior pituitary powder helps in the maintenance of testis growth associated with the growth of the sex cords,with an effect on their diameter as well as on their somatic and germinal cell populations. Germ cells even differentiate into primary spermatocytes. However, it should be noted that there is a wide individual variability of response. In the most favorable cases, there is a strong stimulation with a high testicular weight increase and the establishment of spermatogenesis in the whole organ. Spermatids have even been obtained in the maturation phase, that is, in the ultimate phase of their formation in the seminiferous epithelium (3). In this case, cellular associations observed in the seminiferous epithelium resemble those described for the adult. This indicates that spermatogenesis takes place at the same rhythm as that in the normal individual. The constant speed of the spermatogenetic process has already been demonstrated in different conditions of hormonal balance (18, 19). In only one instance has this concept been questioned because of slight variations (20). The results obtained with impuberal testes are logical. There is no acceleration of spermatogenesis, but rather an early beginning of spermatogenetic activity due to pituitary hormones. Precocity and acceleration are two very different things, and only the first one may be obtained for spermatogenesis before it starts.

The search for active factors in the anterior pituitary preparation led to separate supplementation with ovine FSH or LH (ICSH) (Table 2). It was thus observed that LH has the most clearly measurable action on the testis of the hypophysectomized lamb, i.e. organ weight increase and enlargement of sex cord diameter. However, one of the two gonadotropins maintains the supporting cell reserve but the two hormones seemed separately to have no clear quantitative effect on the germ cells (same levels as the hypophysectomized controls, Table 2). Nevertheless, they also allowed the differentiation of some spermatogonial cells into primary spermatocytes as did the anterior pituitary powder but to a lesser degree. This important action of the two gonadotropins on the onset of spermatogenesis is less conspicuous than that related to the supporting cells. It is rather difficult to observe because it affects only a small number of cells in a way similar to that observed at the onset of normal spermatogenesis. When both hormones are administered simultaneously to the hypophysectomized lamb, there is a synergistic effect leading to a stronger testis response which resembles that obtained with anterior pituitary powder. This response concerns all criteria studied: organ weight, tubule diameter, and even germ cell reserve; which is significantly increased as spermatogenesis commences (Table 2).

Some cases of gonadotropic treatment in boys deprived of a functional pituitary gland have been reported in the literature (patient operated on for craniopharyngioma). A 3-month treatment of pure FSH, 3700 U 2nd IRP, does not seem to definitely stimulate the testis (17). On the other hand, testis stimulation is provoked by more complex supplementation with HMG, which has both FSH and LH activities, or with HCG (11). The Sertoli cells mature and spermatogenesis unobtrusively commences (shown by the presence of some

Table 2. Effect of Hormone Supplementation on the Hypophysectomized Lamb Testis.

Treatment and Dose (mg)	No. of Animals	Testis Weight (g)	Sex Cord Diameter (μ)	Supporting Cells/Testis x 10^6	Spermatogonial Cells/Testis x 10^6
FSH (4.5)[1,4]	4	2.9 ± 0.2[2]	39 ± 2.5	2570 ± 75[+]	65 ± 9 NS
LH (2.4)	3	3.8 ± 0.5	53 ± 0.7	2370 ± 350[+]	49 ± 12 NS
FSH + LH (4.5 + 2.4)	4	8.9 ± 0.6	64 ± 3.1	5465 ± 104[+]	91 ± 8 NS
LH + cyproterone acetate [4]	3	3.2 ± 0.2	52 ± 1.7	2010 ± 192[+]	44 ± 9 NS
Cyproterone acetate (20)	3	1.7 ± 0.2	31 ± 2.3	1200 ± 160	40 ± 5
Testosterone (3.75) [3]	7	2.2 ± 0.3	38 ± 1.4	1810 ± 220	55 ± 10
Initial Control	19	3.4 ± 0.1	49 ± 1.0	2540 ± 134	37 ± 4
Hypox. Control	22	1.9 ± 0.1	36 ± 0.6	1680 ± 147	53 ± 6

[1] Dose given twice a day for 15 days. FSH-CNRS-P 15 (1.06 FSH-NIH-S3) LH-CNRS-P8 (0.67 LH-NIH-S3).

[2] m(± s_m). The level of significance is determined in relation to the hypophysectomized control (NS, non-significant; + significant $P \leqslant 0.05$).

[3] Stronger doses have no greater effect.

[4] FSH and LH were kindly supplied by the Endocrinology Coordination Committee of the National Center for Scientific Research (CNRS), which is gratefully acknowledged. The author also wishes to thank Schering AG for supplying the Cyproterone acetate.

primary spermatocytes) in conditions somewhat similar to those reported in the hypophysectomized lamb with FSH or LH. However, these supplementations, even when given over a long period, do not establish complete spermatogenesis in these boys.

In the normal lamb, gonadotropins have the same effects on the impuberal testis as in the hypophysectomized animal, but stimulation is stronger, and FSH then becomes the most efficacious hormone, causing a higher testis response than that obtained with LH (21). The cause of this may be a synergy effect of the gonadotropins injected with those secreted by the animal's own pituitary gland under the effect of the treatment.

The impuberal testis of the normal boy responds to gonadotropic stimulation in the same manner. While the administration of HMG to unilaterally cryptorchidic boys may have no effect on the non-functioning testis, it does stimulate the scrotal testis. The latter presents "histological changes similar to those observed at approximately the second phase of normal puberty" (11). The diameter of the tubules increases, as does the number of their spermatogonial cells. Sertoli cell differentiation begins as well as that of the spermatogonia and primary spermatocytes at the pachytene stage. In boys with genital infantilism, the situation seems to be more complicated because one can obtain stimulation of the seminiferous tubule with HMG or HCG, the best results appearing with simultaneous administration of both hormones, but there are also some failures with these various treatments (5-10).

When the mechanism of action of FSH and LH is analyzed, it appears that the hormones probably have a direct effect on the sex cords of the impuberal testis (7) (Table 2). In the hypophysectomized lamb, FSH acts without stimulating the interstitial gland, for the accessory glands are umodified. LH action on the supporting cells is the result of direct hormonal action on these cells. It does not come from the increased testosterone secretion of the interstitial gland under the effect of the gonadotropin; even injecting a very strong dose of testosterone does not stimulate the supporting cells. Moreover, administering an antiandrogen (cyproterone acetate) simultaneously with LH does not significantly reduce gonadotropic effect on the supporting cells (21).

GONADOTROPIC SUPPLEMENTATION IN THE PREPUBERAL MALE

The prepuberal rat (often referred to as an immature, a juvenile or an impuberal animal) has been used in most studies analyzing the effects of gonadotropins on the testis during the establishment of spermatogenesis. Therefore, we shall take this animal as an example, comparing parallel results obtained in pathological human cases where spermatogenesis cannot progress to term. Ovine FSH stimulates development, or partially corrects post-operative testis regression without any accessory gland reaction in the prepuberal hypophysectomized rat (not older than 40 days), treated subcutaneously immediately, or after a given delay (Table 3) (22). On the other hand, even at a dose (8 μg/100 g body weight) twice that effective in the adult hypophysectomized rat, ovine LH does not either maintain nor restore the testis in the prepuberal hypophysectomized rat. The seminiferous tubules do not present an aspect different from that of the hypophysectomized controls for LH treatment, while with FSH there is stimulation

Table 3. Effect of Ovine FSH and LH on the Maintenance of the Genital Organ Weight in the Prepuberal Hypophysectomized Male Rat.

Treatment and Dose (μg/D)	No. of Animals	Testis Weight (mg)	Seminal Vesicles Weight (mg)
Initial Control	5	269 ± 10	16.1 ± 0.8
Terminal Control	5	589 ± 11	30.8 ± 3.5
Hypox. + Saline	4	67 ± 4	4.9 ± 0.3
Hypox. + FSH (15)	4	330 ± 36	6.3 ± 0.9
Hypox. + LH (5)	4	126 ± 6	10.8 ± 1.2
Hypox. + FSH + LH (15 + 5)	3	466 ± 42	13.2 ± 4.4

Hypophysectomy at 27 days - 12 day treatment with FSH-CNRS-M (5.86 FSH-NIH-S3) and LH-CNRS-M_1 (1.83 LH-NIH-S3).

From Ortavant, R., Courot, M. and de Reviers, M.M., In La Specificite Zoologique des Hormones Hypophysaires et leurs Activites, CNRS ed., Paris, p 369, 1968.

or partial restoration of spermatogenesis, which is less advanced than in the normal animal (Table 4). In cases of experimental or pathological imbalance, an appropriate hormonal supplementation should re-establish conditions in the environment which prevent partial cellular degeneration. This permits spermatogenetic evolution to proceed to term. Thus, when spermatogenesis is established, hormones do not accelerate the process, but prevent cellular degeneration.

Quantitative histological analysis of spermatogenesis shows that FSH acts particularly on the first part of the spermatogenetic cycle (Table 4). FSH permits a large restoration (about 2/3 of the normal control) of spermatogonial division and of meiotic prophase efficiency, at least until the pachytene stage. However, the following critical stages are only partially overcome by the administration of ovine FSH; the transition of primary spermatocytes from the pachytene to the diplotene stage (42 per 100 normal control for diplotene primary spermatocytes), and the maturation divisions (16 per 100 of normal control for young spermatids). After that, there are no longer enough cells to measure cellular yield accurately. It may be that the combined administration of FSH and LH helps to overcome the critical stages (analysis in progress) as it generally improves the spermatogenetic yield. We already know the synergic effect of the mixture of these two hormones on testis weight (Table 3).

Thus, the separate, subcutaneous administration of FSH or LH shows that FSH is the gonadotropic hormone having the most effect on

Table 4. Efficiency of Spermatogenesis in the Prepuberal Hypophysectomized Rat, Supplemented with FSH or LH after 24-day Post-Operative Regression (1).

Treatment (2)	No. of Rats	PRIMARY SPERMATOCYTES L*	P**	D†	SPERMATIDS Round	In Elongation	Elongated	Sertoli Cells
Terminal control (3)	4	9.0 (0.6)	8.5 (0.4)	8.5 (0.5)	35.8 (0.4)	46.8 (1.2)	31.9 (3.8)	115
Hypox.+ Saline (4)	4	12% (0.3)	3% (0.1)	1% (0.1)	<1% (0.1)	0	0	55%
Hypox. + FSH (4)	4.	61% (0.5)	62% (0.4)	42% (0.7)	16% (1.3)	5% (1.5)	<1% (0.2)	68%
Hypox.+ LH (4)	3	14% (0.3)	4% (0.1)	2% (0.1)	1% (0.2)	0	0	57%

(1) Adapted from Ortavant et al (14), 24-day treatment, (2): hormones and doses, see Table 3, L*: Leptot. , P**: Pacyht., D†: Diplot., (3): terminal control: results are expressed in daily production for germ cells (x 10^6), and in testis content for Sertoli cells (x 10^6). (4): treated animals: results are expressed in per 100 of the terminal control; ( ): s_m of the original value.

The leptotene primary spermatocytes permit the measurement of the overall yield of spermatogonial divisions. Note the lack of LH efficiency and the decrease of FSH efficiency with progression of spermatogenesis.

spermatogenesis in the prepuberal animal. This agrees with overall results reported in the literature (see review 20), in spite of some studies which seem to have contradictory conclusions, but in which the histological pictures appear to support the results reported here. It should be emphasized that only a correct, quantitative histological analysis gives objective and solid conclusions.

The results reported in men having incomplete spermatogenesis (who may be parallelled to the individuals with prepuberal testis) seem more complicated than those obtained in the rat. After treatment with HMG, complete spermatogenesis and viable sperm in post-treatment ejaculates have been obtained in patients with hypogonadism (9). Positive results of spermatogenesis stimulation have also been reported after treatments with HCG alone (6), especially if there is already a preexisting although small spermatogenetic activity. However, the best results are obtained after a combination of FSH and LH (5-8, 10,23).

A tentative explanation for the variability in the human results might be the existence of variable final FSH to LH ratios. An optimum might exist for the ratio but it is still disputed (24). In supplementation with exogenous hormones, this ratio has to be considered, taking into account the patient's own gonadotropic balance. One might also point out that in the human it could be a relationship between the physiological state of the testis and its responsiveness to gonadotropic treatment as is the case in the rat where the importance of age in relation to spermatogenetic response to gonadotropins has been demonstrated (22). After puberty and in the adult, the main hormone is LH whereas it is FSH in the prepuberal rat, this transition occurring during the post puberal period (22). Most often, this observation explains the various conclusions in the literature concerning endocrine control of spermatogenesis.

CONCLUSION

Thus, in addition to the information about the endocrine balance of the patient, a good knowledge of the state of the abnormal testis is necessary to propose an adapted treatment. However, it should be remembered that combined hormonal action always gives the best results, provided it is administered for an appropriate period of time. It is at present the most often proposed treatment for spermatogenetic accidents in man.

SUMMARY

This short analysis shows that testis seminiferous tubules are under early pituitary control, when there is still no spermatogenetic activity (impuberal testis). They respond to hypophysectomy or to gonadotropic supplementation. Pituitary LH or/and FSH is necessary to the onset of spermatogenesis (differentiation of spermatogonial cells). FSH appears to play a leading role in the prepuberal testis, while LH is the principal hormone after puberty, but there is always synergy between the two hormones. This article also emphasizes the importance of somatic cells in the seminiferous tubules and their dependence in relation to the pituitary hormones, either before (supporting cells) or after their differentiation (Sertoli cells).

ACKNOWLEDGMENT

This work was supported by the French National Institute for Agronomic Research (I.N.R.A.).

REFERENCES

1. Courot, M., Hochereau-de Reviers, M. T., Ortavant, R., In The Testis, Vol. I, Chap. 6, Eds. Johnson, A.D., Gomes, W.R., Van Demark, N. L., Academic Press (in press).

2. Smith, P.E., In Les Hormones Sexuelles, ed. Brouha, L., Hermann, Paris, p 201, 1938.
3. Courot, M., J. Reprod. Fertil., Suppl. 2: 89, 1967.
4. Ortavant, R., and Courot, M., Arch. Anat. Micr. Morph. Exp. (Paris), 56: (Suppl. 3-4) 111, 1967.
5. Heller, C. G. and Nelson, W. O., J. Clin. Endocr., 8: 345, 1948.
6. Paulsen, C.A. In Proc. 6th Pan Amer. Congress Endocrinol., Mexico City, 1965, Excerpta Medica Foundation ICS 112: 398, 1966.
7. Davies, A.G. and Crooke, A.C., Proc. Roy. Soc. Med. 58: 580, 1965.
8. Johnsen, S.G., Acta Endocr. (Kobenhavn), 53: 315, 1966.
9. Lunenfeld, B. In Recent Research on Gonadotrophic Hormones, Proceedings 5th Gonadotrophin Club Meeting, Edinburgh 1966, eds. Bell, E. T. and Loraine, J.A., E & S Livingstone Ltd., p 284, 1967.
10. Crooke, A.C., Davies, A.G. and Morris, R., J. Endocr., 42: 441, 1968.
11. Rosemberg, E., Mancini, R.E., Crigler, J.F. and Bergada, C. In Gonadotropins 1968, ed. Rosemberg, E., Geron-X, Inc., Los Altos, California, p 527, 1968.
12. Mancini, R.E., Seiguer, A.C. and Perez-Lloret, A., J. Clin. Endocr., 29: 467, 1969.
13. Courot, M. and Courte, M.T., unpublished data.
14. Ortavant, R., Courot, M. and de Reviers, M.M., to be published.
15. Clermont, Y. and Morgentaler, H., Endocrinology, 57: 369, 1955.
16. Clermont, Y. and Bustos-Obregon, E., Amer. J. Anat., 122: 237, 1968.
17. Mancini, R.E. In Gonadotropins 1968, ed. Rosemberg, E., Geron-X, Inc., Los Altos, California, p 541, 1968.
18. Desclin, J. and Ortavant, R., Ann. Biol. Anim. Biochim. Biophys., 3:329,1963.
19. Clermont, Y. and Harvey, C., Endocrinology, 76: 80, 1965.
20. Boccabella, A.V., J. Reprod. Fertil., Suppl. 2: 139, 1967.
21. Courot, M., to be published.
22. Ortavant, R., Courot, M. and de Reviers, M.M. In La Specificite Zoologique des Hormones Hypophysaires et leurs Activites, C.N.R.S. ed., Paris, p 369, 1968.
23. Heller, C.G., In Estrogen Assays in Clinical Medicine, ed. Paulsen, C.A., University of Washington Press, p 275, 1965.
24. Johnsen, S.G., Rosemberg, E., Lunenfeld, B., Crooke, A.C. In Recent Research on Gonadotrophic Hormones, Proceedings 5th Gonadotrophin Club Meeting, Edinburgh, 1966, eds. Bell, E.T. and Loraine, J.A., E & S Livingstone Ltd. p 301, 1967.

DISCUSSION

SOLARI: Dr. Courot, have you seen signs of nuclear differentiation in the pre-Sertoli cells of the immature testis after the injection of LH and FSH? In the human, the mature Sertoli cell has a nucleolus-chromatin complex which is very characteristic. In the mature Sertoli cells from mice, the nucleolus is flanked by two heteropyknotic, DNA-containing bodies. Are there similar structures in your material?

COUROT: I performed some observations with the electron microscope on the testes of impuberal lambs. It seems to me that in normal lambs, as well as in hypophysectomized animals, nucleoli with associated chromatin are present in the supporting cell nuclei; but I would say that in normal lambs it also appears that the endoplasmic reticulum with associated ribosomes is well developed. After hypophysectomy, what the most important fact seems to be is the disappearance of ribosomes along the endoplasmic reticulum, but as far as the nucleolus is concerned, the postulated changes are very difficult to observe. After supplementation with LH or FSH it seems that the first effects that could be observed concern the endoplasmic reticulum. But these are only preliminary results, this work being now in progress.

BERGADA: Dr. Courot, when you injected FSH and testosterone you did not obtain increases in testicular weight. Have you tried to implant testosterone in the testes simultaneously with FSH administration?

COUROT: No, I have not. Some results with injected exogenous testosterone were reported. I have tried implantation of testosterone crystals but not simultaneous implantation of crystals and injection of FSH.

LIPSETT: Dr. Courot, do you have information as to what sort of plasma testosterone level you achieved with the dose used or about the dose of testosterone with respect to the amount you think an adult ram would normally produce? In other words, were you giving a very large dose or a replacement dose?

COUROT: May I remind you that the animals I am talking about are lambs of 15 kg. body weight. I tested different doses of testosterone and the results presented here have been obtained with 7.5 mg. per day. We have chosen this dosage of testosterone according to the response of the sexual glands i.e. seminal vesicles, and it seems that it is a little too high because with this dose of testosterone we obtained seminal vesicle weights which are a little higher than those of normal animals. With respect to the tubular cell content, we tried a much higher dosage of testosterone, 120 mg. per day, and the effect on the tubules was not different from that obtained with the smaller dosage of 7.5 mg/day. This work is still in progress and I have as yet no results to present with respect to blood plasma concentration of testosterone. I recall that FSH plus testosterone does not parallel the results obtained with FSH plus LH on testis weight, tubular diameter and on the supporting cells. This can be interpreted as a direct effect of LH on this cell category.

A. STEINBERGER: Dr. Courot, could you tell us whether the Sertoli cells normally divide in lambs of the age that were used in these experiments or do they divide only following hypophysectomy and gonadotropin stimulation?

COUROT: Normally, in lambs, the supporting cells divide for a long time after the period at which I operated on the animals. In hypophysectomized animals, the total population of supporting cells decreases rapidly after pituitary removal and then remains at the same level for as long as 8 ½ months; some mitotic figures can be observed in the supporting cell population a long time after hypophysectomy. So it seems that the total population remains quite the same but with some slow replacement of cells.

E. STEINBERGER: What happens to the germinal epithelium in the ram after hypophysectomy? How much cyproterone did you administer and did you have any definite evidence that the cyproterone blocked testosterone at the germinal epithelium level?

COUROT: I have hypophysectomized adult rams and some animals have been maintained without gonadotropic supplementation for 120 days after surgery. In such animals I can observe some young round nuclear spermatids at a stage of evolution corresponding to the beginning of spermiogenesis, but in very very small number. Hence, in the adult hypophysectomized animal spermatogenesis seems to develop at a very low quantitative level until the formation of the young spermatids. This is in opposition to the young animals, where hypophysectomy performed before any spermatogenetic activity is observed prevents development of spermatogenesis. As regards your other question, in one experiment, I used 20 mg. per day and in a second experiment 40 mg. per day of cyproterone acetate in animals of 15 kg. body weight. Cyproterone acetate was injected intramuscularly twice a day. We obtained a complete inhibition of testosterone effect on the vesicles. We do not have to report relative to the effect of this compound at the tubular level.

VILAR: Dr. Courot, since when you talk about stimulation you show no increase in the number of Sertoli cells, could you explain what you mean when you refer to stimulation? What parameter did you use? Is it a kind of maturation of differentiation of the Sertoli cells as we see in the human?

COUROT: I have been wrong with the expression stimulation, because effectively when we compared results in animals supplemented immediately after surgery with those obtained in normal animals, we maintained the number of supporting cells at about the same level. The results were expressed as the total population of cells. We counted the number of cells per cross section of tubules and calculated the total population considering testis weight, diameter of tubules, and relative percentage of seminiferous tubules. I was then able to calculate the total population of supporting cells in the testis.

JUTISZ: Dr. Courot, you did not mention the dosage of FSH and LH used in your work or the ratio of the two hormones in the case of combined injections. I recall an old assay method for FSH in which the weight of the testis of hypophysectomized rats was used as a criterion. Your results show that FSH alone increases the weight of the testis to a very small extent and that there is a synergy between FSH and LH.

COUROT: I used preparations obtained from your laboratory. I adapted the dosage in order to give the equivalent of 10 mg. per animal per day of NIH FSH S1 and 2.5 mg. of NIH LH S1, either in separate or in simultaneous administration of the gonadotropins. The gonadotropins were injected subcutaneously twice a day, beginning immediately after hypophysectomy. With respect to the second question, I would say that the bioassay you referred to was developed on young rats. As you know young rats present a spermatogenetic activity while lambs have no spermatogenetic activity. These are two different physiological situations.

ULTRASTRUCTURAL AND CHEMICAL EFFECTS OF LH UPON THE SEMINIFEROUS TUBULE[1]

Mario H. Burgos, F. L. Sacerdote[2], R. Vitale-Calpe[3] and D. Bari[4]

The interstitial cells have been pinpointed as the only target of LH action on the testis. Greep and Fevold and Lacy et al. (1,2) suggest that any tubular action of this hormone is mediated through the androgen produced by the Leydig cells in response to LH. On the other hand, recent studies on the effect of associated gonadotropins (FSH and LH) have demonstrated that LH is necessary to maintain spermatogenesis (3-6) independently of the presence of androgens. The latter have been shown to inhibit this effect (7,4).

The evidence for a direct action of LH on the seminiferous tubules has received additional support from the comparative study done in our laboratory on the mechanism of spermiation in amphibia (8) and in mammals (9,10). In these studies we have shown that following endogenous or exogenous administration of LH the seminiferous tubule is able to change the ultrastructural characteristics of those Sertoli cells related to the last stages of spermatid differentiation and to induce the release of late spermatids into the tubular lumen. This mechanism of spermiation is characterized in amphibia and mammals by cytoplasmic swelling and vacuolization of the Sertoli cells followed by outburst of apical bubbles into the

---

1 This work was supported by grant M-63-121 from the Population Council, Inc.

2 Member Scientific Career Consejo Nacional de Investigaciones Cientificas y Tecnicas, Argentina.

3 Research Assistant Population Council, Inc. USA.

4 Member of Technician Career, Consejo Nacional de Investigaciones Cientificas y Technicas, Argentina.

tubular lumen, increase in testicular sodium and water content in amphibia (8) and by increase in testicular fluid as measured in the rete testis in mammals (11).

Since these observations indicated a new target of LH in competent Sertoli cells, and also on the basis of the marked swelling and vacuolization found in electron micrographs, we have assumed that an important portion of the testicular fluid increase evoked by LH should be located in the territory occupied by such Sertoli cells. Inasmuch as more than 80% of the testicular volume is occupied by seminiferous tubules and that approximately 1/4 of the total tubular mass belongs to the Sertoli cells associated with the late spermatids, we thought it of interest to study in testicular homogenates and cell fractions whether this movement of water is accompanied by changes in some enzyme activities. We therefore measured the response of the ATPases to LH. These are known to play a role both in fluid transport and in the energy cycle. We also investigated the effect of LH on mitochondrial respiration and determined whether this hormone acts directly on mitochondrial fluid content. Enzymatic study of testicular homogenates of toads, hamsters and mice showed that the ATPase activity decreased approximately 50% in response to a single dose of LH or to the secretion of endogenous LH during copulation. Similar results were obtained in the study of the oxygen consumption (10). Following this line of work we have studied the ultrastructural characteristics of the Sertoli cell-late spermatic association, the response to LH in the guinea pig and the enzymatic activity of cell fractions of rat testis after addition of LH.

METHODOLOGICAL CONSIDERATIONS

Electron microscopy: Adult male guinea pigs weighing approximately 400 g were distributed in two groups: (1) Controls: kept in cages, 2 or 3 per cage, separated from females; (2) Animals mated with females in estrus and killed one hour after the beginning of copulation.

The testes of Nembutal anesthetized animals were fixed by 5% glutaraldehyde in s-collidin buffer, according to the perfusion method of Aoki and Vitale-Calpe (12). The tissue was cut in thin slices, washed in buffer and refixed in cold 1.33% OsO_4 in s-collidin buffer with the addition of sucrose and calcium (13). Blocks dehydrated with acetone were embedded in Epon-Araldite (14). Thin sections were examined in a Siemens Elmiskop I after uranyl acetate and lead citrate stain (15). One-micron sections stained with toluidine blue were studied with the light microscope for orientation and photomicrography.

Chemical determinations: Adult male rats weighing approximately 250 g were decapitated and the testis homogenized in 0.44 M sucrose-EDTA (Fig. 1); the mitochondrial and microsomal pellets were used for

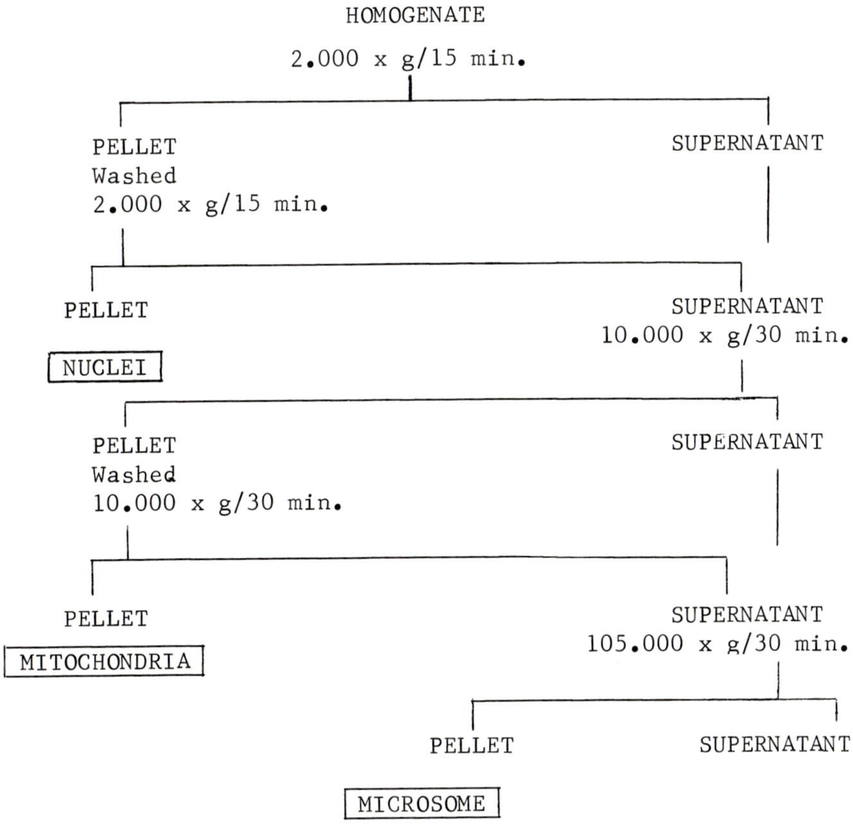

Fig. 1. Fractionation method of rat testis homogenized in 0.44 M sucrose-EDTA.

the enzyme measurements. Total ATPases were assayed in both pellets in a medium containing Na^+, K^+, Mg^{++} and Ca^{++} by measuring the liberated phosphorus (16) both in controls and in the presence of 50 or 100 μg/ml LH (Ovine LH, lot NIH-LH-S-12 was kindly supplied by the Endocrinology Study Section of the National Institutes of Health.)

Respiration of mitochondria in succinate was measured polarographically in a Gilson model KM oxygraph according to the method of Stoppani and Vallejos (17) with and without LH, 50 μg and 100 μg per ml of substrate.

The optical densities of mitochondrial suspensions in 0.25 M sucrose were read over 30 min. in a Beckman DU spectrophotometer at 520 mμ after the addition of LH (100 μg/ml) and after the addition of a well-known mitochondrial swelling agent such as 3 x 10^{-3}M phlorizin (18).

In some preliminary experiments 0.1 ml serum obtained from control or copulating rats was added to the substrate for ATPases and to the substrate for respiratory enzymes and its effect assayed by the above mentioned methods in the presence of testicular mitochondria or microsomes.

RESULTS

Ultrastructure of Sertoli Cell-Late Spermatid Association in the Guinea Pig

1) Control group. As described in the hamster only the last stage of the Sertoli cell-late spermatid association presents the characteristics of spontaneous spermiation. This is stage number 7 in the guinea pig and corresponds to number 8 in the hamster. The main characteristics of this stage are the focal swelling of the apical endoplasmic reticulum, the concomitant release of late spermatids and the retention of the residual bodies (Fig. 2).

2) Experimental group (one hour after starting copulation). It has been shown in the rat (19) and in the hamster (20) that copulation is associated with a marked secretion of pituitary LH. The Sertoli cells related to the stages V, VI and VII (Fig. 3) show a marked swelling of the apical cytoplasmic matrix, associated with vacuolization and distension of the apical endoplasmic reticulum. The apical recesses become erased and the spermatids are released together with the residual bodies. Large bubbles expel into the lumen a fluid which helps the spermatids move toward the rete testis (Fig. 4). We have measured in the hamster rete testis the increase in fluid coming from the testis in response to intravenous injection of LH (11).

Biochemical Observations

<u>Optical density of mitochondria.</u> The addition of LH (100 μg/ml) to a mitochondrial suspension produces a significant decrease in optical density in less than 10 minutes (Fig. 5) which continues for 20 minutes. This effect is comparable to the mitochondrial swelling produced by 3×10^{-3}M phlorizin.

<u>ATPase activity.</u> The addition of 50 μg/ml or 100 μg/ml LH to the substrate in the presence of isolated testicular mitochondria increases ATPase activity by approximately 25% or 35% respectively; the addition of LH inactivated by boiling for 10 minutes in a water bath causes no increase (Fig. 6). Experimental serum as compared to control serum also increases mitochondrial ATPase activity by 25%.

On the other hand, microsomal ATPase activity shows a moderate depression after 100 μg/ml of LH (Fig.6) .

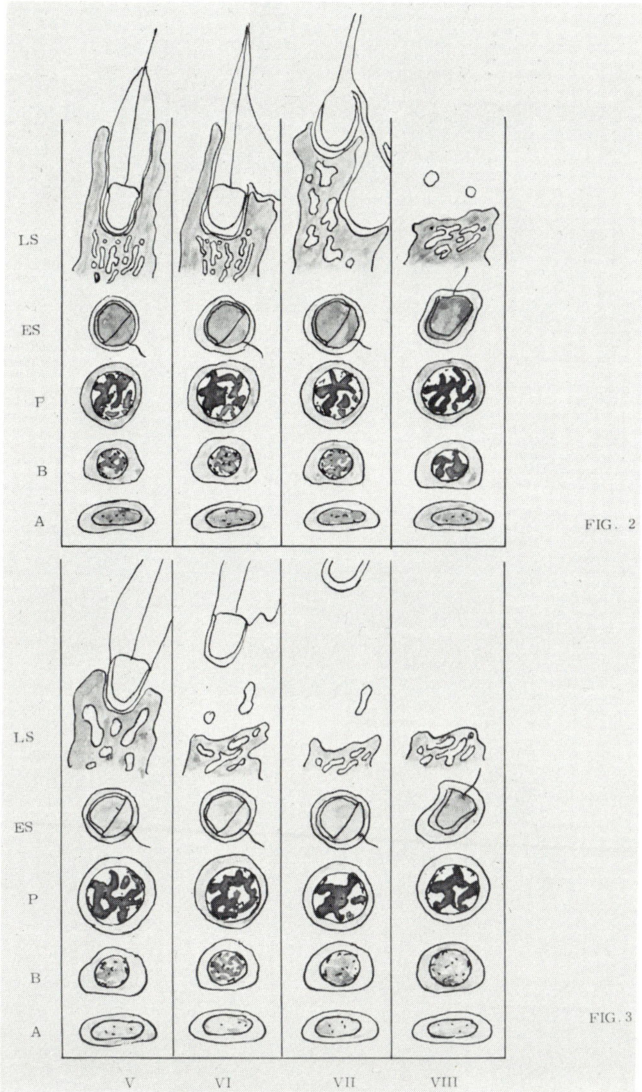

Figs. 2 and 3. Schematic representation of stages 5 to 8 of guinea pig spermatogenesis. Fig. 2 shows the spontaneous spermiation of stage 7 with the retention of the residual body and release of the spermatid . Fig. 3 shows the post-coital spermiation, with release of spermatids in stages 5,6 and 7 without retention of residual bodies. In both figures the apical cytoplasm of the Sertoli cells (in grey) shows swelling and vacuolization during spermiation of late spermatids (LS). The other cell types are: A spermatogonium A; B spermatogonium B; P - primary spermatocyte, pachytene; ES-early spermatid.

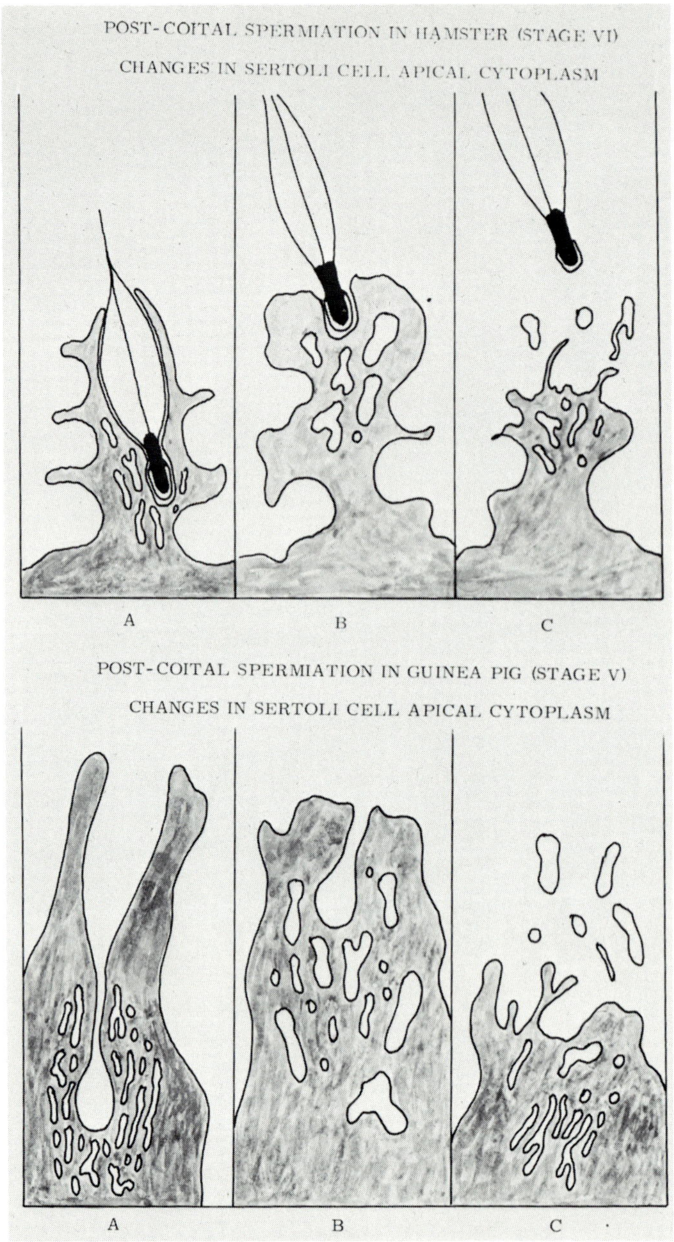

Fig. 4. Schematic representation of post-coital spermiation in the hamster (stage VI) and in the guinea pig (stage V). A shows the beginning, B the middle and C the end of the mechanism of spermiation. The apical recesses become erased by swelling of the cytoplasmic matrix and endoplasmic reticulum, and late spermatids together with the residual bodies are released.

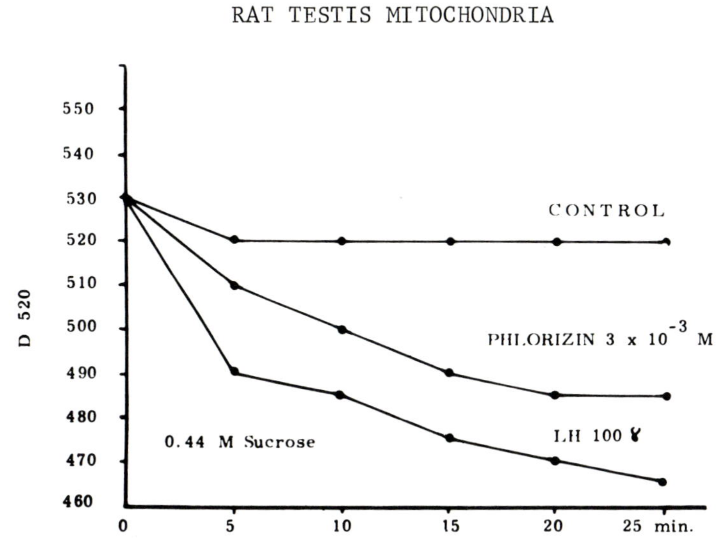

Fig. 5. Optical density of a mitochondrial suspension. It shows the mitochondrial swelling produced by addition of LH or phlorizin.

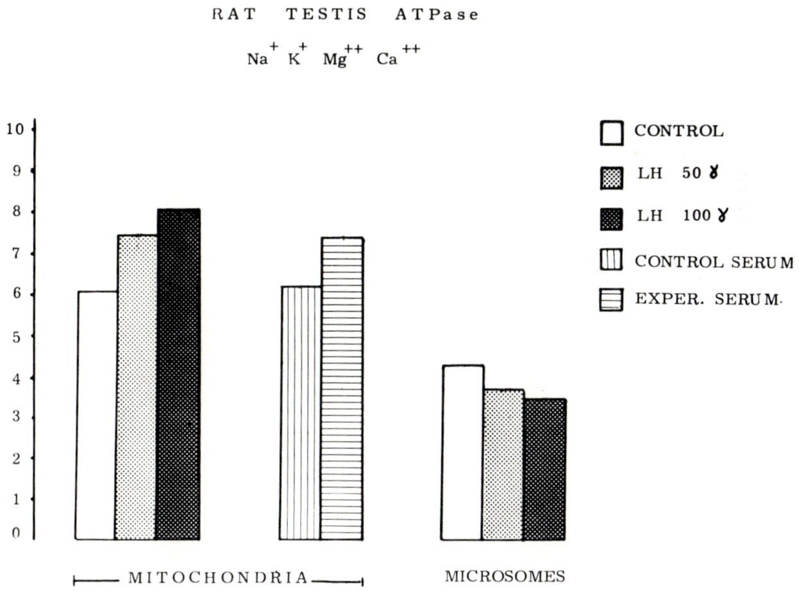

Fig. 6. A typical experiment in isolated mitochondria shows the increase in ATPase activity after addition of LH or post-coital serum. Isolated microsomes show a moderate depression after LH.

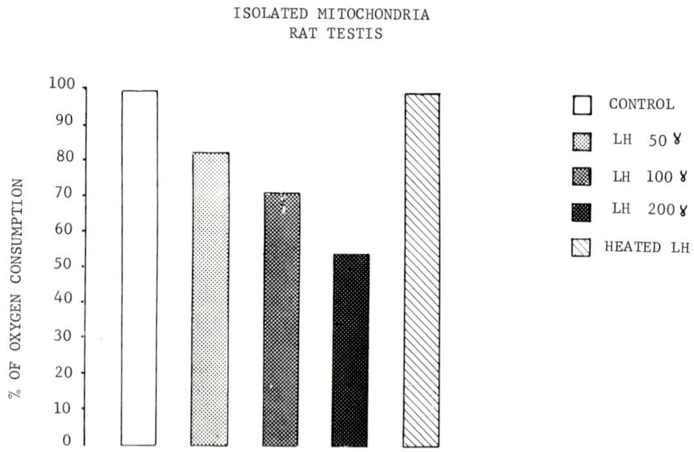

Fig. 7. A typical experiment on oxygen consumption. Mitochondrial respiration is markedly depressed after 200 μg LH. A similar dose of heated LH produces no effect.

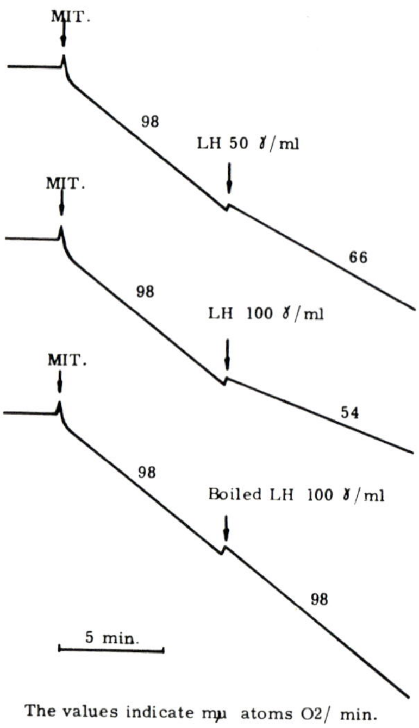

Fig. 8. Polarographic record of the respiratory response of isolated mitochondria in succinate substrate, after the addition of LH.

Oxygen consumption. The addition of LH to the succinate substrate decreases mitochondrial respiration by about 25% (Figs. 7 and 8).

The mitochondrial and microsomal fractions were always checked in the electron microscope and were consistently free of contamination by microsomes and mitochondria, respectively.

DISCUSSION AND CONCLUSIONS

Post-coital changes in the seminiferous tubules of the guinea pig are comparable to those already described in the hamster (9). In the guinea pig from stages V to VII, the apical conglomerate of smooth endoplasmic reticulum of the Sertoli cells swells markedly and forms large vacuoles and dilated cisternae. The rest of the tubule shows no significant changes. The present observations therefore offer additional evidence in favor of our hypothesis that the Sertoli cell-late spermatid association is a target of LH action on the tubule. More specifically, the target is the apical cytoplasm of those competent Sertoli cells.

The enzymatic mechanisms involved in such action remain obscure but some evidence has been presented that the sodium pump (Na^+ dependent ATPase) is related to the LH action and to the swelling of the Sertoli cells (10).

Experiments with total homogenates (10) showed that the activity of Na^+ dependent ATPase is blocked by LH approximately 50%. The results presented in this report prove that the microsome fraction is also depressed, but to a much lesser extent than the total homogenate. This may indicate that most of the LH sensitive ATPase is located in the cell membrane fraction (first pellet). On the other hand, the mitochondria, which only contribute 10% of the total ATPase activity of testis homogenates, contain an ATPase which is significantly stimulated by LH.

Isolated testis mitochondria swell in the presence of LH. This phenomenon is associated with an increase in fluid uptake and with a fall in mitochondrial ATP concentration. The fact that in the work reported here LH inhibits respiration and at the same time stimulates ATPase activity agrees perfectly with the mitochondrial swelling after LH. Other hormones have been also found to produce mitochondrial swelling (oxytocin, vasopressin,insulin, thyroxine,21).

In conclusion, the ATPase sensitive to LH is mainly related to the cell membrane fraction.LH is able to induce mitochondrial swelling directly.

Both effects can help the understanding of the testicular fluid increase evoked by LH in mammals.

REFERENCES

1. Greep, R.O. and Fevold, H.L. Endocrinology, 21: 611, 1937.
2. Lacy, D., Vinson, G.P., Collins, P., Bell, J., Fyson, P., Pudney, J. and Pettitt, A.J., Proc. 3rd Int. Congress Endoc., Mexico, Excerpta Med. Found., 1019, 1969.
3. Lostroh, A.J. Endocrinology, 85: 438, 1969.
4. Heller, C. G., Lalli, M.F. and Rowley, M.J., Ciba Found. Colloq. on Endocr., 16: 1967.
5. Courot, M., J. Reprod. Fertil., Suppl. 2: 89, 1967.
6. Mancini, R. E., Seiguer, A. C. and Perez Lloret, A., In Gonadotropins 1968, ed. Rosemberg, E., Geron-X, Inc., Los Altos, California, p 503, 1968.
7. Rosemberg, E., Mancini, R.E., Crigler, J. F. and Bergada, C. In Gonadotropins 1968, ed. Rosemberg, E., Geron-X, Inc. Los Altos, California, p 527, 1968.
8. Burgos, M.H. and Vitale-Calpe, R., Amer. J. Anat., 120: 227, 1967.
9. Vitale-Calpe, R. and Burgos, M.H., J. Ultrastruct. Res., 1969 (in press).
10. Burgos, M.H., Vitale-Calpe, R. and Russo, J., In Gonadotropins 1968, ed. Rosemberg, E., Geron-X, Inc., Los Altos, California, p 213, 1968.
11. Burgos, M.H., Vitale-Calpe, R., Proc. 3rd Int. Congress Endoc., Mexico, Excerpta Med. Found., 1030, 1969.
12. Aoki, A. and Vitale-Calpe, R., personal communication, 1969.
13. Burgos, M.H., Vitale-Calpe, R. and Tellez De Inon, M.T., J. Microsc., 6: 457, 1967.
14. Mollenhauer, H., Stain Techn., 39: 111, 1964.
15. Reynolds, E'S., J. Cell Biol., 17: 208, 1963.
16. Fiske, Ch.H. and Subbarow, H., J. Biol. Chem., 66: 375, 1925.
17. Stoppani, A.O.M. and Vallejos, R.H., Arch. Biochem. 117: 573, 1966.
18. Burgos, M.H., Aoki, A. and Sacerdote, F.L., J. Cell Biol., 23: 207, 1964.
19. Taleisnik, S., Caligaris, L. and Astrada, J., J. Endocr. 79: 125, 1966.
20. Donoso, A.O. and Santolaya, R.C., Acta Physiol. Lat. Amer., 19: 70, 1969.
21. Lehninger, A.L., The Mitochondrion, Benjamin, New York, 1964.

DISCUSSION

JOHNSEN: Dr. Burgos, Dr. Mancini showed that whereas FSH enters the tubule, LH does not.

BURGOS: When we inject LH, there are changes in the later stages of spermatids associated with Sertoli cells.

CLERMONT: Dr. Burgos, you are probably aware that, in recent studies by Dr. Fawcett, he does not observe any vacuolization or any loss of cytoplasm at the time of spermiation. Secondly, in our own laboratory we have never succeeded in provoking premature release of spermatozoa from the seminiferous epithelium of hypophysectomized or normal rats injected with various hormones. In your electron microscopic study, have you observed any sign of premature maturation of spermatids in your LH-injected animals?

BURGOS: I am aware of the work of Dr. Fawcett on spontaneous release of spermatids at stage 8 in the guinea pig. I think that, in his preparations, there is some swelling of the cytoplasmic projections of the Sertoli cells. However, we work at much earlier stages. We have studied testicular preparations between 30 minutes and one hour after copulation or after injection of the hormone, and we never have found release of any other type of cell apart from late spermatids.

BIOLOGIC EFFECT OF HUMAN PITUITARY LUTEINIZING HORMONE AND HUMAN CHORIONIC GONADOTROPIN

E. Rosemberg, J. F. Crigler, Jr., W. F. Jan, G. Bulat, R. Nakano and S. G. Lee

Medical Research Institute of Worcester, Inc., Worcester City Hospital, Worcester, Massachusetts and The Harvard Medical School, Boston, Massachusetts

Bioassay [ovarian ascorbic acid depletion (OAAD) and ventral prostate weight (VPW) assays] and radioimmunoassay of Human Pituitary Luteinizing Hormone (HLH) and of Human Chorionic Gonadotropin (HCG) indicate differences in biologic activity and immunologic reactivity of these preparations. Information concerning the comparative effect of these gonadotropin materials in the human testes is meager. Hence, it was decided to conduct acute studies with HLH and HCG in four normal adult male volunteers, and in two adolescent male subjects with immature testes.

MATERIAL AND METHODS

The preparations used in this study were a commercial preparation of HCG (Follutein, Squibb) with an activity of 10,000 IU HCG per vial (biologic potency) and a purified HLH preparation supplied by the National Pituitary Agency (Lot A1, LER 856-1) with an LH activity of 200 IU 2nd IRP per vial; the FSH contamination was 2.5 IU 2nd IRP per vial (biologic potency).

ASSAYS

Plasma testosterone levels were determined by the competitive protein binding assay (1). The LH activity in plasma was determined using the double antibody radioimmunoassay described by Odell et al. (2). All samples from an individual subject were assayed in the same assay at two dose levels. The reference materials used in all assays were: LER 907 (distributed by the NPA, USA); the Second International Reference Preparation for Human Menopausal Gonadotropin (2nd IRP); LER 856-1, and HCG Second International Standard (2nd IS).

All reference preparations were tested at four dose levels. Radioimmunoassay results were calculated by appropriate computer programs for parallel line assays. In our assay system, the immunoreactivity of 1 milli International Unit (mIU) of biological activity of the 2nd IRP is equivalent to that of 3.2 ng of LER 907, 0.63 ng of LER 856-1, and 0.28 mIU of biological activity of HCG-2nd IS; 10.6 mIU of biological activity of HCG-2nd IS is equivalent to that of 1 μg of LER 907. In this discussion all concentrations will be expressed in terms of μg of LER 907 per milliliter of plasma.

SUBJECTS

Four normal male volunteers of ages ranging from 26 to 35 years, and two sexually immature male patients were selected for these studies. The first patient (P.R.), aged 16 years, presented bilateral undescended testes at birth. At adolescence, he became concerned about the lack of sexual development and was referred at age 13 7/12 years to the Childrens Hospital Medical Center, Boston for evaluation. His height and bone age corresponded to a chronological age of 13 years, and his weight was 108.2 lbs. Lack of sexual development was observed i.e., the penis was small with a stretched length of 5.3 cm and a diameter of 1.4 cm and the testes were not felt in the scrotal region or in the inguinal canal. Axillary and pubic hair were absent. Bilateral orchidopexy was performed at age 14. The testicular biopsy obtained at that time revealed the presence of small tubules with arrest of spermatogenesis at the spermatocyte stage, presence of immature Sertoli cells, and absence of Leydig cells. Prior to the present studies the patient was never treated with gonadotropin preparations.

The second patient (J.K.) age 18 6/12 years, was referred to the Childrens Hospital Medical Center at 8 years of age because of short stature. On examination, his height age was 4 6/12 years, his bone age 3 2/12 years, his weight 40.2 lbs. and his genitalia were normal for his age. The usual laboratory procedures revealed deficiences in GH, TSH and ACTH and a diagnosis of idiopathic hypopituitarism was made. The patient was treated with l-thyroxine (T_4), 0.1 to 0.15 mg per day from age 10 3/12 years to age 11 9/12 years. At 13 years of age, the patient was treated with human growth hormone (2 mg q.o.d.); T_4 was re-started while on growth hormone at age 15 3/12 years. Both medications were given continuously until the time of the present studies. At 18 years of age, the patient did not show secondary sexual development. On examination, the testes measured 3.8 x 2 cm, the phallus measured 5.3 x 1.8 cm, and axillary and pubic hair were absent. A testicular biopsy performed at 18 years of age revealed the presence of small tubules without a lumen, arrest of spermatogenesis at the spermatocyte stage, immature Sertoli cells, some thickening of the tubular wall and a diminished number of Leydig cells. Prior to the present studies, the patient was never treated with gonadotropin preparations.

EFFECT OF HLH IN NORMAL MALE SUBJECTS

This study was designed to determine the effect of a single dose administration of HLH. Each of the four subjects received a dose of 2,000 IU HLH given intramuscularly at 9:00 a.m. Blood samples were drawn prior to HLH administration and at intervals of 15'; 45'; 75'; 2 hr 15'; 3 hr 15'; 4 hr 15'; 5 hr 15'; 6 hr 15'; 24; 28 and 31 hours following HLH administration.

Fig. 1 depicts the LH concentration in plasma and the plasma testosterone levels after a single dose of 2,000 IU HLH (IM) on each of the four subjects.

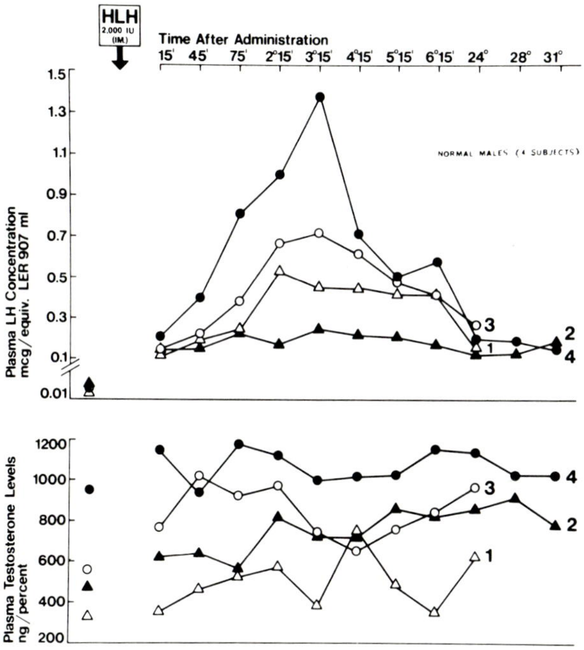

Fig. 1. Plasma LH concentration and plasma testosterone levels after a single dose administration of 2,000 IU HLH to four normal male subjects.

Plasma LH concentration increased to 3 to 6 times the control levels in all subjects 15 minutes after HLH administration. Except for one (subject 2), who did not show significant changes in LH concentration throughout the period of observation, all other subjects showed maximum plasma LH concentration (22 to 40 times control values) 3 hours and 15 minutes after HLH administration. The concentration of LH in plasma remained above control levels (3 to 9-fold) in all subjects 24 hours after HLH administration and 3 to 5 times control values in two subjects (subjects 2 and 4), 31 hours after HLH administration. Testosterone levels, although remaining above control levels throughout the period of observation, varied from subject to subject. However, all subjects showed increased testosterone levels 24 hours after HLH administration. Testosterone levels in two subjects (subjects 2 and 4) were above control levels 28 and 31 hours after HLH administration, respectively.

Fig. 2 depicts the mean increase in plasma LH concentration, and the mean percent increase in testosterone levels in the four subjects studied.

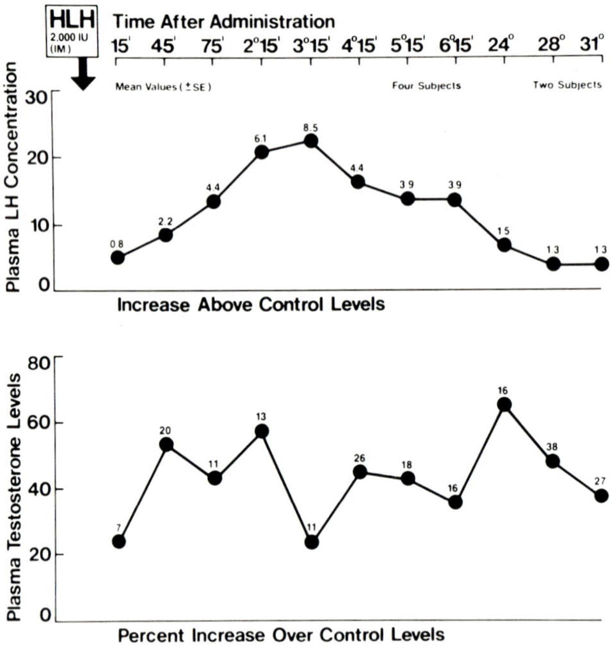

Fig. 2. Mean values (four subjects). Plasma LH concentration and plasma testosterone levels after a single dose administration of 2,000 IU HLH.

Maximum plasma LH concentration was observed 3 hours and 15 minutes after HLH administration. The LH concentration declined steadily throughout the period of observation. However, LH levels in all subjects were 6 times the control values 24 hours after HLH administration. In two subjects LH levels showed a 4-fold increase compared with control levels 28 and 31 hours after HLH administration. Testosterone levels were increased 15 minutes after HLH administration, and remained elevated (65% above control), 24 hours after HLH administration. In two subjects (2 and 4) testosterone levels were 90.6 and 5.4% above control, and 66.4 and 5.5% above control 24 and 21 hours after HLH administration, respectively.

EFFECT OF HLH AND HCG IN THE IMMATURE TESTIS

Patients P.R. and J.K. received four identical courses of medication. During the first course, 5,000 IU of HCG was given as a single intramuscular injection each day for three consecutive days; during the second course, 5,000 IU of HLH was given intramuscularly in three divided doses each day for three consecutive days; during the third course HLH was administered using the dosage and mode of administration used in the second course. During the fourth course HCG was administered using the dosage and mode of administration used in the first course. Each course of medication was separated by an interval of two to four weeks. Blood samples were drawn three times daily at 8:30 a.m., 2:30 p.m. and 8:30 p.m., the day prior to initiation of medication, during medication days and for two days after cessation of therapy. A final blood sample was obtained at 8:30 a.m. on the third day after withdrawal of medication.

Fig. 3 shows the plasma gonadotropin concentration and testosterone levels observed during each of the four courses of medication given to patient P.R. There was no significant variation between samples in a 24 hour period. Hence mean values for a 24 hour period for both plasma gonadotropin concentration and testosterone levels will be reported in the present discussion (Patients P.R. and J.K.)

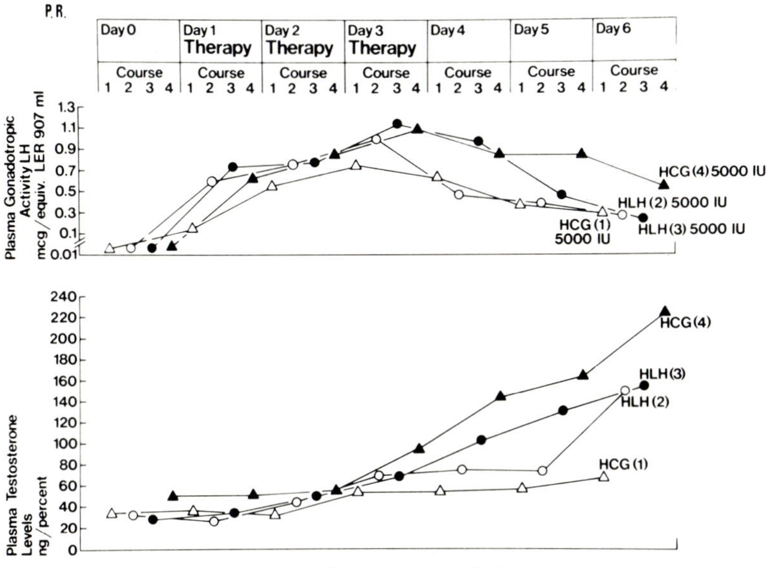

Fig. 3. Patient P.R. Plasma gonadotropic activity (LH) and plasma testosterone levels during four courses of medication with HCG, HLH, HLH and HCG, respectively.

During each of the four courses of therapy, plasma gonadotropin concentration increased to 11 to 37 times the control levels on the first day of therapy; 16 to 43 times on the second day of therapy; 18 to 47 times and 10 to 28 times on the first and second day after withdrawal of medication, respectively. Plasma gonadotropin concentrations remained elevated (6 to 20-fold) on the morning of the third day after cessation of therapy. Plasma testosterone levels were not significantly elevated until the first day after cessation of therapy (courses 2, 3 and 4). Increased testosterone levels were observed on the second day after withdrawal of medication (courses 2, 3 and 4) and on the morning of the third day after cessation of medication (all courses).

It should be remembered that this patient exhibited undescended testes until age 14, at which time the testicular biopsy revealed absence of Leydig cells. Hence, it is important to note that two years after orchidopexy, successive courses of medication steadily increased the response of the Leydig cells to gonadotropin stimulation.

Fig. 4 depicts the plasma gonadotropin concentration and testosterone levels observed during each of the four courses of medication given to patient J.K.

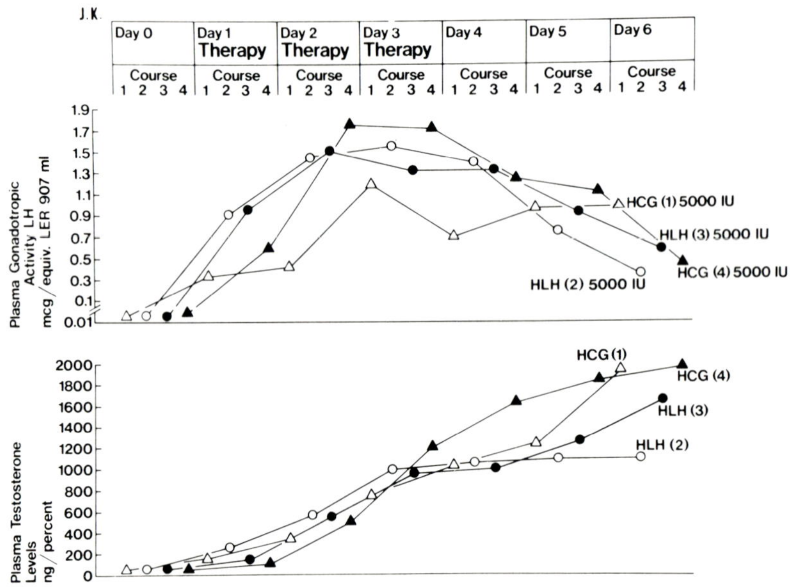

Fig. 4. Patient J.K. Plasma gonadotropic activity (LH) and plasma testosterone levels during four courses of medication with HCG, HLH, HLH and HCG, respectively.

Plasma gonadotropin concentration increased in a manner similar to that observed in patient P.R. The response to gonadotropin administration as judged by the plasma testosterone levels was quite striking. During each of the four courses of medication, testosterone levels were significantly increased (10 to 18%) over control levels on the second day of therapy. Plasma testosterone concentration increased steadily thereafter: 25 to 38% on the second day of therapy, 28 to 52% and 29 to 63% on the first and second day after cessation of medication. Testosterone levels were still elevated (29 to 99%) on the morning of the third day after withdrawal of medication.

COMMENTS

The data suggest that both HLH and HCG at the dosage given induced stimulation of the Leydig cells in two subjects with immature testes. Increased testosterone levels were observed in both subjects and were maintained 60 hours after the last HLH injection and 72 hours after the last HCG injection. However, the magnitude of the increase in plasma testosterone levels differed in each subject. The difference in response could be attributed to differences in the functional state of the end organ in each individual patient, and also to the fact that patient J.K. had received growth hormone medication for over three years prior to and throughout the course of the present studies. The possibility exists, therefore, that human growth hormone may exert a stimulatory action on the testis complementing that of HLH. In both patients, successive courses of medication steadily increased the response of the Leydig cells to gonadotropin stimulation.

The pattern of gonadotropin concentration in plasma during the four courses of medication given was similar in both subjects. The slow disappearance of plasma immunoreactive gonadotropin (HLH and HCG) was coupled with a steady increase in testosterone levels after withdrawal of both hormones. It could be postulated, therefore, that the immunoreactive circulating gonadotropins exerted a prolonged biologic effect on the Leydig cells.

Our studies showed that in normal subjects, plasma levels of immunoreactive HLH remained above control levels 31 hours after the administration of 2,000 IU of HLH given as a single intramuscular dose. Testosterone levels were also increased over control levels 31 hours after HLH administration.

The disappearance rate of endogenous or of exogenously administered gonadotropins has been studied in the human by several investigators. These data are summarized in Table 1.

Table 1

DISAPPEARANCE RATE OF ENDOGENOUS AND EXOGENOUS GONADOTROPINS

Material	ENDOGENOUS	EXOGENOUS Mode of Administration	t 1/2	METHOD	Investigator
HLH		iv	1 hr	Bioassay	Parlow (1965, Ref 3)
		iv	1.16 hr	RIA	Schalch et al. (1968, Ref 4)
		iv	30-60' (initial component)	RIA	Kohler et al. (1968, Ref 5)
	After hypox.	-	21' (initial component) 3.9 hr (second component)	RIA	Yen et al. (1968, Ref 6)
HFSH		iv	3 hr	Bioassay	Parlow (1965, Ref 3)
	After hypox.	-	3.9 hr (initial component) 70.4 hr (second component)	RIA	Yen et al. (1970, Ref 7)
HCG		iv	8 hr	Bioassay	Parlow (1965, Ref 3)
		iv	5.1- 5.6 hr (initial component) 23.6-23.9 hr (second component)	RIA	Rizallah et al. (1969, Ref 8)
		iv	8 hr	RIA	Wide et al. (1968, Ref 9)
	After delivery	-	11 hr (initial component) 23 hr (second component)	RIA	Yen et al. (1968, Ref 6)
	After delivery	-	8.9 hr (initial component) 37.3 hr (second component)	RIA	Midgley-Jaffe (1968, Ref 10)
		IM (10,000 IU)	32 hr	RIA	Midgley-Jaffe (1968, Ref 10)
		IM (10,000 IU)	30.1 hr (maximum at 6 hr)	RIA	Rizallah et al. (1969, Ref 8)

The studies utilizing the i.v. infusion of a tracer dose of hormone indicate that the half life ($t\frac{1}{2}$) of HLH is approximately 1 hour, that of HFSH (human follicle stimulating hormone) is approximately 3 hours, and that the $t\frac{1}{2}$ of HCG shows a fast and slow component of approximately 5 and 23 hours, respectively. The study of the disappearance rate of endogenous gonadotropins indicates that the $t\frac{1}{2}$ of HLH has a fast and slow component of 21 minutes and 3.9 hours, respectively, and the $t\frac{1}{2}$ of HFSH has a fast and slow component of 3.9 and 70.4 hours, respectively. The $t\frac{1}{2}$ of HCG has a fast and a slow component of 8 to 11 hours and 23 to 37.3 hours, respectively. The calculations of metabolic clearance rates (MCR) (5 and 8) of HLH and HCG indicate that the MCR of HCG is approximately 1/10 that of HLH.

Because of the apparent difference in the metabolism of these hormones it was of interest to note that the only two reported studies on the disappearance rate of intramuscularly administered HCG showed a disappearance rate of approximately 30 hours, which is similar to that observed in the present studies after a single intramuscular dose of HLH. The slow release of HLH and HCG into the circulation could provide an explanation for these findings. The only support for this explanation could be found in experiments (11) in which the kinetics of HCG-^{131}I adsorption after intramuscular injection were studied, showing that 50% of the radioactivity disappeared from the injection site in 110 minutes, while 10% remained in the site of injection six hours after the HCG-^{131}I administration. However, it remains to be shown that the kinetics of HLH-^{131}I adsorption after intramuscular injection are similar to that of HCG.

ACKNOWLEDGEMENTS

This work was supported by Grants AM-07564 and RR 00128, USPHS, National Institutes of Health, Bethesda, Maryland, and by a Grant from the Theodore Schulze Foundation, New York, New York.

We are indebted to the National Institutes of Arthritis and Metabolic Diseases, NIH, and to the National Pituitary Agency, Baltimore, Maryland for the supply of immunologic reagents and the supply of HLH and HGH used in this study. We wish to thank Dr. E. C. Reifentstein, Jr., the Squibb Institute for Medical Research, New Brunswick, New Jersey for the gift of Follutein (human chorionic gonadotropin), and Dr. D. R. Bangham, Department of Biological Standards, Medical Research Council, Mill Hill, London for the gift of HCG 2nd IS and the 2nd IRP.

REFERENCES

1. Mayes, D. and Nugent, C. A., J. Clin. Endocr., 28: 1169, 1969.
2. Odell, W. D., Ross, G. T. and Rayford, P. L., J. Clin. Invest., 46: 248, 1967.

3. Parlow, A.F., Recent Progr. Hormone Res., 21: 201, 1965 (Discussion).
4. Schalch, D.S., Parlow, A.F., Boon, R.C. and Reichlin, S., J. Clin. Invest., 47: 665, 1968.
5. Kohler, P.O., Ross, G.T. and Odell, W.D., J. Clin. Invest., 47: 38, 1968.
6. Yen, S.S.C., Llerena, O., Little, B. and Pearson, O.H., J. Clin. Endocr., 28: 1763, 1968.
7. Yen, S.S.C., Llerena, L.A., Pearson, O. H., and Littell, A.S., J. Clin. Endocr., 30: 325, 1970.
8. Rizkallah, T., Gurpide, E. and Vande Wiele, R.L., J. Clin. Endocr., 29: 92, 1969.
9. Wide, L., Johannisson, E., Tillinger, K.-G., and Diczfalusy, E., Acta Endocr. (Kobenhavn), 59: 579, 1968.
10. Midgley, A.R. and Jaffe , R. B., J. Clin. Endocr., 28: 1712, 1968.
11. Parker, M.L., Utiger, R.D. and Daughaday, W.H., J. Clin. Invest., 41: 262, 1962.

DISCUSSION

TROEN: Dr. Rosemberg, do you have comparable data on the pattern of the blood levels of FSH after intramuscular injection of HMG or HFSH?

ROSEMBERG: No, we do not.

PAULSEN: We have studied a normal male who received an intramuscular injection of 450 IU of FSH and 450 IU of LH. Serum LH was increased significantly two hours after injection. Within twenty-four hours, the serum LH levels had returned to control levels. However, the FSH levels remained elevated at 24 hours. These data agree in general with information obtained by Dr. Ross's laboratory. They demonstrated that the metabolic clearance rate for LH is essentially twice that observed for FSH.

ROSEMBERG: Dr. Paulsen, you realize that the amount of LH given contained in the HMG administered was only 450 IU. We administered 2000 IU. If pituitary LH (HLH) and urinary LH follow the same metabolic pathway, then, after a single injection of a much higher dose of HLH, circulating levels of HLH will remain elevated 24 hours after the administration of HLH. We have to bear in mind the dose and type of hormone being given.

PAULSEN: Yes, I agree. I will show you later this morning data which indicate that the pituitary HLH at a maximum dose of 400 IU is cleared fairly rapidly.

ROSS: I have no data on the disappearance from plasma when Pergonal is given intravenously to the human subject. However in validating the use of iodinated human pituitary extract LH preparations as a tracer in our studies of metabolic clearance rates, we examined the disappearance of this radioactively labelled tracer material and of Pergonal given intravenously simultaneously to rhesus monkeys. We showed essentially identical kinetics of disappearance of the radioactively labelled human pituitary extract and the LH component of Pergonal.

SAVARD: I believe there are two lines of thought running through our discussion. One is the fate of the gonadotropin as it circulates peripherally. The other is the fate of the gonadotropin as it sits in the binding sites of the target cells. Are these one and the same thing? I do not believe so. I believe that it is possible to have all kinds of peripheral changes in concentration, clearance, and so forth; while all target cells are very happily saturated with molecules of the tropic hormone. It seems to me that once above a critical plàsma concentration, most variations are of little consequence to the target cell. I think that, in attempting to relate gonadotropin to cellular function, we must look to the half-life of the gonadotropin at the cell site. This is no easy problem at the present time.

LUNENFELD: In answer to Dr. Savard, Mrs. Eshkol and myself have actually tested this problem; we tested the pattern of HCG exchange between the ovaries and the circulation in mice. Four phases of HCG uptake in the ovary were identified: a) during the first hour only inflow of HCG was detected, b) between 60 and 90 minutes inflow from the circulation was greater than the outflow from the ovary to the circulation, c) between 90 and 180 minutes inflow was equal to outflow and in the fourth phase between 3 and 6 hours the outflow was greater than the inflow. I think it is these kind of experiments which could answer the questions which you have asked. (Eshkol, A . and Lunenfeld, B., In Gonadotropins, 1968, p 188).

BERGADA: Dr. Rosemberg, I was very enthusiastic about the results of plasma testosterone on your two patients, in whom testosterone levels increase after treatment with HCG. In our experience, before puberty, we have not seen this result. In one case, after five days of 5,000 IU of HCG daily, plasma testosterone rose and came down on the third day after HCG was discontinued. In some patients treated for five days with HCG followed by 1,000 units weekly, after one or two months the testosterone level was less than after the acute HCG test. I wonder whether the testis before puberty responds, as far as steroid synthesis is concerned, equally as well as after puberty. I am referring to the testis of a 7- or 8-year-old boy as opposed to that of a 16- or 17-year-old boy with or without pituitary function.

ROSEMBERG: In our cases, we know that the patients did see endogenous gonadotropins; they had measurable levels prior to administration.

This means that, although histological evidence indicated that Leydig cells were absent or immature, the testis, however, had been exposed to some gonadotropin stimulation. Both responded to medication. One responded better than the other. This is the patient receiving growth hormone throughout these studies. We cannot state that a prepubertal testis has never seen gonadotropin. Dr. Ross is here to testify that there is measurable gonadotropin in prepubertal children. So, I really do not have an explanation for your findings.

BERGADA: With regard to the human growth hormone administration together with HCG, we have experience with three patients: one with a congenital idiopathic hypopituitarism and two with organic lesions. We administered HCG during a period of three or four months, and did not obtain any androgen response. In idiopathic congenital hypopituitarism, when we added human growth hormone to HCG we obtained development of secondary sexual characteristics.

ROSEMBERG: It is possible then to conceive that growth hormone acts synergistically with LH on the Leydig cells.

DICZFALUSY: I have a question and a comment, Dr. Rosemberg. Is there any information available on the amount of LH which is excreted in the urine following a single injection? We have estimated both by bioassay and by radioimmunoassay the amount excreted in the urine and it was around 20% with both methods. Actually, the half-life time was between 8 and 11 hours. The results of bioassays and radioimmunoassays showed a close agreement.

ROSEMBERG: We are in the process of completing all the urinary studies on the LH excretion after administration of LH.

OHNO: If the patient himself was making the mutant FSH or LH, the normal FSH or LH would serve as an antigen and he would start making the antibodies against it. Have you had any cases where patients started making the antibodies against the injected LH or FSH?

ROSEMBERG: We did not study this problem.

THE EFFECT OF GONADOTROPINS ON THE PREPUBERTAL TESTIS

Cesar Bergada

Servicio de Endocrinologia, Hospital de Ninos, Buenos Aires, Argentina

The response of the infantile testis to the exogenous administration of gonadotropins has been occasionally studied in detail in the human (1-6) as it is reported as a functional test in isolated cases. This is understandable as there is no justification for the administration of gonadotropins to a child unless it is necessary to study testicular function in cases with a probable diagnosis of primary hypogonadism, abnormality of sexual differentiation (6-8), or in the presence of bilateral or unilateral cryptorchidism (1,6, 7,9). This latter condition has been considered as the ideal situation in which to study the effect of gonadotropins on the prepubertal testis and its capacity to secrete testosterone and differentiate the germinal epithelium. These studies not only increase understanding of the role of different gonadotropins in testicular maturation but also permit investigation into the pathogenesis and behavior of some diseases before puberty; such as cryptorchidism associated with primary or secondary hypogonadism, Klinefelter's syndrome, congenital or acquired hypopituitarism, delayed or precocious puberty, male pseudohermaphroditism, etc.

Before discussing the effect of gonadotropins in children, it is necessary to review briefly normal differentiation of the human testis and its relation to sexual development.

During early embryonic life, at approximately the sixth week, the gonad in the male begins its differentiation into the testis (10,11). The interstitial cells of the primitive gonad reveal marked 3 β-ol-dehydrogenase enzymatic activity suggesting steroid synthesis (12-15), and simultaneously the embryonic cords, composed of primitive coelomic cells and primary gonocytes, differentiate into seminiferous tubules. At the same time, testicular hormones induce masculinization of the wolffian ducts and external genitalia. All these changes occur at the time of maximal development of Leydig cells thereby demonstrating their active participation in the development and differentiation of the testis and genitalia which terminates at approximately the fourth to fifth month of pregnancy. From this time on, the number of Leydig cells decreases but some remain until a few weeks after birth when the stimulus of the chorionic gonadotropin disappears (16). During infancy and childhood the interstitial tissue is composed only of fibroblasts and for this reason the endocrine function of the testis remains apparently inactive during this period. The urinary excretion of testosterone glucuronide remains very low before puberty, approximately from 5 to 11 μg/24 hrs. with no difference observed between boys and girls (17-20). Plasma testosterone concentration has been recently determined by several authors with somewhat similar results. Frasier and Horton (21) postulate that testosterone production in children of either sex is low and plasma concentration prior to the onset of puberty is not dependent either on age or sex; their values being of 42$\pm$ 9 mμg/100 ml. in prepubertal children. Saez and Bertrand (22) obtained values of 31.8 $\pm$ 10 mμg/100 ml in normal boys aged from two to thirteen years. August et al. (23) obtained 18 mμg/100 ml. with a range between 10 and 75 mμg for boys between one and twelve years. More recently, Rivarola et al. (24) determined plasma testosterone levels by a competitive protein binding method in children between four and eight years and obtained values of 21.8 $\pm$ 28 mμg/100 ml and in boys aged between nine and 12 years the levels were 73.4 $\pm$ 44 mμg/100 ml.

With regard to the seminiferous tubules, after the complete differentiation of the testis they increase their size and at birth reach a diameter of approximately 50μ. After birth, no important changes are observed until puberty when hypophyseal gonadotropins induce their development and stimulate the germinal epithelium (25). During this prepubertal period, the tubules are composed of sustentacular cells, precursors of Sertoli cells, and germ cells. The nuclei and cytoplasm of these spermatogonia acquire different aspects during fetal and postnatal life receiving different names by some investigators (1,25-29) who attributed this to different stages of cell activity. Two different types of Sertoli cells have also been demonstrated by Johnsen (30). The significance of this is at present difficult to explain. At approximately five to six years of age, a tubular lumen appears without significant changes in the germinal or Sertoli cells. Although this spermatogonial activity is not really marked and no variation in the tubular diameter is observed before puberty, whether or not the small amount of circulating gonadotropins detected during infancy and childhood could be responsible for this cellular process remains to be clarified. Both LH and FSH have been detected in the urine of prepubertal children either by biological or radioimmunological assays (31-34). Simultaneously several authors measured these gonadotropins in the plasma of children by radioimmunoassay (35-41). Most of these investigators gave similar results for LH plasma levels ranging between 1.5 and 15 mIU/ml in boys and girls under eight years of age. Yen et al. (40) reports higher amounts for girls than boys after age eight. FSH was found in much higher amounts than was LH (37,41).

As a consequence of the lack of change in the size of the seminiferous tubules and the inactivity of the fibroblasts of the interstitial tissue, the size of the testes do not vary much from infancy to puberty. At this time, and before any other sexual or somatic signs appear, the testes increase their volume which coincides with the rise of plasma and urinary gonadotropins and testosterone, and usually precedes the growth spurt. Tanner clinically classified the sexual development of boys in five stages (42): Stage 1: preadolescent: testes, scrotum and penis are about same size and shape as in early childhood. Stage 2: testicular enlargement begins with some scrotal changes. Stage 3: penis is slightly enlarged, testes and scrotum are further enlarged and pubic hair appears. Stage 4: penis, testes and scrotum are further enlarged and sexual hair is now adult in type but its area is still considerably smaller than in the adult. Stage 5: the genitalia and sexual hair are adult in size and shape. Johnsen (43) mentioned that he found the first appearance of gonadotropins in the urine of boys two and a half years before their change of voice. He also pointed out that growth of the testes comes first, followed by signs of androgen activity. Hudson et al. (44) demonstrated a significant rise in plasma testosterone levels about six months to one year prior to the beginning of sexual maturation. On the other hand, Albert (45,46), in testes obtained at autopsy, observed that the seminiferous tubules develop before Leydig cell maturation. Mancini et al. (16,47) pointed out that the first change observed in the testis is an active proliferation of the interstitial fibroblasts, precursors of Leydig cells, and then enlargement of the seminiferous tubules occurs followed by maturation of the germinal epithelium and appearance of mature Leydig cells. In a study of the urinary excretion of gonadotropins, Rifkind et al. (32) observed that during childhood the testis is exposed to some FSH stimulation. At puberty both FSH and LH increase significantly, stimulating the seminiferous tubules and the interstitial cells, respectively. More recently Yen et al. (41), studying plasma gonadotropins by radioimmunoassay, detected a progressive rise in LH and FSH concentration as sexual maturity was reached. The rise in LH was more marked than in FSH. Therefore in boys he found that the FSH:LH ratio decreases around puberty from 9 to 2 accompanied by a progressive rise in plasma testosterone. Raiti et al. (34) have recently correlated the plasma and urinary FSH determined by radioimmunoassay with the clinical stages of sexual development mentioned by Tanner (42). In the urine of preadolescent boys at Stage 1, they found 2.2 IU of 2nd IRP-HMG $\pm$ 1S.D. 1.1 IU/24 hr. In Stage 2, when testicular enlargement begins, the level was 4.4 $\pm$ 2.5 IU/24 hr and in Stage 3, with sexual hair and penis enlargement it was 7.1 $\pm$ 3.0 IU/24 hr.

On the basis of all these findings we may conclude that growth of the seminiferous tubules, stimulated by FSH which causes the increase in the size of the testis, takes place before complete maturation of the interstitial cells, induced by LH, and before full androgen development occurs.

Administration of gonadotropins to prepubertal boys would permit evaluation of the response capacity of an immature testis in order to appreciate more specifically the role of FSH and LH on the seminiferous tubules and interstitial cells not previously exposed to gonadotropic stimulation.

THE EFFECT OF HUMAN CHORIONIC GONADOTROPIN (HCG) ON THE PREPUBERTAL TESTIS

Treatment of cryptorchidism with HCG has been widely used and in the experience of more than 1500 patients treated in the Department of Endocrinology of the Hospital de Ninos of Buenos Aires, 30 to 40% of the cases with unilateral or bilateral cryptorchidism were cured with gonadotropin therapy. This is in accordance with data reported in the literature. Clinical, endocrinological and histological studies of the testes which did not descend with this treatment and underwent surgery, were considered an ideal situation in which to evaluate the effect of different gonadotropins on the immature testis.

Intramuscular administration of HCG at a dose of 1,000 to 1,500 IU weekly provokes, at any age, clinical signs of androgen activity, such as congestion of the scrotum and penis and erections, after the first or second week of treatment. This reaction is considered a good sign to be taken into account when HCG is given to a boy with no palpable testes since the lack of any response would suggest an anorchidism (6-8). This effect demonstrates that the interstitial cells are able to respond before puberty despite the age of the child (1-7).

In 1967 Lipsett (48) observed that very young children are able to increase their testosterone following HCG administration. Saez and Bertrand (22) gave 1,500 IU of HCG every two days for 15 days to 16 children aged from two to thirteen years, and the plasma testosterone level increased from 31.8 ± 10 to 554 ± 121 mμ g/100 ml. More recently Rivarola et al. (24) measured plasma testosterone in 18 boys with cryptorchidism aged from four to twelve years before and after daily injections of 800 to 5,000 IU of HCG for only five days. From control values of 26.3 ± 27 mμg/100 ml., the testosterone rose to 378.9 ± 188 mμg/100 ml. (range: 84-678). Some children under six years of age reached values above 500 mμg/100 ml. with only 800 IU daily for five days. The same study performed in boys with clinical signs of androgen activity such as slight testicular enlargement or scanty pubic hair, revealed higher testosterone levels in the basal state and a more marked response to HCG was observed in some patients.

Intramuscular administration of HCG for evaluation of plasma testosterone response should be given daily or every other day due to the short life of this gonadotropin. Rizkallah et al. (49) gave 10,000 IU of HCG i.m. in a single injection and obtained a maximal plasma concentration of this gonadotropin, 2,000 IU/ml, at 6 hr. The half-life of the tail part of the curve was approximately 30 hr. in their experiments. When 5,000 IU was injected daily for four days, a maximal plasma concentration of HCG was noted each day, six hours after injection. The values achieved ranged from 1200 to 1800 IU/ml.

Microscopic examination of the interstitial tissue of the testes treated with short term HCG therapy, despite the androgen signs, did not demonstrate full maturation of the Leydig cells, suggesting that the precursor cells may be able to synthesize steroids (50). Histological studies performed in the scrotal testes of patients with unilateral cryptorchidism treated with a prolonged series of gonadotropins were selected to evaluate the effect of these hormones in the normal immature testis (51). Administration of HCG (Elea Laboratories, Buenos Aires) to children between six and nine years of age at a dose of 1,000 to 1,500 IU weekly for periods ranging from three to six months, produced marked stimulation of the interstitial tissue with development of immature and mature Leydig cells. Tubular diameter was markedly increased to 70 or 90 μ. The normal median for these ages is 53 μ. Thickness of the tubular wall was not observed even in a case treated for six months. Germinal epithelium was also markedly stimulated up to the appearance of primary spermatocytes, being more marked with the more prolonged treatment. The same occurred with the Sertoli cells. Cytochemical and cytoenzymatic studies revealed an increase in the enzymatic activity of the interstitial cells, more marked in the scrotal than in the cryptorchidal testes (52). The clinical signs of androgen activity observed were congestion of the skin of the scrotum and penis, and erections. No sexual hair appeared during or after treatment.

THE EFFECT OF PREGNANT MARE SERUM GONADOTROPIN (PMS) IN THE PREPUBERTAL TESTIS

This preparation has seldom been used in children with cryptorchidism because it primarily exerts an FSH activity which does not induce testicular descent. For this reason PMS is not indicated in the treatment of cryptorchidism. We had the opportunity to study three boys aged between six and nine years with unilateral cryptorchidism associated with visible hernia in whom surgical procedure was indicated (51). PMS (Elea Laboratories, Buenos Aires) was given in daily or weekly injections in total doses ranging between 7,500 and 28,000 IU over 15 to 60 days. Absolutely no clinical signs of androgen activity were observed. Microscopic examination of the testes revealed a slight increase in tubular diameter, up to 77 μ in one case. Germinal epithelium was also slightly stimulated as well as the Sertoli cells. In the nine year old patient treated for 60 days some spermatocytes were observed. A very small effect was seen in the interstitial cells. Appearance of anti-PMS in the serum of these patients was not investigated.

EFFECT OF HCG PLUS PMS IN PREPUBERTAL TESTIS

Combined administration of both HCG and PMS provoked greater effects than HCG alone (51). Five patients from six to nine years of age were treated for one to six months with total doses of FSH between 1,254 and 2,508 IU of 2nd IRP-HMG and of LH between 6,520 and 19,308 IU. The FSH and LH activity of the HCG used was checked using the augmentation test and ascorbic acid depletion technique. One IU of HCG contains 0.001 IU of FSH and 0.924 IU of LH (53). The FSH:LH ratio was completely different with higher amounts of LH. The FSH:LH ratio of 1:8 employed in three patients produced more changes than ratios with less amounts of LH. Marked stimulation of the Leydig cells, increased tubular diameter and marked stimulus of the Sertoli cells and germinal epithelium up to spermatocytes were seen. These changes were more marked when both gonadotropins were administered simultaneously instead of subsequently. Again no thickness or hyalinization of the tubular wall was observed. Clinical signs were identical to the cases treated with HCG alone.

EFFECT OF HUMAN MENOPAUSAL GONADOTROPIN (HMG) IN PREPUBERTAL TESTIS

With the results previously mentioned, it was decided to employ a preparation with both FSH and LH activity. In 1968, Rosemberg et al.(54) reported the effect of Pergonal with different FSH:LH ratios in four boys with unilateral cryptorchidism aged six to seven years who were treated for periods ranging from 16 to 75 days. FSH:LH ratios varied from 1.2 : 1 to 2 : 1. Stimulation of the interstitial cells was observed, but more marked changes were seen at the seminiferous tubules. Tubular diameter increase up to 90 μ and meiotic spermatocytes reaching the pachytene stage were observed even in the case treated for only 16 days. Since treatment was prolonged in the longest case to two and a half months, it was questioned whether the dose or duration of treatment was not sufficient to bring about full spermatogenesis.

EFFECT OF HMG PLUS HCG IN THE PREPUBERTAL TESTIS

Several authors have reported better results in restoring spermatogenesis with the combination of HMG and HCG (55,53). In order to induce a greater stimulation of the testes in children with cryptorchidism, administration of both gonadotropin preparations with varied FSH:LH ratios was performed in seven children with unilateral undescended testis aged from six to nine years (51). Treatment lasted from three and a half to eight months. Patients received doses of FSH from 3,100 to 8,400 IU of 2nd IRP-HMG and of LH from 14,200 to 43,400 IU with FSH:LH ratios between 1 : 5 and 1 : 25. The interstitial tissue showed marked stimulation with development of mature Leydig cells comparable to adult testes. Tubular diameter was markedly increased up to 110 μ and active development of the tubular wall was observed without signs of hyalinization. Germinal epithelium showed more marked stimulation than with previous treatments, as far as spermatogonia and spermatocytes are concerned, since full spermatogenesis was not obtained in any case. Some spermatids were occasionally seen in the patient who received the highest dose of LH (43,380 IU) with 1,800 IU of FSH (FSH:LH ratio of 1 : 25) and who was treated for a period of six months. Another patient treated for eight months with 37,968 IU of LH and 8,432 IU of FSH, with a ratio of approximately 1 : 5, showed very marked stimulation of the interstitial cells and germinal epithelium although spermatogenesis was only developed up to the spermatocytes. Plasma testosterone was markedly increased after several months on treatment in accordance with the stimulation of the Leydig cells, although the level reached was not so high as the values obtained during the acute test of gonadotropin stimulation. In the two patients mentioned above, plasma testosterone reached values of 450 and 620 mμg/100 ml. respectively.

CONCLUSIONS

Administration of gonadotropins to prepubertal boys induced changes in their testes which confirm previous concepts that FSH stimulates the germinal epithelium and LH stimulates the interstitial cells. However, the response capacity of these two structures in the prepubertal testis varied greatly with that of the pubertal or adult testis.

These investigations have determined that the inactive fibroblasts of the interstitial tissue of the prepubertal testis are capable of synthesizing testosterone within 48 to 72 hours after the administration of daily injections of HCG, with a 15 to 20-fold increase in plasma testosterone levels (22,24) even before they differentiate completely to mature Leydig cells. At the onset of puberty, when endogenous LH begins to increase and stimulates these cells, testosterone production also increases and the exogenous administration of HCG produces more marked response in plasma testosterone. In both instances mature Leydig cells and adult levels of plasma testosterone could be induced.

The seminiferous tubules do not respond in the same manner. These studies have determined that combined administration of small amounts of FSH and LH are able to produce changes in the size of the tubules and initiate spermatogenesis. However, in all our studies performed in normal prepubertal boys using different ratios of FSH and LH for prolonged periods of time up to eight months, full spermatogenesis was not induced. It appears that the germinal epithelium may be stimulated up to first meiotic division very easily, but despite the dose of gonadotropin employed or the duration of treatment, it was impossible to stimulate the spermatogenic process any further. In only one case (51) a few spermatids were observed with 43,380 IU of LH and 1,800 IU of FSH over six months. Perhaps the ideal FSH:LH ratio has not been found, but it seems that the prepubertal testis should acquire some sort of maturation associated with adequate steroid synthesis and be stimulated by a proper FSH:LH ratio in order to develop full spermatogenesis. Data reported here suggest that in the immature human testis small amounts of FSH would first stimulate the seminiferous tubules with minimal steroid function of the interstitial tissue, and then, gradual increase of both FSH and LH with predominance of LH would produce active stimulation of the Leydig cells whose steroids will contribute to complete spermatogenesis (already stimulated by FSH) from meiotic spermatocyte up to spermatozoa.

Finally, it should be pointed out that in studies performed in a group of adult men who were treated for cryptorchidism during their childhood (56), all the patients with unilateral cryptorchidism who received treatment with HCG and surgery with testicular biopsy are fertile.

ACKNOWLEDGEMENT

This work was performed in part with grants from the Fundacion de Endocrinologia Infantil and from Consejo Nacional de Investigaciones Cientificas y Tecnicas, Buenos Aires, Argentina.

REFERENCES

1. Charny, C.W. and Wolgin, W. In Cryptorchidism, Hoeber-Harper, New York, p 80, 1957.
2. Loras, B., Ollagon, C. and Bertrand, J., Pediatrics 21: 455, 1966.
3. Paulsen, C.A., In Endocrinology, ed. Williams R.H., W. B. Saunders Co., p 441, 1968.
4. Folk, R.L., Taulor, J.N., Sotos, J.F., Vorys, N. and Wieland, R. G., Amer. J. Med. Sci., 225: 221, 1968.
5. Mancini, R.E., Cullen, M., Andrada, J.A., Vilar, O., Lavieri, J. C. and Saraceni, D.J., V Panamer. Congress of Endocrinology, Lima, 1961, p 150 (Abstract).
6. Bergada, C., In Genital Anomalies, eds Nabil Rashad, M and Morton, W.R.M., Charles C. Thomas, Springfield, Ill. p 591, 1969.
7. Cullen, M., Bergada, C., Mora, H. and Soubie, C., Rev. Argent. Endocrinol., Suppl. 1: 70, 1957.
8. Bergada, C., Cleveland, W.W., Jones, H.W., Jr. and Wilkins L., Acta Endocr. (Kobenhavn) 40: 493, 1962.

9. Bongiovanni, A.M., Pediatrics, 36: 786, 1965.
10. Witschi, E., Carnegie Inst. Wash. Publ. 209, Contrib. to Embryol., 32: 67, 1948.
11. Gillman, J., Carnegie Inst. Wash.Publ. 209. Contrib. to Embryol., 32: 81, 1948.
12. Bloch, E., Tissenbaum, B., and Benirschke, K., Biophys.Acta 60 182, 1962.
13. Baillee, A.H., Niemi, M. and Ikonen, M.,Acta Endocr. (Kobenhavn) 48: 429, 1965.
14. Goldman, A.S., Yakovac, W.C. and Bongiovanni, A.M., J. Clin. Endocr., 26: 14, 1966.
15. Schlegel. R.J., Farias, E.,Russo, N.C., Moore, J.R. and Gardner, L.I., Endocrinology, 81: 565, 1967.
16. Mancini, R.E., Vilar, O., Lavieri, J. C., Andrada, J. A. and Heinrich, J.J., Amer. J. Anat., 112: 203, 1963.
17. Rosner, J.M., Conte, N.F., Briggs, J.H., Chao, D.Y., Sudman, E. M. and Forsham, P.H., J. Clin. Endocr., 25: 95, 1965.
18. Vermeulen, A., In Androgens , Vermeulen, A. and Exlev, D., eds. Excerpta Med. Found. Amsterdam, 1966.
19. Knorr, D., Acta Endocr. (Kobenhavn) 54: 457, 1967.
20. Gupta, D and Butler, H., Steroids, 14: 343, 1969.
21. Frasier, S.D. and Horton, R., Steroids, 8: 777, 1966.
22. Saez, J.M. and Bertrand, J.,Steroids, 12: 749, 1968.
23. August, G.P., Tkachuk, M. and Grumback, M.M., J. Clin. Endocr., 29: 891, 1969.
24. Rivarola, M.A., Bergada, C., and Cullen, M., IX Meeting of the Latinoamerican Society for Pediatric Research, Valdivia, Chile, 1969, J. Pediatrics (in press) (Abstract) 1970.
25. Albert, A., In Sex and Internal Secretions 3rd Ed. Williams and Wilkins, Baltimore, p 305, 1961.
26. Evertt, N.B., Biol. Rev., 20: 45, 1945.
27. Roojen-Runge, E.C., Barlow, F.D., Amer. J. Anat., 93: 143, 1953.
28. Clermont, Y., Amer. J. Anat. 112: 35, 1963.
29. Mancini, R.E., Narbaitz, R. and Lavieri, J.C., Anat. Rec.,136: 477, 1960.
30. Johnsen, S.G., Acta Endocrinol. (Kobenhavn), 61: 111, 1969.
31. Fitschen, W. and Clayton, B.E., Arch. Dis. Child., 40: 16, 1965.
32. Rifkind, A.B., Kulin, H.E. and Ross, G.T., J. Clin. Invest., 46: 1925, 1967.
33. Faiman, C., Ryan, R.J. and Albert, A., J. Clin. Endocr., 28: 1078, 1968.
34. Raiti, S.M.B., Light, C. and Blizzard, R.M., J. Clin. Endocr., 29: 884, 1969.
35. Odell, W.D., Rossi, G.T. and Rayford, P.L., J. Clin. Invest., 46: 248, 1967.
36. Schalch, D.S., Parlow, A.F., Boon, R.C. and Reichlin, J., J. Clin. Invest., 47: 665, 1968.
37. Taymor, M.L., Aono, T. and Pheteplace, C., In Gonadotropins, 1968. ed. Rosemberg, E., Geron-X, Inc., Los Altos, Calif., p 349, 1968.

38. Raiti, S., Johanson, A., Light, C., Migeon, C.J. and Blizzard, R.M., Metabolism, 18: 234, 1969.
39. Saxena, B.B., Demura, H., Gandy, H.M. and Peterson, R.E., J. Clin. Endocr. 28: 519, 1968.
40. Yen, S.S.C., Vicic, W.J. and Kearchner, D.V., J. Clin. Endocr., 29: 382, 1969.
41. Yen. S., Vicic, W., Wieland, R. and Pohlman, C., Fifty-first Meeting Endocrine Society, New York, 1969 (Abstract).
42. Tanner, J.M., In Growth at Adolescence, 2nd ed., Blackwell Sci. Publ., Oxford, England p 32, 1962.
43. Johnsen, S.G., In Gonadotropins 1968, ed. Rosemberg, E., Geron-X, Inc., Los Altos, Calif. p 542, 1968.
44. Hudson, B., Coghlan, J.P. and Dulmanis, A., Ciba Found. Colloq. Endocr. Vol. 16, p 140, 1967.
45. Albert, A., Mayo Clinic Proceedings, 28: 409, 557 and 698, 1953.
46. Albert, A., Mayo Clinic Proceedings, 29: 131, 317 and 368, 1955.
47. Mancini, R.E., Cullen, M., Rosemberg, E., Lavieri, J.C., Vilar, O. and Bergada, C., J. Clin. Endocr., 25: 927, 1965.
48. Lipsett, M.B., IV International Congress in Endocrinology, Mexico, 1967.
49. Rizkallah, T., Gurpide, E., Vande Wiele, R.L., J. Clin. Endocr., 29: 92, 1969.
50. Mancini, R. E., In Gonadotropins 1968, ed. Rosemberg, E., Geron-X, Inc., Los Altos, Calif. p 543, 1968.
51. Bergada, C and Mancini, R.E., in press.
52. Seilicovich, A and Perez Lloret, A., XIV Meeting of the Soc. Arg. Invest. Clin., Bariloche, December 1969, Medicina, 1970 in press (Abstract).
53. Mancini, R.E., Seiguer, A.C. and Perez Lloret, A., J. Clin. Endocr., 29: 467, 1969.
54. Rosemberg, E., Mancini, R.E., Crigler, J.F. and Bergada, C. In Gonadotropins 1968, ed. Rosemberg, E., Geron-X, Inc. Los Altos, Calif. p 527, 1968.
55. Paulsen, C.A., In Gonadotropins 1968, ed. Rosemberg, E., Geron-X, Inc., Los Altos, Calif. p 491, 1968.
56. Zamudio, R., Bergada, C. and Cullen, M.,Meeting of the Soc. Arg. Invest. Clin., Bariloche, Medicina 1970, Chile, December 1969, in press (Abstract).

DISCUSSION

SCHIRREN: Dr. Bergada, we know that in most cases of unilateral cryptorchidism, the scrotal testis shows a histologic picture similar to that of the undescended testicle. This has been our experience in 300 cases, where we demonstrated in 80 percent of our cases hypoplasia of the scrotal testis. In evaluating results, one should consider the age of the patients. For example, would a high dose of HCG cause damage to the testes of a four year old child?

BERGADA: The lesion of the scrotal testis in unilateral cryptorchidism in our experience is minimal in comparison with the total population of cryptorchid children. We are studying the fertility pattern in patients treated for cryptorchidism in our department for the last ten years. Of 21 of our patients with unilateral cryptorchidism treated before puberty, all but one are fertile at the present time. With respect to the dosages of HCG administered; we did not observe any damage as far as testicular histology is concerned.

CHAPTER V

TESTICULAR STEROIDOGENESIS

STEROID SECRETION BY THE HUMAN TESTIS

Mortimer B. Lipsett

National Cancer Institute, Endocrinology Branch,

National Institutes of Health, Bethesda, Maryland 20014

To prove the secretion of a steroid, one must show that the venous effluent from the gland has a higher concentration of the steroid than has peripheral blood. This rigorous criterion is necessary since there is conversion among steroids in peripheral tissues as well as secretion by the adrenal cortex and gonads. There are, of course, important inferences that can be obtained about secretion without sampling the venous effluent by devising appropriate experimental conditions both in vitro and in vivo. For example, the failure to demonstrate 11β-hydroxylation in the normal testis and ovary under any conditions almost surely places the origin of the 11β-hydroxysteroids in the adrenal cortex. Suppression of adrenal cortical function in men does not alter plasma testosterone levels; thus testosterone must either be secreted by the testis or be a product of peripheral metabolism of another steroid secreted by the testis. This sort of inference has been made extensively and has been confirmed on many occasions. It should be clear however that the demonstration that a particular steroid is synthesized in vitro or in vivo from a radioactive precursor gives no information about secretion. One further caution is necessary; there are differences in the testicular secretory patterns among species so that extrapolation to man may not be warranted.

It is appropriate here to state two hypotheses that have not as yet been contradicted. First, in normal men, testosterone is the single important plasma androgen and second, the single important function of the Leydig cell is the synthesis and secretion of testosterone. Testosterone was isolated from the testes during the infancy of steroid endocrinology (1) and 22 years later it was identified in human spermatic venous blood (2). Subsequently, there have been many measurements of testosterone in spermatic venous blood (3-7). The data of Jeffcoate et al. (6) and Dupre et al. (5) yield an average spermatic venous testosterone level of 50 μg/100ml with a very wide range. In older men, the level was 17 μg/100 ml (7) again with a wide range. If testosterone secretion rates of 8 and 5 mg daily are assumed for young and old men respectively, then an estimate can be obtained for testicular blood flow (Table 1). The total testicular blood flow was estimated at 21 to 33 ml/min or 0.5 to 0.8 ml/g/min. These are reasonable estimates since Hudson et al. (8) reported blood flows of 7 to 20 ml/min per testis in man, and in the rat an adrenal cortical blood flow of 2 ml/g/min has been reported (9). In the subsequent discussion a value of 25 ml/min for testicular blood flow will be assumed.

Table 1. Testicular Blood Flow

	Young Men	Old Men
Testicular Venous Plasma T	50 μg/100 ml	17 μg/100 ml
Hematocrit	47%	40%
Testicular Venous Blood T	27 μg/100 ml	10 μg/100 ml
T Blood Production Rate	5.5 μg	3.5 μg/min
Total Testicular Blood	21 ml/min	33 ml/min

T = testosterone

The testis probably secretes testosterone in fetal life although the evidence is entirely inferential. Fetal Leydig cells are prominent from the ninth week of gestation in man (10); the human fetal testis has the capacity to synthesize testosterone (11) and testosterone produces development of external genitalia in the orchiectomized animal fetus (12). Within a few months of birth the Leydig cells dedifferentiate not to appear again until shortly before the beginning of pubescence.

There are no data in man about the secretion of testosterone by the immature testis. The studies of Lindner (13,14) have shown that testes of the lamb, calf, and piglet secrete testosterone at rates one-tenth to one-fiftieth those of the adult. Similarly Resko (15) and we (16) found that the testes of the 20-day-old rat secrete testosterone. In our study, a few atypical Leydig cells were present at this time. It may be surmised that in man, the testis secretes small amounts of testosterone before the start of pubescence since plasma testosterone levels (17) are higher in boys than in girls. The identification of luteinizing hormone in the blood (18, 19) and urine (20) of prepubertal boys supports the contention that there is a constant low level of a trophic hormone necessary for Leydig cell function.

In the above discussion we have assumed that the blood production rate of testosterone in men is a consequence solely of secreted testosterone.[1] Since the testicular blood flow in man is not know from independent measurements, the absolute secretion rate of testosterone cannot be calculated. However, quantitative studies of the peripheral transformation of such possible precursors of testosterone as androstenedione (21), 17-hydroxyprogesterone (22) dehydroepiandrosterone (23) and its sulfate (24) make it unlikely that significant amounts of plasma testosterone in normal men are derived from any or all of these steroids (Table 2). Another possible precursor, androstenediol[2], has not been studied but the conversion of other compounds such as dehydroepiandrosterone (23) and 17-hydroxypregnenolone (25) containing the Δ^5-3 β-hydroxy function to a Δ^4-3-ketosteroid is low so that it is improbable that androstenediol could be an important peripheral precursor of plasma testosterone in man.

Table 2. Testicular Secretion Rates and Transfer Constants

Testosterone	mg/24 hr	P_{BB}^{X-T}*	Fraction of T blood production rate (%)
Testosterone	7		
Androstenedione	3	0.05	2
Androstenediol	(1-3)**	(0.02-0.1)**	Small
17-Hydroxyprogesterone	2	<0.01	low
17-hydroxypregnenolone	1	<0.01	low
Dehydroepiandrosterone	7	0.006	0.4

*Transfer constant of blood steroid precursor to blood testosterone

**Best estimate

The steroid-synthesizing glands probably secrete each steroid that lies in the biosynthetic sequence from pregnenolone to the chief secretory product. It is our concept that this is an epiphenomenon secondary to the process of steroid synthesis and has been dubbed a consequence of the "leaky" gland by Short (26). The

---

[1] Production rate signifies the total rate of entry of the steroid from all sources into the blood compartment. This would include secretion from the glands and entry from such organs as liver and skin. Secretion rate refers solely to the rate of entry of the steroid from a gland.

[2] The following trivial names have been used for steroids:

Androstenedione =	androst-4-ene-3,17-dione
Androstenediol =	androst-5-ene-3β,17β-diol
17-hydroxyprogesterone =	17α-hydroxy-5β-pregn-4-ene-3,20-dione
17-hydroxypregnenolone =	3β,17α-dihydroxypregn-5-ene-20-one
Dehydroepiandrosterone =	3β-hydroxyandrost-5-en-17-one

amounts of steroids secreted will depend on such variables as the activity of the several biosynthetic pathways and the velocity of reaction of each enzymatic step of synthesis. Although steroid synthesis will be discussed in a subsequent paper an outline of the several steps in the biosynthetic sequences leading to testosterone is shown in Fig. 1. We propose to discuss the secretion rates of each of these steroids where data are available.

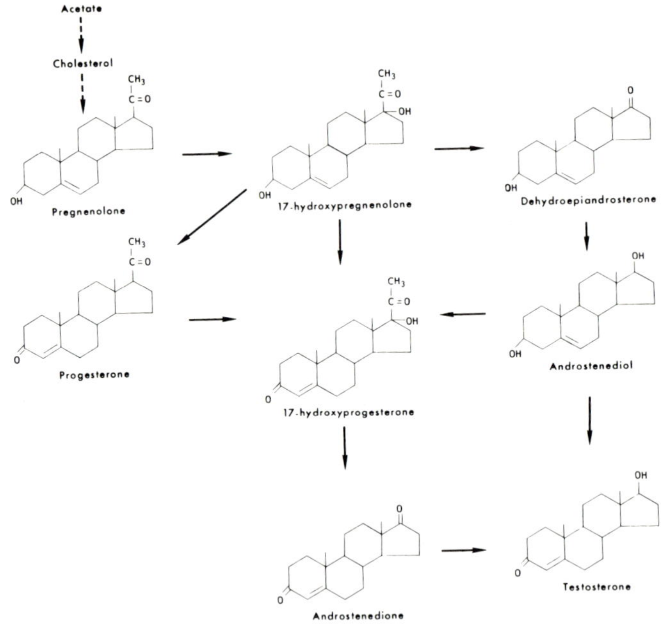

Fig. 1 Pathways of testosterone biosynthesis in the Leydig cell.

Androstenedione, a proximate precursor of testosterone, is secreted by the Leydig cell. Since its spermatic venous concentration is about one-tenth that of testosterone in man (7) and in other species (13,14), the secretion rate by the human testes would be about 700 μg/day. Using the transfer constant of 5.0% (10), only 35 μg of the testosterone production rate would originate with testicular androstenedione. It is significant that in the calf (13), piglet (14), and prepubescent rat (15) the spermatic venous androstenedione level equaled the testosterone level. Thus, in the nonstimulated state, androstenedione is as important a secretory product as is testosterone. The change with pubescence then lies not only with increased secretion of these steroids but in a major shift in the relative amounts secreted. How the equilibrium of the androstenedione-testosterone 17-oxido reductase system is affected by pubescence is not clear.

Androstenediol, the other possible proximate precursor of testosterone, has not been measured either in peripheral or spermatic venous blood. Androstenediol was identified in canine spermatic vein blood after HCG stimulation at levels 1/2 to 1/20 those of testosterone (27). If a similar concentration were present in man, the secretion rate could be several milligrams daily. Since the transfer constants for the conversion of dehydroepiandrosterone to androstenedione (6%) (23) and 17-hydroxypregnenolone to 17-hydroxyprogesterone (2-11%) (25) are low, it is unlikely that androstenediol could be an important precursor of plasma testosterone in man.

There is considerably more information about the testicular secretion of another Δ^5-3β-hydroxysteroid, dehydroepiandrosterone. It was identified in canine testicular venous effluent by Ibayashi et al. (28). Its secretion in man was established by Gandy and Peterson (7) who reported a spermatic venous gradient ranging from 0.13 to 11 μg/100 ml, the mean being approximately 1.3 μg/100 ml. Using the earlier estimates of testicular blood flow, the estimated secretion rate would be about 400 μg/24 hr or 6% of the estimated dehydroepiandrosterone blood production rate. Thus, their finding that orchiectomy did not alter plasma dehydroepiandrosterone levels is in accord with these estimates since a small decrease would not have been detected. Rivarola et al. (29) reported considerably higher gradients of dehydroepiandrosterone in patients with testicular feminization. If their data were accepted, then the testes in these subjects would be the most important source of dehydroepiandrosterone.

17-hydroxyprogesterone is a precursor of androstenedione in the testis and there is now considerable evidence bearing on its secretion rate. Its blood production rate was estimated at 2 mg/24 hr (30). Since suppression of LH by an exogenous androgen reduced plasma levels and production rates by 90%, and adrenal cortical suppression had little effect, it was concluded that the testis was the source of most of the plasma 17-hydroxyprogesterone (30). The possibility that 17-hydroxypregnenolone was secreted in large enough amounts and converted peripherally to 17-hydroxyprogesterone to account for its production rate was ruled out by studies showing that no more than 200 μg could originate in this way (25). Thus, there must be a high testicular secretion of 17-hydroxyprogesterone. The older findings of an increase in urinary pregnanetriol in response to HCG (31) suggested that the origin of this metabolite was 17-hydroxyprogesterone secreted by the testis.

17-Hydroxypregnenolone may be the precursor of 17-hydroxyprogesterone or dehydroepiandrosterone within the Leydig cell or after secretion in peripheral tissues. We have estimated that only 30-40% of the blood production rate of 2 to 3 mg daily is secreted by the testis (25). The larger moiety is clearly due to adrenal cortical activity.

Pregnenolone and progesterone have not been measured in spermatic venous blood and there is no evidence regarding their secretion. Progesterone plasma levels are so low in men (30) that suppression studies are difficult to interpret. Our preliminary estimates of plasma pregnenolone concentration show it to be present at about 60 ng/100 ml so that the amount secreted by the testis must be small. The secretion rates of the steroids by the testis and their transfer constants to testosterone are summarized in Table 2.

CONJUGATES

The roles of steroid sulfates as intermediates in the biosynthetic process and as secretory products of the adrenal cortex (32, 33) led to similar studies of the testis. Although a sulfokinase has been identified in the human testis (34), the secretion of dehydroepiandrosterone sulfate has not been demonstrated conclusively. In the syndrome of testicular feminization, Morris and Mahesh (35) and Pion et al. (36) found high spermatic venous levels of the sulfate whereas Rivarola et al. (29) and Lastikainen et al. (37) reported similar levels in peripheral and spermatic venous blood. In one in vivo perfusion of a normal human testis, the secretion of dehydroepiandrosterone sulfate was not shown (38). The best evidence for secretion of this conjugate is the finding that HCG treatment for 14 days increased peripheral dehydroepiandrosterone sulfate levels threefold in young children (39) but this stimulation did not occur in older children (30) or in adults (40). These data and the findings in testicular feminization suggest that the testis has the capacity to secrete dehydroepiandrosterone sulfate but that in normal men, the secretion rate is very low.

The human testis has the capacity to synthesize testosterone sulfate (34). Laatikainen et al. (37) found the spermatic venous plasma level to average 1.5 μg/100 ml. This would be equivalent to a secretion rate of 270 μg/24 hr. The peripherial testosterone sulfate concentration was about 0.1 μg/100 ml (37,41). Since Baulieu et al. (33) reported that testosterone sulfate is not metabolized further, it should not be a precursor of plasma testosterone. The identification of testosterone sulfate in the urine in very small amounts (42,43) suggests that perhaps the route of excretion is other than the urine if no metabolism is possible.

Androstenediol monosulfate has been identified in peripheral blood (44) at a level of several micrograms per 100 ml. The origin of this steroid, a putative precursor of testosterone, has not been examined.

ESTROGENS

The complex problems associated with the secretion of estrogens by the testis are derived from observations that HCG increased urinary estrogens in men (45-49) and that castration caused a marked fall in their excretion. These data proved that the testis secreted estrogens or their precursors. The synthesis of estrogens from acetate (50,51), cholesterol (52), testosterone (52) and androstenedione (53) has been demonstrated in the testes of several species including the human. In all cases, the conversions even from the immediate precursors, such as androstenedione, were low. The identification of estrone and estradiol in spermatic venous blood from the normal human testis at concentrations higher than in peripheral blood has not been made. The early observations of Steinach and Kun (54) and the later studies of West et al. (55) showed that testosterone could be converted to estrone and estradiol in man. There were many subsequent reports of the conversion of radioisotope labelled androgens to urinary estrogens (56-59) and to blood estrogens (60,61). The sites of conversion were not defined by these studies but human liver (62,63) has been shown to synthesize estrogens from androgens in vivo. There is suggestive evidence that human mammary cancer (64) and rat liver and kidney (65) may also be able to aromatize androstenedione to estrone. Since aromatization of androstenedione took place in an ovariectomized adrenalectomized woman (59), it is not necessary to postulate that the process of aromatization of androgens normally occurs in the adrenal cortex or gonads.

MacDonald et al. (59) reported the first complete quantitative studies of the source of estrogens in men. After infusing tritiated androstenedione and labelled estrone and measuring the conversion of androstenedione to urinary estrone, they concluded that 1.3% of blood androstenedione was converted to blood estrone, thereby accounting for 18 μg or an important fraction of the daily estrone production rate. Longcope et al. (61) and we (66) found essentially the same transfer constants (1.5%) between blood androstenedione and estrone. From our estimates of blood androstenedione production rates, we (61,66) concluded that 30 to 40 μg of estrone entered the blood compartment daily as a result of conversion from blood androstenedione. Since the metabolic clearance rate of estrone is about 2000 1/24 hr (67,68) and the 9:00 a.m. plasma estrone concentration was 6 ng/100 ml (69), the calculated blood estrone production rate was 120 μg/24 hr. However, there is a diurnal variation of blood estrone in men (69) most probably related to the diurnal variation of androstenedione secreted by the adrenal cortex (70). Thus a mean 24 hour plasma estrone level would be closer to 4 ng/100 ml and the 24 hour production rate about 80 μg. If this is the case then androstenedione blood production would account for one-half of estrone production.

The possibility then remains that some estrone is secreted by the testis. Baird (71) demonstrated that there is a small adrenal cortical secretion of estrone but this could account for only a small fraction of the estrone blood production rate. Other possible precursors such as dehydroepiandrosterone are unimportant sources of estrogens in men (72). We would thus conclude that the testis secreted about 40 μg of estrone daily. From the estimate of testicular blood flow, a plasma estrone concentration of about 0.3 μg/100 ml should be present in spermatic venous blood. Methods of requisite sensitivity have not been applied as yet to this problem. Only in testicular feminization have estradiol and estrone been identified as testicular secretory products (36,73) and the testis in this syndrome can scarcely be equated with the normal testis.

The conclusion that the testis secretes estrone depends critically on the estimate of the estrone blood production rate. Data obtained by several workers using urinary isotope dilution methods place the estrone production rate considerably lower than that estimated from the blood level and clearance rates. Based on these lower estimates, the testicular estrone secretion would be negligible. This question will be settled by analysis of spermatic venous estrogen levels.

The contribution of blood testosterone to blood estradiol has been examined similarly, and the transfer constant was considerably lower, values of 0.4% (59) and 0.6% (66) being reported. Using a testosterone blood production rate of 7 mg/24 hr., we estimate that 35 μg of estradiol is derived from blood testosterone. In addition, the estrone-estradiol blood transfer constant is 15% (67) so that an additional 12 to 15 μg of estradiol would originate from plasma estrone. This accounts for all of the estimated estradiol production in men. Thus, there is no need to assume appreciable secretion of estradiol by the normal testis. These data are summarized in Fig. 2 and 3.

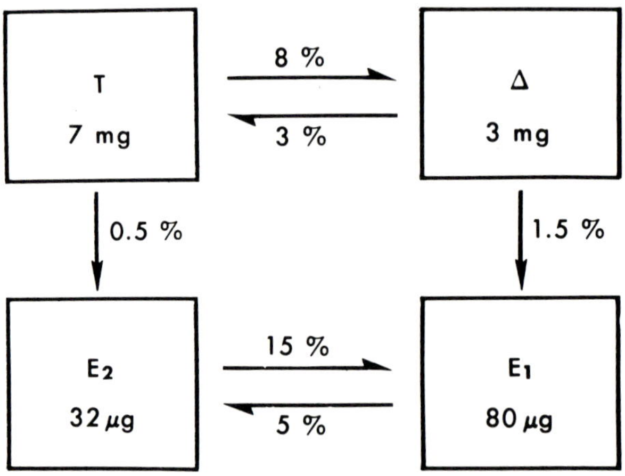

Fig. 2 Transfer constants and blood production rates of estrogens and their precursors. The numbers within the blocks give the estimated daily blood production rates and the transfer constants between compartments are shown with the appropriate arrows.

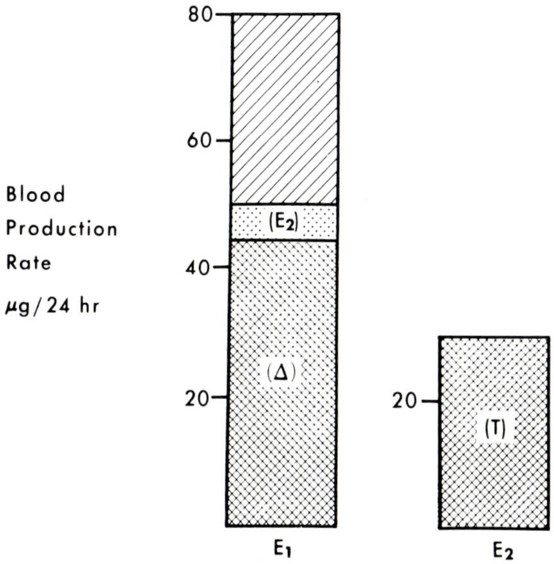

Fig. 3 Contribution of androgens to estrogen production rates in men. The amount of estrone derived from blood androstenedione and estradiol is shown within the total estrone production. All of the blood estradiol is derived from blood testosterone.

In summary then, there is no evidence that the testis secretes any steroid other than testosterone in amounts sufficicient for significant biologic effects. None of the steroids secreted can be converted with high enough efficiency in target tissues to exert important androgenic or estrogenic activity. It is probable that estradiol is not secreted by the testis whereas estrone may be. All of the intermediates in steroid biosynthesis may escape the biosynthetic process and thereby be secreted by the testis.

REFERENCES

1. David, K., Dingmanse, E., Freud, J., and Laqueur, E., Physiol. Chem., 233: 281, 1235.
2. Lucas, W.M., Whitmore, W.F., Jr., and West, C.D., J. Clin. Endocr., 17: 465, 1957.
3. Hollander, N., and Hollander, V.P., J. Clin. Endocr., 18: 966, 1958.
4. Hudson, B., Coghlan, J., Dulmanis, A., Wintour, M., and Ekkel, I., Aust. J. Exp. Biol. Med. Sci., 41: 235, 1963.
5. Dupre, J., Brooks, R.V., Hyde, R.D., London, D.R., Prunty, F.T.G., and Selp, J.B., J. Endocr., 29: vii, 1964.
6. Jeffcoate, S.L., Brooks, R.V., Lim, N.Y., London, D.R., Prunty, F.T.G., and Spathis, G.S., J. Endocr., 37: 401, 1967.

7. Gandy, H.M. and Peterson, R.E., J. Clin. Endocr., 28: 949, 1968.
8. Hudson, B., Coghlan, J.P., Dulmanis, A., and Wintour, M., Proc. Second Intern. Congr. Endocr., 2: 1127, 1964.
9. Kramer, R.J. and Saperstein, L.A., Endocrinology, 81: 403, 1967.
10. Van Wagenen, G. and Simpson, M.E., Embryology of the Ovary and Testis, Yale University Press, New Haven, 1965.
11. Bloch, E., Endocrinology, 74: 833, 1964.
12. Jost, A., Recent Progr. Hormone Res., 8: 379, 1953.
13. Lindner, H.R., J. Endocr., 23: 139, 1961.
14. Lindner, H.R., J. Endocr., 23: 171, 1961.
15. Resko, J.A., Feder, H.H. and Goy, R.W., J. Endocr., 40: 485, 1968.
16. Knorr, D., Vanha-Perttula, T., and Lipsett, M.B., Endocrinology, in press.
17. Frasier, S.O. and Horton, R., Steroids, 8: 777, 1960.
18. Johanson, A.J., Guyda, H. Light, C., Migeon, C.J., and Blizzard, R.M., J. Pediat., 74: 416, 1969.
19. Sciarra, N., Leone, V., and Pastorino, G.F., J. Endocr., 42: 167, 1968.
20. Rifkind, A.B., Kulin, H.E., and Ross, G.T., J. Clin. Invest., 46: 1925, 1967.
21. Horton, R. and Tait, J.F., J. Clin. Invest., 45: 301, 1966.
22. Camacho, A.M. and Migeon, C.J., J. Clin. Invest., 43: 1083, 1964.
23. Horton, R. and Tait, J.F., J. Clin. Endocr., 27: 79, 1967.
24. Slaunwhite, W.R., Jr., Burgett, M.J., and Sandberg, A.A., J. Clin. Endocr., 27: 663, 1967.
25. Bermudez, J.A., Strott, C.A., and Lipsett, M.B., Clin. Res., 17: 587, 1969.
26. Short, R.V., Biochemical Soc. Symposia, 18: 59, 1960.
27. Yamaji, T., Motohashi, K., Tanioka, T., and Ibayashi, H., Endocrinology, 83: 992, 1968.
28. Ibayashi, H., Nakamura, M., Uchikawa, T., Murakawa, S. Yoshida, S., Nakao, K., and Okinaka, S., Endocrinology, 76: 347, 1965.
29. Rivarola, M.A., Saez, J.M., Meyer, W.J., Kenny, F.M., and Migeon, C.J., J. Clin. Endocr., 27: 371, 1967.
30. Strott, C.A., Yoshimi, T., and Lipsett, M.B., J. Clin. Invest., 48: 930, 1969.
31. Landau, R.L. and Lanes, M.L., J. Clin. Endocr., 19: 1399, 1959.
32. Vande Wiele, R.L., MacDonald, P.C., Gurpide, E., and Lieberman, S., Recent Progr. Hormone Res., 19: 275, 1963.
33. Baulieu, E.E., Corpechot, C., Dray, F., Emiliozzi, R., Lebeau, R., Mauvais-Jarvis, P., and Robel, P., Recent Progr. Hormone Res., 21: 411, 1965.
34. Dixon, R., Vincent, V., and Kase, N., Steroids, 6: 757, 1965.
35. Morris, J. McL. and Mahesh, V., Amer. J. Obstet. Gynec., 87: 731, 1963.
36. Pion, R.J., Dignam, W.J., Lamb, E.J., Moore, J.G., Frankland, M.V., and Simmer, H.H., Amer. J. Obstet. Gynec., 93: 1067, 1965.
37. Laatikainen, T., Laitinen, A., and Vihko, R., J. Clin. Endocr., 29: 219, 1969.

38. Oertel, G.W., Wendlberger, F., Menzel, P., Treiber, L., and Knapstein, P., Europ. J. Steroids, 2: 299, 1967.
39. Saez, J.M. and Bertrand, J., Steroids, 12: 749, 1968.
40. Yamaji, T., and Ibayashi, H., J. Clin. Endocr., 29: 273, 1969.
41. Dray, F., Mowszowicz, I., and Ledru, M.J., Steroids, 10: 501, 1967.
42. Dessypris, A., Drosdowski, M.A., McNiven, N.L. and Dorfman, R.I., Proc. Soc. Exp. Biol. Med., 121: 1128, 1966.
43. Tamm, J., Volkwein, V., and Voigt, K.D., Experientia, 23: 299, 1967.
44. Sjovall, J. and Vihko, R., Steroids, 7: 447, 1966.
45. Leach, R.B., Maddock, W.O., Tokuyama, I., Paulsen, C.A., and Nelson, W.O., Recent. Progr. Hormone Res., 12: 377, 1956.
46. Jayle, M.F., Baulieu, E.E., Scholler, R., Lisboa, B.P., and Savoie, J.C., Rev. Franc. Etud. Clin. Biol., 3: 455, 1958.
47. Givner, M.L., Bauld, W.S., Hale, T.R., Vagi, K., and Nilsen, M., J. Clin. Endocr., 20: 665, 1960.
48. Morse, W.I., Clark, A.F., MacLeod, S.C., Ernst, W.A., and Gosse, C.L., J. Clin. Endocr., 22: 678, 1962.
49. Jayle, M.F., Scholler, R., Sfikakis, A., and Heron, M., Clin. Chim. Acta, 7: 212, 1962.
50. Rabinowitz, J.L. and Oleksyshyn, O., Arch Biochem. Biophys., 64: 285, 1956.
51. Rabinowitz, J.L. and Dowben, R.M., Biochim. Biophys. Acta, 16: 96, 1955.
52. Rabinowitz, J.L., Atompraxis, 4: 85, 1958.
53. Bedrak, E. and Samuels, L.T., Abstracts Third Intern. Congr. Endocr., 1: 35, 1968.
54. Steinach, E., and Kun, H., Lancet, 2: 845, 1937.
55. West, C.D., Damast, B.L., Sarro, S.D., and Pearson, O.H., J. Biol. Chem., 218: 409, 1969.
56. Braun-Cantilo, J.A., LaRoche, G., Novitsky, M., and Lawrence, J.H., Acta Isotop., 1: 351, 1961.
57. Breuer, H., Acta Endocr., 40: 111, 1962.
58. Epstein, B.J., Raheja, M.C., Prow, E., and Morse, W.I., Canad. J. Biochem., 44: 971, 1966.
59. MacDonald, P.C., Rombaut, R.P., and Siiteri, P.K., J. Clin. Endocr., 27: 1103, 1967.
60. Fishman, L.M., Sarfaty, G.A., Wilson, H., and Lipsett, M.B., Ciba Found. Colloq. Endocr., 16: 156, 1967.
61. Longcope, C., Kato, T., and Horton, R., J. Clin. Invest., 48: 2191, 1969.
62. Bolt, W., Ritzl, F., and Bolt, H.M., Munchen Med. Wschr., 108: 875, 1966.
63. Bolt, W., Ritzl, F., and Bolt, H.M., Verh. Deutsch Ges. Inn. Med. , 72: 461, 1966.
64. Adams, J.B., and Wong, M.S.F., J. Endocr., 41:41, 1968.
65. Frieden, E.H., Patkin, J.K., and Mills, M., Proc. Soc. Exp. Biol. Med., 129: 606, 1968.

66. Hembree, W.C., Bardin, C.W., and Lipsett, M.B., Abstracts Third Intern. Congr. Endocr., 1: 181, 1968.
67. Longcope, C., Layne, D.S., and Tait, J.F., J. Clin. Invest., 47: 93, 1968.
68. Hembree, W.C., Bardin, C.W., and Lipsett, M.B., J. Clin. Invest., 48: 1809, 1969.
69. Baird, D.T. and Guevara, A., J. Clin. Endocr., 29: 149, 1969.
70. Crafts, R., Llerena, L.A., Guevara, A., Lobotsky, J., and Lloyd, C.W., Steroids, 12: 151, 1968.
71. Baird, D.T., Uno, A., and Melby, J.C., J. Endocr., 45: 135, 1969.
72. Baird, D.T., Horton, R., Longcope, C., and Tait, J.F., Recent Progr. Hormone Res., 25: 611, 1969.
73. French, F.S., Baggett, B., Van Wyk, J.J., Talbert, L.M., Hubbard, W.M., Johnston, F.R., Weaver, R.P., Forchielli, E., Rao, G.S., and Sarda, I.R., J. Clin. Endocr., 25: 661, 1965.

DISCUSSION

JOHNSEN: Dr. Lipsett, I would like to comment on your statement that most or all of the estrone/estradiol in men is derived from peripheral conversion of androgens. I would say, that if there were only one significant testicular hormone we would be unable to understand testicular function since we have two different gonadotropins both being regulated more or less independently by fee[illegible]ack mechanisms from the testis. Next, if most or all of the e[illegible]ns were derived from the androgens, one would would expect [illegible] certain correlation between the levels of these two hormo[illegible]le. We have been unable to find such a correlation. In 2[illegible]aged 20 to 40 years we performed, under continuous suppre[illegible] adrenals with dexamethasone, a HCG stimulation test an[illegible]ed the rise of urinary estrone/estradiol and the rise of urina[illegible]ndrosterone/ etiocholanolone which we believe to be a good parameter for testicular androgen during adrenal suppression. We have made a plot of the log value of the rise of androsterone/etiocholanolone (i.e. the stimulation value minus the value before stimulation) versus the log value of the rise of urinary estrone/estradiol. There was no correlation. The correlation coefficient was 0.28 (P value >0.1). This is surprising because both parameters show a wide variation so that a correlation could easily show up. At one end we have a man with a 160% rise in androgen but only a 36% rise of estrogen. At the other end there is a man with only a 38% rise of androgen but a 157% rise of estrogen. For statistical reasons we have excluded three extreme values. If these are included the correlation coefficient drops to 0.14 and there is one man with 104% androgen rise but only 14% estrogen rise and another with only 14% androgen rise but no less than 210% estrogen rise. One may speculate as to where the estrogens came from. We think that the lack of correlation between androgen and estrogen levels in the male speaks against the concept that most or all of the estrogen is derived from peripheral conversion of androgen. We even think that the lack of correlation, particularly between the rise of androgen and estrogen after HCG, is an indication that these two may not have the same testicular cellular origin. Dr. Lipsett, did you ever try to correlate the levels of androgen and estrogen in the male?

LIPSETT: No, we have not tried to correlate the levels of androgen and estrogen. Very rough correlations have been obtained by many workers showing that when the level of androgen is low the level of estrogen is low and so on. In terms of looking at correlations between plasma testosterone and plasma estradiol, this has not been done. I cannot comment on the question of two hormones of the testis. However, with estrone and estradiol there are at least three groups, all of whom have essentially the same data, which show all of plasma estradiol can be accounted for by conversion from testosterone. Now, as I indicated, the picture with estrone is not nearly as clear, because it depends not only on some problems of measurement of secretion and production rates but also on what figure one uses for the androstenedione level. There is a diurnal variation of androstenedione much of it coming from the adrenal cortex. In six cases of feminizing testis syndrome, secretion of either estradiol or estrone has in fact been shown.

TROEN: In covering the steroid secretion very nicely, I wonder whether Dr. Lipsett would also care to discuss briefly the role of conjugated steroids in biosynthetic processes in the testis. Dr. Uanaihara and I have been studying the synthesis of testosterone in minces of testicular tissue obtained at orchiectomy for prostatic cancer, during herniorrhaphy or because of severe testalgia. One gram of tissue was incubated for one hour in a standard incubation mixture to which labelled steroid precursors were added. After incubation with DHA, identification of the metabolites revealed the major free compounds to be Δ^5-androstenediol and testosterone, with only a small amount of Δ^4-androstenedione. In the approximately 5% conjugated fraction, with labelled dehydroepiandrosterone sulfate and Δ^5-androstenediol sulfate, additional incubations with mixed precursors were performed. When labelled Δ^5-androstenediol was incubated with either labelled DHA or DHA sulfate, Δ^5-androstenediol sulfate was found from all three. The tritium/C^{14} ratios indicate that Δ^5-androstenediol sulfate is formed more readily from Δ^5-androstenediol than from either DHA or DHA sulfate. From mixtures of DHA and DHA sulfate the Δ^5-androstenediol sulfate preponderantly comes from DHA. In addition there is far greater conversion of DHA to Δ^5 androstenediol than DHA sulfate to Δ^5-androstenediol sulfate. These findings indicate that the pathway is DHA to Δ^5-androstenediol to Δ^5-androstenediol sulfate. To determine the role of Δ^5-androstenediol sulfate in the biosynthesis of testosterone, particularly since no testosterone sulfate was identified, additional studies were performed. The effect of added carrier Δ^5-androstenediol or Δ^5-androstenediol sulfate on the conversion of labelled DHA to testosterone was determined. The addition of the conjugated material had no inhibitory effect on the conversion of DHA to testosterone whereas a progressive and marked inhibition of conversion resulted from the addition of the free compound. These data suggest that Δ^5-androstenediol sulfate may function as an available reservoir but not as a significant precursor in the biosynthetic pathway to testosterone.

LIPSETT: Well, it is clear that there is a sulfokinase in the testis and sulfation of testosterone has been clearly shown by Mason and Payne. DHA sulfate has been synthesized by the testis. DHA sulfate has been shown to be a poor precursor by Eik-Nes and his co-workers on perfusion of the testis, however, the fact is that no matter what one says about the biosynthetic sequence, DHA sulfate does not seem to be a secretory product. There is a report by Saez and Bertrand concerning children who, when treated with HCG for 14 days, show a rise in DHA sulfate, whereas it does not increase in the adult. You mentioned that you had some difficulty showing synthesis of testosterone sulfate, but I think the data of Vihko and Laatikinin using both gas chromatography and mass spectrometry very clearly show its secretion. Thus we may always find some discrepancies between a particular set of in vitro incubation results and measurement of a steroid in peripheral blood or in the venous effluent from a gland.

ROSEMBERG: I am very glad that both Dr. Lipsett and Dr.Hudson brought up the question of diurnal variation of testosterone correlated to levels of plasma LH as measured by radioimmunoassay. Dr. Hudson mentioned the report from Dr. Saxena's group which points to some diurnal variation in testosterone level. I would like to ask both Dr. Lipsett and Dr. Hudson if there is enough data from various laboratories which will indicate one way or another that there is indeed some diurnal variation of LH levels, as measured by radioimmunoassay and if there is some variation in testosterone levels at least in a 24-hour period. Dr. Lipsett, when you presented the effects of HCG, how much HCG was given and how soon did you record the increase in testosterone levels?

LIPSETT: It is now the consensus that there is a small decrease in plasma testosterone in the evening as compared to early morning. I would agree that this occurs in some patients and not in others, and when one averages them out one finds some small decrease. No one has found the large decreases that were reported by Dr. Saxena.

HUDSON: We first reported on the study of the diurnal variation of testosterone in 1964 in an experiment done with Dr. Bartter when he was visiting our laboratories. We used nine normal male medical students, and when we averaged the data we were unable to find any circadian rhythm in plasma testosterone. Because a number of groups, in particular Eik-Nes and Resko, Drey and others found evidence to the contrary, we repeated this experiment with another group of medical students. On this occasion, LH was also estimated simultaneously. Analysis of this data showed a small diurnal variation with high morning and low evening values for both LH and testosterone in some individuals only. The changes in LH preceded those for testosterone and were of a magnitude of from plus to minus 17% around the mean. I believe we must look at this data realistically. We are asking quite a lot from our methods, I believe,that methods can measure 10 to 15% changes in these compounds. However, despite all the care that is taken in the laboratory, within assay variation can be at least plus or minus 10%, and this is what I mean by methodological "noise" and biological "signal."

TESTOSTERONE PLASMA LEVELS IN NORMAL AND PATHOLOGICAL CONDITIONS

Bryan Hudson, H.G. Burger, D.M. de Kretser,

J. P. Coghlan and H.P. Taft

Departments of Medicine and Anatomy, Monash University, Medical Research Centre Prince Henry's Hospital and Howard Florey Laboratories of Experimental Physiology, University of Melbourne, Melbourne, Australia

The purpose of this paper is to review what is now a fairly substantial body of knowledge about the concentration of testosterone in human plasma both in normal and abnormal conditions. For the most part, this review will be directed to testosterone in the male; however, other closely related steroids such as androstenedione and dehydroepiandrosterone (DHEA) will be discussed in so far as these are relevant; likewise, plasma levels of all these steroids in the female will be discussed particularly when it may be appropriate to compare and contrast them between the two sexes. This presentation will thus aim to synthesize this knowledge, and will draw upon many contributions from different laboratories, including our own.

The reason why there is now such a substantial body of knowledge is undoubtedly related to the existence of methods for the measurement of testosterone in plasma and other biological fluids. This paper cannot possibly review the many methods that now exist (1 - 14), but clearly methods that depend upon the interaction between testosterone and macromolecules have now displaced earlier procedures because of their relative simplicity, adequate specificity and reasonable precision.

TESTOSTERONE IN NORMAL ADULT MALES

In the normal, sexually mature, adult male, there is good agreement that the concentration of testosterone in peripheral plasma is between 3.5 and 10.5 μg/l. These data, which are not generally disputed, have been derived from many different laboratories using most of the methods that have been mentioned. In round numbers, these values are about 10 times those found in the normal adult female.

About 10 years ago Slaunwhite and Sandberg (15) and later Chen et al. (16) suggested that testosterone was bound to plasma proteins. Since then, many workers have independently confirmed these observations and have done much to characterize the nature of this binding protein (17-23). Although testosterone in plasma is bound to albumin, this binding is relatively weak and non-specific in comparison with the binding to what is probably a β-globulin which has a high affinity not only for this steroid but also for estradiol, with which it probably shares a common binding site (or sites). Rivarola et al. (23) have shown by in vitro studies that in the male 92.8$\pm$ 1.6% is bound, a figure that is significantly different from the female in whom about 95.5$\pm$ 1.2% is bound. Treatment with estrogens, and pregnancy, further increase this binding, so that a value of 99$\pm$ 0.2% is observed under these conditions. The biological implication of these in vitro observations is that in the male, the unbound and presumably active form of testosterone circulates in a concentration of about 80 ng/1. The comparable value for the adult female is between 4 and 5 ng/1. Extensive studies on the nature of this testosterone binding affinity have also been made by August et al. (24) who have shown that a fairly wide spectrum of affinities exists under physiological conditions; pregnancy plasma showing the highest affinity and umbilical venous plasma the lowest.

Blood levels of testosterone reflect the momentary balance between entry into and removal from the blood. In the male, about 1000 liters of plasma are cleared of testosterone each day. This figure is significantly correlated with liver blood flow; the fact that it is only about 60-70% of liver plasma flow is presumed to reflect the degree to which the steroid is normally bound to protein, a presumption which is supported by the finding that in the female, in whom protein binding is greater, the clearance rate is less, and in both sexes may be further reduced by treatment with estrogen (25-30).

Although the liver is undoubtedly the principal organ responsible for the metabolic removal of testosterone from plasma, extrahepatic metabolism of testosterone certainly occurs (31,32), but the precise contribution by skin, muscle and other tissues to testosterone clearance has not been precisely determined. It may be, for instance, that reduced clearance in the female not only reflects increased protein binding but also a lower extrahepatic metabolism by such sensitive tissues as skin, muscle and sexual structures. With plasma levels ranging between 3.5 and 10.5 μg/1, and clearance rates of between 900 and 1200 1/day, the rate of entry of testosterone into blood may be calculated, assuming a steady state, to be between 3 and 13 mg/day. This statement begs two further questions: first, is the state steady, and, second, is the rate of entry synonymous with secretion?

It seems likely that the state is not entirely steady. In the past there has been some controversy as to whether the level of this steroid changes within the day or between days (11,33-36). The weight of evidence would now suggest that within the day there is a variation, with higher morning and lower evening values; the amplitude of these swings is probably small when compared, for instance, to that of cortisol. A possible reason for past uncertainty is that the methodological noise has tended to obscure biological signals. Several authors (37,38) have been unable to show that a significant circadian rhythm exists for luteinizing hormone (LH) or follicle stimulating hormone (FSH), although in a recent report Saxena and Gandy (39) have shown a circadian rhythm of large amplitude for LH and FSH to which is entrained a rhythm of much smaller amplitude for testosterone. In limited longitudinal studies on normal males, we have been unable to demonstrate systematic variations in the plasma concentration of testosterone over a period of five weeks; in fact values were found to range widely in an apparently random fashion (40).

The original studies of Tait and Horton (25,41), which have now been clearly substantiated, have shown that in the adult male more than 95% of testosterone in blood is secreted as such, the remaining 5% being derived as a peripheral conversion product mainly from androstenedione(27,42). This whole subject has been extensively reviewed by Baird et al. (43). It is also clear that the testosterone secreted originates from the testis and not from the adrenal cortex. Thus, following adrenocortical suppression or after adrenalectomy, or in patients with Addison's disease, testosterone levels are not significantly different from other normal males (40); further, the administration of ACTH to some normal male patients is associated with a significant decrease in plasma levels of testosterone (27). Why this should be so is not entirely clear. Is it that ACTH exerts a direct effect on the testis, or is it that increased blood levels of adrenal androgens, androstenedione and DHEA, or adrenal estrogens act to inhibit the secretion of tropic hormones?

Methods for the measurement of testosterone in plasma have now made it possible to examine more formally those proposals previously shown by classic techniques in endocrinology that the testis and the anterior lobe of the pituitary constitute an endocrine axis, and that the secretion of testosterone is directly regulated by the hypothalamus acting through the anterior pituitary. The pituitary hormone responsible is the interstitial cell stimulating hormone (ICSH) for which there is putative evidence of a common identity with pituitary LH. A similar action is also shared by human chorionic gonadotropin (HCG) which, when administered parenterally, is associated with prompt elevations in the level of plasma testosterone in normal, hypophysectomized and prepubertal males and as such provides a useful method for the evaluation of Leydig cell function. Administration over a three or four day period is almost certainly a more discriminatory procedure than a single injection and the measurement of changes within a few hours of this stimulus (44-46). Although there is good evidence that FSH acts on the seminiferous epithelium, it seems unlikely that this gonadotropin plays a role in the regulation of Leydig cell function and the secretion of testosterone (47,48). It is of interest, however, that Steinberger and Duckett (49) have described depletion of pituitary FSH and a rise in plasma FSH following castration in the male rat, changes that can be reversed by the administration of testosterone.

The neuro-endocrine mechanisms involved in the regulation of testosterone secretion appear to be of the usual type; high levels of plasma testosterone inhibit the secretion of LH (11,36), while low levels are associated with an increased secretion of this hormone (40). There is good evidence that the receptor sites of this neuro-endocrine loop are hypothalamic, and are susceptible to exogenous influences that may stimulate or inhibit the formation or secretion of releasing factors. The anti-estrogen clomiphene, when given in doses of 200 mg/day over a five-day period to normal subjects has been shown to cause rises in both plasma LH and testosterone to between 80 and 160% of basal values, an action that can be blocked by fairly substantial doses (80 mg/day) of the synthetic androgen fluoxymesterone. Bardin and others (50) have proposed this as a useful test of hypothalamic and pituitary function and have shown that these changes do not result from the diminished disposal of the steroid or from a direct effect of the compound on testicular steroidogenesis. In addition to androgens, estrogens (51,52) and progesterone analogues (53) cause a fall in the levels of plasma LH and testosterone. This inhibition of LH secretion, which has useful therapeutic implications, is achieved only relatively slowly (as compared, for instance, with ACTH) thus, following the administration of substantial inhibitory doses of estrogens or androgens, LH levels fall over the course of three or four days; likewise, plasma levels of testosterone also take several days to reach a nadir and from our own studies the secretion of neither hormone is completely suppressed even after weeks of such treatment (51).

INFANCY, CHILDHOOD, ADOLESCENCE AND OLD AGE

At the extremes of life there are distinct differences from the normal adult male pattern of testosterone secretion. In the immediate neonatal period, plasma levels are elevated in both male and female infants, but there is no significant sex difference (23,54). Both are significantly lower than the levels found in maternal plasma, but testosterone binding affinity is low in umbilical venous plasma and high in maternal plasma. From the data of Grumbach and his colleagues (24), it is not readily possible to calculate the proportion bound to protein, but presumably the level of free testosterone in fetal plasma is higher than is reflected by the total level. The fact that there should be no sex difference in plasma levels of testosterone at birth is of interest, taking into consideration the intense stimulation of the Leydig cells of the fetal testis that occurs during the second trimester. In one series there was a significant difference between male and female neonates in the levels of androstenedione, the values being higher in the former (54). If conventional male sex hormones are responsible for influencing the development of the male or female brain, then it can only be presumed that these influences have operated at an earlier stage of fetal development. Immediately after birth, plasma levels fall to values that are at, or below, the normal female range, and remain at this level until puberty. Frasier and Horton (55) have shown that during this period plasma levels of androstenedione are of the same order as is found in the adult male, that the androstenedione/testosterone ratio is the order of two or thereabouts, and that about 40% of testosterone is derived by conversion from androstenedione.

As puberty approaches in the male there is a gradual increase in the level of testosterone in plasma, a rise which follows the secretion of LH at that time (44,56,57). These measurable chemical changes precede by many months the physical manifestations of this metamorphosis, and can usefully be employed in the management of those adolescents about whom there is some concern for their sexual maturation. The finding of plasma levels of testosterone above the prepubertal but below the adult male range usually indicates that puberty is likely to proceed normally, and that watchful expectancy is the appropriate medical management.

At the other extreme of life, there is no abrupt fall in the level of plasma testosterone that might be taken to indicate the existence of a male climacteric, although low levels are sporadically encountered in septa-, octo- and nonogenarians. An interesting study in this context is that of Kent and Acone (58) who showed that the clearance of testosterone from blood fell progressively with advanced years; mean plasma levels of testosterone were also lower in older men, so that it would seem that Leydig cell activity does become impaired with age, and there is a fall in the secretion of testosterone. Is it possible that this reduced clearance might also be taken to imply a lower extrahepatic metabolism by which normally sensitive tissues are utilizing less testosterone with advancing years?

ABNORMALITIES OF TESTOSTERONE SECRETION

In the male, an apparent clinical deficiency of androgen secretion is more commonly encountered than androgen excess. Low levels of plasma testosterone can result from disorders that primarily and directly affect the testis and Leydig cell function, or from conditions in which these tissues are secondarily affected. Sometimes this is a consequence of a more generalized endocrine disorder, but at others the primary disease is not identifiably endocrine in origin.

Patients with Testicular Disorders

Following castration, the concentration of testosterone in plasma falls to very low levels within two or three days, and although testosterone can be measured in the plasma of these patients, there is reason to believe that it is derived by conversion from androstenedione. Patients with anorchia show similar findings (59).

Low levels of plasma testosterone are observed in patients with bilateral cryptorchidism, but these values are not usually as low as those found in the castrate or anorchic male. Although Leydig cell function in the cryptorchid male is normally reduced, or apparently absent, significant changes in the level of plasma testosterone can be observed following treatment with HCG, indicating the presence of Leydig cells or their precursors that are normally responsive to LH. The practical significance of this observation is that it may be used to indicate that testicular tissue is present outside the scrotum should surgical removal be contemplated.

Numerous studies have been made on the levels of plasma testosterone in Klinefelter's syndrome, the most common cause of male hypogonadism (36,45,46,60). These have shown that a fairly wide range of values may exist in this disease, from those found in the normal female to those observed in the adult male. Attempts by a number of workers to correlate testosterone levels with the chromatin pattern have not yielded useful correlates; that is, patients who were chromatin negative showed no consistent differences from those who were chromatin positive; nor was there any systematic correlation between plasma levels of testosterone and the presence of mosaicism or with an XXXY karyotype. We have attempted to correlate plasma levels with interstitial cell morphology, but have not found this to be helpful. Paulsen et al. have also pointed out the difficulty of correlating plasma levels of testosterone with the degree of secondary sexual development (46). It is of interest that in the few studies that have been made, plasma androstenedione appears to be normal in this disorder.

A number of studies have demonstrated the damage inflicted on the germinal epithelium by the presence of an additional X chromosome; what has yet to be satisfactorily explained is the morphology of the Leydig cells which frequently appear nodular, clumped or hyperplastic, the high levels of plasma LH and the lower than normal levels of plasma testosterone. One might well speculate that the additional X chromosome is also injurious to these cells, but that their biosynthetic capacity is not irreparably damaged. Is it that these cells need greater stimulation than normal in order to secrete testosterone? This could explain the high levels of LH and the hyperplastic appearance of these cells, the hormonal output of which may or may not be adequate, but still does not account for those patients with normal levels of testosterone and high levels of LH. Whatever the explanation, it seems clear that in these patients the biosynthetic capacities of the Leydig cells are reduced; the administration of additional exogenous HCG over a three or four day period may sometimes produce an increment in the level of plasma testosterone seen in the normal subject, but in some patients there is no such increment (46, 60).

Although not primarily a testicular disorder, it would seem relevant to refer to a number of studies that have been undertaken on males with an XYY chromosomal complement. Although these subjects may show distinctive physical and psychological features, abnormalities of testicular function do not appear to be present. We have investigated several such subjects and have found plasma levels of testosterone and LH to be normal (61,62). Other investigators have measured the rate of urinary excretion of testosterone glucuronide and have found it to be elevated (63,64). Methodological differences may explain these apparent discrepancies, particularly as plasma levels were not measured in the latter two studies.

Primary disorders of the testicle other than those that have been mentioned do not commonly show abnormalities of testosterone secretion. We have now investigated in excess of 40 patients with infertility associated with oligo- or azoospermia without apparent clinical abnormalities of androgen secretion. These patients have been shown to have germinal cell aplasia (the Sertoli cell only syndrome), germinal cell arrest, and other disorders of spermatogenesis, the nature of which was often quite obscure. Commonly, levels of plasma testosterone in these patients are within the normal range and respond appropriately to normal stimuli. In about 25% of these patients, however, plasma levels of testosterone are lower than normal (less than 300 ng/100 ml) and in this group the common morphological change is that of germinal cell aplasia. Such patients have high levels of FSH but normal LH. (65).

The testes may fail to mature because of primary gonadotropic failure or following removal of the gonadotropic stimulus before puberty; regression may also occur following removal of this stimulus after puberty. In such patients plasma levels of testosterone are usually lower than normal, the ultimate level depending upon the extent and duration of the failure of gonadotropic secretion. In patients with the rather unusual disorder of primary hypogonadotropic hypogonadism, plasma levels are in the female range and fail to respond to clomiphene; patients with hypopituitarism likewise show levels which vary from very low normal to normal, levels that generally correlate with the output of LH which is not invariably lost in all patients.

Disorders not Primarily Affecting the Testis.

Plasma levels of testosterone have been found to be abnormal in a variety of disorders that are not normally regarded as being primarily testicular in origin, although the testis may be involved incidentally in the disorder. Perhaps the best recognized of these is liver cirrhosis in which the triad of spiderangiomata, testicular atrophy and gynecomastia is well recognized, particularly when the disorder results from the ravages of alcohol. It has long been speculated that an excess of circulating estrogen is present and that plasma androgens may be normal or reduced in amount. Shaver et al. (66) have reported studies which suggested that blood levels of estrogen were elevated and Zumoff et al. (67) have shown that the metabolism of estradiol was abnormal in cirrhosis. Only recently have these suggestions been confirmed by the direct measurements made by Korenman et al. (68) who found that levels of plasma estradiol in men with cirrhosis were almost twice those of normal men. It is relevant that Tarvenetti et al.(69) have shown that the plasma binding of this steroid was increased in male and female patients with cirrhosis. Plasma levels of testosterone have been found to be low in patients with alcoholic cirrhosis (59). It has also been observed that levels of gonadotropins are lower than normal (71) and that the response to HCG appears to be blunted in this condition. These observations suggest that in cirrhosis the elevation of circulating estrogen levels inhibits testosterone secretion either directly or by reducing gonadotropin secretion, and it is the combination of high circulating estrogens and low testosterone which combine to produce the classical endocrine abnormalities of this disorder. The pathogenesis of this condition has yet to be proved formally.

Diminished sexual potency, features of hypogonadism and testicular atrophy are well recognized features of hemochromatosis. Stocks and Martin (72) have shown that in this disorder plasma levels of testosterone were below normal in about 50% of the subjects they studied; these values correlated well with levels of plasma LH which were also at or below the lower limit of normal, and with the appearance of the testis or biopsy. Tubular atrophy, reduction in the Leydig cell population and a virtual absence of stainable iron in the testis, were other important features. Collectively, these findings indicate that the lesion in this disorder is primarily a failure of pituitary function, a proposition that is supported by other evidence: low plasma thyroxine levels and diminished cortisol and growth hormone responses to hypoglycemic stress. This is thus in contrast to the situation that prevails in liver cirrhosis. Likewise, we have investigated three patients with transfusion hemisiderosis due to iron storage. These were adolescents with severe hypoplastic anemia who had received repeated blood transfusions over many years. All patients showed hypogonadism and testicular atrophy and were found to have abnormally low levels of plasma testosterone, but following the administration of HCG there was an increase in these levels. At necropsy in one patient, extensive deposition of iron was observed in the sinusoids of the anterior pituitary with minimal iron deposition in the testis.

The testicular lesions of leprosy have been known for some years (73), and have been likened to those observed in Klinefelter's syndrome with tubular hyalinization and clumping of Leydig cells. In a series of 10 patients with this disorder, some with gynecomastia, we have found high levels of urinary gonadotropins and low levels of testosterone in plasma, these changes in general correlating with the severity of hypogonadism and gynecomastia(74). At present, the reason for the predilection for tubular involvement in leprosy is obscure, but the hormonal changes would appear to be a direct consequence of testicular involvement in this disease.

ELEVATED PLASMA LEVELS OF TESTOSTERONE

Levels of plasma testosterone that are higher than normal are less frequently encountered. Undoubtedly the most dramatic examples are those unusual patients with sexual precocity, which may result from the inappropriate secretion of LH; idiopathic sexual precocity, from adrenal hyperplasia or tumor, or much less commonly, from interstitial cell tumors of the testis. In patients with inappropriate LH secretion, plasma levels of testosterone are usually elevated but these may vary from below the normal adult male range to values that are within this range. Administered HCG produces a further rise in these levels, while the administration of estrogens or medroxyprogesterone acetate (Provera) will lower the values (36,53). It is of interest that Provera has been found to be associated with a decrease in testosterone binding, and it is possible that while this drug will induce a lowering of total testosterone content in plasma (bound and unbound), the value of the unbound and active moiety may increase, or at least may remain unchanged, and thus may prevent the complete therapeutic efficacy of this compound.

An increased concentration of testosterone in plasma is also found in patients with both salt-losing and non salt-losing forms of congenital adrenal hyperplasia (CAH). Migeon (75) has shown that in all these patients there is a striking increase of the normal testosterone/androstenedione ratio with androstenedione levels of between 0.5 and 5 μg/100 ml. Further studies have shown that the increased concentration of testosterone in patients with CAH not only reflects an increased secretion of testosterone, but also the conversion to testosterone of androstenedione which may contribute up to 60% of the total blood production of testosterone. The abnormal secretion of androstenedione and the production of testosterone can be suppressed by the administration of corticosteroids.

Some solution to the apparent paradox of a normal feminine appearance and normal adult male levels of plasma testosterone in patients with the syndrome of testicular feminization has recently been suggested (76,78). It has been shown that skin taken from patients with this disorder did not convert testosterone to dihydrotestosterone as did normal controls (32,79). These observations provide additional evidence that at a tissue level the active form of testosterone is dihydrotestosterone, a proposition that has been strongly suggested by the work of Wilson et al. (80).

Levels of plasma testosterone have now been measured in a variety of clinical and experimental conditions, many but not all of which have been summarized in this paper. What has emerged from these fairly intensive studies over the past four to five years is that no level or group of levels may be entirely meaningful unless a proper account can be taken of the form in which the steroid is presented to the tissues; that is, unless there is some knowledge of the degree to which the steroid is bound. In this context it is of interest that plasma levels of testosterone have been found to be high in patients with untreated thyrotoxicosis (81,82). It has been shown further that the metabolic clearance of testosterone in these patients is reduced, an observation that has been related to an increased testosterone binding affinity of the plasma in these patients. The importance of steroid binding is further emphasized by the studies of Southren et al. (83) who showed that in hirsute female patients with the syndrome of polycystic ovaries and elevated levels of plasma testosterone, metabolic clearance was increased and binding reduced, so that by extrapolating in vitro studies as much as a six-fold rise in the unbound levels of testosterone might be predicted. In the reverse situation in the hypogonadal male, it is possible that simple measurement of the level of testosterone in blood may not yield a full measure of the androgenic stimulus unless some account is taken of the level of free or unbound steroid which, of course, may be significantly reduced if plasma levels of estrogen (known to increase binding) are also increased. From these studies it would seem important to point out that while measurements of plasma testosterone have been of material value in understanding some of the problems of the normal and disordered physiology of androgen secretion, future endeavors must be directed to determining the levels at which testosterone is present in the free or unbound form in the circulation and of the tissue or plasma levels of conversion products such as dihydrotestosterone.

ACKNOWLEDGEMENTS

This work has been supported by grants from the Australian National Health and Medical Research Council, and from the Anti-Cancer Council of Victoria.

REFERENCES

1. Murphy, B.E.P., Canad. J. Biochem., 46: 299, 1968.
2. Kato, T. and Horton, R., Steroids, 12: 631, 1968.
3. Mayes, D. and Nugent, C.A., J. Clin. Endocr., 28: 1169, 1968.
4. Hallberg, M.C., Zorn, E.M. and Wieland, R.G.Steroids, 21: 241, 1968.
5. Rosenfield, R.L., Eberlein, W.R. and Bongiovanni, A.M., J. Clin. Endocr., 29: 854, 1969.
6. Niswender, G.D. and Midgely, A.R., Proc. 51st Meeting Endocrine Society, 1969,(Abstract No. 22).
7. Finkelstein, M., Forchielli, E. and Dorfman, R.I., J. Clin. Endocr., 21: 98, 1961.
8. Hudson, B., Coghlan, J.P., Dulmanis, A., Wintour, M. and Ekkel, I., Aust. J. Exp. Biol. Med. Sci., 41: 235, 1963.
9. Riondel, A., Tait, J.F., Gut, M., Tait, S.A.S., Joachim, E.and Little, B., J. Clin. Endocr., 23: 620, 1963.
10. Burger, H.G., Kent, J.R. and Kellie, A.E., J. Clin. Endocr., 24: 432, 1964.
11. Kirschner, M.A., Lipsett, M.B. and Collins, D.R., J. Clin. Invest., 44: 657, 1965.
12. Rivarola, M.A. and Migeon, C.J., Steroids, 7: 103, 1966.
13. Gandy, H.M. and Peterson, R.E., J. Clin. Endocr., 28: 949, 1968.
14. Brownie, A.C., Van der Molen, H.J., Nishizawa, E.E. and Eik-Nes, K.B., J. Clin. Endocr., 24: 432, 1964.
15. Slaunwhite, W.R. and Sandberg, A.A., J. Clin. Invest., 38: 384, 1959.
16. Chen, D.S., Mills, I.H. and Bartter, F.C., J. Endocr., 23: 129, 1961.
17. Mercier, C. and Beaulieu, E.E., Ann. Endocr. (Paris), 29 (Suppl): 159, 1968.
18. Pearlman, W.H. and Crepy, O., J. Biol. Chem., 242: 182, 1967.
19. Rosner, W., Christy, N.P. and Kelly, W.G., Biochemistry (Wash), 8: 3100, 1969.
20. Vermeulen, A. and Verdonck, L., Steroids, 11: 609, 1968.
21. Kato, T. and Horton, R., J. Clin. Endocr., 28: 1160, 1968.

22. Barlow, J.J., MacLaren, J.A. and Pothier, L., J. Clin. Endocr., 29: 767, 1969.
23. Rivarola, M.A., Forrest, M.G. and Migeon, C.J., J. Clin. Endocr., 28: 34, 1968.
24. August, G.P., Tkachuk, M. and Grumbach, M.M., J. Clin. Endocr., 29: 891, 1969.
25. Horton, R. and Tait, J.F., J. Clin. Invest., 45: 301, 1966.
26. Hudson, B., Dulmanis, A., Coghlan, J.P. and Wintour, M., Aust. Ann. Med., 15: 236, 1966.
27. Rivarola, M.A., Saez, J.M., Meyer, W.J., Jenkins, M.E. and Migeon, C.J., J. Clin. Endocr., 26: 1208, 1966.
28. Bardin, C.W. and Lipsett, M.B., J. Clin. Invest., 46:891, 1967.
29. Southren, A.L., Gordon, G.G., Tochimoto, S., Pinzon, G., Lane, D.R. and Stypuckowski, W., J. Clin. Endocr., 27: 686, 1967.
30. Bird, C.E., Green, R.N. and Clark, A.F., J. Clin. Endocr., 29: 123, 1969.
31. Gomez, E.C. and Hsia, S.L., Biochemistry (Wash), 7: 24, 1968.
32. Wilson, J.D. and Walker, J.D., J. Clin. Invest., 48: 371, 1969.
33. Dray, F., Reinberg, A. and Sebaun, J.C.R., C.R. Seanc. Acad. Sci., 261: 573, 1965.
34. Southren, A.L., Gordon, G.G. and Tochimoto, S., J. Clin. Endocr., 25: 1441, 1965.
35. Resko, J.A. and Eik-Nes, K.B., J. Clin. Endocr., 26: 573, 1966.
36. Hudson, B., Coghlan, J.P. and Dulmanis, A., Ciba.Found. Colloq. Endocr., Endocrinology of the Testis, 16: 140, 1967.
37. Faiman, C. and Ryan, R.J., Nature, (London) 215: 85, 1967.
38. Peterson, N.T., Midgley, A.R. and Jaffe, R.B. J. Clin. Endocr., 28: 1473, 1968.
39. Saxena, B.B. and Gandy, H.M., Symposium on in vitro Procedures with Radioisotopes in Clinical Medicine and Research. Vienna 1969.
40. Burger, H.G., Brown, J.B., Catt, K.J., Hudson, B. and Stockigt, J.S., In Protein and Polypeptide Hormones, ed. Margoulies, M., Excerpta Medica Foundation International Congress Series, Amsterdam, 161: 412, 1968.
41. Tait, J.F. and Horton, R., Steroids, 4: 365, 1964.
42. Korenman, S.G. and Lipsett, M.B. J. Clin. Invest., 43: 2125, 1964.
43. Baird, D.T., Horton, R., Longcope, C.T., Tait, J.F., Perspect. Biol. Med., 11: 384, 1968.
44. Hudson, B., Coghlan, J.P., Dulmanis, A. and Wintour, M. Excerpta Medica Foundation International Congress Series, Amsterdam., 83: 1127, 1967.
45. Lipsett, M.B., Davis, T.E., Wilson, H. and Canfield, C.J., J. Clin. Endocr., 25: 1027, 1965.

46. Paulsen, C.A., Gordon, D.L., Carpenter, R.W., Gandy, H.M. and Drucker, W.D., Recent Progr. Hormone Res., 24: 321, 1968.
47. Means, A.R. and Hall, P.F., Endocrinology, 81: 1151, 1967.
48. de Kretser, D.M., Taft, H.P., Brown, J.B., Evans, J.H., and Hudson, B., J. Endocr., 40: 197, 1968.
49. Steinberger, E. and Duckett, G., Acta. Endocr., (Kobenhavn) 57: 289, 1968.
50. Bardin, C.W., Ross, G.T. and Lipsett, M.B., J. Clin. Endocr., 27: 155, 1967.
51. Alder, A.B., Burger, H.G., Davis, J., Dulmanis, A., Hudson, B. Sarfaty, G.A. and Straffon, W., Brit. Med. J., 1: 28, 1968.
52. Young, H.H. and Kent, J.R., J. Urol., 99: 788, 1968.
53. Rivarola, M.A., Camacho, A.M. and Migeon, C.J. J. Clin. Endocr., 28: 679, 1968.
54. Mizuno, M., Lobotsky, J., Lloyd, C.W., Kobayashi, T. and Murasawa, Y., J. Clin. Endocr., 28: 1133, 1968.
55. Frasier, S.O. and Horton, R., Steroids, 8: 777, 1966.
56. Boon, D.A., Keenan, R.E., Slaunwhite, W.R. and Aceto, T. Excerpta Medica Foundation International Congress Series, Amsterdam, 157: 52, 1968 (Abstract).
57. Johanson, A.J., Guda, H., Light, C., Migeon, C.J. and Blizzard, R.J., J. Pediat . 74: 416, 1969.
58. Kent, J.R. and Acone, A.B., In Androgens in Normal and Pathological Conditions, eds.Vermeulen, A. Exley, D., Excerpta Medica Foundation International Congress Series, Amsterdam, 101: 31, 1966.
59. Coppage, W.S. and Cooner, A.E., New Eng. J. Med. 273: 902, 1965.
60. Lipsett, M.B., Wilson, H., Kirschner, M.A., Korenman, S.G., Fishman, L.M., Sarfaty, G.A. and Bardin, C.W., Recent Progr. Hormone Res., 22: 245, 1966.
61. Wiener, S., Sutherland, G., Bartholomew, A.A. and Hudson, B., Lancet, 1: 150, 1968.
62. Hudson, B., Burger, H.G., Wiener, S., Sutherland, G. and Bartholomew, A.A., Lancet, 2: 699, 1969.
63. Ismail, A.A., Harkness, R.A., Kirkham, K.E., Loraine, J.A., Whatmore, P.B. and Brittain, R.P., Lancet, 1: 220, 1968.
64. Rudd, B.T., Galal, O.M. and Casey, M.D., J. Med. Genet., 5: 286, 1968.
65. de Kretser, D. M., Studies on the Structure and Function of the Human Testis . M.D. Thesis, Monash University, 1968.
66. Shaver, J.C., Roginsky, M.S. and Christy, M.P.,Lancet, 2: 335, 1963.
67. Zumoff, B., Fishman, J., Gallagher, T.F. and Hellman, L., J. Clin. Invest., 47: 20, 1968.
68. Korenman, S.G., Perrin, L.E. and McCallum, T., Proc. 61st Meeting American Society Clin. Invest., 1969, (Abstract No.144).
69. Tarvenetti, R.R., Rosenbaum, W., Kelly, W.G., Christy, N.P. and Roginski, M.S., J. Clin. Endocr., 27: 920, 1967.

70. Taft, H.P., Seah, C.S., Burger, H.G. and Hudson, B., Unpublished Observations.
71. Rosselin, G. and Dolais, J., Press Med., 75: 2027, 1967.
72. Stocks, A.E. and Martin, F.I.R., Amer. J. Med. Sci., 45: 839, 1968.
73. Grastbald, H. and Swan, L.L., J.A.M.A., 149: 1287, 1952.
74. Martin, F.I.R., Maddocks, I., Brown, J.B. and Hudson, B., Lancet, 2: 1320, 1968.
75. Migeon, C.J., Ann. Intern. Med. , 68: 1329, 1968.
76. Southren, A.L., Tochimoto, S., Carmody, N.C. and Isurugi, K., J. Clin. Endocr., 25: 1441, 1965.
77. Deshpande, N., Wang, D.Y., Bulbrook, R.D. and McMillan, M., Steroids, 4: 437, 1965.
78. French, F.S., Van Wyk, J.J., Baggett, B., Easterling, W.E., Talbert, L.M., Johnston, F.R., Forchielli, E. and Day, A.C., J. Clin. Endocr., 26: 493, 1966.
79. Northcutt, R.C., Island, D.F. and Liddle, G.W., J. Clin. Endocr., 29: 422, 1969.
80. Wilson, D.J., Bruchovsky, N. and Chatfield, J.H., Excerpta Medica Foundation International Congress Series, Amsterdam, 184: 17, 1968.
81. Dreyfus, G., Sebaoun, J., Delzant, G., Dray, F., Ledru, M.J. and Crepy, O., Excerpta Medica Foundation International Congress Series, Amsterdam, 157: 55, 1968.
82. Gordon, G.G., Southren, A.L., Tochimoto, S., Rand, J.J. and Olivo, J., J. Clin. Endocr., 29: 164, 1969.
83. Southren, A.L., Gordon, G.G., Tochimoto, S., Olivo, J., Sherman, D.H. and Pinzon, G., J. Clin. Endocr., 29: 1356, 1969.

DISCUSSION

PAULSEN: Dr. Hudson, is the basis for the discrepancy between plasma testosterone and serum HLH levels in patients with Klinefelter's syndrome known? Do you have any data which indicate that there may be a difference in testosterone binding in the plasma of these patients as opposed to the normal male?

HUDSON: We do not, but in a paper by Vermeulen and Verdonk in the Journal of Clinical Endocrinology (November, 1969) they report that binding in hypogonadal males was increased. I am not certain that patients with Klinefelter's syndrome were included among these.

SAVARD: Dr. Hudson, in your values for testosterone secretion in the prepubertal and the neonatal children, did you make concomitant measurements of androstenedione? In other words, is testicular function in the youngsters reflected in a more abundant production of androstenedione? Your data showed at least in the prepubertal children that a substantial amount of testosterone was derived from androstenedione. The testis itself in its prepubertal state may conceivably be elaborating androstenedione as its major product. I think that this has certainly been observed in animals by Lindner.

HUDSON: I do not have that data from my own laboratory, but in a paper from Lloyd's group in which levels of androstenedione in cord blood were estimated, they showed high levels for this steroid in males.

DICZFALUSY: Dr. Hudson, would you consider that in cord blood you will find some testosterone because the placenta secretes androstenedione and this is converted by the fetal liver to testosterone?

HUDSON: Yes, I would consider this.

LIPSETT: In the prepubertal child Fraser and Johnson showed that testosterone levels are higher in boys than in girls although androstenedione levels were the same. We have recently performed studies in the rat. At 20 days of age when there is absolutely no evidence of increase in secondary sexual characteristics in prostate or seminal vesicle weight, there are only few Leydig cells, but one can clearly demonstrate testosterone secretion, although peripheral testosterone levels still remain unmeasurable. Only subsequently does Leydig cell activity increase and peripheral values of testosterone begin to rise.

BERGADA: We have treated prepuberal boys with HCG. Three groups of patients were treated. We gave 800 IU of HCG daily in one group, 2,000 and 4,000 in the others, and the mean response in three groups was approximately the same with a large range. It seems that there is no dose response relationship with an HCG stimulation test given for five days.

HUDSON: I am very interested in those data, because there has been some discussion about what is the appropriate dose of HCG. We have used 1500 IU of HCG daily for four days. It would seem that this is an adequate dose as a test of testicular function, and this is the reason we have used it.

E. STEINBERGER: I would like to make a comment on Dr. Hudson's paper. He stressed the "methodological" noise interference in detection of fine changes in testosterone production. I would just like to add one more noise, namely the "patient noise". Doctors Persky and Smith of our group obtained data on a group of college students, aged 17 to 22 years, who were given a series of psychologic tests to determine the levels of aggression and hostility. The psychological test scores were plotted against testosterone production rates. An excellent positive correlation between these two parameters was observed ($R= + 0.66$; $p < 001$, for 17 dt). The predicted testosterone production rates of these patients based on their psychologic scores again showed an excellent correlation. These results suggest an additional parameter related to testosterone production rate.

RELATION OF IN VITRO METABOLISM OF STEROIDS IN HUMAN TESTICULAR TISSUE TO HISTOLOGIC AND CLINICAL FINDINGS

E. Steinberger, M. Ficher and K.D. Smith

Division of Endocrinology and Reproduction, Research Laboratories, Albert Einstein Medical Center, Philadelphia, Pa. 19141

INTRODUCTION

The first definitive evidence for androgen secretion by the human testis was provided by experiments demonstrating the formation of radioactive testosterone and androstenedione in spermatic venous effluent following perfusion of the testis with acetate ^{14}C (1). Lucas et al. (2) isolated testosterone from spermatic vein blood, and subsequently a number of investigators demonstrated conversion of suitable steroidal precursors to androgens by human testicular tissue in vitro (3-7). Deficiency of the side-chain cleaving enzyme in testicular tissue of an older man was shown by Axelrod (5). Carstensen (3) demonstrated in vitro an increased conversion of 17α-hydroxypregnenolone to testosterone in the presence of ICSH. He suggested that the side-chain cleaving enzyme may be activated by gonadotropins. A suppression of the activity of the side-chain cleaving enzyme and the 17α-hydroxylase, but no change, or possibly an increase, in the activity of 17 β-hydroxysteroid dehydrogenase was demonstrated in the microsomal fraction of testicular tissue from a patient with prostatic carcinoma treated with estrogens (8). If the assumption is made that estrogen suppressed patients' endogenous gonadotropins, the decrease in 17-20 lyase may be interpreted as confirmation of Carstensen's findings.

On the other hand, Schoen (7), also utilizing testicular tissue from prostatic cancer patients treated with estrogens, demonstrated suppression of testosterone formation from androstenedione and concluded that gonadotropins may be essential for the activity of 17 β-hydroxysteroid dehydrogenase. Similarly, Slaunwhite et al. (4), utilizing testicular tissue from patients with prostatic carcinoma, showed that long-term estrogen therapy prevented the reduction of androstenedione to testosterone, but did not affect the conversion of 17α-hydroxyprogesterone to androstenedione.

The above briefly summarized studies clearly indicate that human testicular tissue can incorporate simple precursors like acetate into the steroid molecule and convert suitable steroidal precursors to androgens. Also, these studies have elucidated, at least in part, the biogenetic pathways leading to formation of androgens in human testicular tissue. However, information concerned with the hormonal control of this biosynthetic process is still controversial and fragmentary. Furthermore, most studies reported to date were performed on testicular tissue from elderly patients with carcinoma of the prostate. Consequently, almost no information is available on the steroid biosynthetic activity of testes from patients of reproductive age, with various spontaneously occurring disorders of testicular function. Since the only practical way to obtain testicular tissue in such patients is by means of surgical biopsy, techniques for study of steroid biosynthesis in small amounts of testicular tissue are required.

Danezis (9) and Schoen (7) have shown that it is possible to demonstrate in vitro conversion of steroidal precursors to androgens in as little as 20 mg. of testicular tissue. In the study reported here, we re-evaluated the feasibility of utilizing small amounts of human testicular tissue and made an attempt to correlate the pattern of progesterone metabolism in testicular tissue, obtained either by orchiectomy or surgical biopsy, with the histologic appearance of the testes, the clinical picture of the patient, and in some instances, with in vivo biochemical parameters of androgen secretion.

MATERIALS AND METHODS

A. Source of testicular tissue. The age and diagnosis for each patient are summarized in Tables 1 and 2.

B. Hormonal studies: Urinary levels of FSH were determined by the Steelman-Pohley technique (10), and LH by the rat ovarian ascorbic acid depletion technique (11). Plasma testosterone (P.T.) levels were determined by the technique of Horton et al. (12), and the testosterone production rates (T.P.R.) by the technique of Rivarola et al. (13).

C. Chromosomal studies: A micro-technique employing whole blood was utilized (14).

D. Steroid biosynthetic studies: Minced testicular tissue was incubated with ^{3}H-progesterone (20×10^6 dpm, 3 mμ mole, dissolved in 1.5 ml of incubation medium) for 3 hr. in a Dubnoff shaker at 37°C in an atmosphere of 95% air and 5% CO_2. The incubation was terminated by the addition of 10 ml ethyl acetate. At this point, appropriate ^{14}C labelled tracers (40,000 dpm of each) were also added to the incubate in order to correct for losses in subsequent manipulations. The material was then frozen until further processing. Com-

Table 1. Testicular Tissue Obtained at Orchiectomy

Case	Age	Diagnosis
A	71 years	Carcinoma of the prostate
B	65 years	Carcinoma of the prostate
C	79 years	Carcinoma of the prostate
D	22 years	Testicular feminization

Table 2. Testicular Tissue Obtained at Biopsy

Case	Age	Diagnosis
E	24 years	Klinefelter's syndrome
F	26 years	Carcinoma of contralateral testicle
G	36 years	Azoospermia and impotence
H	32 years	Azoospermia and impotence
I	18 years	Oligospermia and gynecomastia
J	35 years	Oligospermia and varicocele
K	29 years	Oligospermia and liver disease
L	26 years	Oligospermia
M	25 years	Oligospermia

position of incubation medium (for total volume of 1.5 ml);

1 ml Hank's balanced salt solution
125 µl 1.3% $NaHCO_3$
175 µl NADP,Na solution (3.257 µmole/ml)
175 µl G-6-P,Na_2 solution (36.17 µmole/ml)
25 µl ethanol

The extraction procedure and the techniques of separation and identification of the steroid metabolites have been described elsewhere (15). The final identification and quantitation of some of the steroids was accomplished by the technique of derivative formation and isotopic dilution and crystallization to constant $^3H/^{14}C$ ratio or constant specific activity.

RESULTS

1) Metabolism of Progesterone by Various Amounts of Testicular Tissue

Tissue from Case A was utilized in amounts varying from 10 to 100 mg. per incubation flask, providing for approximate ratios of substrate to tissue from 1:15,000 to 1:100,000. The results obtained after first chromatography in a Bush A system are summarized in Table 3. No significant difference was observed at tissue ratios varying from 1:30,000 to 1:100,000; a diminution in capacity to metabolize progesterone was observed at the ratio of 1:15,000.

About 50% of the precursor was converted to metabolites with the chromatographic mobility of testosterone and 17α-hydroxyprogesterone. This material was further worked up and the percent conversion to testosterone and 17α-hydroxyprogesterone determined (Table 3). No significant differences in conversion of progesterone to testosterone were observed at ratios 1:30,000 to 1:100,000.

Small amounts of progesterone were converted to material with the chromatographic mobility of 20α-dihydroprogesterone and androstenedione, and about 20% to highly "polar" metabolites. The identity of 20α-dihydroprogesterone and androstenedione was confirmed by repeated chromatography in several systems and isotopic dilution and crystallization to constant specific activity.

2) Progesterone Metabolism in Testicular Tissue of Patients with Carcinoma of the Prostate

In all cases, progesterone was actively metabolized. However, differences in the amounts of progesterone converted to specific metabolites were observed (Table 4). Utilization of ^{14}C labelled tracers and crystallization to constant $^{3}H/^{14}C$ ratios permitted relatively precise determination of the percent conversions of progesterone to testosterone and 17α-hydroxyprogesterone. The tissue from Case A was very actively converting progesterone to 17α-hydroxyprogesterone (50% was converted), but only 1.0 percent of progesterone was converted to testosterone. Low level metabolism of progesterone was observed in tissue from Case B, and fairly active metabolism was observed in tissue from Case C. In all cases, in addition to 17α-hydroxyprogesterone and testosterone, 20α-dihydroprogesterone and androstenedione were formed. These metabolites were identified by isotopic dilution and crystallization to constant specific activity. The "polar" materials in tissues from Cases A and C were rechromatographed, utilizing thin layer technique. Material with the chromatographic behavior of 17 β-estradiol was detected. Its identity was confirmed by isotopic dilution and crystallization to constant specific activity (Table 5). Microscopic examination of the biopsies revealed spermatogenic activity, including mature spermatozoa in all specimens (Fig.1). The Leydig cells in the biopsies varied markedly, and did not correlate with the biochemical data. Tissue with the greatest capacity for conversion of progesterone to 17α-hydroxyprogesterone and testosterone (Case A) showed only sparse but well formed Leydig cells (Fig. 1a), while tissue showing the least conversion (Case B) revealed the largest masses of Leydig cells (Fig. 1b).

Table 3. Metabolism of Progesterone by Various Amounts of Testicular Tissue*

METABOLITES	SUBSTRATE TO TISSUE RATIOS						
	1:15,000	1:30,000		1:50,000		1:100,000	
		p	pc	p	pc	p	pc
"Polar Compounds	13	27		15		17	
Testosterone	20	39	0.7	52	0.9	53	1.0
17α-hydroxyprogesterone			38.0		50.0		50.0
20α-dihydroprogesterone	6	5		9		6	
Androstenedione	1	1		2		2	
Progesterone (unconverted substrate)	60	28		21		21	

p - percent of radioactivity recovered in respective zones after the first chromatography in Bush A system

pc -percent conversion of progesterone to testosterone and 17α-hydroxyprogesterone

* - tissue from Case A (see Table 1) was used

Table 4. Conversion of Progesterone by Testicular Tissue From Patients with Carcinoma of the Prostate

METABOLITES	SOURCE OF TISSUE					
	A		B		C	
	p	pc	p	pc	p	pc
"Polar" compounds	17		13		23	
Testosterone	53	1.0	8	0.3	29	2.0
17α-hydroxyprogesterone		50.0		8.0		26.0
20α-dihydroprogesterone	6		13		10	
Androstenedione	2		3		2	
Progesterone (unconverted substrate)	21		37		27	

p - percent of radioactivity recovered in respective zones after the first chromatography in Bush A system

pc - percent conversion of progesterone to testosterone and 17α-hydroxyprogesterone

Table 5. 17β-Estradiol Crystallization to Constant $^{3}H/^{14}C$ Ratio

		Case A	Case C	Case E
Crystallization #1	xls[a]	0.86[b]	0.86[b]	1.04[b]
Crystallization #2	xls	0.96[b]	0.82[b]	1.09[b]
Crystallization #3	xls	0.88[b]	1.06	0.97[b]
MEAN ± S.E.		0.90±0.03	0.84±0.02	1.03±0.035

a - crystals
b - $^{3}H/^{14}C$ ratio used for calculation of the mean ± S.D.

3) Metabolism of Progesterone in Testicular Tissue Obtained by Means of Surgical Biopsy

Unfortunately, we do not have data on progesterone metabolism in testicular tissue from perfectly normal individuals. Thus, no absolute comparisons can be made. However, the information obtained, when related to the data on plasma testosterone levels and testosterone production rates of the same patients and compared with the P.T. levels and T.P.R. of normal individuals, provides interesting information (Table 6)

a) Azoospermia. Two patients (G and H) with spontaneously occurring azoospermia and a gradual onset of impotence of three to four years' duration, and one patient (E) with azoospermia associated with Klinefelter's syndrome were studied. The laboratory data are summarized in Table 7. Unfortunately, no P.T. levels or T.P.R. are available for the patient with Klinefelter's syndrome. Both patients with impotence (G and H) showed markedly depressed P.T. levels, while no urinary gonadotropins were detected in Case H. Histologic study of the testis showed almost complete degeneration of seminiferous tubules in Case G, with masses of Leydig cells forming "pseudoadenomas" in some areas (Fig. 1d). Case H showed immature seminiferous tubules lined with "supporting cells" and no evidence of Leydig cells (Fig. 1e). Testes from the patient with Klinefelter's syndrome (Case E) revealed occasional seminiferous tubules containing germinal epithelium cells and large masses of Leydig cells (Fig. 1f).

Results of steroid studies are summarized in Table 8. In incubates of tissue from Case G, most of the progesterone (71%) remained unmetabolized, in spite of the fact that the tissue contained masses of Leydig cells and the levels of gonadotropins were elevated. This low steroid metabolic activity of the tissue was also reflected by the extremely low P.T. levels and T.P.R. Similarly, low levels of steroid metabolism were observed in testicular incubates from Case H, also reflected by low P.T. levels and T.P.R., but associated with atrophy of Leydig cells. In incubates of testicular tissue

Table 6. Plasma Testosteoone Levels and Production Rates, Urinary LH and FSH Levels in a Group of Normal Males 18 to 26 Years of Age with Sperm Counts Over 80 Million

	P.T. mμg/100 ml	T.P.R. mg/24 hrs.	LH* I.U./24 hrs.	FSH* I.U./24 hrs.
MEAN	685	10.1	7.4	1.8
S.D.	195	3.6	4.8	1.4
N	18	18	25	24

*LH and FSH expressed in terms of 2nd I.R.P.

Table 7. Summary of Laboratory Data for 3 Patients with Azoospermia

Case	P.T. mμg/100 ml	T.P.R. mg/day	LH I.U./24 hrs.	FSH I.U/24 hrs.	Karyotype
G	303	1.82	52.3	14.9	46/XY
H	196	1.52	*not detect.	*not detect.	46/XY
E	-	-	1.2	12.5	47/XXY

*Tested in 24 hr. aliquots of urine
Gonadotropins expressed in terms of 2nd I.R.P.

Table 8. Metabolism of Progesterone by Biopsies from Patients with Azoospermia (G and H), Klinefelter's Syndrome (E) and Testicular Feminization (D)

METABOLITES	Case G p	Case G pc	Case H p	Case H pc	Case E p	Case E pc	Case D p	Case D pc
"Polar" compounds	0		15		29		40	
Testosterone	18	0.7	18	0.7	43	9.0	27	12
17α-hydroxyprogesterone		8.3		1.2		30.0		22
20α-dihydroprogesterone	5		4		3		3	
Androstenedione	1		1		2		2	
Progesterone (unconverted substrate)	71		59		10		15	

p- percent of radioactivity recovered in respective zones after first chromatography in Bush A system

pc- percent conversion of progesterone to testosterone and 17α-hydroxyprogesterone from the patient with Klinefelter's syndrome (Case E), progesterone was avidly metabolized and readily converted to testosterone (Table 8). The identity of the small amounts of materials with chromatographic mobilities of androstenedione and 20α-dihydroprogesterone was confirmed by isotopic dilution and crystallization to constant specific activity.

b) Oligospermia. Six patients with oligospermia were studied. Except for Case F, with carcinoma of the contralateral testicle, the oligospermia was of unexplained origin. The laboratory findings in these patients, except for Case F, are summarized in Table 9. The appearance of biopsies is illustrated in Fig. 2. The distribution of radioactivity after first chromatography in Bush A system is illustrated in Table 10. Again, a marked difference in the capacity of the tissues from the different patients to metabolize progesterone can be seen. In two patients (Iand J), we were able to obtain P.T. levels and T.P.R. It is of interest to note that patient J had both depressed P.T. levels and T.P.R. and no elevation of gonadotropin levels. His testicular tissue metabolized progesterone avidly, but the conversion to testosterone was very low, only 1.1%. In the Bush A system, the bulk of the material showing the Rf value of testosterone and 17α-hydroxyprogesterone did not turn out to be either of these two metabolites. The identity of this metabolite and the metabolite migrating like androsterone are presently being investigated. Patient I's testosterone production rates and plasma levels were within normal limits for this age male (Table 9), and while his testicular tissue did not metabolize progesterone as avidly as J, it formed testosterone more readily and converted progesterone to 17α-hydroxyprogesterone very actively.

In spite of the biochemical differences, the histological appearance of the testicular biopsies of patients I and J was similar (Fig. 2b,c). Both show spermatogenic activity, and the Leydig cells in Case I seem to be actually less prominent than in Case J, the latter showing large clumps of Leydig cells in the interstitial area. Comparison of biopsies from Cases K, L and M and the biochemical data again reveals lack of correlation. The most active metabolism of progesterone and highest conversion to testosterone was observed in tissue from Case M. Histological examination of the biopsies, however, showed well developed Leydig cells in Cases K and L, and only sparsely distributed Leydig cells in Case M (Fig. 2e,d, f). The least active progesterone metabolism observed in Case F was associated with numerous Leydig cells forming large clumps in the biopsy tissue (Fig. 2a).

4) Metabolism of Progesterone by Testicular Tissue from a Patient with the Syndrome of "Testicular Feminization"

The histologic appearance of the biopsy is illustrated in Fig. 3. The tubules are lined with Sertoli cells and surrounded by mas-

Table 9. Laboratory Data on Patients with Oligospermia

Case	mμg/100 ml	mg/24 hrs.	I.U./24 hrs.	I.U./24 hrs.	Sperm Count million/ml
I	981	9.82	1.7	2.1	<1
J	343	5.74	1.0	3.9	18-50
K	-	-	74.0	3.2	8-37
L	-	-	38.5	6.2	10-40
M	-	-	-	-	4-10

ses of Leydig cells. Distribution of radioactivity in a Bush A chromatogram and percent conversion to testosterone and 17α-hydroxyprogesterone are summarized in Table 8. The progesterone was actively metabolized (15% remained unconverted) and considerable amounts of 17α-hydroxyprogesterone (22%) and testosterone (12%) were formed. A large proportion of progesterone (40%) was converted to highly polar metabolites. Thin layer chromatography of the polar metabolite revealed material with the mobility of 17 β-estradiol. Its identity was confirmed by crystallization to constant specific activity (Table 5).

DISCUSSION

In most instances the etiology of spermatogenic defects in the human male still falls into the category of "idiopathic". A number of reasons are responsible for this. Our understanding of the mechanisms involved in hormonal control of mammalian, and particularly human, spermatogenesis is meagre (16). There are a lack of precise techniques for quantitative evaluation of sperm production by the testes, and the techniques for assessment of testicular androgen production are difficult. While it has been clearly established that gonadotropins are essential for testicular function, the role of androgens, particularly in human spermatogenesis, remains obscure. The possibility that steroids other than testosterone may play an important role in spermatogenesis has been suggested.

Techniques for relatively precise measurements of testosterone plasma levels and production rates are now available. However, the problems of extratesticular conversion of testosterone precursors, as well as testosterone and its metabolites, create difficulties in studies of lesions in the steroid biogenetic pathways.

A technique permitting an investigation of pathways leading to the biogenesis of androgens in testicular tissue has been applied in the present study in an attempt to look for possible enzymic lesions in testes with various forms of spermatogenic abnormalities. This

TABLE 10. METABOLISM OF PROGESTERONE BY TESTICULAR TISSUE FROM PATIENTS WITH OLIGOSPERMIA

	PATIENTS											
	I		J		K		L		M		F	
METABOLITES	p	pc	p	pc	p	pc	p	pc	p	pc	p	pc
"Polar" compounds	18				47		15		21		12	
Testosterone	49	3.0	50	1.1	23	1.2	30	1,2	44	2.0	12	0.6
17α-hydroxyprogesterone		32.0		2.0		16.0		18.0		-		11.0
20α-dihydroprogesterone	2		4		10		6		6		2	
Androstenedione	1		2		2		1		0.6		1	
Androsterone	-		33		-		-				-	
Progesterone (unconverted substrate)	29		6		41		36		28		59	

p - percent of radioactivity recovered in respective zones after first chromatography in Bush A system

pc - percent conversion of progesterone to testosterone and 17α-hydroxyprogesterone technique can only provide information concerning the presence or activity of the various enzymes involved in the steroidogenic pathway, and its quantitative aspects are difficult to evaluate when information concerning endogenous pools of the steroid precursors and metabolites is not available. Concentrations of the various steroids in testicular tissue, their production rates or the secretory activity of the tissue cannot be assessed by this technique. Furthermore, utilization of progesterone in experiments described here limits the evaluation of the pathways and provides no information concerning the capacity of tissue to synthesize the steroid nucleus de novo from acetate, nor its capacity to convert cholesterol to C-21 and C-19 compounds. In spite of these limitations, this technique provides a sensitive tool for in vitro studies of the enzymes involved in steroid biosynthesis.

A positive correlation between plasma levels and production rate of testosterone and the in vitro capacity of testicular tissue to metabolize progesterone to testosterone has been demonstrated. In patient I, the normal testosterone production rate and plasma level were associated with the active conversion of progesterone to testosterone. In patients G and H, the markedly depressed testosterone production rates and plasma levels were associated with marginal conversion of progesterone to testosterone in vitro.

The isolation and identification of 17α-hydroxyprogesterone, androstenedione, 20α-dihydroprogesterone and testosterone indicate the presence of 17α-hydroxylase, 17-20-lyase, 17β-hydroxysteroid dehydrogenase and 20α-hydroxysteroid dehydrogenase in testicular tissues of older males, males of reproductive age with various forms of oligospermia, and patients with Klinefelter's syndrome and testicular feminization. Also, the capacity to aromatize ring A and form 17β-estradiol by tissues from elderly individuals and a patient with testicular feminization was demonstrated.

The above mentioned enzymic activities have been amply demonstrated to occur in testicular tissue from a variety of mammalian species. However, except for a number of studies with testicular tissues from patients with testicular feminization, only a limited number of experiments with non-tumorous human testicular tissue has been reported (3,5,6,8); and those reported, except for study of one specimen of tissue from a 16-year old male, were performed on older individuals suffering with carcinoma of the prostate.

In studies with immature rats treated with HCG, Steinberger and Ficher (17) called attention to the lack of correlation between the histological appearance of Leydig cells and the ability of the tissue to convert progesterone to testosterone. The studies reported here demonstrated a similar lack of correlation in human testicular tissue. Of partial interest is the biopsy from patient G showing masses of Leydig cells in the form of "pseudoadenomas", but only marginal capacity for in vitro metabolism of progesterone, with low plasma levels and production rates of testosterone, associated with elevated urinary levels of gonadotropins.

Similar lack of correlation was observed in biopsies of patients with oligospermia. This can be illustrated by comparing Cases I and J. The tissue from Case J shows large clumps of Leydig cells, while Case I shows a small number of dispersed Leydig cells. Both tissues metabolize progesterone avidly, but in an entirely different manner, tissue from patient I converting progesterone more readily to 17α-hydroxyprogesterone and testosterone, while tissue from patient J was almost unable to perform 17α-hydroxylation.

These findings clearly demonstrate a dichotomy between morphological characteristics and steroid biogenetic capacity of Leydig cells, a phenomenon not appreciated in the past, but one which provides further evidence for the concepts of steroid biosynthetic lesions in Leydig cells. Furthermore, these observations suggest that microscopic interpretation of testicular biopsies needs to be tempered with considerable caution when judgments concerning the secretory capacity of the Leydig cells are made.

Studies with tissue from the patient with Klinefelter's syndrome (Case E) demonstrated its capacity to convert progesterone to 17α-hydroxyprogesterone, androstenedione and testosterone. In fact, it showed the greatest capacity for testosterone formation of all tissues studied, except for that from testicular feminization. These studies suggest that the pathway of progesterone to testosterone is intact in the testis of a patient with Klinefelter's syndrome. Since, to our knowledge, this is the first report of such a study in Klinefelter's syndrome, evaluation of further cases will be necessary before a generalization can be made.

Demonstration of an active steroid biogenetic pathway in the testis from a case of testicular feminization in this study confirms a number of similar findings in the literature. The detection of 17β-estradiol confirms the findings of some investigators (18-21), but not of others (22-24).

In summary, we have demonstrated that it is feasible to utilize minute amounts of human testicular tissue obtainable by means of surgical biopsy for the study of steroid biogenetic pathways. Formation of testosterone from progesterone was demonstrated in testicular tissue of elderly individuals with carcinoma of the prostate and in the testicular tissue of man of reproductive age suffering with azoospermia, oligospermia, Klinefelter's syndrome and testicular feminization. In some cases, the lack of correlation between the ability of the testicular tissue to form testosterone and the microscopic characteristics of the Leydig cells was observed. In cases where it was studied, a correlation between the ability of testicular tissue

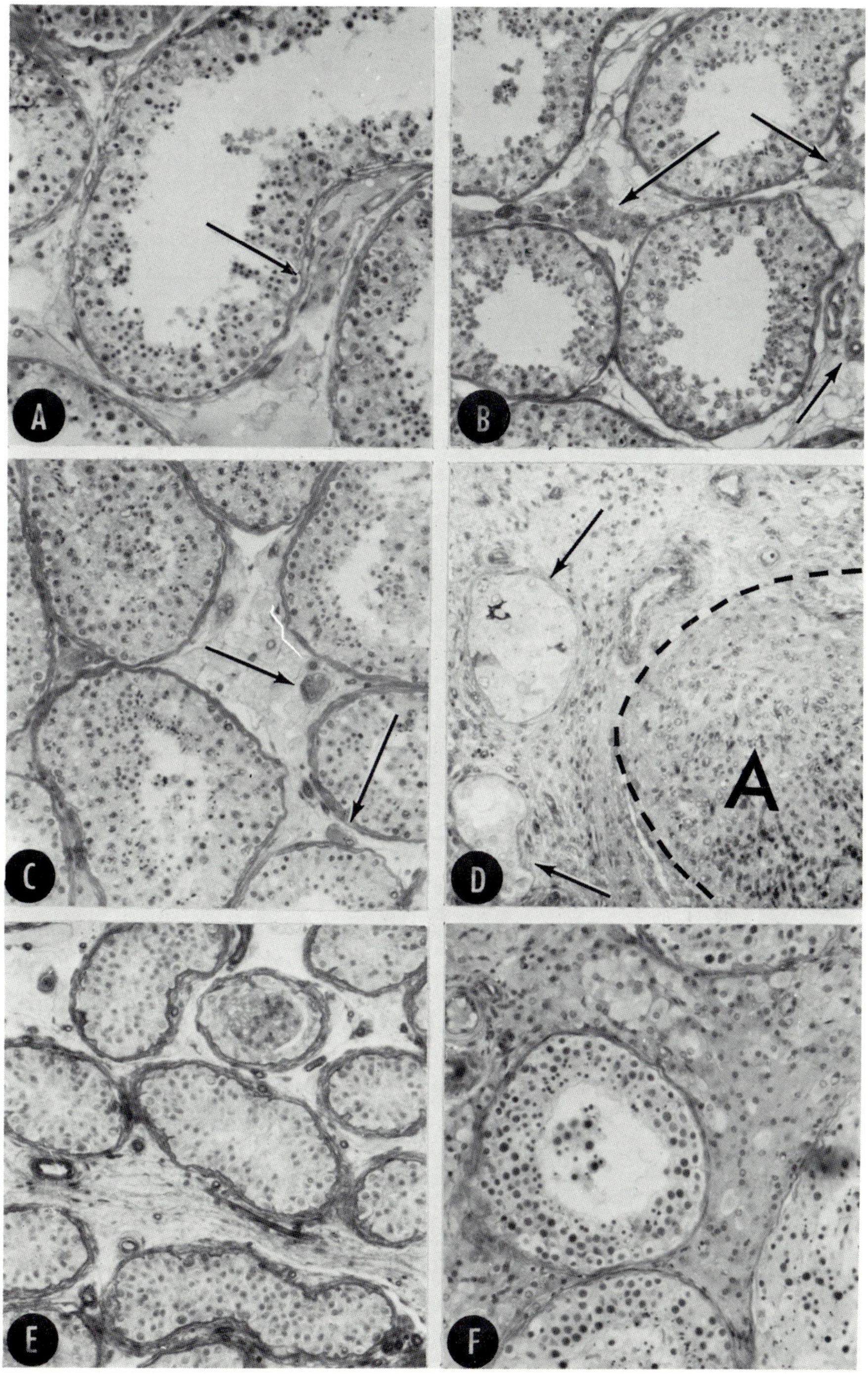

Fig. 1. A-F

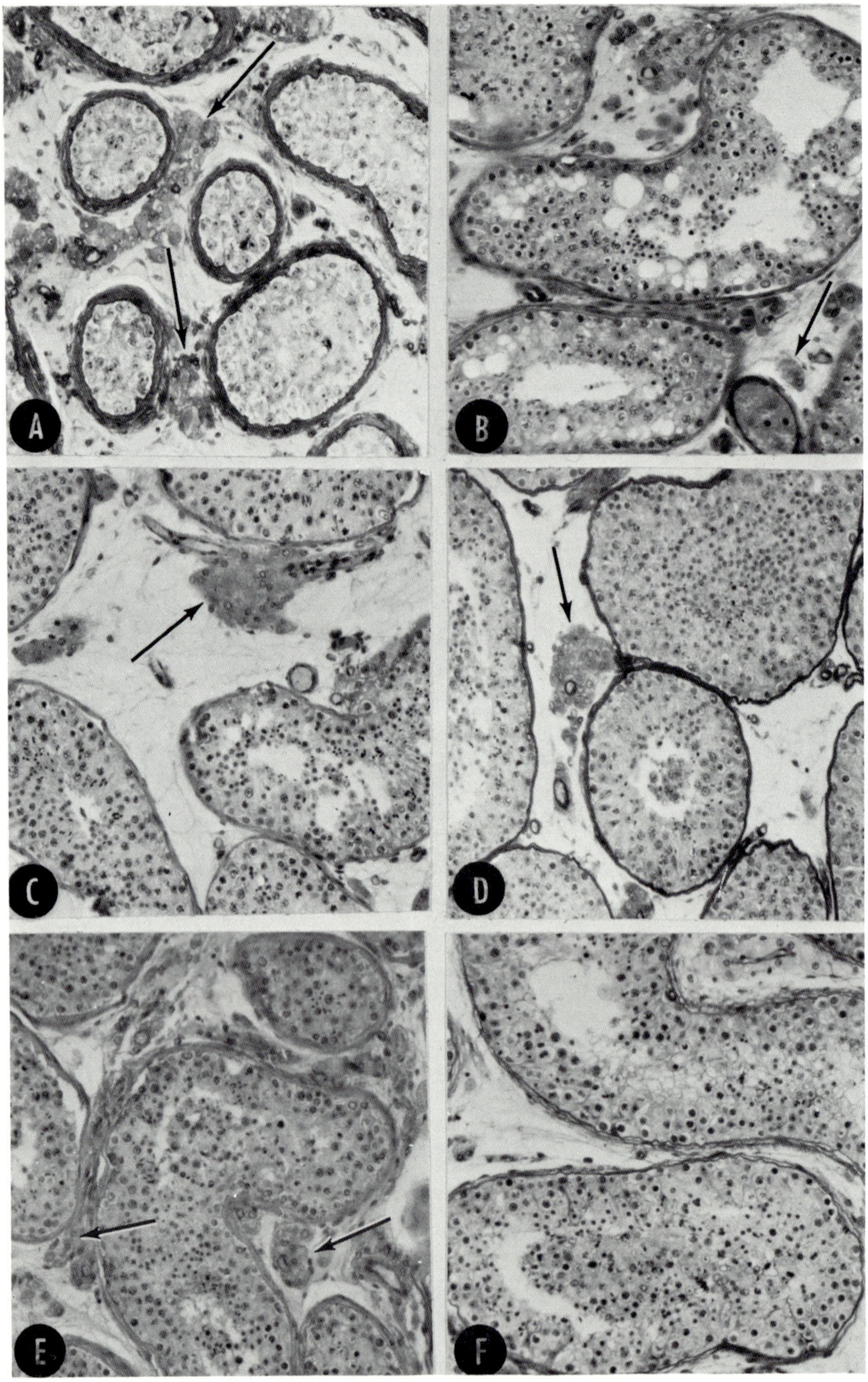

Fig. 2. A-F

Fig. 1. A) Case A - note presence of spermatogenesis, including mature spermatids and a small group of Leydig cells (arrow). B) Case B - note presence of spermatogenesis, including mature spermatids and a number of large clumps of Leydig cells (arrows). C) Case C - note presence of spermatogenesis, including mature spermatids and occasional small groups of Leydig cells (arrows). D) Case G - note two completely atrophic seminiferous tubules (arrows) and a Leydig cell "pseudoadenoma" (see A). E) Case H - note immature seminiferous tubules lined by Sertoli cells and primitive spermatogonial cells and lack of Leydig cells in the interstitial areas. F) Case E - note seminiferous tubules containing germinal cells, including advanced spermatids and masses of large Leydig cells in the interstitial areas.

Fig. 2. A) Case F - note seminiferous tubules containing Sertoli cells and spermatogonia, and masses of Leydig cells in the interstitial area (arrows). B) Case I - note spermatogenic activity in seminiferous tubules and occasional small groups of Leydig cells (arrow). C) Case J - note spermatogenic activity and large clumps of Leydig cells (arrow). D) - Case K - note spermatogenic activity and clumps of Leydig cells (arrow). E) - Case L - note spermatogenic activity and clumps of Leydig cells (arrows). F) Case M - note spermatogenic activity and sparsity of Leydig cells.

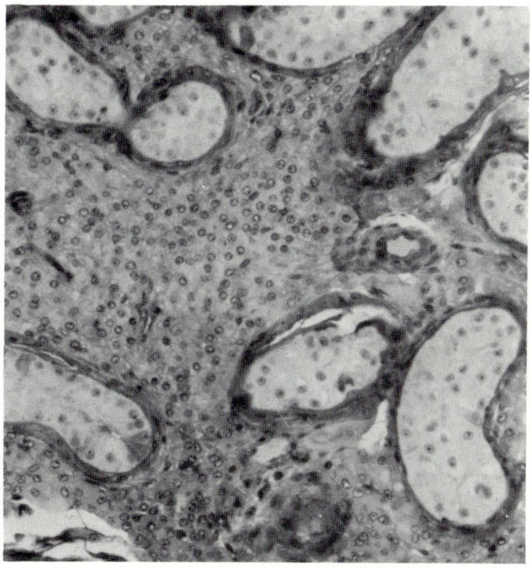

Fig. 3. Note immature seminiferous tubules lined with Sertoli cells embedded in a mass of Leydig cells.

to convert progesterone to testosterone and plasma testosterone levels and production rates was demonstrated. A variation in the steroid biosynthetic pathways in testicular tissue from different patients with oligospermia was demonstrated. The observations support the concept of steroid biosynthetic lesions in some cases of testicular disorders.

ACKNOWLEDGEMENTS

This study was supported by a grant from the Ford Foundation. The excellent technical assistance of A. Gdowik and O. Luckyj is gratefully acknowledged. Acknowledgement to Drs. A.L. Schneeberg, J.M. Schneeberg and Dr. R. Klaus for providing the tissues of patients undergoing orchiectomy and for performing surgical biopsies.

REFERENCES

1. Savard, K., Dorfman, R.I. and Poutasse, E., J. Clin. Endocr., 12: 935, 1952.
2. Lucas, M., Whitmore, W.F. Jr. and West, C.D., J. Clin. Endocr., 17: 465, 1957.
3. Carstensen, H.C.H., Acta Soc. Med. Upsal., 66: 129, 1961.
4. Slaunwhite, W.R. Jr., Sandberg, A.A., Jackson, J.E. and Staubitz, W.J., J. Clin. Endocr., 22: 992, 1962.
5. Axelrod, L.R., Biochim. Biophys. Acta, 97: 551, 1964.
6. Sharma, D.C., Racz, R.I. and Schoen, E.J., Acta Endocr. (Kobenhavn), 56: 726, 1967.
7. Schoen, E.J., Acta Endocr. (Kobenhavn), 56: 56, 1967.
8. Tamaoki, B.I. and Shikita, M., In Steroid Dynamics, eds. Pincus, G., Nakao, T. and Tait, J.F., Academic Press, New York, p. 493, 1966.
9. Danezis, J., Folia Bioch. et Biol. Graeca, 3: 41, 1966.
10. Steelman, S. and Pohley, F.M., Endocrinology, 53: 604, 1953.
11. Parlow, A.F., In Human Pituitary Gonadotropins, ed. Albert, A., Charles C. Thomas, Springfield, Ill., p. 300, 1961.
12. Horton, R., Kato, T. and Sherrins, R., Steroids, 10: 245, 1967.
13. Rivarola, M.A., Saez, J.M., Meyer, W.J., Jenkins, M.E. and Migeon, C.J., J. Clin. Endocr., 26: 1208, 1966.
14. Steinberger, A., Smith, K.D., Steinberger, E. and Perloff, W.H., J. Albert Einstein Med. Center, 12: 5, 1964.
15. Steinberger, E. and Ficher, M., Steroids, 11: 351, 1968.
16. Steinberger, E., Physiol. Rev., 1970 (in press)
17. Steinberger, E. and Ficher, M., Biol. Reprod. 1: 119, 1969.
18. Sharma, D.C., Dorfman, R.I. and Southren, A.L., Endocrinology, 76: 966, 1965.
19. Neher, R., Kahnt, F.W., Roversi, G.D. and Bompiani, A., Acta Endocr. (Kobenhavn), 49: 177, 1965.
20. Kase, N. and Morris, J. McL., Amer. J. Obstet. Gynec., 91: 102, 1965.
21. Rice, B.F., Cleveland, W.W., Sandberg, D.H., Ahmad, N., Politano, V.T. and Savard, K., J. Clin. Endocr., 27: 29, 1967.

22. Griffiths, K., Grant, J.K. and Whyte, W.G., J. Clin. Endocr., 23: 1044, 1963.
23. David, R.R., Wiener, M., Ross, L. and Landau, R.L., J. Clin. Endocr., 25: 1393, 1965.
24. Wade, A.P., Wilkinson, G.S., Davis, J.C. and Jeffcoate, T.N.A., J. Endocr., 42: 391, 1968.

DISCUSSION

HUDSON: Dr. Steinberger, I was intrigued that the patient with Klinefelter's syndrome had a normal value for plasma LH. Secondly, in one of the patients, there was a testosterone production rate of 5.7 mg. per day and a plasma level of 343 nanograms per 100 ml. I think these are correctly quoted. A rough calculation would give a metabolic clearance rate of about 1700 liters per day. This is certainly well outside the limits of normal males. Thirdly, in one of the incubation studies, 33% pregnenolone and 4% 20-α -hydroxy-progesterone was found. This is of relevance in view of the paper by Lacey and Petit in the British Medical Bulletin (Jan. 1970) in which they gave a clear indication that Sertoli cells have two metabolic pathways, one leading to testosterone and the other leading to reduced metabolites of progesterone. I wonder whether in your study this represented Sertoli cell activity.

E. STEINBERGER: In answer to your first question; yes, the urinary LH levels in the patient with Klinefelter's syndrome were within normal levels and FSH was elevated. In answer to the second question, I do not recall offhand what was the specific patient's clearance rate but the value in our laboratory for a group of 18 normal men was about 1500 $\pm$ 100 (S.E.) liters per day. Recently Lipsett et al. reported a clearance rate of over 1200 liters and Southern et al. a rate of about 1300 liters in normal individuals. These values are very close to your "rough" calculation. In answer to your third question, I have not read Dr. Lacey's paper and cannot comment on the possibility that the reductase activity resides in the Sertoli cells. However, as a sheer speculation, I would doubt this since in rat Leydig cell cultures we can detect 5-α -reductase while in organ cultures composed primarily of Sertoli cells we do not.

CHANDLEY: Dr. Steinberger, you were quite emphatic in stating that your four or five Klinefelter patients showing spermatogenesis in the testis were in fact not mosaics. I wonder how many tissues you actually looked at to establish this fact. It is much easier to say that a patient is a mosaic than to say that he is not, until you have looked at almost every cell in the body. I know that there have been one or two previous reports claiming spermatogenesis in Klinefelter's syndrome; but there has always been the doubt expressed that these may be XY/XXY mosaics.

E. STEINBERGER: I agree with you fully. As you recall, in our first paper on Klinefelter's syndrome with spermatogenesis published about five years ago, we analysed only blood and we found no mosaic in that case. Since that time we studied a case where blood, skin and testicular tissue were analysed and again no mosaic was found. However, you can always come back and argue the point that we did not look at all cells and have missed cells with XY. Unfortunately one is limited, particularly when studying tissue like the testis, in the number of good metaphases when dealing with a biopsy specimen. So I did not mean to be emphatic that these patients are not mosaics. I meant to state emphatically that we were unable to prove mosaicism in these patients.

PAULSEN: In one of our patients with Klinefelter's syndrome we had to examine 209 metaphase plates from testis tissue culture before finding a single example of XXY configuration. It is essential to have sufficient metaphase plates for study before one can disprove the existence of mosaicism.

FORD: My point is also concerned with the possibility of mosaicism in the Klinefelter patients. I would like to raise the possibility of a rather special kind of mosaicism involving the germ cells, but not the soma, arising out of the observations on the XXY human males. I believe I am right in saying that 15 cases have been examined so far and, in 14 of the 15, the spermatocytes were all XY, one of the Y chromosomes had been lost. In the other, the majority of the spermatocytes were XY. So, may I suggest the possibility of a parallel process occurring sometimes in the Klinefelter with loss of one of the two X chromosomes to give normal XY cells?

E. STEINBERGER: I think that we should bear in mind that study of karyotypes in cultured testicular tissue should not be taken as synonymous with study of karyotypes of germinal cells because most likely we are not looking at karyotypes of germinal cells but probably of fibroblasts. So your point is very well taken, the germ cell may very well exhibit a different karyotype.

MANCINI: Dr. Steinberger, as far as I know, this is the first time there has been an in vitro demonstration of a disturbance in the conversion of progesterone to testosterone in oligospermic patients. In terms of the relationship between spermatogenesis and in vitro steroidogenesis I would like to know if you have had the chance to study the "fertile" eunuch, because in this condition it has been claimed that Leydig cells cannot be identified morphologically, but that spermatogenesis is almost complete.

E. STEINBERGER: It is a fascinating question. I did not have the opportunity to study a case of "fertile" eunuch. Incidentally, the patient you mentioned was treated with Pergonal. We elected this form of therapy because we felt that by simply increasing the rate of steroid production we might elevate testosterone production. On therapy the patient's sperm count increased to 150 million and his wife became pregnant. The other patient with oligospermia and low gonadotropin levels was also treated with Pergonal with good results. Thus in a group of six oligospermic patients we were able to make a specific diagnosis in two and both of them responded to treatment.

LIPSETT: I think Dr. Steinberger's findings may be very important. I therefore want to comment a little critically about them. First, I would like to ask you why you decided to use a low substrate to enzyme concentration? If one wants to test the enzymes, one would like to use a concentration of substrate to enzyme that is 100:1 or 200:1, because when one uses a low ratio, one may be affecting many factors, such as pool size, rate of penetration and so on, which can be overcome by using very high levels.

E. STEINBERGER: In response to your comment concerning substrate to tissue ratios, I would like to state that the ratio we employed was comparable to that used by most workers who studied steroid metabolism in testicular tissue slices or minces. Furthermore, your concern of possible lack of saturation of the enzyme system by substrate in our incubates is well taken. However, since we had considerable quantities of unconverted substrate remaining in the flask by the end of the incubation period this concern may not be warranted. We should also keep in mind the problem of substrate inhibition.

LIPSETT: You are not limited by that, because you can always increase the amount of substrate and have a higher substrate to tissue ratio.

ROSEMBERG: Dr. Steinberger, I wondered what was your rationale for using Pergonal in oligospermic patients? You mentioned that they had a normal production rate of testosterone. Now if they did, did you want to see the effect of FSH plus that LH in the patients? How much Pergonal did you use? What was the total FSH and LH activity given and how soon did you obtain satisfactory results?

E. STEINBERGER: The reason why we used Pergonal was as follows: Since we did not know how much testosterone the testes would produce in response to the gonadotropins, we were worried that the testosterone levels might become sufficiently high to block the patient's own FSH and thus possibly interfere with spermatogenesis. By giving Pergonal we were assured of the presence of at least exogenous FSH. As far as the doses are concerned, we used two ampoules three times weekly for about six months. He responded within a month with the first increase in sperm count.

CHRISTENSEN: One of the generalities that seemed to emerge from

Dr. Steinberger's presentation was that the apparent number of interstitial cells does not seem to correlate very well with the level of androgen production from progesterone in vitro. In fact, it seemed inversely correlated. I wonder whether this is really surprising. If interstitial cells are not performing as they should, then the pituitary will respond by producing LH, which may cause some interstitial cell hyperplasia which would be in line with your findings.

E. STEINBERGER: I agree with you, but I would like to correct one point. I did not mean to correlate testosterone production rate and Leydig cells, but only the pattern of steroid metabolism, which really can not be very well correlated with the production rate.

SUBCELLULAR STRUCTURE AND SYNTHESIS OF STEROIDS IN THE TESTIS

Kenneth Savard

Endocrine Laboratory, Department of Biochemistry and Medicine, University of Miami School of Medicine, Miami, Florids, U.S.A.

It is becoming increasingly evident that subcellular localization of enzymes, substrates, cofactor systems, transport systems for oxygen, electrons, etc. are factors to be considered in the process of elaboration of steroid hormones. The production of the characteristic array of steroids by specific endocrine tissues, and more important, its control by gonadotropin, cannot at the present time be explained exclusively in terms of enzymes alone. Studies of various gonadal tissues in recent years reveal that the same enzymes or families of enzymes (3β-hydroxysteroid dehydrogenase-isomerase, 17-hydroxylase, C17,20-lyase, the 19-hydroxylase-aromatase system, 17β-hydroxysteroid dehydrogenase) are present in testicular tissues, in follicular tissue, in the human corpus luteum and in ovarian interstitial tissue. Yet each of these gonadal elements elaborates its own unique steroidal product.

It seems appropriate at this time to review the field in its present status. It is to be hoped that calling attention to the importance of the subcellular distribution of the enzymes of the steroidogenic pathway will cause an awareness of what is well documented in the testis, what is not clearly established and what work remains to be done.

The overall picture of the process of steroidogenesis in the cell is depicted in Fig. 1. This is a highly idealized generalization which is only partially true for the testis, and some data are drawn from studies of ovarian and adrenal tissues where the process and distribution seem to be largely the same.

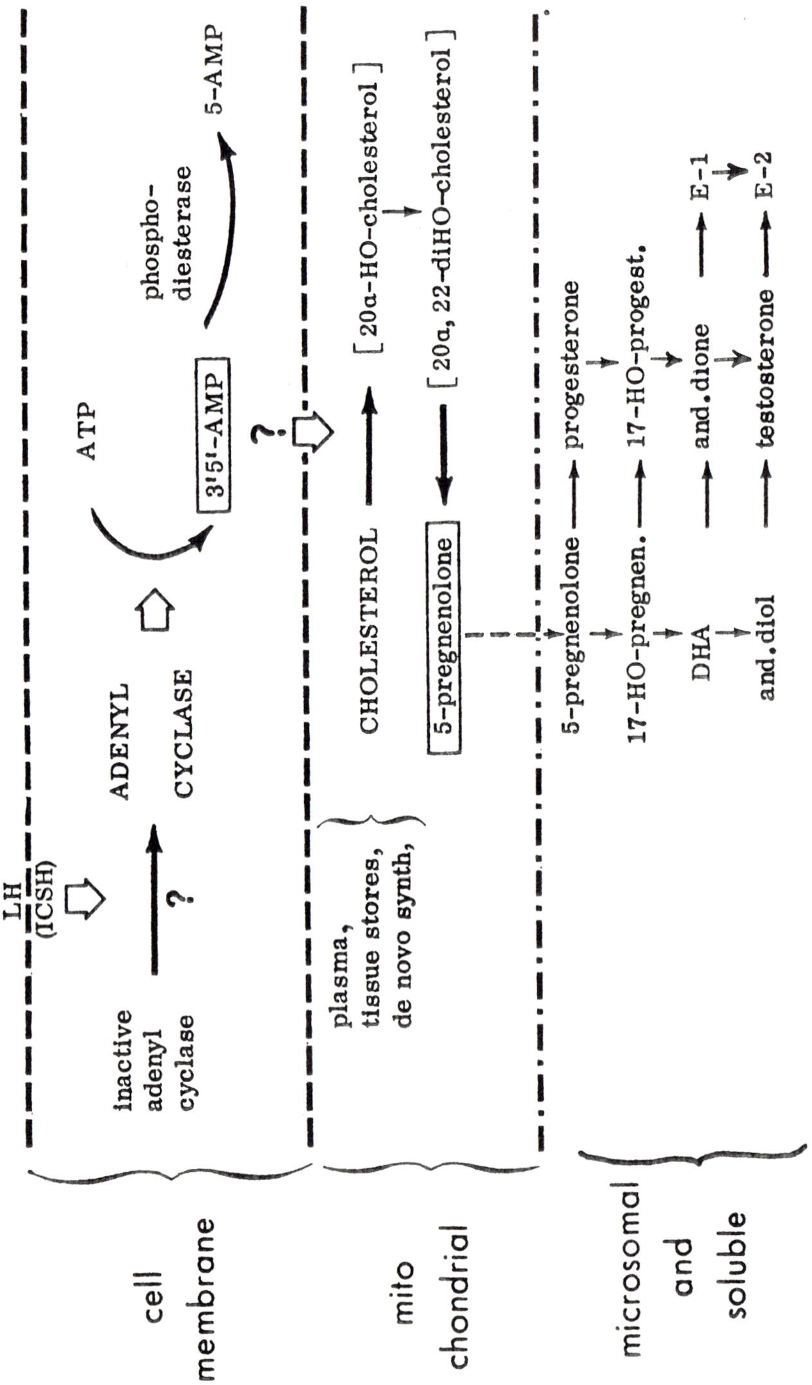

Fig. 1. Steroidogenesis in the testis.

ENZYMES OF THE STEROIDOGENIC PATHWAY

The enzymes involved in the elaboration from pregnenolene of progesterone, androgen, and estrogen appear to be localized largely in the microsomal fraction of testicular homogenates. Much of this important work has been carried out by Tamaoki and his group in Japan, (1-7) and by Samuels and his associates (8,9). The Japanese workers have carefully characterized, by electron microscopy, the purity of their centrifugal fractions and have concluded that except for the 20-hydroxysteroid dehydrogenase, which is in the soluble fraction, the 17-hydroxylase-lyase system, the 19-hydroxylase-aromatase system (7), the 17β-hydroxysteroid-isomerase and the 3β-hydroxysteroid dehydrogenase-isomerase system are microsomal. A review of this literature has appeared (1,10). The Japanese workers have studied this intracellular distribution in the testes of rats (3), mice (4), rabbits (5), guinea pigs (6) and men (7).

It has been reported that seminiferous tubules have the capacity to convert progesterone to androgens in vitro (11); more recent work has shown that only the Leydig cells and not the tubules can convert cholesterol into androgen (12). Both studies however point to the presence of certain enzymes of the biosynthetic pathway in the tubular elements. The physiologic significance of these observations is hard to interpret since the concensus is that the Leydig cells are the major source of androgens in the testis.

THE FORMATION OF PREGNENOLONE

This principal and presumably obligatory precursor of steroid hormones in the testis, as well as in other tissues, is derived from cholesterol (Fig. 1) by the enzyme complex called the "cholesterol side-chain cleavage" enzyme system (12,14). This enzyme complex is totally located in the mitochondria of all steroidogenic tissues examined, including the testis (15), and consists of three discrete enzymes: 20α-hydroxylase, 22-hydroxylase, and C-20,22 lyase (or 20α, 22-dihydroxycholesterol side-chain cleavage enzyme).

This mitochondrial enzyme complex has been studied more thoroughly in adrenal tissue than in the testis, and the sequence of reactions shown in Fig. 1 may not necessarily be the correct one, according to recent studies (16) in homogenates of adrenal tissue.

The "cholesterol side-chain cleavage" enzyme complex of testicular tissue appears to be the limiting step in the rate of overall steroidogenesis in the testis, (17) as it appears to be in adrenal and ovarian tissues. The system is dependent on gonadotropin which restores, or prevents the decline, in the rate of this system following hypophysectomy (17).

Stimulation of steroid hormone production by appropriate tropic hormones, in intact cell preparations of adrenal, corpus luteum, ovarian interstitium (of the rabbit) and testis tissues, is considered to be mediated by the cyclic nucleotide, 3', 5'-AMP. In the testis, the complete picture has not yet been drawn. However, conversion of labelled cholesterol to testosterone by testicular preparations has been reported by several laboratories and is stimulated by gonadotropin (18) and by 3', 5'-AMP (19). In perfused preparations, 3', 5'-AMP, like ICSH-LH, causes increased biosynthesis of the total steroidal product of the testis which includes testosterone, DHA, androstenedione, 17-hydroxyprogesterone, 17-hydroxypreg - nenolone and progesterone (van der Molen and Eik-Nes, quoted in ref. 20). This has also been observed in intact slice preparations (21, 22).

The mechanism by which 3', 5'-AMP stimulates the rate of the transformation of cholesterol to pregnenolone is entirely unknown. It is under investigation in the adrenal (23) and ovarian tissue (24,25) but is relatively unexplored in testicular tissues (26). The stimulating action of 3', 5'-AMP can be inhibited by inhibitors of protein synthesis such as puromycin and chloramphenicol (24,27). The nature of this phenomenon in adrenal (23), ovarian and testicular tissues is unknown.

Although the transformation of cholesterol to steroid is a mitochondrial process, the source of cholesterol is not known. It can be presumed that much of testicular cholesterol originates in the plasma. However, ^{14}C from small molecular precursors like acetate and mevalonate is incorporated into steroids (27,28) and sterols (28) by isolated testicular preparations. De novo synthesis of cholesterol therefore occurs in testicular tissue and in Leydig cells (12,21) although the subcellular component or components involved are not known.

ADENYL CYCLASE AND 3', 5'-AMP

The mediating role of 3', 5'-AMP in the stimulation of steroidogenesis in adrenal. ovarian and testicular tissues is now generally accepted, though its mechanism is not understood. It is also generally considered that the step in the biosynthetic process stimulated is the mitochondrial "cholesterol side-chain cleavage" enzyme system,since this seems to be the rate-limiting step. An early effect of gonadotropin and ACTH (in their respective tissues) would consequently be to cause increased concentrations of endogenous 3', 5'-AMP in the tissue. This has been observed in ovarian (29) and in testicular tissues (30). It is assumed that the tropic hormone activates adenyl cyclase (31,32) in the membrane of the cell, where transformation of ATP to 3', 5'-AMP presumably occurs (Fig. 1). The transport or migration of the newly formed 3', 5'-AMP from the membrane to mitochondria where its steroidogenic effect takes place, is unexplained.

A little light is being shed in the area of the activation of gonadal adenyl cyclase by ICSH-LH, the nature of which is virtually unknown in any tissue. It would now appear that a prostaglandin, PGE_2, may mediate the effect of the gonadotropin on adenyl cyclase. Recent studies by J.M. Marsh of the Endocrine Laboratory in Miami have shown that PGE_2, added to incubating slices of bovine corpora lutea, causes a rapid and significant activation of adenyl cyclase with a presumed concomitant increase in endogenous 3',5'-AMP concentrations (35). This same prostaglandin has been recorded as mimicking both ICSH-LH and exogenous 3',5'-AMP on steroidogenesis in this same tissue (36). This postulated mediating role of PGE_2 on adenyl cyclase will require the demonstration that the gonadotropin will increase concentrations of PGE_2 in the tissue; this has not been done.

EFFECTS OF GONADOTROPIN IN THE TESTIS

It is well known that both testicular weight and protein synthesis are influenced by purified preparations of FSH and ICSH-LH (33,34). It seems however that ICSH-LH is more effective (on a weight basis) than FSH in stimulating steroidogenesis in testicular slices (27); whether the steroidogenic effect of FSH is due to its ICSH-LH contaminant is not clear (27), although it is interpreted to be so (20). Murad and associates (29) have recently reported the stimulation of adenyl cyclase in testicular homogenates by both purified preparations of ICSH-LH and FSH at reasonably low concentrations. The activity of the FSH preparation was greater than could be attributed to its LH content. Murad et al. however point out that their testicular preparation contained elements of connective tissue, tubules, nerves, blood vessels, besides Leydig cells, and that there could be more than one cellular type of cyclase responding to the gonadotropins.

To summarize and perhaps to predict, it would seem that steroidogenesis in the testis is part of a larger natural scheme where the process in the male gland is not unlike that in ovarian and adrenal tissues. Biochemical phenomena in the membrane and the mitochondria are comparable and almost identical, save for the binding sites for ACTH or gonadotropin. Distinctiveness and physiological uniqueness, that of the production of androgen as major product, appears to reside in parameters associated with the endoplasmic reticulum. It is here, in the microsomal fraction, that the enzymes and other factors are localized and determine the course of steroidogenesis leading to androgen formation and secretion by the testicular cell.

The ultra structure of the steroid-forming cell thus is becoming more prominent as knowledge of the subcellular distribution of the enzyme system of the steroidogenic process evolves. The well-established changes in ultrastructure of the cell following hypophysectomy, and their prevention or reversal by treatment with appropriate tropic hormone (reviewed by Christensen and Gillim (10) point to the role of tropic hormone in the maintanance of these fragile structures. It is obvious from Fig. 1 that a high degree of organization and transport in the steroidogenic cell is implied. Even more complicated is the manner by which tropic hormone accelerates steroidogenesis. If the schematic representation of Fig. 1 is true, it is plain why disruption of the cell's integrity by freezing or by homogenization abolishes the stimulatory effects of tropic hormone or of exogenous 3',5'-AMP. It follows then that far more attention and awareness in maintaining and preserving cellular integrity must be given than in the past. Only in this way will biochemical studies in vitro have physiological relevance, and provide further insight into this complex process.

ACKNOWLEDGEMENT

Supported in part by grant HD-03248 National Institute of Child Health and Human Development, U.S. Dept. of Health, Education and Welfare.

REFERENCES

1. Tamaoki, B., Inano, H. and Nakano, H., In The Gonads, ed. McKerns, K.W., Appleton-Century-Crofts, Inc. New York p. 547, 1969.
2. Inano, H., Harl, Y. and Tamaoki, B., In Endocrinology of the Testis, eds. Wolstenholme, G.E.W. and O'Connor, M. J. and A. Churchill Ltd. London p. 105, 1967.
3. Shikita, M. and Tamaoki, B., Endocrinology, 76: 563, 1965.
4. Murato, S., Shikita, M. and Tamaoki, B., Steroids, 5: 509,1965.
5. Tamaoki, B. and Shikita, M. In Steroid Dynamics,eds. Pincus, G., Nakao, T. and Tait, J.F., Academic Press, New York, p. 493, 1966.
6. Inano, H., Egusa, M. and Tamaoki, B., Biochim. Biophys. Acta, 144: 165, 1967.
7. Murato, S., Shikita, M. and Tamaoki, B., Biochim. Biophys. Acta, 117: 241, 1966.
8. Mahajan, D.K. and Samuels, L.T., Fed. Proc.,21: 209, 1962.
9. Matsumoto, K. and Samuels, L.T., Endocrinology, 85: 402, 1968.
10. Christensen, A.K. and Gillim, S.W. In The Gonads, ed. McKerns, K.W., Appleton-Century Crofts, Inc., New York, p. 415, 1969.
11. Christensen, A.K. and Mason, N.R., Endocrinology, 76: 646, 1965.
12. Hall, P.F., Irby, D.C. and de Kretser, D.M., Endocrinology, 84: 488, 1969.
13. Shimizu, K., Hayano, M., Gut, M. and Dorfman, R.I., J. Biol. Chem., 236: 695, 1961.
14. Shimizu, K., Gut, M. and Dorfman, R. I., J. Biol. Chem., 237: 966, 1962.
15. Toren, D., Menon, K.M.J., Forchielli, E. and Dorfman, R.I., Steroids, 3: 381, 1964.

16. Burstein, S. and Gut, M., Steroids, 14: 207, 1969.
17. Forchielli, E., Menon, K.M.J., and Dorfman, R.I., In The Gonads, ed. McKerns, K.W., Appleton-Century-Crofts, Inc. New York, p. 519, 1969.
18. Hall, P.F., Endocrinology, 78: 690, 1966.
19. Sandler, R. and Hall, P.F., Endocrinology, 79: 647,1966.
20. Connell, G.M. and Eik-Nes, K.B. In The Gonads, ed. McKerns, K.W., Appleton-Century-Crofts, New York p. 491, 1969.
21. Rice, B.F., Cleveland, W.W., Sandberg, D.H., Ahmad, A., Politano, V.T. and Savard, K., J. Clin. Endocr., 27: 29, 1967.
22. Leymarie, P. and Savard, K., unpublished
23. Garren, L.D., Vitamins and Hormones, 26: 119, 1968.
24. Marsh, J.M. and Savard, K., J. Reprod. Fertil. Suppl., 1: 133, 1966.
25. Dorrington, J.H. and Kilpatrick, R., Biochem. J., 104: 725, 1967.
26. Sandler, R. and Hall, P.F., Endocrinology, 79: 647, 1966.
27. Hall, P.F. and Eik-Nes, K.B., Biochim. Biophys. Acts, 63: 411, 1962.
28. Tsai, S.E., Ying, B.P. and Gaylor, J.L., Arch. Biochem. Biophys. 105: 329, 1964.
29. Marsh, J.M. Butcher, R.W., Savard, K. and Sutherland, E.W., J. Biol. Chem., 241: 5436.
30. Murod. F., Chi, Y.M., Rall, T.W. and Sutherland, E.W., J. Biol. Chem., 237: 1233, 1962.
31. Murod, F., Strauch, B.S. and Vaughn, M., Biochim. Biophys. Acta, 177: 591, 1969.
32. Marsh, J.M., J. Biol. Chem., in press (1970).
33. Tanoka, K., Wilson, W.O. and McFarland, E.Z., Amer. J. Vet. Res., 27: 1067, 1966.
34. Means, A.R. and Hall, P.F., Endocrinology, 83: 597, 1968.
35. Marsh, J.M., FEBS Letters, in press (1970)
36. Speroff, L. and Ramwell, P.W., J. Clin. Endocr. in press (1970).

DISCUSSION

JOHNSEN: Dr. Savard, you made reference to a patient with testicular fibrosis without production of estrogens. Did this fact surprise you or did it have anything to do with the fact that there was testicular fibrosis?

SAVARD: The patient was a case of incomplete testicular feminization, and therefore virtually consisted of a pure Leydig cell preparation, but we were very pleased that we had data that seemed to be in agreement with Dr. Lipsett; that the Leydig cells are a very poor source of estrogen, because the quantities of both estradiol and estrone combined are extremely small.

CHAPTER VI

NON-HORMONAL FACTORS INFLUENCING SPERM PRODUCTION AND TRANSPORT

THE BIOCHEMICAL CHARACTERISTICS OF SPERMATOZOA AND SEMINAL PLASMA

Thaddeus Mann

Director, Unit of Reproductive Physiology and

Biochemistry, University of Cambridge,

Cambridge, England

Semen is made up of two components, viz. the spermatozoa and seminal plasma, which differ from each other physiologically as well as chemically. Moreover, the physiological and chemical properties of these two components of semen do not remain constant but undergo characteristic changes in the course of the period of sperm passage from the testes to the site of final destination in the female reproductive tract.

TESTICULAR SEMEN

Testicular semen is a dilute suspension of testicular spermatozoa which can be obtained by means of a catheter from the rete testis (1). It has few properties in common, physiologically or chemically, with ejaculated semen. Testicular spermatozoa are immotile and incapable of effecting fertilization. Their immaturity is also reflected in structural pecularities, such as the persistent occurrence of kinoplasmic droplets as well as in certain chemical and metabolic properties, best illustrated by the behavior of sperm phospholipids.

In ejaculated ram spermatozoa the principal phospholipid is the choline-based plasmalogen, that is, phosphatidalcholine, which in the course of endogenous sperm respiration yields oxidizable fatty acids (2,3). In both testicular and ejaculated ram spermatozoa the amount of phosphatidalcholine appears to be approximately the same, but the concentration of other phospholipids, such as phosphatidylcholine (lecithin), phosphatidylethamolamine and phosphatidalethanolamine (ethanolamine-based plasmalogen) is distinctly higher in testicular spermatozoa, and the fatty acids extracted from these phospholipids include more palmitic acid and less myristic acid (4). When incubated with (U-^{14}C) glucose, testicular ram spermatozoa exhibit a much higher rate of radioactivity incorporation into the glycerol component of phospholipids and neutral lipids than the ejaculated spermatozoa. However, none of that radioactivity appears in phosphatidalcholine. Like the biosynthetic ability, so too the rate of metabolic breakdown of lipids differs in testicular and ejaculated ram spermatozoa. Thus for example, ram testicular spermatozoa are much less active than ejaculated spermatozoa in hydrolysing either added ethanolamine phosphoglycerides or added lecithin (5).

Equally pronounced are the differences between testicular and ejaculated seminal plasma. A review listing recent findings pertaining to testicular plasma, that is the fluid collected directly from the rete testis (mainly from rams) has been published by Setchell, Scott, Voglmayr and Waites (6). It is evident that although testicular plasma has the same osmolality as other body fluids, the rete testis fluid is watery so that its content of protein (measured as biuret-reactive material) is only 0.28 g/100 ml. Its total mineral (ash) content, on the other hand, is similar to that of blood plasma; but the ionic composition is not the same, there being less sodium but about three times as much potassium in the testicular fluid. Most of the free amino acids are present in lower concentration in the rete testis fluid than in either testicular lymph or blood plasma. An exception in this respect is the behavior of glutamic acid and aspartic acid; these two amino acids are present in testicular plasma in concentrations which exceed about tenfold those of testicular lymph or blood plasma. There is no glucose or fructose in the rete testis fluid. An interesting chemical feature of that fluid is the occurrence of free inositol.

Inositol has been known for some time to be a characteristic constituent of mammalian seminal plasma. Its concentration is particularly high in the boar, where it is produced in the seminal vesicles. The fluid secreted by the boar seminal vesicles may contain as much as 3 g inositol/100 ml, and it is from that fluid that inositol was isolated in a pure crystalline state (7). Though in much smaller concentrations, inositol occurs also in the seminal plasma of other mammals, including ram and man (8,9). More recently it has also been shown to occur in the rete testis fluid, in concentrations ranging from 0.97 to 0.15 g/100 ml (10).

Of much interest is yet another recent observation pertaining to the chemical composition of ram rete testis fluid, namely the occurrence in that fluid of testosterone (11,6), in quantities comparable to those in testicular blood and lymph (12). If future studies should prove conclusively that the plasma of testicular semen collected from the rete testis does, in fact, originate in the seminiferous tubules, and furthermore, if one accepts as valid the view that testosterone is generated in the intertubular tissue (that is not inside but outside the seminiferous tubules), then the inescapable conclusion is that testosterone can pass through the wall of the seminiferous tubule and enter its lumen. The movement of testosterone, or for that matter of any other organic material, across the wall of the seminiferous tubules is, as yet, poorly understood. High molecular weight substances at any rate, such as serum proteins, seem to be unable to pass into the seminiferous tubules, in spite of the fact that testicular interstitial blood capillaries are unusually permeable to serum proteins and that such proteins tend to accumulate readily and at a high rate in extravascular spaces (13,14). Nor is there much information with regard to the possible involvement of Sertoli cells in the movement of substances across the wall of seminiferous tubules, but of some significance in that respect may be the observation that Sertoli cells are able to take and transport peroxidase from blood (15). We shall know more about the formation of the testicular plasma when the ultrastructural relations between the elements which compose the walls of the seminiferous tubules and those which compose the intertubular tissue are cleared up. In this connection there may be significance in the recent finding (16) that in the guinea-pig and chinchilla the testicular interstitium contains in addition to blood capillaries an extensive system of sinusoidal lymphatics, located in close proximity on one side to the Leydig cells, and on the other side to the tunica propria of the seminiferous tubules.

EPIDIDYMAL SEMEN

During the period of about two weeks which the spermatozoa require to pass along the epididymis, they undergo a number of changes, described as "maturation" or "ripening". In addition, the epididymus also plays a part in the disposal of aged, that is, superfluous spermatozoa. Ripening is associated with morphological and physicochemical changes. The former include the phenomenon of kinoplasmic droplet migration as well as ultrastructural changes in both the acrosome and mitochondrial sheath (17,20). The latter involve a process of progressive dehydration and a rise in both specific gravity and permeability as well as changes in sperm composition, particularly in the lipid constituents. As spermatozoa pass along the epididymis of the ram, the concentration of total phospholipid and non-esterified cholesterol gradually decreases (21). This may be due either to the metabolic activity of the spermatozoa themselves or to the influence exerted by the epididymal tissue. It is by no means certain in what measure the changes associated with sperm ripening depend on reactions within the sperm cells themselves, and to what extent they are triggered off by extraneous factors originating in the epididymal epithelium. Apart from phospholipids, epididymal and ejaculated spermatozoa differ in other properties, and one of the most interesting differences is the much higher level of pyridine nucleotides in epididymal than in ejaculated spermatozoa, a phenomenon discovered by the Italian research-workers, Bistocchi, d'Allessio and Leone (22).

The fluid medium for the spermatozoa within the epididymis is the "epididymal plasma": together, the epididymal sperm and plasma constitute epididymal semen. Chemically the epididymal plasma is distinct from both the testicular fluid and the ejaculated seminal plasma. This is particularly striking in respect of the ionic composition. When the sodium and potassium ions are measured at different levels of the bovine epididymis, the K/Na ratio is distinctly higher in the corpus epididymis than at the point of sperm entry from the efferent ducts into the caput. In the cauda epididymidis, however, the combined contents of K and Na are lower than in the corpus, some of the osmotically active ions having been replaced by organic substances (23,24). Among the organic constituents of epididymal plasma two deserve special mention on account of their unusually high concentration, namely glycerylphosphorylcholine (25) and carnitine (26).

Glycerylphosphorylcholine occurs in such a high concentration in the epididymis that in some species at least, notably ram, bull, boar and stallion, a determination of glycerylphosphorylcholine in semen can be used as a criterion for the evaluation of the epididymal contribution to the whole ejaculate. Glycerylphosphorylcholine also occurs in human semen but its concentration does not exceed 400 μmoles or 100 mg/100 ml, i.e. ten times less than in the ram. On the other hand, human seminal plasma is much richer in another choline derivative, phosphorylcholine, than the semen of either ram, bull, boar or stallion. However, phosphorylcholine is probably derived from accessory organs other than the epididymis. Like most secretory products of the male reproductive tract glycerylphosphorylcholine formation is under the influence of the male sex hormone; its formation is arrested by castration, but can be stimulated by exogenous testosterone (27).

Carnitine (β-oxy-γ-butyrobetaine, $C_7H_{15}O_3N$), together with acetylcarnitine, has so far been studied mainly in the rat reproductive tract. The cauda epididymidis of adult rats contains nearly 100 μmoles carnitine, as well as about 5 μmoles acetylcarnitine, per g dry weight tissue. Most of that carnitine seems to be derived from the epididymal secretion (26). Whether the high content of carnitine arises from synthesis de novo, or from accumulation by the epididymal epithelium, is not known for certain. Much more is known about the intermediary reactions in carnitine formation. In that respect investigations on the relationship between the occurrence in edpdidymal plasma of carnitine and glutamic acid could be of much interest, particularly in relation to the possibility of carnitine arising by decarboxylation of glutamic acid, via γ-aminobutyric acid and butyrobetaine. The high level of carnitine in the epididymal plasma, and the high level of activity of the enzyme carnitine acetyltransferase in the spermatozoa, both strongly suggest that carnitine and acetylcarnitine may play an essential role in semen metabolism, perhaps in the oxidation of fatty acids.

EJACULATED SEMEN

Practically all that is known at present about the testicular and epididymal semen derives from studies on species other than man. But our knowledge of the biochemistry of ejaculated semen includes a great deal of information on human semen. The account below is intended as a brief introduction to the biochemistry of the human ejaculate, and provides an outline of certain chemical methods which are applicable to human semen.

The intracellular constituents of human spermatozoa appear to be similar to those encountered in sperm cells of other mammals. The human sperm nucleus is haploid and contains only half the amount of deoxyribonucleic acid which one would expect to find in the diploid cells of somatic cells; its average content appears to vary slightly within the narrow range of 2.2 to 2.6 x 10^{-9} mg DNA/sperm cell (28). This constancy, however, characterizes only normal human spermatozoa; in subfertile and sterile men (or animals) the DNA content is said to be much more variable (29-31). The intracellular enzymes present in human spermatozoa also resemble those found in animals. Human spermatozoal lactate dehydrogenase (LDH) shares with the animal LDH the occurrence of the unusual LDH_{IV} or X isozyme This isozyme appears to be testis-specific for man and animals alike. In the species that have been investigated its formation is linked up with the process of spermatogenesis. The isozyme first appears during the late spermatogonial or spermatocyte stage, but not before. Its substrate specificity and certain other properties are quite distinct from the other lactate dehydrogenase isozymes (32-37). Another enzyme characteristic of spermatozoa and of the mature testis, but not present in the pre-pubertal testis, is ketose reductose (sorbitol dehydrogenase). Discovered in ram spermatozoa and purified from that material (38), this enzyme was later shown also to occur in testicular homogenates of a variety of other animals, and in man (39).

At one time the human spermatozoa as present in ejaculated semen were erroneously believed to differ from animal spermatozoa by being incapable of respiring. However, in the light of numerous studies carried out during the last decade (40-47), this view can no longer be sustained. It is now certain that human spermatozoa possess marked respiratory activity. They also contain, in common with other species, the complete cytochrome system (48,49). The variations, however, which one encounters in the metabolic rates of human spermatozoa, appear to be much greater than in animal semen. This variability characterizes not only respiration but also the anaerobic metabolism, that is fructolysis.

Human seminal plasma represents the combined secretions of the epididymis, vas deferens, ampulla, seminal vesicle, prostate gland, and the glands of Cowper and Littre. In chemical composition it differs quite significantly from the seminal plasma of other mammals. Among its unusual and characteristic components are nitrogenous bases, such as choline, spermine and spermidine; a whole range of specific proteolytic enzymes, which are associated with the process of semen coagulation and liquefaction and responsible for the breakdown of large molecular weight proteins to smaller peptides and free amino acids; various other oxidative and hydrolytic enzymes, including the powerful acid phosphatase and 5'-nucleotidase; and many other organic substances, including at least thirteen prostaglandins, a large group of free as well as bound carbohydrates, and organic acids such as citric, lactic and ascorbic acid.

The prostaglandins are a group of unsaturated C_{20}-fatty acids, characterized by the presence of a cyclopentanone ring which broadly speaking can occur in four forms, known as E, F, A and B. The

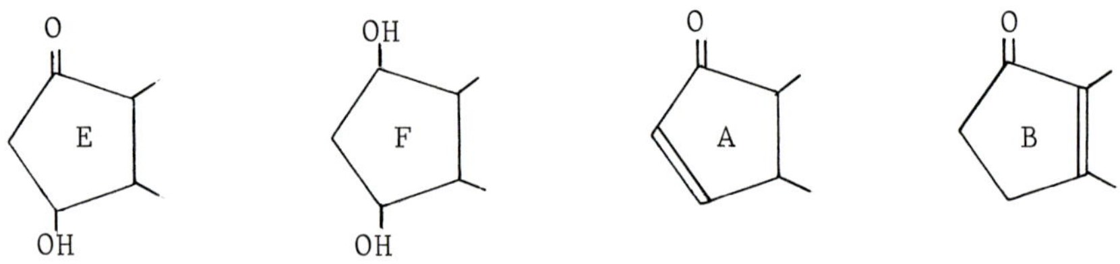

extensive literature on prostaglandins was summarized by Pike and Weeks (50) in their "Prostaglandin Bibliography", and the whole field has been reviewed by several authors (51-53). The currently held views on prostaglandins in relation to the reproductive functions in both the male and female were discussed in recent reviews by Ingelman-Sundberg (54) and Horton (55). Of the thirteen prostaglandins so far detected in human 'seminal plasma', the two most prominent ones are prostaglandin E_1 (11α 15-dihydroxy-9-keto-prosta-13-enoic acid and prostaglandin E_2 (11α 15-dihydroxy-9-keto-prosta-5,13-dienoic acid), each present at a concentration of approximately 2 mg/100ml. So far as is known at present, prostaglandins account for practically the whole of the smooth-muscle stimulating activity of human seminal plasma. Serotonin (5-hydroxytryptamine) which at one time was believed to account for at least one part of the 'oxytocic' activity of semen, has been shown to be absent from human seminal plasma (56).

The carbohydrates of human seminal plasma are partly free and partly bound to proteins. The principal free sugar is fructose (57) but in addition, human seminal plasma contains small amounts of various other free carbohydrates, including sorbitol, inositol, glucose, ribose and fucose. The bound carbohydrate is composed chiefly of amino sugar, sialic acid and orcinol-reactive material which on acid hydrolysis yields galactose, mannose and fucose, but only a trace of glucose. Glycogen occurs in human semen in traces; the bulk of bound carbohydrate is present in the form of glycoproteins (58).

In addition to the glycoproteins human seminal plasma contains various other proteins, some of which break down during storage of semen into smaller fragments (59-61). According to one recent estimate (62), based on optical density measurements of polyacrylamide columns prepared by disc electrophoresis, out of a total of 5.8 g protein/100 ml seminal plasma, 13% was present as prealbumin (a fraction migrating ahead of albumin), 14% as albumin, 36% as α_1-globulin, 15% as α_2-globulin, 8% as β_1-globulin, 6% as β_2-globulin, and 7% in the form of immunoglobulins; plasma separated from semen samples with sperm counts below 20,000/µl contained more prealbumin and β_1-globulin but less albumin. Another significant deviation from the pattern of protein distribution in human seminal plasma has been reported by Herrmann (63): in two cases of hypogonadism he could find no evidence for the occurrence of the so-called 3,72S-protein (mol. wt. 50,000) which according to this author, is normally secreted by the seminal vesicles.

Among the organic acids secreted in seminal plasma, citric acid deserved special attention because of its high concentration in human semen (up to 0.5%, or even more), and its origin in the prostate, it provides a good indicator of prostatic function. Just as fructose can serve as a quantifiable criterion of ampullary and vesicular activity, so citric acid, and also acid phosphatase, represent a similarly sensitive and reliable indicator of prostatic activity. A combined citric acid - fructose determination can be particularly useful, e.g. as a diagnostic aid for the detection of defects in the male reproductive tract such as bilateral aplasia of the seminal ducts and vesicles or occlusion of the ejaculatory ducts. In cases of this kind, there are no spermatozoa and no fructose in the ejaculates which, however, show at the same time an abnormally elevated concentration of citric acid (64). There are other instances in which the chemical analysis of semen can be applied as a diagnostic aid of reproductive failure in man (65). One to which we are directing our special attention at present concerns chemical methods of semen analysis in the detection of disturbances in the ejaculatory process (66). Interference with the normal nervous mechanism which controls the pattern of ejaculation, caused e.g. by the administration of certain drugs, can seriously disturb the order in which the various seminal fractions are ejaculated. In such conditions the chemical characteristics of the so-called split ejaculates, that is, of the pre-sperm, sperm-rich, and post-sperm fractions, are markedly altered, and the characteristic sequence with which the various fractions are normally voided, is upset or even altogether reversed.

REFERENCES

1. Voglmayr, J.K., Scott, T.W., Setchell, B.P. and Waites, G.M.H., J. Reprod. Fertil, 14: 87, 1967.
2. Hartree, E.F. and Mann, T., Biochem. J., 71: 423, 1959.
3. Hartree, E.F. and Mann, T., Biochem. J., 80: 464, 1961.
4. Scott, T.W., Voglmayr, J.K. and Setchell, B.P., Biochem. J., 102: 456, 1967.
5. Scott, T.W. and Dawson, R.M.C., Biochem. J., 108: 457, 1968.
6. Setchell, B.P., Scott, T.W., Voglmayr, J.K. and Waites, G.M.H., Biol. Reprod. Suppl., 1: 40, 1969.
7. Mann, T., Proc. Roy. Soc. (Biol.) 42: 21, 1954.
8. Hartree, E.F., Biochem. J., 66: 131, 1957.
9. Nixon, D.A., J. Reprod. Fertil.,8: 419, 1964.
10. Setchell, B.P., Dawson, R.M.C. and White, R.W., J. Reprod. Fertil.,17: 219, 1968.
11. Voglmayr, J.K., Waites, G.M.H. and Setchell, B.P., Natrre, 210: 861, 1966.
12. Lindner, H.R., J. Endocr., 25: 483, 1963.
13. Everett, N.B. and Simmons, B., Circ. Res., 6/3, 307, 1958.
14. Mancini, R.E., Vilar, O., Alvarez, B. and Seigner, A.C., J. Histochem. Cytochem., 13: 376, 1965.
15. Reddy, J.K. and Svoboda, D.J., J. Cell Biol., 35: 379, 1967.
16. Fawcett, D.W., Heidger, P.M. and Leak, L.V., J. Reprod. Fertil, 19: 109, 1969.
17. Fawcett, D.W. and Hollenberg, R.D., Z. Zellforsch., 60: 276, 1963.
18. Bedford, J.M., J. Anat., 99: 891, 1965.
19. Nicander, L. and Hellstrom, B., Exp. Cell Res., 48: 622, 1967.
20. Fawcett, D.W. and Phillips, D.M., J. Reprod. Fertil.,Suppl. 6: 405, 1969.
21. Quinn, P.J. and White, I.G., Aust. J. Biol. Sci., 20: 1205, 1967.
22. Bistocchi, M., d'Alessio, G. and Leone, E., J. Reprod. Fertil., 16: 223, 1968.
23. Crabo, B. and Gustafsson, B., J. Reprod. Fertil.,1: 337, 1964.
24. Wales, R.G., Wallace, J.C. and White, I.G., J. Reprod. Fertil., 12: 139, 1966.
25. Dawson, R.M.C., Mann, T. and White, I.G., Biochem. J., 65: 627, 1957.
26. Marquis, N.R. and Fritz, I.B., J. Biol. Chem., 240: 2197, 1965.
27. Dawson, R.M.C. and Rowlands, I.W., Quart. J. Exp. Physiol., 44: 26, 1959.
28. Meyhofer, W., Arch. Klin. Exp. Derm., 216: 556, 1963.

29. Leuchtenberger, C., J. Dairy Sci., 43: (Suppl.), 31, 1960.
30. Meyhofer, W., Arch. Klin. Exp. Derm., 219: 925, 1964.
31. Joel, C.A., Fertil. Steril., 17: 374, 1966.
32. Goldberg, E., Science, 139: 602, 1963.
33. Goldberg, E., Arch. Biochem. Biophys., 109: 134, 1965.
34. Goldberg, E. and Hawtrey, C., J. Exp . Zool., 165: 309, 1967.
35. Zinkham, W.H., Blanco, A. and Kupchyk, L., Pediatrics, 37: 120, 1966.
36. Stanbaugh, R. and Buckley, J., J. Biol. Chem., 242: 4053, 1967.
37. Schatz, L. and Segal, M.L., J. Biol. Chem., 244: 4393, 1969.
38. King, T.E. and Mann, T., Proc. Roy. Soc. Biol., 151: 226, 1959.
39. Bishop, D.W., Testicular enzymes as fingerprints in the study of spermatogenesis. In Reproduction and Sexual Behavior ed. Diamond, M., Indiana University Press, p. 261, 1968.
40. Rothschild, Lord, Proc. Roy. Soc. Biol. 152: 298, 1960.
41. Terner, C., Amer. J. Physiol., 198: 48, 1960.
42. Terner, C., In Spermatozoan Motility. Amer. Ass. Advan. Sci. Publ. No. 72, 89, 1962.
43. Nevo, A.C., J. Reprod. Fertil.,11: 19, 1966.
44. Murdoch, R.N. and White, I.G., J. Reprod. Fertil.,16: 351, 1968.
45. Eliasson, R., Murdoch, R.N. and White, I.G., Acta Physiol. Scand., 73: 379, 1968.
46. Peterson, R.N. and Freund, M., J. Reprod. Fertil.,17: 357, 1968.
47. Peterson, R.N. and Freund, M., Biol. Reprod., 1: 238, 1969.
48. Mann, T., Biochem. J., 48: 386, 1951.
49. Mann, T., Biochemistry of Semen and of the Male Reproductive Tract, Methuen., London, 1964.
50. Pike, J.E. and Weeks, J.R., Prostaglandin Bibliography. The Upjohn Company (Kalamazoo, Michigan, 1969.
51. Bergstrom, S. and Samuelsson, B. (ed), Prostaglandins. Nobel Symposium 2, held in Stockholm. Interscience Publishers, New York, 1966.
52. Pickles, V.R., Biol. Rev., 42: 614, 1967.
53. Euler, U.S. and Eliesson, R., Prostaglandins. Academic Press, New York and London, 1967.
54. Ingelman-Sundberg, A., In Progress in Infertility eds. Behrman, S.J. and Kistner, R.W. Little, Brown & Co., Boston, 1968.
55. Horton, E.W., Physiol. Rev., 49: 122, 1969.
56. Mann, T., Seamark, R.F. and Sharman, D., Brit. J. Pharmacol., 17: 208, 1961.
57. Mann, T., Biochem. J., 40: 481, 1946.
58. Mann, T. and Rottenberg, D.A., J. Endocr ., 34: 257, 1966.
59. Shulman, S. and Bronson, P., Fertil. Steril., 19: 549, 1968.
60. Quinlivan, W.L.G., Arch. Biochem., 127: 680, 1968.
61. Herrmann, W.P. and Hermann, G., Arch. Klin. Exp. Derm., 234: 100, 1969.
62. Quinlivan, W.L.G., The Physiologist, 12, No. 3, Aug., 1969.

63. Herrmann, W.P., Der Hautarzt, 19: 365, 1968.
64. Marberger, M., Marberger, E., Mann, T. and Lutwak-Mann, C., Brit. Med. J., i, 835, 1962.
65. Mann, T., Chemical analysis of semen as a diagnostic aid in reproductive failure. Proc. World Congr. Fertil. Steril., Tel-Aviv, 1969.
66. Mann, T., J.Reprod. Fert. Suppl., 4: 101, 1968.

DISCUSSION

DICZFALUSY: Dr. Mann, is there new information regarding the factors which initiate sperm motility in the epididymis? This question came up recently in a recent scientific group of WHO. It was felt that, if it were possible to interfere with sperm motility specifically, we would probably have an ideal male contraceptive.

MANN: Unfortunately, we do not know for certain what initiates motility in the epididymis, apart from oxygen. At one time it was believed that the migration of the kinoplasmic droplet forms a very important prerequisite. But now we know that that is not necessarily so. Even a sperm-flagellum severed from the sperm-head can still be motile. For example, we have at the Animal Research Station in Cambridge, a bull which is completely fertile, and ejaculates decapitated spermatozoa, that is sperm heads and flagellae separated from each other. These flagellae consist of midpieces and tails which although completely decapitated, are perfectly motile. Epididymal plasma per se is also unable to induce motility, but ejaculated seminal plasma can induce motility of immotile but viable spermatozoa not only aerobically but also anaerobically, since it contains fructose.

E. STEINBERGER: I seem to recall that Dr. Clermont reported some years ago motile flagellae in immature spermatids in the testis.

MANN: Yes, indeed one can occasionally observe some motility even in testicular spermatozoa, but these are very weak oscillatory movements. There is no progressive motility.

COUROT: Dr. Mann, is there something known about the factors involved in the initiation of the fertilizing ability of spermatozoa?

MANN: We know that the spermatozoa in the caput epididymidis at least in the rabbit, bull and ram, are still non-fertile; in the cauda epididymidis, however, they become fertile (though not fully capacitated). Fertilizing ability must be acquired, therefore, during the epididymal passage, however, not necessarily simultaneously with motility. We know that under certain conditions, motility and fertilizing ability can be dissociated from each other. For example, by exposing a sample of ram semen to a heavy dose of x-rays, so much so that the glass of the test-tube acquires a brownish color, one can render the spermatozoa completely infertile without disturbing their motility. So, again, we do not know what renders the spermatozoa fertile in the epididymis. We do know, however, that during the epididymal passage the spermatozoa change as regards their ultrastructure, metabolism and composition. As regards the chemical changes,we know, for instance, that the chemical character of the protein which complexes with nucleic acid changes during the epididymal passage.

MACLEOD: Dr. Mann, would you agree that the first substrate that would be utilizable for motility is probably not met until the spermatozoa reach the ampulla of the ductus deferens, where clearly there is production of fructose by the epithelium of that organ?

MANN: Yes, the first chance that the spermatozoa have to acquire motility anaerobically occurs in the ampullae when they come in contact with fructose. There is no fructose, however, in the epididymis. Epididymal spermatozoa depend, therefore, not on fructose, but on their aerobic endogenous respiration for induction of motility. The endogenous sperm respiration requires oxygen and it depends mainly on the oxidation of fatty acids liberated from phospholipids. The RQ (the oxidation quotient) is 0.7, as one would expect, in the absence of fructose. In the presence of fructose, it becomes 1.

PAULSEN: Discounting a blockage in the ductile system, where one observes an absence of fructose, do you recognize any specific or unique biochemical change in the seminal fluid plasma of androgenically normal but oligospermic males?

MANN: Not really.

MANCINI: Are there any data related to the appearance of sorbitol dehydrogenase in the cells of the germinal epithelium, and at which cell stage?

MANN: David Bishop at Baltimore investigated the behavior of sorbitol dehydrogenase not only in ejaculated spermatozoa, as we did, but in the immature and mature testis. He established convincingly that sorbitol dehydrogenase appears at the time when the testis becomes spermatogenically active. The appearance of sorbitol dehydrogenase is, therefore, dependent on spermatogenesis. But the same applies to certain other sperm enzymes, for example, lactate dehydrogenase. Among the isozymes of that enzyme is the so-called LDH IV (thus named because it migrates in electrophoresis as no. 4). This particular enzyme also appears at the time of spermatogenesis. In general, the formation of intracellular sperm enzymes must be regarded as a process which depends on spermatogenesis.

OHNO: In man, a number of genetic defects,such as Gauchey's disease, Nieman-Pick's and Marfan's syndrome are now known to be due to the deficient lysosomal enzymes, such as beta-glucosidase and beta glucosaminidase. I was wondering if the study of the sperm of these patients might give us pertinent information as to which acrosomal enzyme is essential for fertility.

MANN: It is our hope to relate some of the forms of male infertility in animals to enzyme abnormalities. The question which you raised, Dr. Ohno, is indeed very important.

THE SIGNIFICANCE OF DEVIATIONS IN HUMAN SPERM MORPHOLOGY

John MacLeod[1]

Department of Anatomy, Cornell University Medical College,

New York, N.Y.

If the premise is accepted that the spermatozoa released from the germinal epithelium do not, in the light microscope at least, undergo marked changes in head-structure in their subsequent passage through the duct system to the ejaculate; and if it is further assumed that, under physiological conditions, the germ cells are not absorbed in numbers by the ductal epithelium, then the cellular components of the ejaculate can be accepted, qualitatively and quantitatively, as truly representing the output of the germinal epithelium. It is certain that the spermatozoa in all species studied do undergo further maturation in the epididymis and possibly in the ductus deferens. The size, shape and internal structure of the acrosome are modified (1,2) as is the organization of the mitochondria of the middle piece (3). In confirming earlier work that the capacity for motility increases as the spermatozoa pass through the epididymis, Blandau (4) and Gaddum (5) have shown in the rabbit that this potentiation of motility is produced partly by an alteration in the head-tail relationship of the cell. Undoubtedly chemical changes in the cells occur in the epididymal transit which, in turn, may induce changes in their metabolic properties and an increasing capacity for the ultimate utilization of substrates.

However in man, and probably in other species, it seems reasonably certain that the gross shape and size of the sperm head is not modified to an appreciable degree between release from the germinal epithelium and the appearance of the cells in the ejaculate.

---

[1]Career Scientist, Health Research Council of the City of New York.

The authors were fortunate in having access to a variety of populations (medical students, patients, prisoners) in which the cellular content of serial ejaculates obtained over extended periods could be examined in relation to all aspects of semen quality. Only sperm morphology will be discussed here.

The validity of the sperm morphology examination is dependent upon at least two essentials. The first is that the same although arbitrary criteria of cell classification be followed throughout. The second is that a single observer perform all examinations. These conditions have been followed in all the studies presented below and have been described in detail elsewhere (6). Figs. 1 and 2 are diagrammatic representations of the dominant types of cells in the human ejaculate under normal and pathologic conditions. Table 1 shows a laboratory work sheet and the cell classifications in four hypothetical patients. The system of cell classification used may not suit all experienced workers in the field but it has proved valuable in this study. It is believed that the major changes in seminal cytology found as a result of trauma, illnesses, the use of antispermatogenic compounds, etc. occur within these cell classes.

In this study, the "mature" cell is defined arbitrarily as possessing a head, middle-piece and tail, regardless of aberrations in any of these structures. When structural defects in head-shape or size are found and cannot be classed as oval, large, small or tapering or bicephalic (Table 1) they are put in the amorphous category.

The spermatids and other immature cells form a single class and the ratio is expressed as a percentage of the total number of germinal cells in the ejaculate. This percentage is not additive in the mature-cell ratios.

EXPERIMENTAL RESULTS

Under stable environmental conditions the morphology of the germinal cells in the human ejaculate, in terms of the cell classification in Fig. 1 and Table 1, is remarkably constant (Table 2). In men of known fertility and otherwise normal semen quality the dominant cell is the "oval" form. The mean head-length of this cell is approximately five microns but it may vary from 2.5 to 10 microns, in which case the cell is classified in the "small" or "megalo" class. We have considered the "oval" form to be the "normal" cell in terms of potential fertility although it is quite certain that pregnancies can occur when other cell types predominate in the ejaculate. For example, in certain individuals of known fertility, the "small" form ratio may be as high as 60%. But since "oval" forms of normal dimensions are present in these ejaculates and since no one yet has been privileged to observe directly the types of human spermatozoa capable of fertilization, one cannot

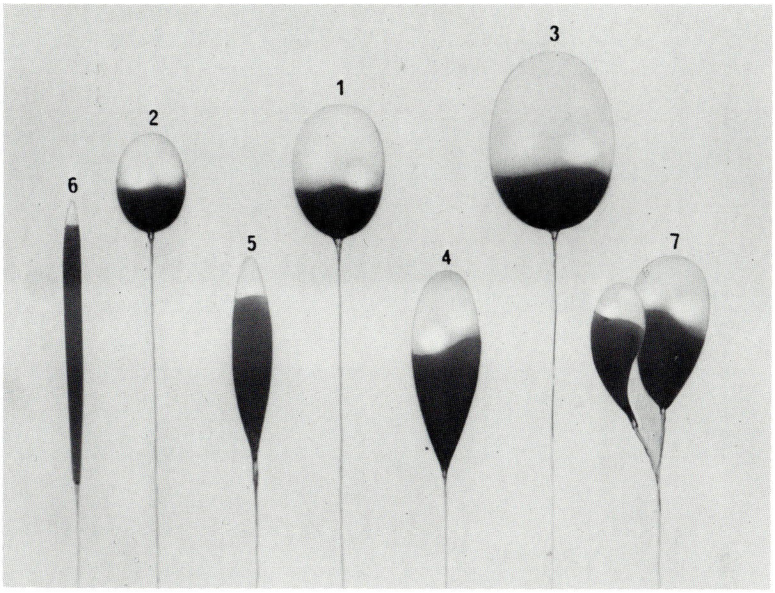

Fig. 1. Major types of spermatozoa in human ejaculate.
1) Normal; 2) Small; 3) Megalo; 4) Pyriform; 5) Tapering; 6) Acutely-tapering ("stress" cells); 7) Bicephalic.

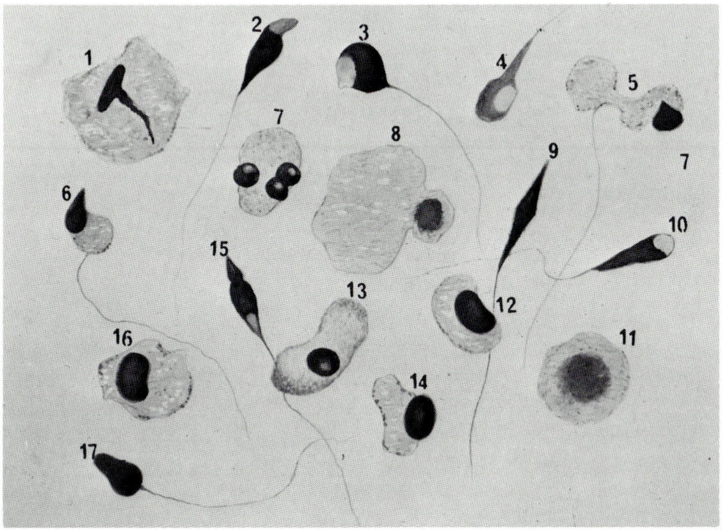

Fig. 2. Abnormal spermatozoa and immature cells in human ejaculate
1) Immature form with abnormal chromatin;
2,3,4,5,6,17 Types of amorphous forms; 7, Three spermatid nuclei in common cytoplasm; 8,11 "spermatid" "ghosts" -nuclei extruded; 9,10,15 Bizarre tapering and pyriform cells; 12,13,14,16 Mononuclear spermatids.

Table 1

MORPHOLOGY WORK SHEET							
PATIENT	OVAL (NORMAL)	LARGE	SMALL	TAPERING	AMORPHOUS	DOUBLE HEAD	IMMATURE (spermatids aberrant)
A	80	9	5	3	2	1	
B	20		60		20		
C	29	19	5	29	14		4
D	21	1	2	52	9	2	13

A typical work sheet of differential germ cell enumeration on 4 hypothetical cases.

Table 2. Sperm Morphology Readings on Same Individual Over 4 Year Period.

Date	Oval	Large	Small	Taper.	Amorph.	Biceph.	Immature (Spermatids)
12-27-62	43	3	8	12	17	17	4
1-18-63	38	3	2	18	19	20	16
12-3-63	38	7	2	10	23	20	6
11-4-64	34	4	6	17	19	20	6
*5-19-66	38	3.2	5.85	16.8	7	29	2.5

*1000 cells counted

speculate unduly on fertility in relation to head-shape and size.

The important facts are that each individual has a characteristic pattern of sperm morphology, whether it be perfection or one in which certain deviations in head-shape are found in constant ratios. Table 2 demonstrates this point in the semen of a medical student over a four-year period. In his freshman year, this young man had emotional problems but he also was found to have a large varicocele. His sperm morphology featured an unusually high percentage of bicephalic forms although other deviations were present (tapering, amorphous and immature forms). It will be seen that over a four-year period (he refused the varicocele ligation) the ratios of these cell types fell constantly within a narrow range. The ratio of immature forms varied and at the end of 3½ years the bicephalic ratio was higher than before although the basic pattern of spermatogenesis throughout the study was essentially the same.

This stability in sperm morphology can be demonstrated in large populations. In recent years our laboratory has been fortunate in its access to large clinical populations (husbands in sterile marriages) and to prison populations participating in studies of antispermatogenic compounds. Medical students also have been studied over extended periods. Table 3 presents data from over 900 prisoners in four penitentaries, from 1500 patients seen in sequence during a randomly-selected period and in 146 patients in whom varicocele had been found. It will be seen that the sperm morphology of the prisoners not only is good in terms of the "oval" forms but that the ratios of the various cell types are very similar in the group from each penitentiary. It can be said at this time that the prisoner morphologies show a remarkable lack of pathology.

In contrast, the patient groups, while quite similar numerically within themselves in so far as cell types are concerned, show much fewer "oval" forms. The ratio shift is towards the "large", tapering and amorphous forms and is accompanied by a nearly 10-fold increase in the presence of spermatids. The conjunction of the latter cells with the tapering and amorphous forms we have come to recognize as the response of the testes to a variety of stresses (7,8, 9). It is found after certain illnesses, (Table 4) allergic reactions (Table 5),and can be produced experimentally by antispermatogenic compounds (Table 6). In all of these instances too, spermatogenesis is severely depressed in the quantitative sense but both the sperm count and the morphology eventually return to the control levels after periods ranging from several weeks to months. The deviations in the sperm morphology may appear before the count depression and usually are gone before the count fully recovers.

The same "stress pattern" (tapering and immature forms) is found to a striking degree in the presence of varicocele. Indeed, it is diagnostic of varicocele if the individual does not give a clinical history which could otherwise account for the seminal picture. When this pattern is found in varicocele it persists in constant ratios until the varicocele is removed and may continue at a diminished level of pathology thereafter. It has also been found that bicephalia is common in the presence of varicocele. Table 7 illustrates a case of bilateral varicocele in which the semen quality was followed before and after the bilateral ligation. This husband was close to the sterile level. His seminal cytology showed the classic "stress" picture (tapering, amorphous and immature) plus a high percentage of bicephalic forms. Within six weeks after operation, a marked improvement in sperm motility was found although the sperm count remained low. In addition, the seminal cytology showed a marked drop in the ratios of bicephalic and immature forms. Five weeks later or about 11 weeks post-operatively, the sperm count had risen sharply to 62 million/ml, the motility remained at a good

Table 3

SEMINAL CYTOLOGIES OF PRISONERS AND PATIENTS

Location & Number		Oval %	Large %	Small %	Taper %	Amorph %	Bicephalic %	Spermatids % of Total Germinal
Prisoners								
Oklahoma	625	73.0	3.0	9.0	6.0	8.0	1.0	0.30
San Quentin	125	73.0	3.0	9.0	6.0	8.0	1.0	0.10
Atmore	103	73.0	2.0	8.5	5.5	10.0	1.0	0.40
Oregon	91	73.0	2.6	8.0	7.0	8.4	1.0	0.80
Patients in Sequence as seen 1-11-61 to 5-16-62								
1st	500	56.0	7.0	11.0	12.0	12.5	1.5	4.00
2nd	500	58.6	3.1	9.5	13.6	13.7	1.5	4.60
3rd	500	57.0	5.7	10.3	12.8	12.4	1.8	3.50
Varicocele								
	146	34.0	5.0	10.0	23.0	25.0	3.0	16.00

Patterns of sperm morphology in prison, infertile marriage and varicocele populations.

Table 4

EFFECT OF VIRAL INFECTION ON CYTOLOGY OF THE EJACULATE

Date 1961	Oval %	Large %	Small %	Taper %	Amorph %	Double Head %	Immature %
11-12	17	6	3	25	46	3	47
11-21	42	10		38	8	2	3
11-28	22	9	1	53	15	0	6
12-6	32	3		60	5	0	2
12-11	51	14	1	29	5	0	1.5
12-13	40	18	2	34	6	0	2.0
12-23	77	4	3	9	4	1	0.3
12-30	52	6	2	31	8	1	2.5
1-8-62	64	4	3	27	1	1	0
1-13	56	5	0	37	2	0	0
2-8	77	12	0	8	2	1	0

Effect of viral infection on sperm morphology following acute stage and during recovery.

level and the bicephalic forms remained relatively low. The "stress" picture, particularly the exfoliation of spermatids, virtually had disappeared. A conception occurred about this date and a normal pregnancy ensued. This case offers an excellent example not only of the initiation of fertility but of a virtually complete reversal of testicular pathology.

DISCUSSION

We believe these data show that the human testes are extremely sensitive to changes in their environment and that this sensitivity can be measured in the cellular components of the ejaculate with a considerable degree of precision. That the response of the testes to a variety of trauma is non-specific probably means that a particular level of spermatogenesis is vulnerable. Since the "tapering" forms and the spermatids in the ejaculate are prominent cells in the "stress" reaction, a strong argument can be made that the early and middle stages of spermatid development are peculiarly susceptible. The premature exfoliation of spermatids seems to occur predominantly between the Sb_1 and Sb_2 levels. The "tapering" form appears to be a cell which has undergone a marked over-elongation of the nucleus at and beyond the Sb_2 level where the normal elongation process occurs. Harvey (11), however, believes that the "tapering" (spindle)

Table 5

SPERMIOGRAM - BEFORE, DURING AND AFTER SEVERE ALLERGIC REACTIONS

Days	Vol. (ml)	Count ml (millions)	Total Count (millions)	Motility Index	Oval %	Large %	Small %	Tapering %	Amorph. %	Biceph. %	Immature %
Control (12 specimens)	4.20	360	1512	303	87	2	2	4	4	1	0.7
After start of reaction 35 days	3.0	115	345	0	47	7	3	7	35	1	17
49	3.2	6	19	0	50	12	10	11	15	2	31
77	4.0	6	24	3	31	20	3	32	12	2	30
90	2.6	7	18	150	53	3	6	12	23	3	20
106	2.0	175	350	388	68	3	9	7	9	4	3.0
126	3.2	309	989	270	82	1	2	7	6	2	0

Table 6

6-MEDROXY-PROGESTERONE ACETATE

AVERAGE SEMEN QUALITY OF FOUR MEN BEFORE AND AFTER

INJECTION OF 1000 MGMS IN A SINGLE SITE

Days After Injection	Vol. (ml)	Total Sperm Count (Millions)	Mot. Index	% Oval	% Large	% Small	% Taper	% Amorph	% Dup	% Sp.
	2.20	1200	212	82	3	5	4	6		1
	3.35	1029	104	71	4	5	7	13	1	2
Controls	2.55	669	320	84	3	2	2	8	1	0
	2.35	390	309	81	1	11	4	3	0	0
	2.45	619	230	76	4	9	3	7	1	0
7	2.80	391	220	81	2	9	2	6	0	0.5
28	2.10	229	248	54	3	6	9	17	1	2
49	2.10	51	49	14	2	20	23	40	1	8
70	2.10	5	2	12	4	16	20	47	1	5
80	1.72	4	0	20	6	13	33	26	2	12
98	2.30	10	66	29	4	16	22	28	1	14

The effect on sperm morphology of antispermatogenic agent (6-medroxy progesterone acetate).

Table 7

SEMEN QUALITY BEFORE AND AFTER VARICOCELE LIGATION

Date	Vol/ml	Count 10^6/ml	Total Count (millions)	Mot. Index	Oval	Large	Small	Taper	Amorph	Biceph	Spermatids
11-12-65	3.0	1.0	3	5	10		4	32	26	28	57
12-9-65	2.0	3	6	20	24		1	25	25	25	32
12-21-65	L I G A T I O N P E R F O R M E D										
2-4-66	2.8	4	11	225	45		9	23	17	6	10
*3-10-66	3.0	62	186	225	38	2	10	12	30	8	1

*conception occurred about this date

form is a result of abnormal behaviour of the chromosomes at both the first and the second maturation divisions. In this regard, one cannot preclude the possibility that the predilection towards the "tapering" form is laid down at a pre-spermatid level. But the premature exfoliation of spermatids from the Sertoli cell which so often appears in conjunction with the "tapering" form is more likely to be a pathologic reaction in spermiogenesis and may perhaps be the result of a traumatic assault directly upon the Sertoli cell.

The spermatids which appear in the ejaculate are usually mononuclear but often are found in clusters sharing a common cytoplasm (Fig. 2). These concretions of spermatid nuclei do not appear to be related to the presence of intercellular bridges at the spermatid level described by Fawcett et al. (12) in which groups of spermatids are joined one to the other in protoplasmic continuity. It seems more probable that the normal syncytial process described by these authors either has not occurred or has broken down. The difficulty still lies in explaining how the spermatid nuclei are lost from the parent cells and find themselves in a common cytoplasm apparently as discrete entities.

A further point of interest is that in the mononuclear and in the multi-nucleate cells, the nuclei are usually located peripherally near or contiguous to the cell border (Fig.2), a position they would occupy in normal spermiogenesis just prior to the first stage of elongation of the nucleus. Indeed, they often appear to be in the process of extrusion. In examining these cells in the seminal plasma, this peripheral positioning of the nuclei is obvious, and in certain cases, we actually have seen obvious bulging of the cell surface and extrusion as if the nuclei were being forced outwards by internal pressure. It is surprising not only that these cells survive the long passage through the duct system (at least 15 days from testes to the ejaculate) without undue degeneration but that these nuclear positions are retained in the ejaculated cells as they were when they first were exfoliated into the lumens of the seminiferous tubules.

In conclusion, it should be emphasized that while severe pathology in the germinal epithelium and the cellular contents of the ejaculate can be produced experimentally, by illnesses, etc. hese changes are fully reversible. And in this regeneration and restoration, the pattern of spermatogenesis, as seen in the ejaculate, prior to the trauma, is retained. In other words, each individual has an inherent pattern of spermatogenesis which possibly may be determined at the level of the spermatogonium.

ACKNOWLEDGEMENTS

The research was supported by Grant HD-00481 from the National Institutes of Health.

REFERENCES

1. Fawcett, D.W. and Hollenberg, R.D., Z. Zellforsch, 60: 276, 1963.
2. Bedford, J.M., J. Reprod. Fertil., 5: 169, 1963.
3. Anberg, A., Acta Obstet. Gynec. Scand. ,36: Suppl. 2 1, 1957.
4. Blandau, R.J. and Rumery, R.E., Fertil. Steril., 15: 571, 1964.
5. Gaddum, P., Anat. Rec., 161: 471, 1968.
6. MacLeod, J., Fertil. Steril., 13: 29, 1962.
7. MacLeod, J., Fertil. Steril., 20: 545, 1969.
8. MacLeod, J., Fertil. Steril., 13: 531, 1962.
9. MacLeod, J., J. and A. Churchill, Ltd. London p. 93, 1965.
10. Heller, C.G. and Clermont, Y., Recent Progr. Hormone Res., 20: 545, 1964.
11. Harvey, C. Studies on Fertility ed. R.G. Harrison, Blackwell, Oxford, p. 8, 1955.
12. Fawcett, D.W. Susumma Ito Slatterback, D., J. Biophys. Biochem. Cytol., 5: 453, 1959.

DISCUSSION

LUNENFELD: We have recently re-investigated Dr. Amelare's findings on the split ejaculate in oligospermic males. In most of the 80 patients which we investigated in the last seven months, the first part of the split ejaculate (0.5 ml. of a 2 ml. ejaculate) was of a significantly better quality than the second part. Could you elaborate on the reasons for these findings?

MACLEOD: The first part of the split ejaculate is richer than the second by nature of the ejaculatory process. It would seem that the ampulla of the ductus deferens is the first to contract and empties into the duct system the spermatozoa which are at that point at the time of ejaculation. I have not observed any real differences in morphology in these two systems; but I have observed that the motility in the first portion is usually much better than in the second. On the other hand, the second part of the ejaculate is usually bad in cellular content.

MANN: Dr. Lunenfeld may be interested in some observations which we made on thoroughbred stallions. Ejaculation in the stallion is a prolonged process, up to half-a-minute, so that it is relatively easy to collect by means of an artificial vagina, several separate fractions of the ejaculate. Normally, when one examines the split ejaculate one finds that the pre-sperm, sperm-rich and post-sperm fraction follow each other in an orderly fashion. However, under certain conditions, e.g. under the influence of drugs, the sequence of ejaculatory events is severely disturbed, and consequently the seminal fractions do not appear during ejaculation in the normal order.

HELLER: I would like to comment on the multinucleated cells that

Dr. MacLeod demonstrated in the ejaculate as well as in the seminiferous epithelium. The explanation for finding groups of cells together was offered some years ago by Dr. Don Fawcett. He found intercellular bridges connecting groups of spermatids. In our laboratory Mavis Rowley has recently demonstrated intercellular bridges between human pachytene spermatocytes. This phenomenon occurs early in the lifetime of spermatogenesis. Type A dark spermatogonia which can be identified because of the presence of vacuoles lying next to the basal membrane are clearly connected by a large intercellular bridge. I think that each of us is struck with the great similarity of cells during the process of spermatogenesis, in other words, we see whole families of cells that look exactly alike in a given cell association. When we look at another cell association and see the same cell, however, it appears slightly different from those in the first cell association but these cells again resemble each other exactly like members of a family. I wish to raise the question if this represents not a rare phenomenon but a usual phenomenon. In other words as these cells multiply they stay together as a family connected together by intercellular bridges. Now, assuming any and all of this, I want to ask Dr. MacLeod if during spermiation he thinks that maybe something goes wrong.

MACLEOD: The observation of intercellular bridges does not completely explain the phenomenon of multinucleated cells in the ejaculate. I agree with Dr. Heller that when one sees these multinucleated cells in the ejaculate, the nuclei are already separated and are located at distinctly separate points in the cytoplasm. The presence of more immature cells with multinucleation may be related to the phenomenon of the intercellular bridges. Similarly, the bicephalic mature spermatozoa are probably a manifestation of disruption late in spermiogenesis. This disruption may involve the bridges. At the present time, I would consider that the late stages in spermatogenesis are most vulnerable to "trauma".

E. STEINBERGER: Dr. MacLeod, do you see patients with oligospermia who do not show histologic abnormalities in the spermatozoa?

MACLEOD: Yes, I am very disappointed indeed when I do not find it. These are the cases which we have now relegated to the category of idiopathic infertility. Since our understanding has improved with respect to the influence of varicocele on spermatogenesis, only a relatively small group of oligospermic males are in the idiopathic category. These cases may exhibit abnormal sperm cytology but not the distinct shift to the right. We associate this with a "stressful" situation.

TROEN: Dr. MacLeod, do the tapering forms which you refer to as stress forms have normal motility?

MACLEOD: Yes, the tapering form may show very good motility and may migrate into the cervical mucus. Indeed, in performing the post-coital examination of the cervical mucus no other abnormal forms are seen aside from the tapering forms.

PHARMACOLOGICAL STUDIES ON THE TESTICULAR CAPSULE IN RELATION TO SPERM TRANSPORT

Joseph R. Davis and George A. Langford[1]

Department of Pharmacology and Therapeutics,
Loyola University Stritch School of Medicine,
Maywood, Illinois

The testicular capsule, which forms the thin outer covering of the testis, has long been considered an inert tissue with no other function than to contain the underlying seminiferous tubular mass. In the course of carrying out in vitro metabolic studies on rat testicular tissue in our laboratory, we have continually peeled off and discarded the capsule of the testis prior to slicing the testis with a Stadie-Riggs microtome. It recently occurred to us, however, that it might be quite easy to prepare and save the capsule of the rat testis as an intact tissue provided one first removed the seminiferous tubules from the interior of the organ (1).

Procedure for the Isolation of the Testicular Capsule.

The testicular capsule has been commonly called the "tunica albuginea", even though the tunica albuginea is but one of three layers comprising the complete capsular membrane. The three layers of the testicular capsule include the tunica vaginalis visceral, which is an outer thin serous layer, the tunica albuginea which forms the substance of virtually the entire capsule and the tunica vasculosa which is a thin delicate layer of loose areolar tissue directly beneath the tunica albuginea. Fig. 1 presents a schematic representation of the procedure that we devised for the isolation of the adult rat intact testicular capsule and its subsequent use as an isolated tissue preparation suitable for pharmacological studies (2). Following sacrifice of the animal, a single testis is removed and placed in Tyrode's solution. A small piece of the inferior end of the testis is cut away. The testicular parenchymal

[1]Predoctoral Trainee, U.S. Public Health Service.

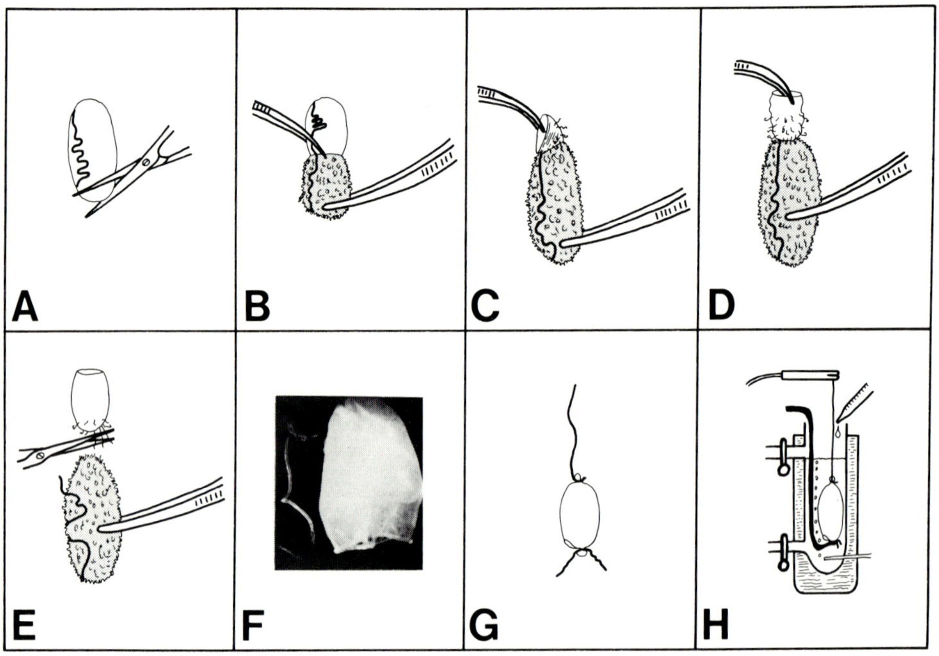

Fig. 1. Schematic representation of the procedure for the isolation of the testicular capsule of the adult rat and its use as an isolated tissue proparation for pharmacological studies. A. Cut a small piece off the inferior end of the testis. B. Grasp both the testicular parenchymal mass protruding through the resulting opening as well as the lower rim of the testicular capsule with forceps and gently pull apart. C. After removing most of the parenchymal tissue mass, turn the testicular capsule inside-out. D. Diagram of the testicular capsule in the inside-out position with only a few seminiferous tubules still attached to its inner surface. E. Cut away the few remaining seminiferous tubules from the testicular capsule, along with the large testicular artery. F. Photograph of the isolated testicular capsule in the inside-out position, illustrating the complete removal of all the interior tissue of the testis. The removed testicular artery is shown on the left. G. Tie the superior end of the testicular capsule with a long piece of silk thread and place a short tie at the inferior end of the capsule, leaving a small portion of the original hole in the capsule open. H. Mount the testicular capsule in a 10 ml isolated tissue bath with the short inferior thread attached to a support rod and the long superior thread leading to a transducer for detection of tissue contractions.

mass protruding through this small hole in the testis is then grasped with a forceps and removed from the interior of the testis. The lower rim of the testicular capsule is then grasped with a second forceps and the capsule is turned inside-out. The testicular capsule is then separated from the testicular parenchymal tissue as well as from the large testicular artery and the few remaining seminiferous tubules still attached to the inside surface of the capsule are carefully cut away. The intact isolated testicular capsule is then tied at its superior end with a long piece of silk thread. A second smaller tie is placed at the inferior end of the testicular capsule with care taken to leave approximately one-fourth of the original small hole in the capsule open. The intact isolated testicular capsule is then mounted in a 10 ml standard isolated tissue bath assembly with the upper long thread leading to a linear motion transducer connected to a suitable recorder.

The resulting isolated testicular capsule of the adult rat was found to resemble a thin hollow sac measuring approximately 2 cm in length and 1 cm in width with an average wet weight of 75 mg. The corresponding dimensions for the isolated testicular capsule of the adult rabbit were quite similar to those of the rat. However, the weight of the rabbit isolated testicular capsule was found to be almost twice that of the rat, averaging 125 mg.

Fig. 2 presents a photograph of the testicular capsule mounted within the complete isolated tissue assembly employed in our laboratory. The physiological salt solution in the isolated tissue bath was Tyrode's solution (3) warmed to a constant temperature and gassed with air. The paper speed of the recorder was 0.25 mm per second. Each drug was dissolved in Tyrode's solution and added to the isolated tissue bath in a volume of 0.1 ml by means of a suitable pipet. Any contraction or relaxation of the isolated testicular capsule then appears as a deflection of the pen on the recorder chart paper.

Pharmacological Studies on the Isolated Testicular Capsule of the Rat.

Now that the testicular capsule of the rat had been obtained as an intact isolated tissue for the first time, it seemed of interest to investigate the possible effects of pharmacological agents on this preparation. It also seemed of interest to compare the possible effects of pharmacological agents on the testicular parenchymal mass which had been obtained in an isolated form during the previously mentioned procedure for the isolation of the testicular capsule. It was therefore a simple matter to attach a superior and an inferior thread to the ends of the isolated testicular parenchymal mass and to mount the entire isolated testicular parenchyma in an organ bath in a manner similar to that just described for the isolated testicular capsule.

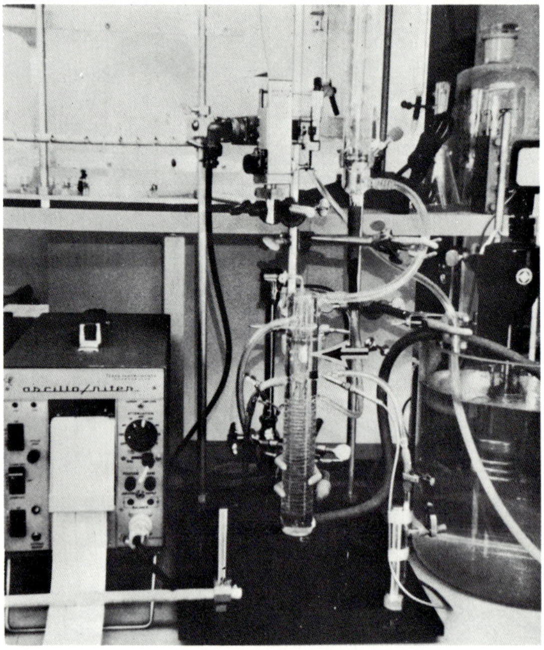

Fig. 2. Photograph of the isolated tissue assembly employed in the authors' laboratory for measurement of contractions of the isolated testicular capsule. The testicular capsule mounted within the isolated tissue bath is indicated by the arrow. A linear motion transducer above the tissue bath is connected to a recorder shown at the left. A constant-temperature water bath, shown at the right, serves to maintain the desired temperature of the isolated tissue bath.

Fig. 3 presents the response of the isolated testicular capsule of the adult rat to various autonomic drugs. Both acetylcholine and norepinephrine were observed to produce a marked contraction of the isolated testicular capsule. In each case, the contractions produced by the neurohumoral agent were found to be dose dependent, with maximal responses occurring at a final organ bath concentration of 1 μg/ml. Maximal contraction of the isolated testicular capsule to both acetylcholine and norepinephrine was reached approximately three minutes following addition of the drug. The testicular capsule was found to relax slowly after it had been caused to contract so that a slight extra weight was added to the initial resting tension load of 100 mg in order to assist its recovery. This procedure was found to conveniently allow doses to be added about once every 15 minutes.

Two additional parasympathomimetic agents, carbachol and pilocarpine, were compared with acetylcholine as to their effect on the isolated testicular capsule of the rat. Carbachol, an example of a

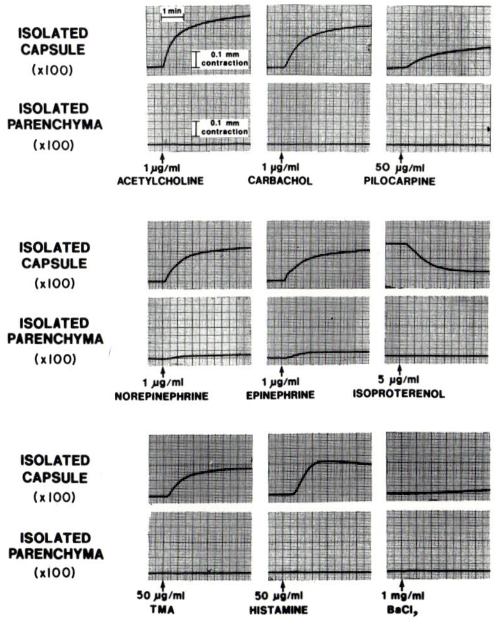

Fig. 3. Comparison of the response of the isolated capsule versus the isolated parenchymal tissue of the adult rat testis to various autonomic drugs. Two large squares shown on the chart paper measure 10 mm. The response magnification was x 100 for both the isolated testicular capsule and isolated testicular parenchyma. The vertical bar represents the actual mm of tissue contraction for each preparation; i.e., for both the isolated testicular capsule and isolated testicular parenchyma, two large squares on the chart paper are equal to an actual tissue contraction of 0.1 mm. In each case, the load on the lever arm was 100 mg. Drug concentrations are expressed per ml of organ bath volume. The temperature of the isolated tissue bath was maintained at 32°C.

synthetic cholinomimetic agent, resembled acetylcholine in producing a marked contraction of the isolated testicular capsule. Pilocarpine, an example of a naturally-occurring cholinomimetic agent, was also found to cause a contraction of the isolated testicular capsule but the response to pilocarpine appeared much less sensitive as compared to acetylcholine. The effects of two additional sympathomimetic agents, namely epinephrine and isoproterenol, were compared with norepinephrine as to their effect on the isolated testicular capsule of the rat. Epinephrine, on the one hand, was observed to cause a contraction of the testicular capsule while isoproterenol, on the other hand, was found to cause a pronounced relaxation of the testicular capsule.

Tetramethylammonium (TMA), which is a ganglionic stimulating agent, was found to produce a contraction of the isolated testicular capsule of the rat. This observation would seem to suggest, for the first time, the possible presence of parasympathetic ganglia located in the testicular capsule. Histamine was also found to cause a marked contraction of the isolated testicular capsule of the rat. However, barium chloride was observed to produce just a slight contraction of the isolated testicular capsule of the rat and only at the extremely high final concentration of 1 mg/ml of organ bath volume.

Fig. 3 also presents a comparison of the response of the isolated testicular parenchymal tissue of the adult rat to the same nine autonomic drugs just mentioned for the isolated testicular capsule. The isolated parenchymal mass of the adult rat testis had a wet weight which averaged 1,450 mg as compared to only 75 mg for the isolated testicular capsule. The load on the lever arm was 100 mg for both the testicular capsule and the testicular parenchyma. Of the nine autonomic drugs studied, only norepinephrine and epinephrine were observed to have any effect on the isolated testicular parenchyma and these two agents caused only a negligible degree of contraction. For example, whereas the addition of 1 μg/ml final concentration of norepinephrine to the isolated testicular capsule produced a tissue contraction of 0.286 mm/100 mg, the same addition of norepinephrine to the isolated testicular parenchyma produced a tissue contraction of only 0.001 mm/100 mg. Whereas 1 μg/ml epinephrine produced a tissue contraction of the isolated testicular capsule of 0.267 mm/100 mg, the same addition of epinephrine to the isolated testicular parenchyma produced a tissue contraction of only 0.002 mm/100 mg.

Pharmacological Studies on the Isolated Testicular Capsule of the Rabbit.

The preparation of the isolated testicular capsule of the adult rabbit is similar to that shown for the rat in Fig. 1 with the exception that it is somewhat more laborious to remove the internal parenchymal tissue of the rabbit testis because of the numerous thin septa extending from the capsule into the testicular parenchyma. In contrast to the adult rat testicular capsule, the isolated testicular capsule of the adult rabbit was observed to undergo marked spontaneous contractions within one hour of mounting in the organ bath and before the addition of any drug. However, it should be kept in mind that while the demonstration of spontaneous contractions employing the rabbit testicular capsule has important physiological implications, the absence of demonstrable spontaneous contractions employing the rat testicular capsule has distinct pharmacological advantages involving assay of drug effects. Indeed, bioassay procedures in pharmacology are often designed to eliminate spontaneous contractions of an isolated tissue in order to determine more accurately the extent of drug-induced contractions. It would seem, therefore, that both the rat and rabbit isolated testicular capsule preparations have their own unique advantages for pharmacological investigations. The amplitude of the spontaneous contractions of the rabbit isolated testicular capsule was found to average a 5 percent shortening of the actual entire length of the mounted capsule and indeed, it was even possible to observe these rhythmic movements of the capsule with the unaided eye. The frequency of the spontaneous contractions of the isolated testicular capsule of the adult rabbit ranged from 3 to 5 per minute.

Fig. 4 presents typical spontaneous contractions recorded from the rabbit isolated testicular capsule as well as from the whole rabbit testis without removal of the capsule. In marked contrast to the periodic spontaneous contractions recorded from both the isolated testicular capsule and the whole testis, no spontaneous contractions of the isolated testicular parenchymal tissue were observed, even at a magnification response of x 100. It would therefore appear that the testicular capsule alone is responsible for the endogenous rhythmic spontaneous contractions observed with the whole rabbit testis. In addition, the fact that the whole testis with its contained seminiferous tubules and interstitial tissue offering a mass of tissue resistance was observed to undergo spontaneous contractions would seem to lend great physiological importance to the contractions described for the isolated capsule alone.

Fig. 5 presents a comparison of the response of the isolated capsule versus the isolated parenchymal tissue of the adult rabbit testis to the same autonomic drugs employed for the adult rat testis. Like the isolated testicular capsule of the rat, the rabbit isolated testicular capsule was found to undergo a contraction following the addition of acetylcholine and norepinephrine. A final concentration of 1 μg/ml of acetylcholine in the organ bath resulted in a contraction of the rabbit isolated testicular capsule which amounted to approximately a 10 percent shortening of the actual entire length of the mounted capsule. A final concentration of 1 μg/ml of norepinephrine in the organ bath produced a 20 percent shortening of the actual entire length of the mounted capsule.

The rabbit isolated testicular capsule was also found to resemble the isolated testicular capsule of the rat in that contractions were produced by the addition of carbachol, epinephrine, tetramethylammonium (TMA) and histamine. The rabbit isolated testicular capsule was found to be unusually sensitive to histamine in that a final concentration of only 5 μg/ml of histamine resulted in a marked contraction. In addition, isoproterenol also produced a prolonged relaxation of the isolated testicular capsule of the rabbit, as well as completely abolishing capsular spontaneous contractions. However, two differences were noted between the isolated testicular capsule of the rat and rabbit in that pilocarpine, in a

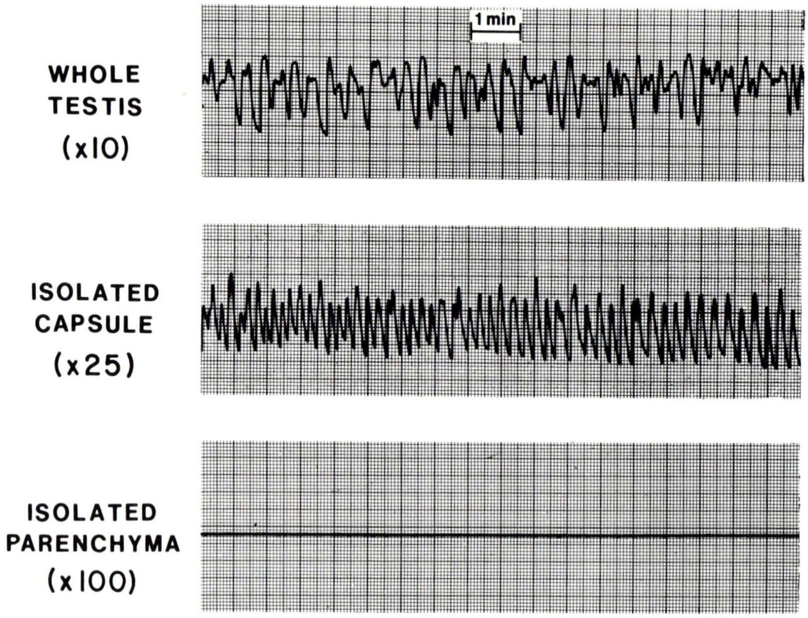

Fig. 4. Spontaneous contractions of the adult rabbit testis in the absence of any added drugs. Two large squares shown on the chart paper measure 10 mm. The top recording was obtained from the whole testis weighing 1,700 mg at a response magnification of x 10. The middle recording was obtained from the isolated testicular capsule weighing 135 mg at a response magnification of x 25. The bottom recording was obtained from the isolated testicular parenchyma weighing 1,550 mg at a response magnification of x 100. In every case, the load on the lever arm was 100 mg. The temperature of the isolated tissue bath was maintained at 37°C.

comparable dose, did not elicit any response while barium chloride, in a comparable dose, produced a very large contraction of the rabbit testicular capsule.

In a similar fashion to that observed in the rat, the isolated testicular parenchymal tissue of the adult rabbit displayed only extremely small and quite negligible contractions with several of the autonomic agents studied, even at a response magnification of x 100. For example, the addition of 1 μg/ml final concentration of both acetylcholine and norepinephrine to the isolated testicular capsule of the rabbit resulted in tissue contractions of 0.975 and 1.185 mm/100 mg respectively. However, similar additions of both acetylcholine and norepinephrine to the isolated testicular parenchyma of the rabbit resulted in tissue contractions which averaged

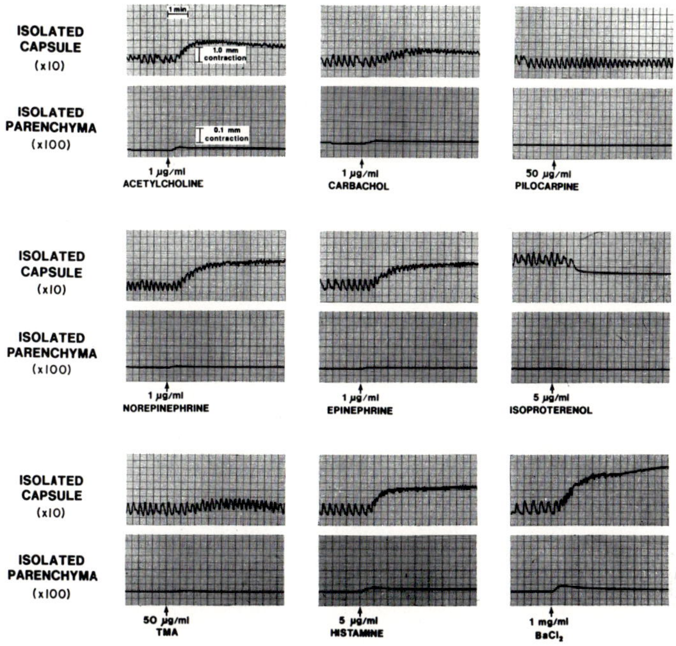

Fig. 5. Comparison of the response of the isolated capsule versus the isolated parenchymal tissue of the adult rabbit testis to various autonomic drugs. Two large squares shown on the chart paper measure 10 mm. The response magnification was x 10 for the isolated testicular capsule and x 100 for the isolated testicular parenchyma. The vertical bar represents the actual mm of tissue contraction for each preparation; i.e., for the isolated testicular capsule two large squares on the chart paper is equal to an actual tissue contraction of 1.0 mm while for the isolated testicular parenchyma two large squares on the chart paper are equal to an actual tissue contraction of only 0.1 mm. In each case, the load on the lever arm was 100 mg. Drug concentrations are expressed per ml of organ bath volume. The temperature of the isolated tissue bath was maintained at 37°C.

not more than 0.001 mm/100 mg.

Pharmacological Studies of the Isolated Testicular Capsule of the Human

The question then arose in our mind as to whether the presently-described pharmacological responses of the isolated testicular capsule of the rat and rabbit would also occur in the human testicular capsule. Segments of normal testes from males aged 60-70 years which had been removed as a therapeutic measure for prostatic carcinoma were brought to our laboratory within 15 minutes of removal of the testis at surgery. Inasmuch as the entire isolated testicular capsule of the human was much too large to be mounted in our organ baths, strips of the testicular capsule were cut and utilized for pharmacological investigations. Each strip of the isolated testicular capsule of the human was cut to an approximate measurement of 20 mm in length and 6 mm in width, with an average wet weight of 400 mg. The strip was then tied with silk thread at both ends and mounted in a 10 ml isolated tissue bath with the upper long thread leading to a transducer connected to a recorder.

Fig. 6 presents the results of our initial pharmacological studies on the isolated testicular capsule of the human. The human testicular capsule was observed to undergo very marked spontaneous contractions which reached an actual tissue contraction of 1.381 mm/100 mg. These extremely strong spontaneous contractions represented a remarkable 39 percent shortening of the actual entire length of the mounted strip of the testicular capsule of the human. The average frequency of these spontaneous contractions of the human testicular capsule was such that one extremely powerful contraction occurred every 13.6 minutes. It is interesting to note that in most instances a large spontaneous contraction was followed by a slightly smaller spontaneous contraction and that the larger contraction was usually biphasic in nature. One might well speculate that spontaneous contractions of the human testicular capsule may occur even more frequently in males who are younger than the ones studied in the present experiments, especially in view of the finding of Mancini et al. (4,5) that the tunica albuginea undergoes hyalinization with increasing age.

Fig. 7 presents the effects of various autonomic drugs on the isolated testicular capsule of the human. Each drug was added to the organ bath shortly after the recording of a spontaneous contraction had returned to baseline so as to be sure that the response was due to the added drug alone. Acetylcholine, carbachol, norepinephrine, tetramethylammonium (TMA) and barium chloride were all observed to induce a contraction of the isolated testicular capsule of the human. The human testicular capsule seemed extremely sensitive to norepinephrine and indeed, norepinephrine was found to induce spontaneous contractions of the testicular capsule at the peak of its effect, which was within two minutes of addition to the organ bath. Whereas norepinephrine was found to produce a shortening of the actual entire length of the mounted capsule of the rat and rabbit testis which amounted to approximately 2 and 10 percent, respectively, norepinephrine produced a 20 percent shortening of the actual entire length of the mounted testicular capsule of the human.

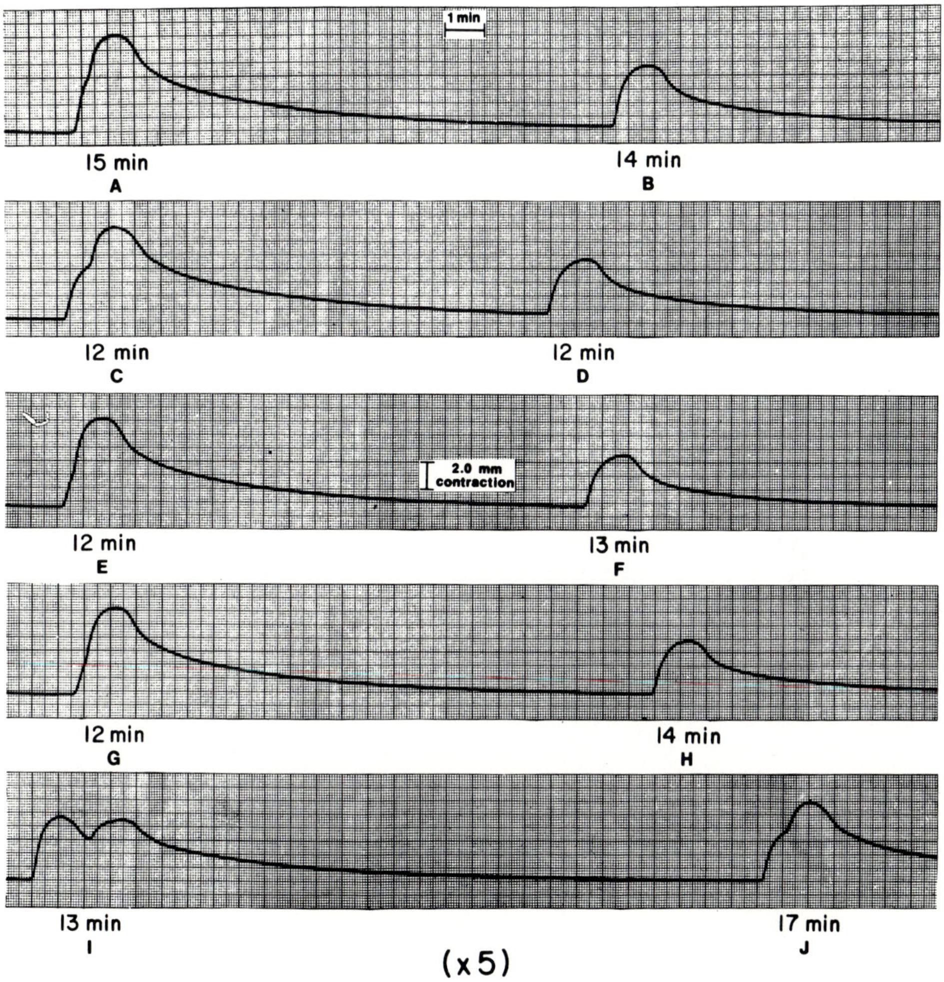

Fig. 6. Spontaneous contractions of the isolated testicular capsule of the human in the absence of any added drugs. Two large squares shown on the chart paper measure 10 mm. The response magnification was x 5. The vertical bar represents the actual mm of tissue contraction; i.e., two large squares on the chart paper equals an actual tissue contraction of 2.0 m. A through J represent consecutive spontaneous contractions observed throughout a time period of 134 minutes. The time beneath each spontaneous contraction represents minutes after the preceding contraction. The temperature of the isolated tissue bath was maintained at 32°C. The preparation employed was a longitudinal strip of the isolated testicular capsule 18 mm in length and 7 mm in width which was obtained from the superior half of the posterior border of the human testis. The load on the lever arm was 250 mg.

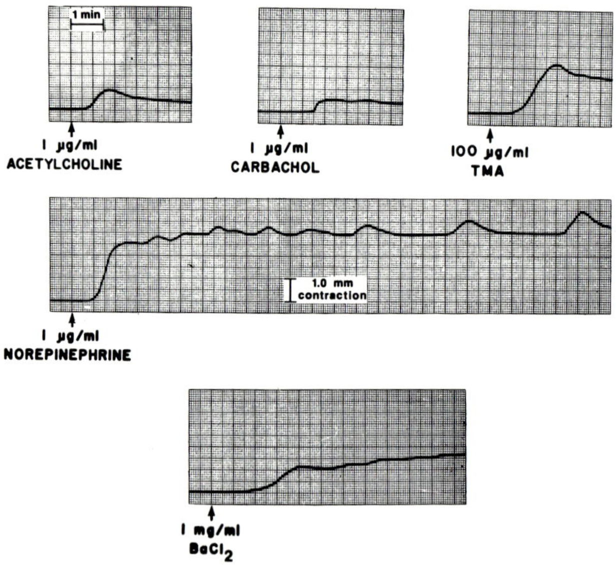

Fig. 7. Effect of autonomic drugs on the isolated testicular capsule of the human. Two large squares shown on the chart paper measure 10 mm. The response magnification was x 10. The vertical bar represents the actual mm of tissue contraction; i.e., two large squares on the chart paper equals an actual tissue contractions of 1.0 mm. Drug concentrations are expressed per ml of organ bath volume. The temperature of the isolated tissue bath was maintained at 32°C. The preparation employed was a circular strip of the isolated testicular capsule measuring 20 mm in length and 6 mm in width which was obtained from the middle third of the medial surface of the human testis. The load on the lever arm was 250 mg.

Histological Studies of the Testicular Capsule of the Rat, Rabbit and Human

Because of the presently-observed pharmacological responses of the isolated testicular capsule of the rat, rabbit and human, it became of particular interest to attempt to ascertain the presence of smooth muscle in the testicular capsule of these three species. Fig. 8 presents typical sections of the testicular capsule obtained from an adult rat, an adult rabbit and a 65-year-old human. By employing Masson's trichrome stain, it was possible to identify occasional smooth muscle fibers as well as smooth muscle nuclei which were located within the collagenous tissue of the rat testicular capsule. In contrast to the sparse amount of smooth muscle present in the testicular capsule of the rat, two distinct layers of smooth

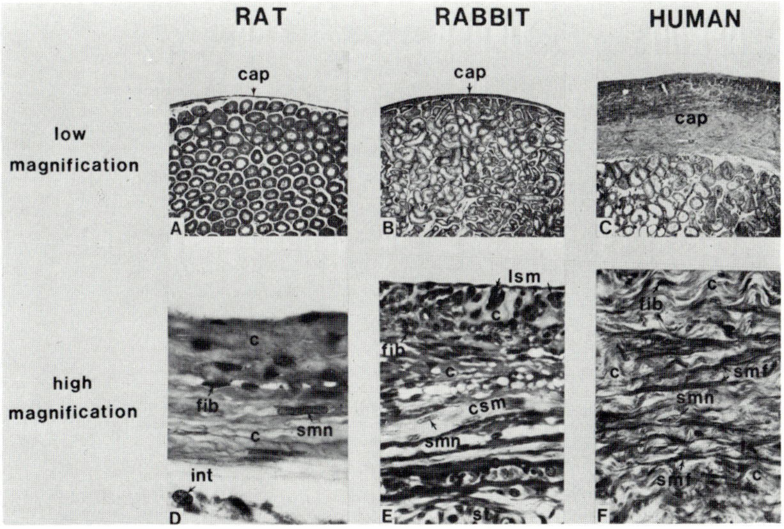

Fig. 8. Representative sections of the testicular capsules of the rat, rabbit and human stained with Masson's trichrome stain illustrating the comparative thickness of each capsule as well as the presence of smooth muscle. A-C. Low magnification of the testicular capsule (cap) surrounding the parenchymal tissue of the rat, rabbit and human testis, respectively (x 22). D. High magnification of the rat testicular capsule demonstrating occasional smooth muscle nuclei (smn) within the collagenous tissue (c) of the tunica albuginea. fib, fibroblast; int, interstitial tissue cell (x 1125). E. High magnification of the rabbit testicular capsule demonstrating the superficial layer of longitudinal smooth muscle (lsm) as well as the deeper layer of circular smooth muscle (csm). st, seminiferous tubule (x 490). F. High magnification of the human testicular capsule demonstrating the abundance of smooth muscle fibers (smf) located within the dense collagenous tissue of the tunica albuginea (x 490).

muscle fibers were found in the tunica albuginea of both the rabbit and the human testicular capsule. A superficial layer of longitudinal smooth muscle appears to run parallel to the long axis of the testis while a second, deeper layer of circular smooth muscle appears to be oriented along the circumference of the testis at right angles to the superficial layer. In addition, numerous fibroblasts were observed within the dense collagenous tissue of the tunica albuginea. A definite relationship appears to exist between the extent of the observed pharmacological responses and the amount of smooth muscle present in the testicular capsules of the three species studied. The fact that the testicular capsule was found to contain smooth muscle seems to offer a reasonable anatomical explanation for both the spontaneous and the drug-induced contractions which have been observed with the isolated testicular capsule.

Pharmacological Studies of the Intact Rabbit Testis In Vivo

While in vitro isolated tissue experiments are known to accurately reflect an actual in vivo situation, it nevertheless seemed of importance to attempt to answer the difficult question of whether spontaneous contractions as well as drug-induced contractions and relaxations of the testicular capsule do indeed occur in a living animal. Fig. 9 presents an in vivo isolated tissue apparatus which we designed to measure spontaneous contractions of the intact rabbit testis in an anesthetized animal. An adult male rabbit weighing approximately 3 kg was anesthetized with urethane and a small incision made through the various layers of the scrotum in order to expose the testis. A long piece of silk thread was carefully placed through the testicular capsule at the superior end of the testis with a second smaller tie placed through the capsule at the inferior end of the testis. The intact testis was then gently drawn through the glass tube in the rubber stopper and anchored to its top lip by means of the inferior tie. The scrotal sac was then sealed around the bottom lip of the glass tube by means of a strong circular tie. A small water-jacketed bath was then placed over the rubber stopper, with the superior thread from the testis leading through a top hole in the bath to a transducer connected to a recorder. The bath was then filled through an inlet tube with 20 ml of Tyrode's solution kept at a constant temperature of 37°C, corresponding to the normal scrotal temperature of the rabbit, in order to prevent the testis from drying out. The intact rabbit testis was completely surrounded by this buffer solution while still being attached via the spermatic cord to the anesthetized animal. It was found that the head of the animal had to be raised slightly to prevent drainage of the buffer solution into the peritoneal cavity. It therefore seemed possible with this apparatus to be able not only to measure spontaneous contractions of the intact testis in vivo, but also to attempt to produce drug-induced responses of the intact testis by injection of a drug into the rabbit ear vein.

Fig. 10 presents the results of our initial in vivo pharmacological studies of the rabbit testis. The photograph illustrates the anesthetized rabbit with its head slightly raised as well as the intact testis inside the temperature-controlled bath simulating an extension of the scrotal sac. As shown in the top recording, spontaneous contractions of the intact rabbit testis were found to occur in vivo with an average frequency of 4 per minute, corresponding almost exactly to our previous in vitro results obtained with the isolated testicular capsule. As shown in the bottom recording, the intravenous injection of 25 μg/kg body weight of carbachol was observed to produce a contraction of the intact rabbit testis in vivo which

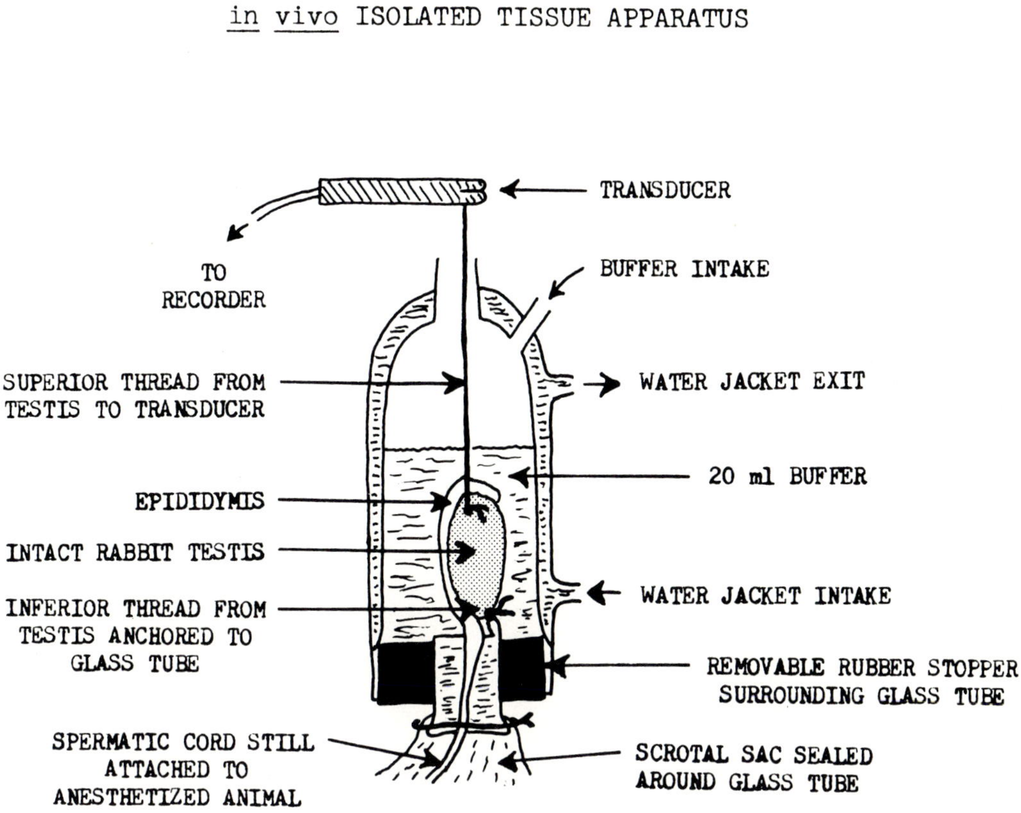

Fig. 9. Schematic representation of the in vivo isolated tissue apparatus designed for measurement of spontaneous and drug-induced contractions of the intact rabbit testis in an anesthetized animal. The intact rabbit testis still attached to the anesthetized animal by the spermatic cord is kept at normal scrotal temperature by a constant-temperature circulating water bath through the outer water jacket. Drugs can be administered intravenously into the systemic circulation of the rabbit by employing either the ear vein or the femoral vein.

was characterized by a marked increase in tone. The intravenous injection of 75 μg/kg body weight of isoproterenol, on the other hand, was found to produce a marked relaxation of the intact rabbit testis in vivo, again confirming our previous in vitro results. These data indicate that both spontaneous contractions as well as drug-induced contractions and relaxations of the rabbit testis related to the testicular capsule can be demonstrated in a living animal using the in vivo isolated tissue apparatus presently described.

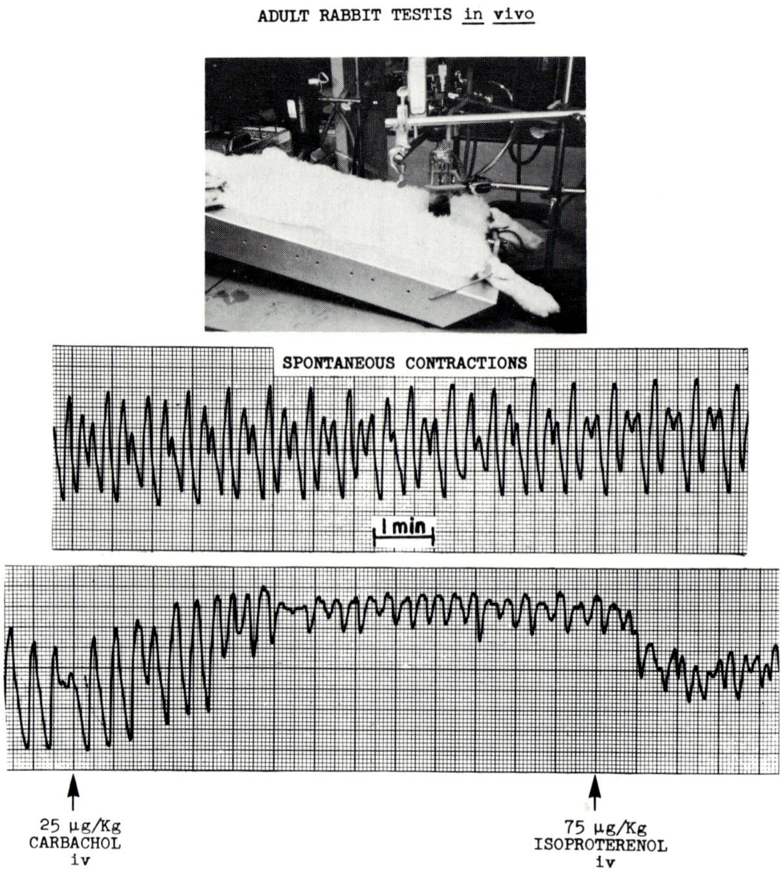

Fig. 10. Spontaneous contractions and drug responses of the intact testis of an anesthetized rabbit employing the in vivo isolated tissue apparatus described in Fig. 9. Two large squares shown on the chart paper measure 10 mm. The response magnification was x 25. The temperature of the circulating water bath was maintained at 37°C. Both carbachol, which produced a sustained contraction of the intact testis, and isoproterenol, which produced a relaxation of the intact testis, were administered intravenously.

Relation of the Testicular Capsule to Sperm Transport

It has long been established that the sperm formed in the seminiferous tubules of the testis are not capable of motility (6) and that the sperm first attain their motility in the epididymis (7). The factors responsible for the initial transportation of non-motile sperm out of the testis and into the epididymis have remained unclear, although a number of possibilities have been offered, including fluid flow resulting from ciliary movements in the rete testis and vasa efferentia (8) and in vitro undulating motions of individual seminiferous tubules involving both Sertoli cells (9) and various forms of peritubular cells (10-13). However, Leeson (14) in investigating the fine structure of the rete testis by electron microscopy concluded that the number of cilia present in the rete epithelium were insufficient to have any effect on sperm transport. In addition, Cross (15) noted that when large coiled masses of seminiferous tubules were viewed directly with a microscope through an incision of the abdominal wall of an anesthetized rabbit, the seminiferous tubules did not exhibit any contractions. Furthermore, there have been suggestions that the testis as a whole organ might be capable of undergoing spontaneous movements, as indicated by rhythmic interstitial pressure changes obtained with a cannula (16) as well as the observation of irregular movements of the entire testis (17). It therefore seems reasonable, in our opinion, to expect something other than ciliary movement or possible minute in vitro undulating motions of the seminiferous tubules as observed with a microscope to be responsible for movements of the entire testis which can be seen with the unaided eye. It would appear, based on the data of the present report, that the responsible factor for testicular movements is the contraction and relaxation of the testicular capsule.

The present finding that the isolated testicular capsule of both the rabbit and the human exhibits periodic and powerful spontaneous contractions in the absence of any added drug would seem to indicate that under normal conditions, the testicular capsule is in a constant state of dynamic movement, capable of exerting great force against the contained seminiferous tubular mass. It seems likely that these rhythmic contractions of the testicular capsule then serve to massage the seminiferous tubules and in so doing provide a pumping action which transports the non-motile sperm from the seminiferous tubules out of the testis and into the epididymis where the sperm can then attain their motility.

The present experiments have also demonstrated that both of the naturally-occurring neurohumoral agents of the autonomic nervous system, namely acetylcholine and norepinephrine, are capable of causing contractions of the isolated testicular capsule of the rat, rabbit and human. The possibility therefore exists that one partial explanation for the loss of fertility in males with sympathetic nerve damage may involve a lack of norepinephrine, thereby resulting in an impairment of testicular capsular contractions necessary to propel sperm into the epididymis. It is interesting to speculate that such cases of male infertility might be corrected if the impaired contractions of the testicular capsule could be artificially stimulated by either a sympathomimetic agent or a parasympathomimetic agent such as carbachol.

On the other hand, one possible approach to male contraception may involve the administration of a drug which can cause a prolonged relaxation of the testicular capsule, thereby preventing the sperm-propelling action of the testicular capsule. It would also seem of interest to explore the possibility that some drugs which are commonly administered to males may have as yet undetected side-effects involving either the stimulation or inhibition of testicular capsular contractions, thereby affecting sperm transport from the testis. Such experiments are now in progress in our laboratory.

SUMMARY

The testicular capsule of the rat, rabbit and human has been prepared for the first time as an isolated tissue suitable for pharmacological investigation. Both cholinergic and adrenergic agents were found to cause a contraction of the isolated testicular capsule. In addition, periodic spontaneous contractions of the isolated testicular capsule have been observed in the absence of any added pharmacological agents. The present experiments have also demonstrated that the testicular capsule contains smooth muscle, thereby offering a reasonable anatomical explanation for both spontaneous and drug-induced contractions of the testicular capsule. It therefore appears likely that the rhythmic contractions and relaxations of the testicular capsule provide a pumping action capable of explaining the transport of non-motile sperm out of the testis and into the epididymis where they can then attain their motility.

ACKNOWLEDGEMENT

This investigation was supported by U.S. Public Health Service Research Grant HD-01573 from the National Institute of Child Health and Human Development.

REFERENCES

1. Davis, J.R. and Langford, G.A., Nature (London), 222: 386, 1969.
2. Davis, J.R. and Langford, G.A., J. Reprod. Fertil., 19: 595, 1969.
3. Tyrode, M.V., Arch. Int. Pharmacodyn., 20: 205, 1910.
4. Mancini, R.E., Arrillaga, F., Vilar, O. and De La Balze, F.A., Rev. Soc. Argent. Biol., 31: 161, 1955.
5. Mancini, R.E., Vilar, O., Perez del Cerro, M. and Lavieri, J.C. Acta Physiol. lat. amer., 14: 382, 1964.
6. Rendenz, E., Wurzb. Abhandl. ges. Med., 24: 107, 1926.
7. Yochem, D.E., Physiol. Zool., 3: 309, 1930.
8. Reid, B.L. and Cleland, K.W., Aust. J. Zool., 5: 223, 1957.
9. Roosen-Runge, E.C., Anat. Rec., 109: 413, 1951.
10. Clermont, Y., Exp. Cell Res., 15: 438, 1958.
11. Lacy, D. and Rotblat, J., Exp. Cell Res., 21: 49, 1960.
12. Ross, M.H. and Long, I.R., Science, 153: 1271, 1966.

13. Niemi, M. and Kormano, M., Ann. Med. Exp. Fenn., 43: 40, 1965.
14. Leeson, T.S., Anat. Rec., 144: 57, 1962.
15. Cross, B.A., In Recent Progress in the Endocrinology of Reproduction, ed. Lloyd, C.W., Academic Press, New York, p. 172.
16. Holstein, A.F. and Weiss, Ch., Z ges. exp. Med., 142: 334, 1967.
17. Wojcik, K., Acta Physiol. Pol., 17: 78, 1966.

DISCUSSION

JOST: Dr. Davis, did you study the effect of oxytocin on the albuginea?

DAVIS: We have just recently begun to investigate the effect of oxytocin and vasopressin on the isolated testicular capsule of the adult rat. Our preliminary experiments have indicated that both are capable of causing contractions of the testicular capsule.

MANN: I am particularly impressed by the regularity of the spontaneous contractions which you observed, e.g. 13 minutes in the human testis capsule. This seems to suggest that some chemical substance must be discharged at the time of spontaneous contraction, and that during the period of relaxation that substance is gradually replenished. Could this phenomenon be explained further by studying the action of, for example, the parasympathetic and sympathic blocking agents, such as atropine, on the spontaneous contractions?

DAVIS: We are presently investigating the effect of a number of autonomic blocking agents on the drugs which we have shown to cause both contraction and relaxation of the isolated testicular capsule. We have found that atropine is capable of blocking acetylcholine-induced testicular capsular contractions in the rat. However, we have not yet investigated the effect of atropine on spontaneous contractions of the rabbit testicular capsule.

TROEN: Dr. Davis, in your in vivo experiments do the contractions cease for a while after ejaculation?

DAVIS: We have not yet attempted to induce ejaculation in the anesthetized rabbits, which were used for our in vivo isolated tissue experiments with the testicular capsule.

BURGOS: I always ask myself how lymphatic vessels drain from the testis as far as they occupy the largest part of the interstitial tissue, so I find reasonable to accept as one of the main functions of the permanent contractions of the capsule to press out the lymph content of the testis.

DAVIS: I think that is a very interesting suggestion and we have also been considering the possibility that testicular capsular contractions may play an important role in the flow of testicular lymphatic fluid. We are also presently contemplating a speculation that testicular capsular contractions and relaxations may result in changes in the interstitial tissue pressure surrounding the Leydig cells, which might possibly influence the secretion of testosterone from the Leydig cells. We are now planning to place a micro pressure transducer in the middle of the testis and to measure interstitial tissue pressure simultaneously with our recordings of testicular capsular contractions. We are also planning to cannulate the rete testis, and following the addition of pharmacological agents which cause contractions and relaxation of the testicular capsule, measure both the flow rate and the sperm content of the rete testis fluid.

MANCINI: Dr. Davis, would you be able to separate the capsule of the testis from that of the epididymis? Anatomically, there is a continuity between the capsule which surrounds the seminiferous tubules and the capsule of the epididymis. If this could be done, you will be able to see if differences in contraction exist. Have you already studied the capsule of the immature testis? In the human testis, there are some differences during development as regards the morphology of the layers and the thickness of the albuginea.

DAVIS: In answer to your first question, the entire epididymis is removed in the process of preparing the isolated testicular capsule. In our in vivo experiments, we are always very careful to anchor the inferior pole of the capsule which eliminates any possible influence of the epididymis on the testicular capsules. In answer to your secone question, we are planning to include the investigation of the effect of age as well as various hormones in our new research program on the pharmacology and physiology of the testicular capsule.

EFFECT OF GONADOTROPINS AND ANDROGENS ON FRUCTOSE AND CITRIC ACID OF SEMINAL FLUID

Juan Carlos Lavieri and Juan C. Calamera

Centro de Investigaciones sobre Reproduccion, Facultad de Medicina, Paraguay 2155, Piso 10, Buenos Aires, Argentina

INTRODUCTION

The existence of a reducing sugar in human seminal fluid was reported many years ago. It was then characterized as glucose (1-4). Afterwards the substance was shown to be fructose (5); later on, Mann (6) identified it as D(-) fructose. These findings were confirmed by others (7). Many papers have been devoted to the occurrence of this substance in both human and animal seminal plasma (8-12); as well as to the site of its origin in different species including man (13-17). In the human species the seminal vesicles are the main source of its production. Moreover, the relationship between androgens and seminal fructose has been established (18), so that the levels of this sugar have been used as indicators of androgenic function (13,19).

Citric acid was found in semen by Schersten who placed its origin in the adnexal genital glands (20). It is secreted by the seminal vesicles in the boar and bull (21) and by the prostate in man (22). As the production of citric acid depends on androgens (15,16, 23,24), both fructose and citric acid determinations were proposed as tests of androgenic activity (25-27).

Considering the importance of semen characteristics in the evaluation of male sterility, the authors carried out both biochemical examination and morphologic studies of animal fluid. Furthermore, the functional capacity of the adnexal glands as well as androgenic effects upon them can be assessed. Low seminal concentrations of fructose have been found in animals and man in hypoandrogenic conditions (26,28,29), and are also seen in inflammatory and infectious diseases of the adnexal glands (28,30,31). Information regarding oligospermic patients of unknown etiology without demonstrable endocrine, metabolic or urologic alteration is fragmentary (28,32,33). Therefore, we considered it important to investigate the levels of these seminial substances in the oligospermic patients and compare these levels with those encountered in normospermic subjects. The action of different hormones upon the level of these substances in seminal plasma was also studied.

NORMOSPERMIC SUBJECTS

Seminal fluid showing the following characteristics was considered normal: over 40 million spermatozoa per ml, 2 ml ejaculate, 60% motility, 80% normal forms and no pus. Fructose (34) and citric acid (35) concentrations were determined in 70 subjects with normal seminal fluid.

Fructose. We found a mean of 266.4 mg % (range of 121-490 mg%); these data were in keeping with those of other workers (26,36-42), (see Table 1) .

Citric Acid. A mean of 421.4 mg %, (range 174-658) mg% was found; these levels were also in keeping with those of other investigators (479 mg % (43), 376 mg % (26) and 347 mg % (42), see Table 1).

Table 1. Seminal Concentration of Fructose and Citric Acid in Normospermic and Oligospermic Subjects.

SUBJECTS	Number of cases	Concentration of FRUCTOSE mg %	Concentration of CITRIC ACID mg %
NORMOSPERMICS	70	266.4 ± 9.2	421.4 ± 14.8
OLIGOSPERMICS	64	286.4 ± 11.6 (P < 0.20)	511.8 ± 22 (P< 0.001

OLIGOSPERMIC PATIENTS

The same investigations were applied to 64 patients with oligospermia not related to either endocrine, metabolic or urologic disturbance. The number of spermatozoa was below 40 million per ml and generally, oligospermia was accompanied by reduced motility. Each specimen was free of signs that indicated infection.

Fructose. A mean 286.4 mg % (range 121-462 mg %) was obtained. Concentrations were similar to those levels found in normal subjects. The means reported by other authors were: 211 mg % (41), 264 mg % (33), 336 mg % (44) and 357 mg % (45), (see Table 1).

Citric acid. There was scarce information about its content in oligospermic semen (32,33). Hence we were especially interested in assessing the level of this substance in this category of patients. We found a mean of 511.8 mg% (range 188-893 mg%). Comparison with normal reveals a significant increase in the mean in oligospermic patients (see Table 1).

HORMONAL EFFECTS

The oligospermic patients were divided into five groups, according to the different hormonal treatment they received. The effect of the hormones was evaluated by the difference in fructose and citric acid concentrations before and after treatment. Hormones administered were: human chorionic gonadotropin (HCG); pregnant mare serum (PMS); human postmenopausal gonadotropin (HMG); testosterone propionate; 17- trimethylsiloxy-4-androsten-3-one ether (SC-16148) (Silandrone. Searle and Co., Chicago, Illinois) (C22 H36 02 Si).

Statistical analysis consisted of: 1) Spot graphs using the horizontal axis for basal values and the vertical axis for differences between basal levels and those levels encountered after hormonal treatment: 2) Calculation of the correlation coefficient. 3) Fitting the regression line of differences from initial values. 4) Construction of 95% confidence intervals for mean differences and regression coefficients. These intervals were equivalent to tests of significance at the 0.05 level. The following results were obtained with the administration of the hormones above mentioned.

HCG. (1000 I.U. given intramuscularly, twice a week for six weeks in each patient. This group comprised 17 cases.) The mean fructose concentrations before and after treatment were not significantly different. However, the negative slope was significantly different from zero. This finding established a relationship between the values obtained with HCG administration and the basal values. It was also observed that the fitted line crossed the horizontal axis near the midpoint of the range of initial values. This suggests that with HCG treatment, low values tended to increase while high values tended to decrease (see Fig. 1).

Results obtained on citric acid levels were similar to those found for fructose (see Fig. 2).

PMS The dose used was 2000 I.U. given intramuscularly, twice a week, for three weeks in each patient. This group comprised 20 cases. With regard to fructose concentration there was no significant difference between the mean values noted prior to and after PMS administration. Since the slope of the line did not differ significantly from the horizontal line, the effect of treatment could not be considered to be altered from the initial values (see Fig. 3).

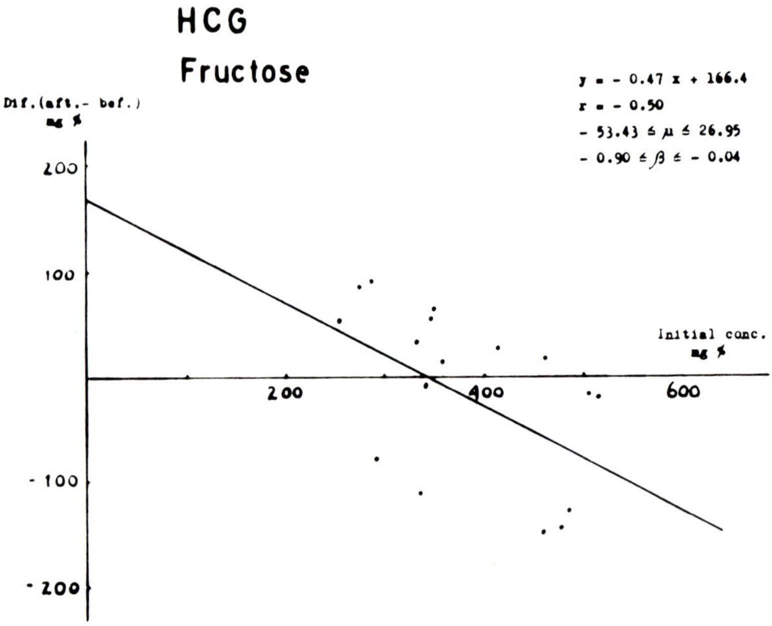
HCG
Fructose
y = - 0.47 x + 166.4
r = - 0.50
- 53.43 ≤ μ ≤ 26.95
- 0.90 ≤ β ≤ - 0.04
Dif.(aft.- bef.)
mg %
200
100
- 100
- 200
200
400
600
Initial conc.
mg %

Fig. 1

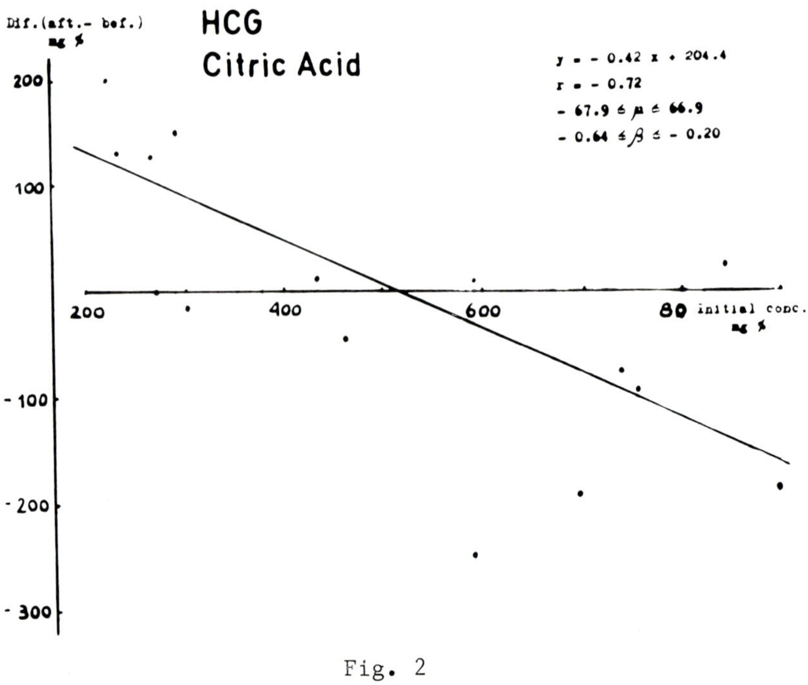
Dif.(aft.- bef.)
mg %
HCG
Citric Acid
y = - 0.42 x + 204.4
r = - 0.72
- 67.9 ≤ μ ≤ 66.9
- 0.64 ≤ β ≤ - 0.20
200
100
- 100
- 200
- 300
200
400
600
80
initial conc.
mg %

Fig. 2

A significant difference in citric acid concentrations between the mean values before and after HCG treatment were noted. However, the slope was not significantly different from zero, indicating that the difference between the increases and basal values was not treatment related (see Fig. 4).

HMG The dose employed was: 1 ampoule (80 μ FSH and 80 μ LH of the 2nd IRP-HMG) given intramuscularly every second day, for 90 days in each patient. This group comprised eight cases. Measurement of fructose concentration revealed no significant differences between the means. According to the confidence interval for the true slope, again, it could not be accepted as an effect of treatment (see Fig. 5).

Results on citric acid concentration were similar to those found for fructose (see Fig. 6).

Testosterone Propionate. The dose used was 25 mg given intramuscularly, once a week, for four or six weeks in each patient. This group comprised 22 cases. With respect to fructose concentration no significant difference was seen between the mean values before and after treatment. Nevertheless the significant negative slope indicated that a relationship existed between final and basal concentrations. Furthermore, the fact that the fitted line crossed the horizontal axis in the vicinity of the mean of initial values, suggested that low initial values increase and high ones decrease under hormonal action (see Fig. 7). Similar results were found with citric acid concentration (see Fig. 8).

Silandrone. The dose employed was 30 mg/day, per os, for 30 days in each patient. This group comprised 15 cases. There was a significant difference between means of fructose concentrations before and after hormonal administration. However, the slope of the straight line did not differ from the horizontal line. In consequence, increases and decreases could not be accepted as being related to treatment (see Fig. 9). Results similar to those on fructose concentration were found for citric acid concentration (see Fig. 10).

COMMENTS

Although we have used a different method for the determination of citric acid our results are comparable with those obtained in normal subjects by other workers (26,42,43). With regard to fructose our technique was the same as previously recommended (26).

The possibility of individual variations must be taken into account (27). However, the subjects under study were requested to adopt a determined sexual rhythm. In this way their seminal fluid did not show major variations in basal conditions in coincidence

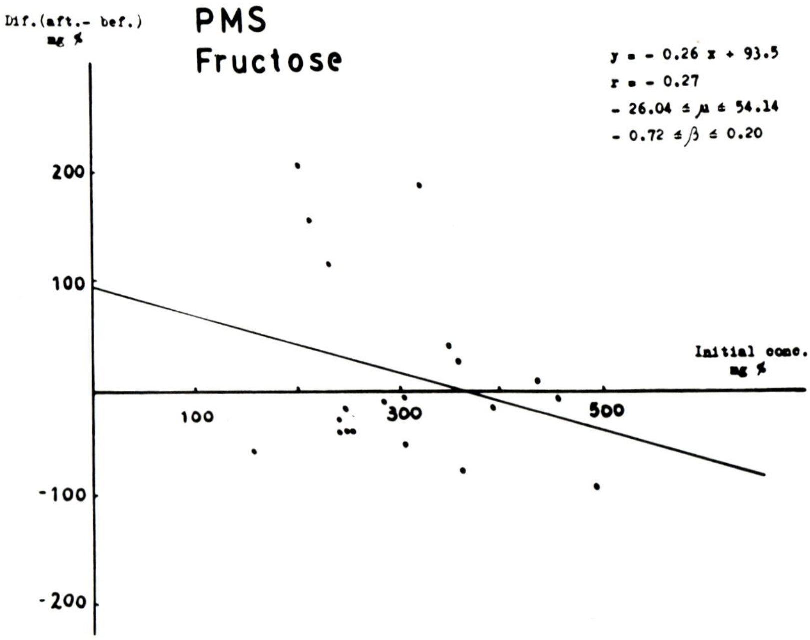
Dif.(aft.- bef.)
mg %
PMS
Fructose
y = - 0.26 x + 93.5
r = - 0.27
- 26.04 ≤ μ ≤ 54.14
- 0.72 ≤ β ≤ 0.20
200
100
-100
-200
100
300
500
Initial conc.
mg %

Fig. 3

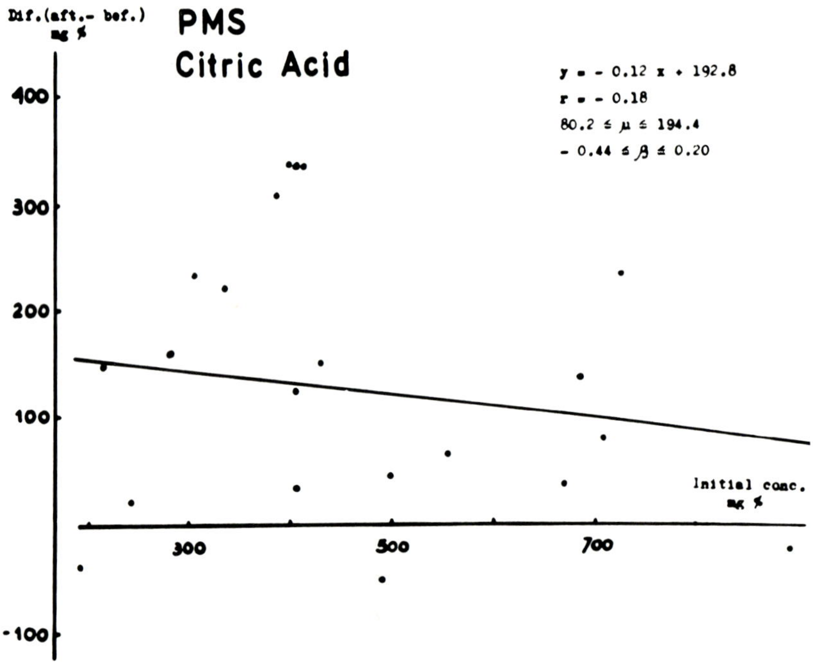
Dif.(aft.- bef.)
mg %
PMS
Citric Acid
y = - 0.12 x + 192.8
r = - 0.18
80.2 ≤ μ ≤ 194.4
- 0.44 ≤ β ≤ 0.20
400
300
200
100
-100
300
500
700
Initial conc.
mg %

Fig. 4

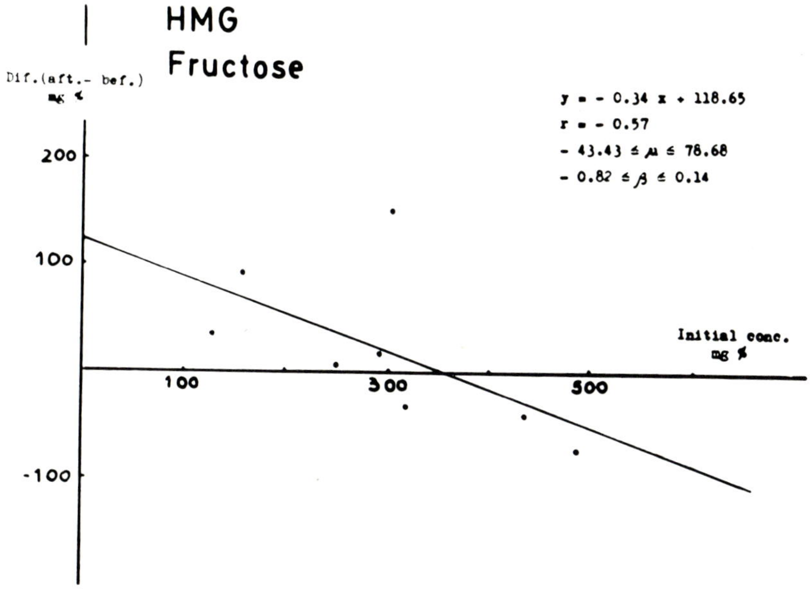
HMG
Fructose
Dif.(aft.- bef.)
mg %
y = - 0.34 x + 118.65
r = - 0.57
- 43.43 ≤ μ ≤ 78.68
- 0.82 ≤ β ≤ 0.14
200
100
-100
Initial conc.
mg %
100
300
500

Fig. 5

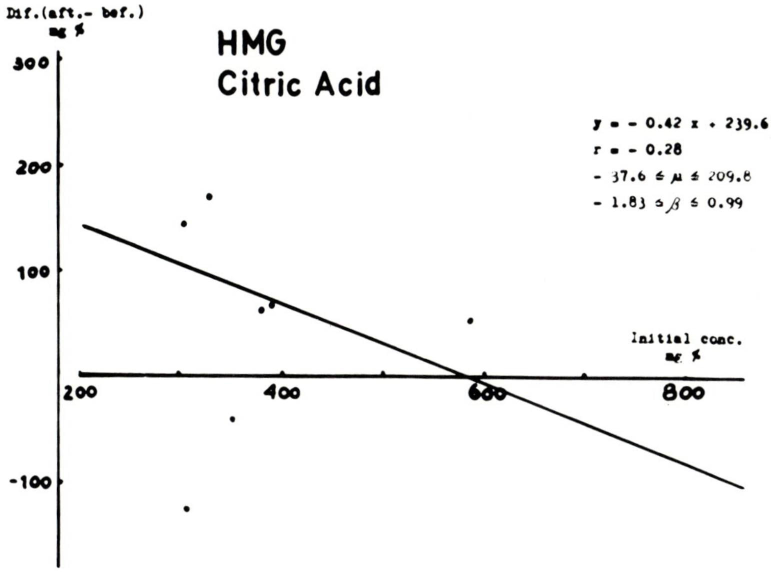
Dif.(aft.- bef.)
mg %
HMG
Citric Acid
y = - 0.42 x + 239.6
r = - 0.28
- 37.6 ≤ μ ≤ 209.8
- 1.83 ≤ β ≤ 0.99
300
200
100
-100
Initial conc.
mg %
200
400
600
800

Fig. 6

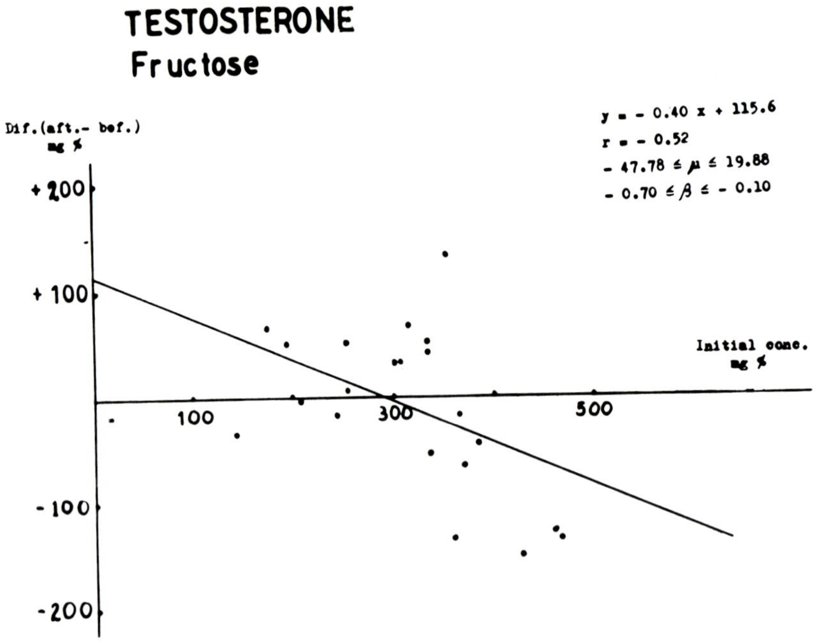
TESTOSTERONE
Fructose
Dif.(aft.- bef.) mg %
y = - 0.40 x + 115.6
r = - 0.52
- 47.78 ≤ μ ≤ 19.88
- 0.70 ≤ β ≤ - 0.10
+200
+100
-100
-200
Initial conc. mg %
100
300
500

Fig. 7

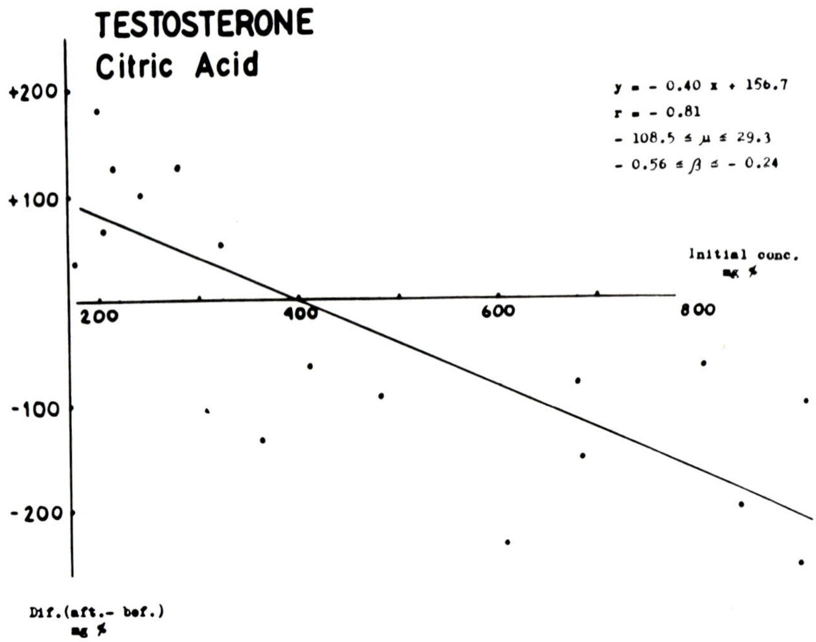
TESTOSTERONE
Citric Acid
y = - 0.40 x + 156.7
r = - 0.81
- 108.5 ≤ μ ≤ 29.3
- 0.56 ≤ β ≤ - 0.24
+200
+100
-100
-200
Initial conc. mg %
200
400
600
800
Dif.(aft.- bef.) mg %

Fig. 8

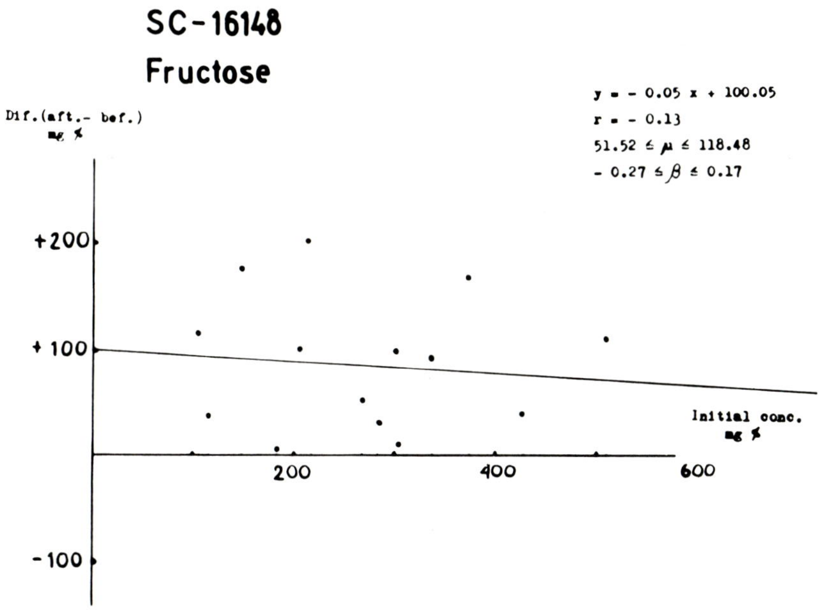
SC-16148
Fructose
y = - 0.05 x + 100.05
r = - 0.13
51.52 ≤ μ ≤ 118.48
- 0.27 ≤ β ≤ 0.17
Dif.(aft.- bef.)
mg %
+200
+100
-100
200
400
600
Initial conc.
mg %

Fig. 9

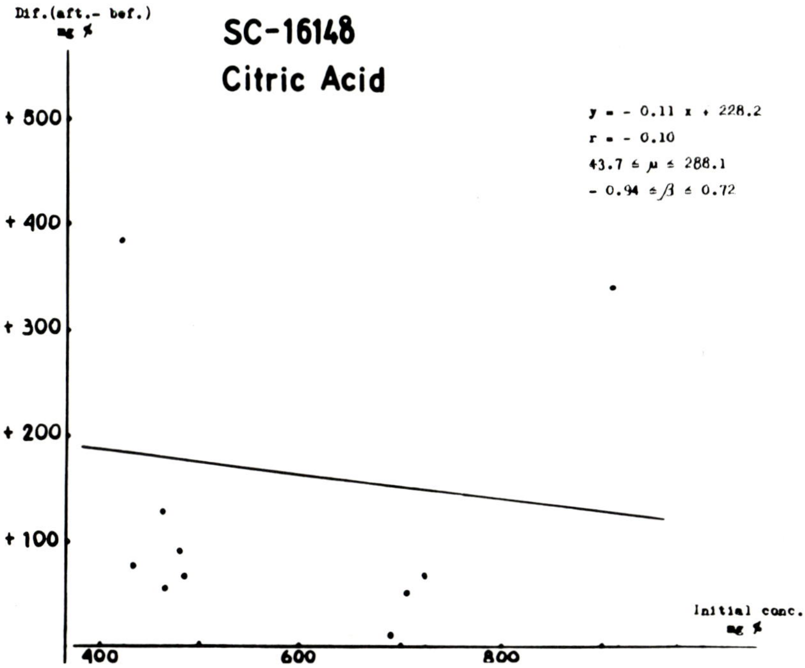
Dif.(aft.- bef.)
mg %
SC-16148
Citric Acid
y = - 0.11 x + 228.2
r = - 0.10
43.7 ≤ μ ≤ 288.1
- 0.94 ≤ β ≤ 0.72
+500
+400
+300
+200
+100
400
600
800
Initial conc.
mg %

Fig. 10

with other investigators (46). When there were such variations the samples were discarded. The initial value was the mean of two or three ejaculates. We would like to emphasize that urinary steroid and gonadotropin assays were not performed in our group of patients.

In oligospermic patients the mean concentration of fructose does not differ from normals. However, the mean of citric acid concentration is significantly increased compared with normals. Within each group there are subjects with low values and others with high values indicating the existence of a wide range. Schirren (28) has already reported several cases of oligospermia with low concentrations of fructose. Kuhnau and Nowakowski (32) have reported other cases with low fructose and high citric acid levels. They postulate that these elevated concentrations might be due to the fact that the seminal vesicles contribute a lesser volume. We feel that while this interpretation might fit the cases with reduced volume of semen it may not be applied to those with normal volumes.

Although the dependence of these seminal substances on testosterone levels has been demonstrated in castrated animals (26), in certain pathological conditions the facts are not quite as clear. In oligospermic patients, the doses of HCG or testosterone used do not produce variations in the mean of fructose and the citric acid, but they do induce an increase in initial low values and a decrease in high values.

In patients with "postpuberal Leydig cell insufficiency and normospermia", methyltestosterone, HCG and methylandrostanolone (mesterolone) increase fructose (29,32) and lower citric acid (32). As the treatment is discontinued, the concentrations return to their initial values. When the treatment is resumed the results are influenced as previously reported (32).

Although in our patients no hormonal steroid levels were determined it could be speculated that the initial low values might be due to an androgenic deficit or that the effectors do not respond to the hormonal stimulus. We are not able to explain initial high values on the same grounds unless we accept that androgens act by regulating the concentration of these substances within given limits. We deem as unsatisfactory the theory of functional exhaustion of glands by overstimulation, since Silandrone further elevates initial high values in similar conditions. Therefore, the mechanism of action still remains undisclosed.

Silandrone induces an increase of both fructose and citric acid. There is still not enough data on its effects in human, but in castrated rats a peak of androgenic stimulation is seen at 20 to 30 days after administration; its effect upon the weight of seminal vesicles and prostate is greater than that of testosterone (Searle, Division of Biological Research. Personal communication). There is also the likelihood that the dose employed by us is more androgenic than that of testosterone. All this would add support to the hypothesis of a direct action upon adnexal glands as is seen in the rat.

PMS was administered for only three weeks in order to prevent the formation of anti-gonadotropins (47,48). No variation in fructose levels was observed with its use. Owing to its low LH activity and predominant FSH action, the dose employed would be insufficient to stimulate steroid production. The unexpected increase of citric acid induced by PMS is by now a matter of mere speculation.

When HMG was used no variations were observed; this fact agrees with its proved inability to produce steroids (49).

Further studies are needed to establish the relationship between the concentration of fructose and citric acid and the concentration of spermatozoa in the seminal fluid under hormonal action.

CONCLUSIONS

1) Fructose and citric acid concentrations found by us in normal subjects agree with those reported by other workers.
2) In oligospermic patients, seminal fructose concentration is similar to that in normals; but citric acid is significantly increased, as reported by other investigators.
3) In oligospermic patients HCG and testosterone tend to regulate the levels of these substances. The marked elevation by Silandrone may be connected to the relationship existing between the concentrations of fructose and citric acid on the one hand and androgenic function on the other hand, as demonstrated by Mann in animals.
4) It is difficult to interpret the mechanism of action of these hormones in the absence of information regarding urinary or plasmatic steroidal levels.

ACKNOWLEDGMENT

The authors wish to express their gratitude to the Centro de Bioestadistica y Demografia, Facultad de Medicina de la Universidad de Buenos Aires for the statistical analysis of our results.

REFERENCES

1. McCarthy, J.F., Stepita, C.T., Johnson, M.B. and Killian, J.A., Proc. Soc. Exp., 25: 54, 1928.
2. Ivanov, E. E., Z. Zucht., B, 20: 404, 1931.
3. Huggins, C.B. and Johnson, C., Amer. J. Physiol. 103: 574, 1933.
4. MacLeod, J. and Hotchkiss, R.S., J. Urol., 48: 225, 1942.
5. Yamada, K., Japan J. Med. Sci. II, Biochem. 2, 93: 245, 1933.
6. Mann, T., Biochem. J., 39: 458, 1945.

7. Pryde, J.,Nature, (London), 157: 660, 1946.
8. Mann, T., Biochem. J., 40: 481, 1946.
9. Mann, T., Advances in Endocrinology, 9: 329, 1949.
10. Mann, T., Recent Progr. Hormone Res., 12: 353, 1956.
11. Mann, T. and Lutwak-Mann, C., Physiol. Rev., 31: 27, 1951.
12. Mann, T. and Wilson, E., J. Endocr., 25: 407, 1962.
13. Davies, D.V. and Mann, T., Nature, (London), 160: 295, 1947.
14. Mann, T., J. Agric. Sci., 38: 323, 1948.
15. Humphrey, G.F. and Mann, T., Nature, (London), 161: 352, 1948.
16. Humphrey, G.F. and Mann, T., Biochem. J.,44: 97, 1949.
17. Bonadonna, T., Zootecnica e Veterinaria, Milano.
18. Mann, T. and Parsons, U., Nature, (London), 160: 294, 1947.
19. Landau, R.L. and Loughead, R., J. Clin. Endocr., 11: 1411, 1951.
20. Schersten, B., Skand. Arch.,58: 90, 1929.
21. Mann, T., Davies, D V. and Humphrey, G.G., J. Endocr., 6: 75, 1949.
22. Huggins, C. and Neal, W., J. Exp. Med., 76: 527, 1942.
23. Lutwak-Mann, C., Mann, T., and Price, D., Proc. Roy. Soc. (Biol), 136: 461, 1949.
24. Mann, T. and Parsons, U., Biochem, J., 46: 440, 1950.
25. Nowakowsky, H. and Schirren, C., Klin, Wschr., 34: 19, 1956.
26. Mann, T., The Biochemistry of the Semen and of the Male Genital Tract. Methuen, London, 1964.
27. Mann. T., Ciba Found. Colloq. Endocr., 16: 233, 1967.
28. Schirren, C., J. Reprod. Fertil., 5: 347, 1963.
29. Schirren, C., 5th World Congress Fertil. Steril., Stockholm, 1966. Excerpta Medica Found. International Congress Series, 133 p. 808, 1967.
30. Eliasson, R., Fredricsson, B., Johannisson, E. and Leander, G., 5th World Congress Fertil. Steril., Stockholm, 1966. Excerpta Medica Found. International Congress Series 133, p. 625, 1967.
31. Eliasson, R., Fertil. Steril., 19: 344, 1968.
32. Kuhnau, J. Jr. and Nowakowski, H., Endokrinologie,40: 1, 1960.
33. Calamera, J.C. and Lavieri, J.C., Bol. Clin. Endocr. Metab., 7: 149, 1968.
34. Roe, J.H., J. Biol. Chem., 105: 15, 1934.
35. Chambon, P., Ann. Pharm. Franc., 21: 78, 1963.
36. Tyler, E.T., Fertil. Steril., 6: 247, 1955.
37. Harvey, C., Proc. Soc. Study of Fertility, 8: 3, 1957.
38. Vaishwanar, P.S., Amer. J. Obstet. Gynec., 75: 139, 1958.
39. Schirren, C., Fertilitatsstrorungen des Mannes. Stuttgart, Enke., 1961.
40. Shet, A.R. and Rao, S.S., Indian J. Med. Sci., 16: 709, 1962.
41. Moon, K.H. and Bunge, R.G., Fertil. Steril., 19: 186, 1968.
42. Ackerman, D.R. and Roussel, J.D., J. Reprod. Fertil., 17: 563, 1968.
43. Harvey, C., Proc. Soc. Study of Fertility, 3: 56, 1951.
44. Abelli, G. and Falagario, M., Attualita Ostet. Ginec., 12: 723, 1966.

45. Pasetto, N., Monitore ost. Gin. di Endocrin. e del Metab., 27: 53, 1965.
46. Eliasson, R., J. Reprod. Fertil,, 9: 331, 1965.
47. Maddock, W., Epstein, M. and Nelson, W.O., Ann. N.Y. Acad. Sci., 55: 657, 1952.
48. Oestergaard, E.- XXI Assisses Franc. de Gynecologie. Clermont Ferrand, 1962.
49. Mroueh, A., Lytton, B. and Kase, N., J. Clin. Endocr., 27: 53, 1967.

IMMUNOLOGICAL ASPECTS OF MALE INFERTILITY

Roberto E. Mancini

Centro de Investigaciones sobre Reproduccion, Facultad de Medicina, Paraguay 2155, Piso 10, Buenos Aires, Argentina.

INTRODUCTION

It is very well known that formation of antibodies in a given organism toward a foreign molecule, virus, bacteria or tissue, constitutes the normal mechanism of defense. Moreover, the concept of an autoimmune response against self tissue antigens in mammals has been widely accepted in the last ten years. Encephalomyelitis, thyroiditis and adrenalitis experimentally induced by sensitizing animals with homologous or autologous antigens extracted from these glands added with adjuvants have met their equivalent in some clinical endocrine diseases. However, the role played by the induced circulating and delayed types of antibodies in conditioning the glandular tissue destruction is still a matter of debate.

Allergic orchitis similarly induced and subsequently followed by azoospermia has been an excellent model to substantiate some cases of male sterility with unexplainable etiology. Consequently, it was admitted that man may be immunized against his own sperm material and a woman against the same antigen from a man. Two reasons may explain why autosensitization is possible in males; firstly the sperm cells are anatomically isolated from the circulation in the genital tract and secondly they develop at puberty long after the neonatal age where immunological tolerance can take place.

In the following sections, the animal experiments and clinical findings supporting this new pathogenic contention in cases of male sterility and the participation of the testis, adnexal glands and semen will be briefly described.

I EXPERIMENTAL BACKGROUND

Testis

It has long been demonstrated that a large variety of animal testicular tissues are antigenic in heterologous sensitization procedures. The "spermotoxic" antisera were capable of immobilizing normal spermatozoa in vitro (1). Nevertheless, an impact in the field of immunologic impairment of reproductive male function was made when selective damage of the germinal epithelium of adult guinea pigs could be obtained after auto- or homo-sensitization with a single dose of testicular homogenate plus complete Freund's adjuvant (2,3).

The allergic response developed between one and eight weeks and was characterized by: a) edema in the intertubular spaces of the gonad and epididymis, foci of perivascular cellular infiltration including mostly plasmocytes and lymphocytes; b) vacuolization and sloughing of the germinal cells, beginning with spermatids, and finally involving spermatocytes and spermatogonial cells. Only Sertoli cells showing striking vacuolization but unchanged nuclei remained; c) no damage was demonstrable in Leydig cells or in other connective tissue cells, such as fibroblasts and scattered mast cells; d) the testicular lesion was accompanied by the appearance of circulating antispermatic and cell-bound antibodies; e) as a consequence of the germinal cell destruction, azoospermia rendered the animal sterile for several months; f) signs of complete recovery of fertility were apparent about 165 days after sensitization and detection of normal motile spermatozoa in the ejaculate occurred after about five months of azoospermia; g) the reaction was not evoked by injections of adjuvant alone, immature testis or even immunologically-damaged testis (4,5). As well as guinea pig, other less susceptible species such as inbred strains of mice (6) or adult rats (7,8) may respond to similar auto or homosensitization. Significant testicular damage in an inbred strain of rats was also accomplished with one injection of testicular antigen incorporated in complete Freund's adjuvant (9). Recently (10) autoallergic orchitis was produced in primates. Rhesus monkeys were auto or isosensitized with testicular homogenates in Freund's adjuvant. After six to eight weeks they developed a patchy lesion similar to that observed in guinea pigs. Circulating antibodies were detected in few animals at very low titers; however, following castration the titers increased. No cell bound antibodies could be detected. The production and pathway of steroid hormones were also studied by in vitro incubation with pairs of the differentially-labelled precursors (11). The rate of production of testosterone by the testicular tissue was somewhat decreased but the results were not statistically significant and were in accordance with the lack of damage of the Leydig cells in the immune process (12).

The need for the simultaneous presence of germinal cell homogenetes and adjuvant in the production of unilateral allergic orchitis has been substantiated by the induction of a local inflammation in the contralateral testis together with an intradermal injection of the adjuvant (13) or by the injection in the contralateral testis of the adjuvant alone (14). In contrast to the admitted role played by complete Freund's adjuvant in conditioning the testicular and antibody response, it was claimed that adult testicular extract,if repeatedly administered in guinea-pigs for three months, may elicit gonadal damage (15), as was shown in other autoimmune diseases such as thyroiditis.

Histology. The vascular and inflammatory changes in allergic orchitis are minimal as compared to the dramatic breakdown of the germinal epithelium. There is general agreement that slight vascular changes and histiocyte-mononuclear cell infiltration appear around the second week and may precede the germinal cell lesion. However, the known sensitivity of this epithelium to different kinds of agents has made controversial the specificity of sloughing and cytolysis of germinal cells (16). Nevertheless, the immunological character of this type of orchitis appears reinforced by its correlation with the presence of both circulating and cell-bound antibodies and by the negative findings in animals injected with other homologous tissue extracts (17).

The cellular basis of the seminiferous tubule lesion has been reinvestigated in our laboratory and the findings of previous authors have been extended to the subcellular level. The dissociation of the unit integrated by Sertoli and germinal cells mediated by the rupture of peripheral areas of Sertoli cells constitutes the main phenomenon of the induced aspermatogenesis. Development of numerous large reticuloendoplasmic vesicles and of dense bodies showing acid phosphatase reaction in the Sertoli cells (lysosomes) coincides with the cytolysis of spermatids and sloughing of spermatocytes and spermatogonial cells. Subsequently, the perinuclear acrosomes appear free in the lumen of the tubules and then in the epididymus, where they are reabsorbed (18). Changes in some other hydrolytic enzymes have been reported (19). The Sertoli cells, acting as a sustentacular and transporting cell system between the intertubular circulation and closely associated germinal cells (20), would permit the antibodies to reach the antigen present in the spermatogenic cells.

The appearance of a bradykinin-like substance in the testicular tissue during the first weeks of the allergic response is also interesting because of its role as mediator in the antigen-antibody interaction in allergic inflammation (21).

Antigens. The heterogeneous nature of testicular homogenates as revealed immunoserologically by the presence of other tissue antigens common to kidney, liver and serum proteins points to the problem of the specific antigens responsible for the antigenicity of the testis (22). Other protein fractions obtained from the testis have been reported as being capable of inducing allergic orchitis, but a testicular polysaccharide-polypeptide complex appears to be a highly potent antigen (23). Recently a glycoprotein substance isolated from guinea pig germinal cells, devoid of hyaluronidase activity or tissue and serum protein contaminants, was able to produce allergic orchitis (24).

The site of localization of the antigens was assessed by the immunofluorescent technique and it was demonstrated that the homologous autologous-antitestis antibodies react specifically with the acrosome of spermatozoa (25) and spermatids (26). This finding and the fact that this structure reacts positively to PAS, together with the polysaccharidic nature of testicular antigens, supports the earlier contention that the later cell stages of spermatogenesis and particularly the spermatids and spermatozoa share the antigenic potency of the testis.

Antibodies. Two types of different immunological significance (circulating and cell bound) have been described in the guinea pig as a result of a complete sensitization. The former are of low titer and may be detected by systemic anaphylaxis, local anaphylaxis (immediate inflammatory skin reaction), passive cutaneous anaphylaxis (PCA), Schultz-Dale, complement fixation, hemagglutination and precipitation. The immune serum also shows in vitro cytotoxic properties such as immobilization and agglutination of motile spermatozoa (27) and a lytic effect on the acrosome of spermatids and spermatozoa (28). The cell bound antibodies are involved in the delayed type of hypersensitivity. These antibodies may be detected by the appearance of a typical granuloma after intradermal injection of the antigen alone.

In spite of the lack of detailed studies it is assumed that the circulating antibodies are inconstant and of low titer and that no strict correlation exists between them and the gonadal lesion. On the contrary, a higher frequency of delayed skin reaction in sensitized animals is generally admitted. Moreover, a sequential follow up of the animals showed that delayed hypersensitivity appears first around the sixth day and circulating antibodies can be detected approximately three days later at the time when tubular damage begins to develop (29,30).

That complete adjuvant is necessary for the allergic orchitis and delayed skin reaction is supported by the fact that testicular tissue alone or with the addition of incomplete adjuvant may only elicit systemic or local anaphylaxis, PCA and immunofluorescent antibodies (31).

Pathogenesis. It has definitely been accepted that induced allergic orchitis may be included in the category of a delayed type of sensitization due to cell bound antibodies. This inference has been drawn from the following facts: a) the use of complete adjuvant is essential; b) testicular lesions are correlated more with delayed skin reaction than with circulating antibodies; c) histology of the testis shows not only typical aspermatogenesis but also mononuclear cell infiltration and weak inflammatory signs; d) mononuclear cells from lymph nodes of sensitized animals are capable of passively inducing skin delayed hypersensitivity when they are transferred to normal receptors (32). Moreover, fetal lesions of "aspermatogenesis" have been evoked by intratesticular injections of lymph node cells obtained from sensitized animals (33). On the contrary, circulating antibodies cannot induce aspermatogenesis passively. Also the immune globulin labelled with fluorescein cannot be detected inside the seminiferous tubules after intravenous injection (33). However intratesticular injection of immune serum may elicit local specific changes (34).

Although the role played by the different types of antibodies remains to be elucidated, the dual necessity for cell bound and circulating antibodies in the pathogenesis of experimental aspermatogenesis has recently been assumed (35). It is possible that among the various antibodies, some may be concerned with damage to the testis (cytotoxic and cell bound) while others are of an anaphylactic type and exert a "protective effect" (36). Nevertheless, a sufficient body of experimental evidence on the significance of all these antibodies as well as on the antispermatic properties of different globulin fractions is still needed.

The prevention of induced allergic aspermatogenesis by thymectomy early in the post-natal period (37) or by the administration of suppressive drugs (38) prior to sensitization has been claimed. On the other hand the induction of immunotolerance early in the postnatal period failed, because germinal cell destruction also develops when the animals reach puberal maturation (39).

Semen

Earlier studies have shown that free spermatozoa or total semen may induce by heterologous sensitization a high titer of sperm immobilizing antibodies.

More recent investigations have emphasized the complexity of semen and the importance of considering sperm and seminal plasma antigens separately. That spermatozoa are mainly responsible for the antigenicity of testis extract was deduced from the production of homologous allergic orchitis using guinea pig seminal or epididymal sperm (40). In addition, cross immunoserological reactions have been observed between testis and epididymal or seminal spermatozoa (41). As in the testis, more than one spermatozoal antigen, which seem to be polysaccharide (42) or glycoprotein substances (43), is able to elicit, with the addition of complete adjuvant, testicular damage and circulating and cell bound antibody response. However, based on serological, immobilizing and agglutinating tests, some discrepancies still stand with regard to sperm species specificity (44). Also three antigens have been recognized after ultrasonic vibration in spermatozoa from various species including man; one in the head, a second in the tail and a third common to both portions (45). Based on the immunofluorescent reaction of spermatozoal acrosomes, it has been shown that isolated acrosomes have an alcohol precipitable fraction rich in aminosugars and sialic acid with a higher antigenic potency than other soluble fractions and residual structures of this cell (46).

The antigenic properties of seminal plasma in heterologous or homologous sensitization procedures are well known. Applying serological techniques and immunoelectrophoresis, several fractions which are immunologically common to serum proteins, epididymal or prostate fluids and to seminal spermatozoa but not to testicular tissues have been studied (47). In contrast to discrepant reports (48), the finding of specific antigens in the seminal spermatozoa which are not of seminal plasma origin was corroborated by direct and cross immunoserological reactions (49). Ejaculated rabbit semen shows about nine antigens, seven of which are common to seminal plasma, two to blood serum and two appeared to be sperm specific and originated in the testis (50). It is then likely that during ductal transit spermatozoa are firmly coated with antigenic material from seminal plasma (51). Indeed washed sperm are considerably less antigenic (52).

Nevertheless, a detailed study of different antibodies induced by both types of spermatozoal antigens, and their relation with those elicited by seminal plasma and testicular antigens, is not complete until now.

Adnexal Glands

The possibility that seminal plasma antigens may be present in the accessory glands before they reach the semen opened a new approach to possible autoimmunological damage of these glands and of sperm cells related to anti-seminal plasma antibodies.

As referred to above, antigens common to seminal plasma, sperm cells, prostate and seminal vesicles secretions have been demonstrated. Also rabbit auto- and isoantibodies have been detected in prostate, seminal vesicles, coagulating and bulbo urethral glands. These antigens are also contained in seminal plasma but absent in testicular tissue (53). Although the isoantibodies do not induce lesions in the glands, those against guinea pig seminal vesicle or prostate agglutinate spermatozoa at lower titer as compared with those against the epididymis (54).

II HUMAN SPERMATIC TISSUE

Testis. Earlier findings showed that extracts of human testicular tissue seem to be antigenic in sensitized animals. A preparation isolated from the human testis containing proteins and carbohydrates has shown antigenic potency in guinea pigs. Antibodies demonstrated by precipitating, Schultz-Dale and immunoelectrophoresis techniques cross react with guinea pig testis antigen (55).

The possible role played by the human testis in the immunologic response to auto- or homosensitization was substantiated trying to induce an allergic orchitis in man, as has already been obtained in animals. Volunteer patients with prostate carcinoma were divided into three groups according to age, previous treatment, general condition and testicular biopsy. Patients of the first group were separately auto- or homosensitized with testicular homogenate, a protein fraction, a mucoprotein preparation provided by Dr. S. Katsh, (Denver, U.S.A.) or a glycoprotein substance obtained from human germinal cells. The second group of patients was sensitized with the same antigens alone or incorporated into complete adjuvants, or with the adjuvants alone. The third group not sensitized at all served as a control. Circulating as well as cell bound antibody determinations and testicular biopsies were performed during and at the end of the experiment, which was followed by therapeutic castration. As compared with the controls, some patients of the experimental group exhibited low titer circulating antibodies (complement fixing, sperm immobilizing, precipitating and passive cutaneous anaphylaxis) and positive skin test as well. Biopsies of the testis showed tubular lesions with sloughing and cytolysis of germinal cells. Immofluorescent techniques using the patient's own sera revealed positive results in the head of spermatozoa and perinuclear area of spermatids (56,57).

More recently another group of similar patients was submitted before castration to a mild unilateral orchitis in order to induce antibodies against spermatic autoantigens emerging from germinal epithelium destruction. However, no immunological response could be detected and no lesions developed in the contralateral gland (58).

Semen and Adnexal Glands. Species specific antibodies were demonstrated by complement fixing, immobilizing and sperm agglutinating tests against these antigens (59). Some experimental evidence indicates that human spermatozoa extracted from spermatocele lack the antigens which characterize the seminal spermatozoa. The possibility that a great part of the antigenic material is taken up during transit, as occurs in animals,was substantiated by direct and cross reactions with heterologous antihuman semen and spermatozoal or seminal plasma antibodies (60). This has been recently substantiated using histoimmunochemical techniques which show several antigenic sites in the head, neck and tail of human seminal spermatozoa whereas only one is demonstrable in testicular sperm cells (61).

Human semen contains at least 16 antigens and the spermatozoa seven, four of the latter being common to seminal plasma (62). Immunochemical analysis of seminal plasma revealed the presence of mucoproteins which seem to have antigenic properties. Prostate specific antigens, as well as cross reaction between this gland or acid phosphatase and seminal spermatozoa have also been shown (63). Also antibodies against seminal plasma and prostate may cause agglutination of seminal spermatozoa and higher hemagglutinating titers than antibodies against testis, epididymis, seminal vesicle or spermatozoa. Cross agar diffusion reactions showed that seminal plasma has a high common antigenicity with prostate and seminal vesicle and a lower one with seminal spermatozoa, testis or epididymis. By immunoelectrophoresis, one of the prostate antigens was identified as acid phosphatase and that of the seminal vesicle as lactoferrin, the latter being claimed as the more potent sperm coating antigen (64). From a comparative study, it has recently been concluded that the immobilizing, agglutinating and cytotoxic properties of antiseminal plasma antibodies are higher than those of antispermatozoal and antitestis antibodies (65).

It is then possible to assume that the testis contributes a few antigens to semen which appear to be sperm specific, as they are present in washed epididymal and seminal spermatozoa but not in seminal plasma, whereas prostate and seminal vesicles provide the major part of secondary sperm antigens.

III CLINICAL FINDINGS

The possibility that some cases of male sterility of unknown etiology have an immunological pathogenesis has attracted the attention of investigators during the past ten years. The interest began when sperm agglutinins were found in human blood and semen in some sterile patients (66). Microscopic and macroscopic agglutination techniques were recommended, and patients' spermatozoa or spermatozoa from normal donors were currently used. With macroscopical agglutination techniques 3.3% of the sera of infertile males were found to be positive while serum samples of fertile males did not show appreciable agglutinins (67). In a random group of 172 azoospermic patients without spermagglutinins in their serum, oligo or azoospermia was found in 94 cases, obstruction in 45, and unqualified in 33 patients (68). Applying the same agglutination technique, 3% was found among cases of oligo and azoospermia (69) whereas 14% of a group of cases of inflammatory diseases of the genital tract was reported (70). Using the supernatant of freeze-thawed spermatozoa as antigen, hemagglutination gives 18% of positive reactions in the sera of infertile men (71). The same technique using washed sperm and seminal plasma as antigens in the hemagglutination technique showed no parallelism with fertility potency in the male (72). It is interesting to note that some cases showing spermagglutinins in their sera do not give a complement fixation response with spermatozoa or seminal plasma but they produce a zone of precipitation with seminal plasma in the gel diffusion technique (73). No strict correlation was observed in a large group of sterile patients, between sperm agglutination and hemagglutination techniques using seminal plasma as antigen. Moreover, blood group isoantigens known to be present in sperm cells or in seminal fluid may induce false positive results when the hemagglutination is used (74).

Applying several immunoserological tests, cases showing a history of retention and of inflammation of the testicle and epididymis gave a 22% positive response with more than one of the tests used (75). The presence of injury, ligation or infection of the vas deferens or epididymis in a high percentage of oligo or azoospermic patients led to the hypothesis that sperm reabsorption into the interstitial tissue could elicit the immunological response (76). However, some patients who had surgical relief of the obstruction continued demonstrating positive spermagglutinin titers and produced pregnancies (77).

Immunofluorescent studies, using serum having spermagglutinins and seminal or testicular spermatozoa, showed positive results. Specific fluorescence appeared to be located in the head and occasionally in the mid-piece or the tail (78). To check the participation of germinal cell destruction during inflammatory conditions of the gonads, antispermatic antibodies were investigated in patients suffering mumps orchitis. Applying complement fixation, gel diffusion, antiglobulin consumption, and skin tests, the presence of antibodies related to delayed hypersensitivity rather than the circulating type was found. Negative results appeared in fertile men, children and in primitive or secondary diseases of the testis having non-developed or involutive germinal epithelium (79).

Although the widely used sperm agglutination techniques do not provide the certainty of an immunological reaction, it has been proved that the same sera may immobilize sperm in the presence of complement and that both antibodies were mainly of the 7S type. Moreover the levels of IgG and IgM were significantly higher in sera from men with sperm antibodies than in control sera (80). Then it is evident that antisperm antibodies may occur in sterile patients, but the independent or combined participation of testis, adnexal glands and seminal plasma in the immunologic response are not yet clarified. Although active germinal cell breakdown in the testis or spermiostasis in the efferent duct may exist, simultaneous presence of an inflammatory process seems necessary in order to initiate the antibody response.

CONCLUSIONS

An evaluation of the immunological factors in the male reproductive process may be made as follows: 1) Alteration of spermatogenesis or impairment of seminal plasma formation may be accompanied by the presence of antispermatic antibodies. 2) Oligo or azoospermia might reflect the immunological destruction of germinal cells whereas immobilization and agglutination of seminal spermatozoa would depend on allergic reaction originating in the adnexal glands. 3) Maturation of spermatozoa appears to be related to differences in their antigenic potency, for antibodies against testis do not affect adnexal glands but may immobilize epididymal spermatozoa, whereas antiseminal plasma antibodies react only with adnexal gland and seminal spermatozoa but not with testicular cells. 4) Acute or subacute inflammatory lesions of gonad and genital tract appear more related to the presence of antibodies than chronic lesions or endocrine diseases of the testis. Thus, the presence of adjuvants added to the antigen in the experimental induction of these antibodies, might be replaced in the naturally occurring diseases of the genital tract by haptens resulting from different kinds of injury to the tissues. 5) While the sperm antigens seem to be of a glycoprotein nature accumulated in the acrosome, neck and intermediate segment, those belonging to the adnexal glands and seminal plasma should be better known. 6) The site of reaction of sperm or adnexal gland antigens with the antibody in the male genital tract, the nature of the phenomenon and its consequence on the reproductive process need to be elaborated. 7) The significance and pathogenic role of detectable antispermatic antibodies in sterile male patients, both circulating and cell bound types, are not yet sufficiently clarified. Their presence, apparently correlated with unexplained cases of infertility, does not necessarily mean that they are specifically responsible for this abnormal state and only would be a reflection of the immunologic process involved.

ACKNOWLEDGEMENT

This work was supported by a grant from The Population Council, Inc. New York.

REFERENCES

1. Metchnikoff, E., Ann. Instit. Pasteur (Paris), 14: 1, 1900.
2. Voisin, G., Delaunay, A. and Barber, M., Ann. Instit. Pasteur (Paris), 81:48, 1951.
3. Freund, J., Lipton, M.M. and Thompson, G.E., J. Exp. Med., 97: 711, 1953.
4. Freund, J., Lipton, M.M. and Thompson, G.E., Proc. Soc. Exp. Biol. Med., 87: 408, 1954.
5. Katsh, S. and Bishop, D., J. Embryol. Exp. Morph., 6: 94, 1958.
6. Pokorna, Z., Vojtiskova, M. and Chutna, J. Folia Biologica (Praha), 9: 203, 1963.

7. Freund, J., Lipton, M.M. and Thompson, G.E., J. Exp. Med., 101: 591, 1955.
8. Mancini, R.E., Davidson, O.V., Vilar, O., Fertil. Steril., 15: 695, 1964.
9. Andrada, J.A., Andrada, E.C. and Witebsky, E., J. Immunology, 1969 (in press).
10. Andrada, J.A., Andrada, E.C. and Witebsky, E., Proc. Soc. Exp. Biol. Med., 130: 1010, 1969.
11. Hoschoian, J.C. and Brownie, A., Steroids, 10: 49, 1967.
12. Andrada, J.C., Proc. First Argentinian Cong. Sterility, 1: 65, 1968.
13. Boughton, B. and Spector, W.G., J. Path. Bact., 86: 69, 1963.
14. Eyquem, A. and Krieg, H., Ann. N.Y. Acad. Sci., 124: 270, 1965.
15. Bishop, D.V., Proc. Soc. Exp. Biol. Med., 107: 116, 1961.
16. Waksman, B.H., J. Exp. Med., 109: 311, 1959.
17. Baum, J., Boughton, B., Mongat, L. and Schild, O.H., J. Immunology, 4: 95, 1961.
18. Mancini, R.E., Proc. 1st. Symp. Intern. Committee Immunol. Reprod. Geneva, p. 55, 1968.
19. Katsh, S. and Aguirre, A., Int. Arch. Allergy, 33: 141, 1968.
20. Mancini, R.E., Vilar, O., Alvarez, B. and Seiguer, A.C., J. Histochem. Cytochem, 13: 376, 1965.
21. Mancini, R.E., Huidobro, H., Fernandez Collazo, G. and Monastirsky, R., Proc. Soc. Exp. Biol. Med., 123: 227, 1966.
22. Alonso, A., Bueno, M.P., Scacciati, I.M., Gonzalez, N. and Mancini, R.E., Acta Europea Fertil., 1: 459, 1969.
23. Bishop, D. and Carlson, G.L., Ann. N.Y. Acad. Sci., 124: 247, 1965.
24. Scacciati, I.M., Gonzalez, N., Bueno, M.P., Alonso, A. and Mancini, R.E., J. Reprod. Fertil., 1970 (in press).
25. Swanson Bech, J., Edwards, R.G. and Young, M.R., J. Reprod. Fertil., 4: 103, 1962.
26. Mancini, R.E., Davidson, O.W., Nemirovsky, M. and Bueno, M.P., Proc. Soc. Exp. Biol. Med., 8: 435, 1962.
27. Voisin, G.A., Toullet, F. and Maurer, P., Ann. N.Y. Acad. Sci., 73: 726, 1958.
28. Mancini, R.E., Monastirsky, R., Fernandez Collazo, E., Seiguer, A.C. and Alonso, A., Fertil. Steril., 70: 779, 1969.
29. Boughton, B., Immunology, 5: 522, 1962.
30. Brown, P.C., Glynn, L.E. and Holborow, E.J., J. Path Bact., 86: 505, 1963.
31. Chutna, J. and Rychlikova, M., Folia Biologica (Praha), 10: 177, 1964.
32. Laurence, K.A., Carpuk, B.A. and Perlabachs, M., Int. Fertil., 10: 13, 1965.
33. Mancini, R.E., Barquet, J. and Alonso, A., Proc. Soc. Exp. Biol. Med., 1970 (in press).
34. Mancini, R.E., Alonso, A. and Barquet, J., Acta Europea Fertil., 1970 (in press).

35. Brown, P.C., Glynn, L.E. and Holborow, E.J., Immunology, 13: 307, 1967.
36. Chutna, J. and Rychlikova, M., Folia Biologica (Praha), 10: 188, 1964.
37. Vojtiskova, M., and Pokorna, Z., Lancet, 21: 644, 1964.
38. Vojtiskova, M., Vikliky, V., Jirsakova, A., Nouza, K. and Pokorna, Z., Folia Biologica (Praha), 11: 364, 1965.
39. Bishop, D., Narbaitz, R. and Lessof, M., Developmental Biology, 3: 444, 1961.
40. Katsh, S., Int. Arch. Allergy, 16: 241, 1960.
41. Maruta, H. and Moyer, D.L., Fertil. Steril., 18: 649, 1967.
42. Katsh, S. and Katsh, G.F., Fertil. Steril., 12: 522, 1961.
43. Voisin, G.A. and Toullet, F., Ann. Instit. Pasteur (Paris), 114: 727, 1968.
44. Pehle, W., J. Immunology, 34: 325, 1928.
45. Henle, W. Henle, G. and Chambers, L.A., J. Exp. Med., 68: 335, 1938.
46. Mancini, R.E., Bueno, M.P., Alonso, A., Fernandez Collazo, E., Scacciati, I.M. and Gonzalez, N., Fertil. Steril., 1970 (in press)
47. Rao, S.S. and Sadri, K.K., J. Compar. Pathol., 70: 1: 1960.
48. Stevens, K.M. and Fost, C.A., Proc. Soc. Exp. Biol. Med., 117: 125, 1964.
49. Hunter, A.G. and Hafs, H.D., J. Reprod. Fertil., 7: 357, 1964.
50. Menge, A.C. and Protzman, W.P., J. Reprod. Fertil., 13: 31, 1967.
51. Weil, A.J., Ann. N.Y. Acad. Sci., 124: 267, 1965.
52. Weil, A.J., J. Reprod. Fertil., 2: 25, 1967.
53. Shulman, S., Yantorno, C., Soanes, W.A., Gonder, M.J. and Witebsky, E., Immunology, 10: 99, 1966.
54. Moyer, D.L. and Maruta, H., Fertil. Steril., 18: 497, 1967.
55. Katsh, S., J. Urol., 87: 896, 1960.
56. Mancini, R.E., Andrada, J.A., Saraceni, A., Bachmann, A.E., Lavieri, J.C. and Nemirovsky, M., J. Clin. Endocr., 25: 859, 1965.
57. Mancini, R.E., Proc. 3rd Int. Pharmacology Meeting, 2: 75, 1966.
58. Mancini, R.E., Andrada, J.A., Guirlanda, A. and Pascale, R., Acta Europea Fertil., 1970 (in press).
59. Popiranov, R. and Vulchanov, V.H., Acad. Bulg. Sci., 17: 865, 1964.
60. Weil, A.J. and Rodenburg, J.M., Proc. Soc. Exp. Biol. Med., 105: 43, 1960.
61. Mancini, R.E., Gutierrez, O. and Fernandez Collazo, E., J. Reprod. Fertil., 1970 (in press).
62. Rao, S.S. and Sadri, K.K., Proc. Sixth Int. Confer. Planned Parenthood, New Delhi, p. 243, 1959.
63. Flocks, R., Bandhauer, K., Patel, C. and Begley, R.J., J. Urol., 87: 457, 1962.
64. Hekman, A. and Rumke, Ph., Fertil. Steril., 20: 312, 1969.
65. Fernandez Collazo, E., Gutierrez, O. and Mancini, R.E., Fertil. Steril., 1970 (in press).

66. Wilson, L., Proc. Soc. Exp. Biol. Med., 85: 652, 1954.
67. Rumke, Ph. and Hellinga, G., Amer. Clin. Path., 32: 357, 1959.
68. Rumke, Ph., Ann. N.Y. Acad. Sci., 124: 696, 1965.
69. Nakabayashi, N.T., Tyler, E.T. and Tyler, A., Fertil. Steril., 12: 544, 1961.
70. Bandhauer, D., Urologica Internationalis, 21: 247, 1966.
71. Rao, S.S., Sadri, K.K. and Sheth, A.K., Proc. Symp. Proteins Central Food Technol. Res. Instit. Mysore, India, 1961.
72. Southam, A.L., J. Reprod. Fertil., 5: 458, 1963.
73. Weil, A.J., Lotsevalov, O. and Wilson, H., Proc. Soc. Exp. Biol. Med., 92: 606, 1956.
74. Schwimmer, W.B., Ustay, K.A. and Behrman, S.J., Amer. Obst. Gynec., 30: 192, 1967.
75. D'Almeida, M., Belaisch, J., Eyquem, A., Guillon, G. and Palmer, R., Cited by Cohen, In Acta Europea Fertil., 1: 193, 1969.
76. Rumke, Ph., Proc. Roy . Soc. Biol., 61: 275, 1968.
77. Phadke, A.M. and Padukone, K., J. Reprod. Fertil., 7: 163, 1964.
78. Feltkamp, T.E.W. and Kruyff, K., Ann. N.Y. Acad. Sci., 124: 702, 1965.
79. Andrada, J.A., Loyzaga, P. and Mancini, R.E., Fertil. Steril., 1970 (in press).
80. Fjallbrant, B., Acta Obstet. Gynec. Scand., 48: 131, 1969.

DISCUSSION

A. STEINBERGER: Dr. Mancini, you have indicated that the testicular antigen is primarily located in the spermatids or spermatozoa. As you have so beautifully illustrated in vitro, fluorescent tagged antibody localizes in the spermatozoa, particularly in the acrosome. How do you explain then the finding that when testicular homogenates are injected in vivo together with complete Freund's adjuvant you not only get degeneration of spermatids and spermatozoa but also degeneration of spermatocytes and spermatogonia? Do you think that there is some immunologic cross reactivity between these cells?

MANCINI: The first cells which degenerate are the spermatids and the spermatozoa in the seminiferous tubules, then the spermatocytes which may appear in the lumen or are phagocytosed by the Sertoli cells. What is most surprising is that also spermatogonial cells may exfoliate and degenerate, in most but not in all of the tubules. With immunofluorescence techniques, the antigen appears located in the acrosome but we do not know if the resolution of the immunohistochemical technique is high enough to detect the precursors of the antigens which may be contained in spermatocytes. This may be a partial explanation. I do not know of any other unless one speculates on possible damage in the sustentacular function of Sertoli cells.

JOHNSEN: Could you indicate how often you find good evidence that immunologic factors are the cause of infertility in males?

MANCINI: I cannot answer your question because I am not yet engaged in exploration of sterile patients with immunological techniques. Various investigators have found spermagglutinins and sperm immobilizing antibodies in the serum of infertile individuals which will increase if an injury such as an inflammatory condition is present in the testis or in the genital male tract. I would like to stress the fact that nobody can explain yet whether or not there is a causal relationship between antigenic antibodies and sterility in men.

JIRASEK: Did you use oxidase labelled or just the fluorescent labelled antibodies for analysis of your sections?

MANCINI: We have used in the last years as label, horseradish peroxides as recommended by Pearse and Nakane. We saw that the horseradish peroxidase, at least in our systems, is very useful and we are able to detect the presence of antigenic areas, which point to the site of interaction with the antibody in human spermatozoa better than the immunofluorescent techniques.

JIRASEK: I refer to the sections. Were the results with the peroxidase identical to those with the fluorescein labelled antibodies?

MANCINI: We did not apply the horseradish peroxides as a label of antibodies in the sections of human testis. If one applies this technique to sections of the human testis, some lipids, located in the Leydig and spermatogonial cells, may react. It is well known that some lipids may have a peroxide activity, and in this sense the reaction will give a false positive reaction.

PAULSEN: I think that the evidence with respect to the immunologic factors in testicular disease presented by Dr. Mancini is exceedingly important. Several years ago we described that after unilateral testicular biopsy (without any clinical evidence of an inflammatory reaction) about 40% of the patients showed a significant reduction in sperm count. Working with Dr. William Clarke's group, we have been able to demonstrate that the sperm from some of these patients following a unilateral biopsy become "tagged" with fluorescent labelled antibodies. This was not present prior to the biopsy. This demonstrates that in some patients you can elicit an antigen-antibody reaction by incising the seminiferous tubules.

MANCINI: In terms of potential antigenicity for antibody formation, it is not necessary that a great amount of antigen should be liberated at the site of the injury. Also, the reactivity of the immune system of the individual is of importance.

ROSEMBERG: The number of patients undergoing testicular biopsy is considerable. What would be then the proportion of individuals who become infertile after a testicular biopsy? Are we justified in asking for it?

PAULSEN: I must emphasize that this is a very transient phenomenon in the majority of patients. It usually clears within 90 days. We do not find a permanent reduction in spermatogenesis as a consequence of testicular biopsy.

MANN: May I be allowed to make a general comment on the antigens and antibodies in semen? We have to draw a very clear distinction between two classes of immunologically active factors, namely those that are coming from the accessory gland secretions, and those that are found in spermatozoa. As regards the first class, these can be identified easily in the accessory secretions, and they can be explored by experiments performed directly on, for example, the prostatic and seminal vesicle secretion. However, I am somewhat doubtful about the true origin of antigens and antibodies which are supposed to occur in spermatozoa. One of the biochemical peculiarities of spermatozoa is the extraordinary ease with which they can be coated with various proteins and mucoproteins and indeed, as Weil has shown, some of the so-called sperm antigens and antibodies have been trapped by the spermatozoa from the accessory secretions. There is, therefore, the possibility that already in the epidididymis, those antigens and antibodies which we find in spermatozoa may have originated in the epididymal plasma. I do feel that progress on the true origin of immunologically active factors in spermatozoa as such, can only be made when testicular spermatozoa become available for that kind of investigation.

MANCINI: Dr. Mann, you raise the question which appeared in Dr. Weil's papers more than ten years ago, related to the existence of intrinsic antigens and coating antigens. Our present studies are confirming what you assumed. It is difficult to separate from the surface of the human spermatozoon, in spite of repeated washing and some other treatment, the coating antigen which depends on the seminal plasma to see what are really the intrinsic antigens. However, using immunohistochemical techniques, testicular spermatocele showed a weak head cap reaction in contact with antihuman testicular antibodies.

DICZFALUSY: Why do you only mention epididymal antigens? I believe that in prostatic secretions, at least three highly specific proteins have been found, which are not present in any other organ.

MANCINI: Yes, the prostate has a strong antigenicity as compared with that of the epididymis. Dr. Rumke has found that one of them is a lactoferrin, which is also present in milk. This antigen is apparently responsible for the antigenicity of the prostate. This of course does not exclude the existence of some other antigenic proteins in this gland.

CHAPTER VII

GONADOTROPIN THERAPY

SECTION 1: TREATMENT OF HYPOPITUITARISM

EFFECTS OF HCG, HMG, HLH AND HGH ADMINISTRATION ON TESTICULAR FUNCTION

C. Alvin Paulsen, Duane H. Espeland and Edward L. Michals

Department of Medicine, University of Washington School of Medicine, Division of Endocrinology, U.S. Public Health Service Hospital, Seattle, Washington

Proper patient selection together with the use of purified gonadotropic hormones having known biologic activity are of paramount importance when experiments are conducted to define the effects of follicle stimulating hormone (FSH) or luteinizing hormone (LH) on human testicular function. This is particularly true when assigning physiologic roles to these gonadotropins.

With regard to patient selection, males who have normal or elevated endogenous FSH and LH levels and present with either oligospermia or azoospermia are unsuitable for such studies irrespective of their testicular histology. This is due to the fact that the involved etiologic and pathologic factors are largely unknown.

Although still not ideal, patients with markedly diminished pituitary gonadotropin secretion are best suited for studies of this nature. Included in this group of patients are males with the genetic disorder, hypogonadotropic eunuchoidism (1) or males who demonstrate in addition to gonadotropin deficiency diminished secretion of one or more than one of the other pituitary tropic hormones.

The human gonadotropic hormones which have been available for study in experimental systems up to the present time have not been optimal agents due to either their lack of purity or to the fact that they contain both gonadotropic hormones, i.e. FSH and LH. For example, human menopausal gonadotropic (HMG) preparations exhibit FSH and LH potencies of varying ratios (2). Even the purest preparations contain both FSH and LH. Also human chorionic gonadotropin (HCG), which behaves like luteinizing hormone (LH) in stimulating the Leydig cells, possesses an unknown FSH or follicle-stimulating factor (FSF) activity in certain animal systems (3,4). Thus the response to HCG can not be directly equated to that which might be obtained with human (HLH) administration.

Despite these limitations, certain working concepts have emerged from clinical studies in patients with hypogonadotropic hypogonadism which in the main correspond to the information derived from animal studies where more pure pituitary gonadotropins of animal origin have been used.

This report will summarize our experience with respect to the testicular response following HMG and HCG administration. Preliminary studies with HLH or human growth hormone (HGH) treatment will also be presented.

A. EFFECT OF HMG ON THE IMMATURE GERMINAL EPITHELIUM

Although FSH and LH act in concert during normal puberty to produce testicular maturation, we desired to determine whether or not FSH could stimulate immature germinal epithelium. Therefore HMG was administered to three hypogonadotropic patients as their initial form of gonadotropic therapy (D.L., C.H., D.D., see Tables 1, 2, 3, 4). The details of these patients' clinical, hormonal and testicular status before and after treatment have been documented previously (5-7). The dose of HMG was adjusted in an attempt to administer that dose of FSH which had been shown to stimulate ovarian follicular growth and later to restore spermatogenesis after hypophysectomy (8). At the same time we endeavored to keep the LH dose low enough to avoid Leydig cell stimulation. This latter point had no precedence since the minimal effective dose for LH action on Leydig cell function is unknown. The daily FSH dose ranged from 27.3 (raised to 81.9 I.U. in patient D.L. after two weeks) to 148.6 I.U. and for LH was 42.5 to 261.2 I.U. Treatment was carried out for five and one-half to six weeks. Essentially two types of response were noted. In patient D.L. the seminiferous tubules remained the same size and no proliferation of the immature germinal epithelium occurred. (See photomicrographs published in reference 5).

On the other hand, in patient C.H. the mean seminiferous tubular diameter increased from 58.6 μ ± 1.5 to 71.0 μ ± 1.4 (5). However no proliferation of germinal cells was noted, e.g. control, 42.7 ± 2.1 cells per tubular cross section and 49.1 ± 2.3 cells per tubular cross section following HMG therapy. C.H.'s LH dosage was the highest of the three patients, ranging from 130.6 to 261.2 I.U. per day. Furthermore his plasma testosterone level increased from a control of 0.05 μg% to 0.11 μg%, which suggests that his interstitial cells were stimulated by the administered LH in his HMG preparation. In patient D.D. two different sized tubules existed before treatment (Table 1). This observation might be related to

Table 1. Seminiferous Tubule Diameter in Normal Adult Males and in Males with Prepuberal Hypogonadotropic Hypogonadism.

Patient	Age (yrs)	Diagnosis	Mean Diameter (μ) of 10 Circular Tubules	
RV 11	27	Normal male	189.6	
RV 16	36	"	185.4	
RV 20	50	"	162.6	
RV 28	30	"	166.6	Group Mean 171.8 ± 12.0 (S.D.)
RV 32	46	"	174.0	
RV 38	24	"	156.6	
RV 53	41	"	168.0	
M.B.	23	Hypogonadotropic eunuchoidism	55.4	
B.S.	25	"	57.3	
J.P.	20	"	62.7	Group Mean 62.1 ± 8.8 (S.D.)
F.H.	19	"	59.3	
C.H.	17	"	58.6	
D.D.	22	Craniopharyngioma [a]	79.5 (96.1)[b]	
E.J.	28	Idiopathic selective pituitary deficiency[c]	66.6	

a. Patient had TSH and gonadotropin deficiency. ACTH secretion was presumed to be normal by testing; HGH secretion presumed normal because of his normal height. He was on thyroid replacement therapy.

b. Two populations of tubules in biopsy specimen. Smaller tubules used for group mean calculations.

c. Sella turcica as well as suprasellar area was normal. Decreased HGH, FSH, LH secretion by radioimmunoassay or bioassay testing. Presumed normal TSH and ACTH secretion by appropriate testing, e.g., RAI uptake, PBI, response to metapirone, 17-ketogenic steroid excretion.

Table 2. Hypogonadotropic Hypogonadism Pretreatment Studies

Patient	Age	Urinary Gonadotropins GGA	Urinary Gonadotropins FSH	Urinary Estrogens	Plasma Testosterone
D.L.	20	<0.7	-	<0.2	-
J.P.	20	<0.7	-	<0.2	-
M.S.[a]	20	-	<3.8, 1.6	<0.2	0.05
H.G.	24	<0.7, 0.9	-	-	0.02, 0.02, 0.15
G.G.[a]	19	<0.7	-	-	-
D.D.	21	<0.7	-	<0.2	-
P.N.	16	<0.7	-	<0.2	-

Hormonal data before treatment. GGA refers to a general gonadotropin assay method which measures the combined effect of FSH and LH. (Normal adult male range 0.7 - 3.8 mg. -eq. per 24 hours). Urinary estrogens determined biologically. (Normal adult male range 0.3 - 3.0 μg. -eq. estradiol benzoate per 24 hours). Plasma testosterone by double isotope derivative method. (Normal adult range 0.28 - 1.44 μg. %.) a Patients with anosmia.

previous therapy with methyl testosterone, since exogenous androgen can stimulate the immature seminiferous tubule to some extent. Only general gonadotropin assays were conducted prior to treatment so that the precise status of his endogenous FSH and LH levels is unknown. Following HMG therapy the mean seminiferous tubular diameter of D.D. increased to 109.3 ± 4.5 μ. At this time an increase in germinal cell numbers was also noted, but maturation had not progressed beyond the cell type noted before treatment, i.e., the pachytene spermatocyte.

These data could be interpreted in the following manner: FSH by itself does not affect the immature seminiferous tubule unless Leydig cells are stimulated by concomitant administration of LH or unless the seminiferous tubules have been previously exposed to endogenous or exogenous testosterone. de Kretser (9) noted early seminiferous tubular maturation and an increase in plasma testosterone levels in a patient with hypogonadotropic eunuchoidism when the FSH/LH dosage was 200/500 I.U. three times weekly for five months. Rosemberg et al. (10) in their studies on prepuberal males with cryptorchidism noted germinal cell stimulation and early Leydig cell maturation following HMG therapy of equivalent or higher FSH and LH doses.

Table 3. Summary of Histologic Findings in Hypogonadotropic Hypogonadism before and after HCG Therapy

Patient	Previous Therapy	Duration HCG Therapy (weeks)	Most Advanced Germ Cell Type	
			Before HCG	After HCG
D.L.	HMG (7 wks)	23	Immature germinal epithelium	Early differentiation of spermatogonia
J.P.	None	59	"	Sd Spermatid
D.D.	1) intermittent methyl testosterone (? yrs) 2) HMG (6 wks)	25	Pachytene spermatocyte	Sd Spermatid
P.N.	None	56	No biopsy	Pachytene spermatocyte
E.J.	1) "Pituitary" shots (1 mo duration, age 14) 2) HGH therapy (15 wks)	10	Pachytene spermatocyte	Sc spermatids

Table 4. Studies to Induce Spermatogenesis in Hypogonadotropic Hypogonadism

		HCG		HCG-HMG		
Patient	Age	Duration of treatment (weeks)	Sperm Count mill/ml	Duration of treatment (weeks)[c]	Sperm Count mill/ml	Highest Sperm Count
J.P.	20	59	Azoo	7	1-2/hpf	39[b]
M.S.[a]	20	16	59	-	-	71[b]
H.G.	22	85	(42)	-	-	(42)
G.G.[a]	19	78	Azoo	5	1/hpf	1-3/hpf
D.D.	22	25	Azoo	15	1-2/hpf	14.7
E.J.	28	30[d]	Azoo	13	0.3	48
P.N.	16	56	Azoo	19	occasional dead sperm	

In patient H.G., the bracket surrounding the sperm count indicates that this was the only specimen obtained. a. Patients with anosmia. b. Patients who were married and achieved a pregnancy. c. Duration in weeks refers to that interval between onset of treatment and the first appearance of sperm in the ejaculate. d. During the last twenty weeks HGH therapy was added.

B. EFFECT OF HCG ON THE IMMATURE TESTIS

Seven patients received HCG therapy at a dosage of 2000-5000 I.U. three times weekly for 16 to 85 weeks. Four patients (D.L., J.P., P.N., G.G.) exhibited the classic form of hypogonadotropic eunuchoidism, i.e., no discernible evidence of effective endogenous gonadotropin secretion. Two of the seven patients (M.S., H.G.) were considered as variants of the syndrome resembling the subcategory "Fertile Eunuch." Both men were devoid of androgen effects and demonstrated very low plasma testosterone levels (see Table 2). On the other hand, urinary FSH excretion was at the lower limit of the normal adult male range on one occasion in patient M.S. Patient H.G. exhibited a normal urinary GGA (general gonadotropin assay) titer on one of two occasions while his control testicular biopsy specimen revealed seminiferous tubular stimulation. The mean tubular diameter was 116.4 $\mu \pm 18.6$ and spermatogenesis had progressed to the Sd spermatid level. The remaining patient, D.D., has been described before (Table 1 and section A).

In the patients who demonstrated positive evidence of endogenous FSH secretion prior to treatment, therapy with HCG alone produced full spermatogenesis including spermatozoa in the ejaculate. This response occurred within 16 and 85 weeks, respectively. Patient H.G. was unable to submit a seminal fluid specimen until the 85th week of treatment. Therefore we are uncertain as to the exact time that full spermatogenesis developed.

The remaining five patients were still azoospermic at the completion of HCG therapy alone. Treatment lasted 25 to 78 weeks (Table 4). Despite the azoospermia, examination of the testicular biopsy specimens in D.L., J.P., D.D., and E.J. revealed that spermatogenesis had been stimulated by HCG therapy in each patient where a pre-HCG biopsy was available for comparison (Table 3, Figs. 2,3). The question as to why HCG therapy by itself should initiate spermatogenesis in these hypogonadotropic "prepuberal" patients remains unclear. The fact that sufficient endogenous FSH secretion existed in patients M.S. and H.G. affords a plausible explanation as to why Leydig cell function plus full spermatogenesis was achieved by only HCG therapy. However no such evidence was present in patients D.L. and J.P. It may be that the "FSF" activity present in HCG permits germinal cell stimulation. On the other hand, it may be that the endogenous testosterone secretion initiated by HCG therapy has a definite but limited action with respect to stimulating spermatogenesis. Lastly it is possible that LH acts directly on the germinal epithelium. Definitive conclusions will have to wait until purified HLH is used in similar patients.

C. EFFECT OF COMBINED HCG-HMG TREATMENT

Five patients received combined HCG-HMG therapy of varying dose schedules when solo HCG treatment of 25 to 78 weeks was still associated with azoospermia (Table 4). The treatment schedule is listed below:

	HCG (I.U., t.i.w.)	FSH (HMG) (I.U.)
J.P.	2000	64.5 - 74.3 daily
D.D.	2000-4000	63.0 - 74.3 daily
G.G.	4000	150 t.i.w.
E.J.	4000	75 t.i.w.
P.N.	4000	75 t.i.w.

The addition of HMG (FSH) to the therapeutic regimen was successful in four out of the five patients as measured by the appearance of spermatozoa in their seminal fluid (Table 4). It required from 5 to 19 weeks of combined HCG-HMG therapy for this event to occur. Seminal fluid specimens were submitted for analysis once weekly. The varying HMG (FSH) dosage did not appear to affect the response to treatment in this limited study. HCG-HMG administration was continued to a maximum of four years (J.P., see reference 6). The highest seminal fluid sperm concentration was achieved in

E.J. (48 mill/ml) after a total of 60 weeks[1] of combined therapy. In J.P., the highest sperm count noted was 39 mill./ml. HMG therapy was discontinued in P.N., D.D. and G.G. after 34, 45 and 32 weeks, respectively.

It is difficult to explain why combined HCG-HMG therapy did not produce numerically greater sperm counts. Fundamental information pertinent to this point is lacking. That is, at what point in time do males attain normal sperm production during their puberal process? Until these data are obtained, we have to consider the following possibilities: 1) treatment did not last long enough, 2) the proper FSH/LH ratio was not employed, 3) HCG exerts an action which is qualitatively different from that exerted by HLH, 4) the testis as well as the pituitary-hypothalamic system is defective in patients with this syndrome. (11)

It is also possible that the multiple biopsies employed to document the response to treatment might have influenced sperm production. However, no testicular biopsy was performed in patient G.G.

Only two patients were married while receiving treatment (J.P., M.S.). J.P.'s wife became pregnant twice and delivered two normal male infants. M.S.'s wife became pregnant once and delivered a normal female infant.

D. EFFECT OF HLH ON LEYDIG CELL FUNCTION

The dose of administered HLH required to produce normal Leydig cell function has not been established. Therefore we initiated studies in our patients with hypogonadotropic eunuchoidism in an effort to obtain this information. Data from our HMG therapy experience (see discussion patient C.H.) suggested that the effective HLH dosage might approximate 200 I.U. per day.

M.S. (Tables 2,4) who had received HCG for over three years was selected for study. His current HCG dose was 2000 I.U. three times weekly and his sexual maturation was essentially complete. Just prior to starting HLH and twenty-four hours after his last dose of HCG blood was sampled for plasma testosterone assay (see Table 5). The value was 1.2 μg % (normal adult male range 0.28 - 1.44 μg % (12)) which confirmed our clinical judgment that he was receiving optimal HCG therapy.

During the four weeks of HLH treatment (400 I.U. three times weekly) M.S. stated that he experienced vasomotor symptons, e.g. hot flashes, on those days he did not receive his medication. Li-

1. There were two periods of therapy, 28 weeks and 32 weeks, with a one-year interval between.

Table 5. Comparison Between HCG and HLH Administration in terms of Leydig Cell Function (Patient M.S.)

Hormone	Dosage Schedule	Duration of Therapy at Indicated Dosage	Time Interval Between Treatment and Blood Sampling (hrs)	Serum HLH Levels[c] (mIU/ml)	Plasma Testosterone (T) Levels[d] (μg %)
HCG[a]	2000 I.U. t.i.w.	43 wks	24	-	1.2
HLH[b]	400 I.U. t.i.w.	4 wks	12	9.4	0.23
HLH	400 I.U./d.	4 d	4	33.0	0.34
HLH	200 I.U./d.	4 d	8½	6.8	0.11
HCG	2000 I.U. t.i.w.	3 wks	24	-	0.63

a. HCG, Ayerst Laboratories; b. HLH-LER 856, lot A-1, 200 I.U./vial (VPW), kindly supplied by the National Pituitary Agency; c. Serum HLH assayed by radioimmunoassay method of Midgley (16); d. Plasma testosterone levels determined by a modification of the displacement technique of Nugent (17).

bido was reported to be normal but his sexual potentia had decreased slightly. Twelve hours after an injection of 400 I.U. HLH, his serum HLH level was 9.4 m.I.U./ml. but his plasma testosterone was 0.23 μg %, which is below the normal male range. His plasma testosterone increased to 0.34 μg % after four days of 400 I.U. HLH per day and dropped to 0.11 μg % after four days of 200 I.U. per day. Serum LH levels were 33 m.I.U./ml four hours after 400 I.U. of HLH and 6.8 m.I.U./ml eight and one-half hours after 200 I.U. He then returned to HCG therapy at his previous dose schedule. Androgen withdrawal symptoms disappeared one week after the resumption of HCG therapy, and his plasma testosterone titer was 0.63 μg % two weeks later.

These preliminary data indicate that for optimal maintenance of Leydig cell function in patients without endogenous LH secretion, HLH therapy using saline as the diluent will have to be administered daily at doses slightly above 400 I.U. These observations as to daily dose requirements are in keeping with the recent data on half-life studies for HCG and HLH (a fast and slow component for each: t 1/2 HCG = 11 hr, 23 hr; t 1/2 HLH = 21 min, 235 min). (13,14,15)

E. EFFECT OF HGH ON TESTICULAR FUNCTION

It has been suggested that when growth hormone and gonadotropin deficiency exist together the testes of prepuberal males are less developed than when only gonadotropin deficiency is present. (18) If this is true, HGH may exert a stimulatory action on the testis.

To evaluate this hypothesis we studied the effect of HGH therapy on patient E.J.'s testicular function (Table 1). This patient demonstrated deficient HGH and gonadotropin secretion with intact thyroid and adrenal cortical function. Testicular biopsy specimens were obtained prior to and following HGH[2] therapy (5mg thrice weekly). Before treatment, examination of his biopsy specimen revealed an immature testis except for an occasional seminiferous tubule containing maturing germinal cells. The most advanced cell type observed was the pachytene spermatocyte (Fig.1). The mean tubular diameter in E.J.'s control biopsy specimen was comparable to that noted for patients with presumably normal HGH but deficient gonadotropin secretion (Table 1), 66.6 μ vs 62 ± 8.8 μ. After fifteen weeks of HGH therapy his biopsy specimen was unchanged (Fig. 2), including the mean tubular diameter (65.9 μ). At this time his plasma testosterone level was 0.04 μg %.[3] Since a control testosterone titer was not obtained, HGH was discontinued for three weeks

2. Kindly supplied by the National Pituitary Agency. Bioassay of this HGH preparation revealed the presence of 2.0 I.U. HLH and 4.0 USP units Prolactin per mg. No FSH activity was detected.

3. Performed by Dr. Hortense Gandy using the double isotope derivative method.

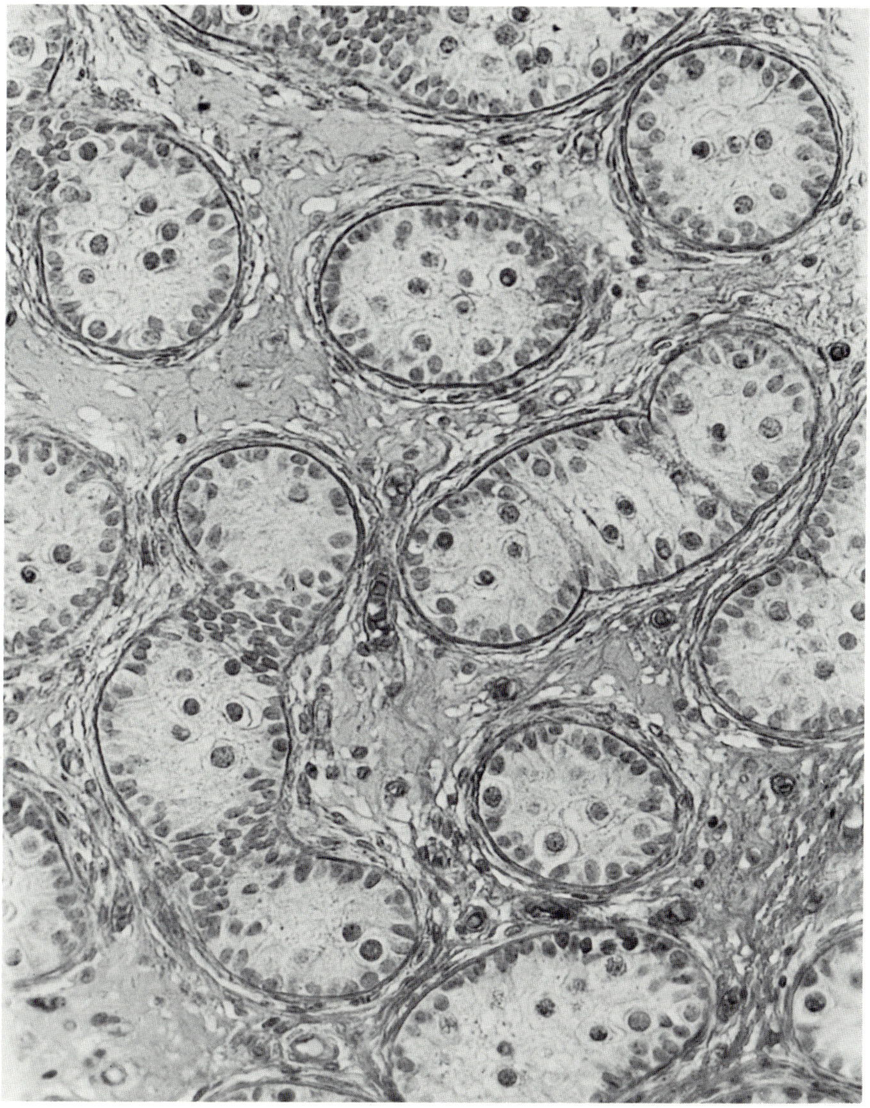

Fig. 1. (x 63.) Testicular biopsy specimen before HGH. Seminiferous tubules contain mainly an immature germinal epithelium with an occasional germ cell undergoing differentiation.

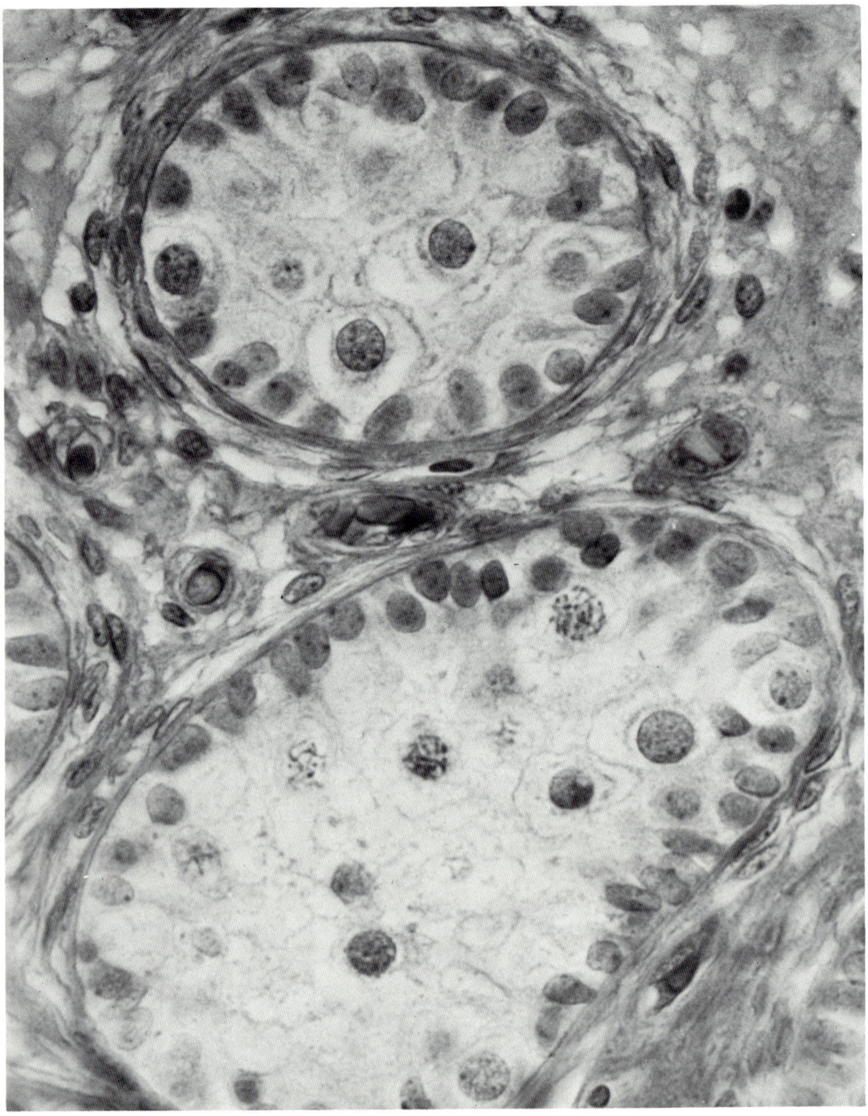

Fig. 1A (x 160.) E.J. before HGH, higher magnification. Note pachytene spermatocytes.

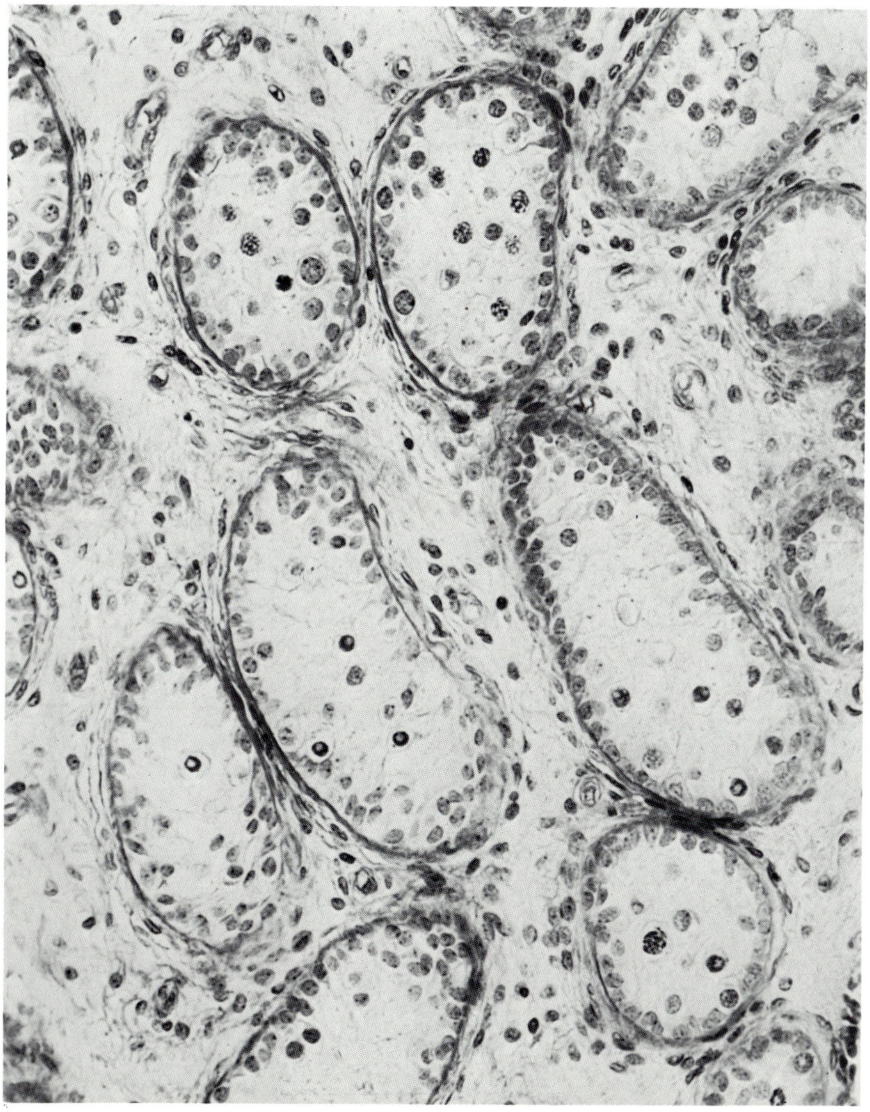

Fig. 2. (x 63.) E.J. testis specimen after HGH. Essentially no change in the number of cells undergoing maturation. Tubules are of the same size as before HGH.

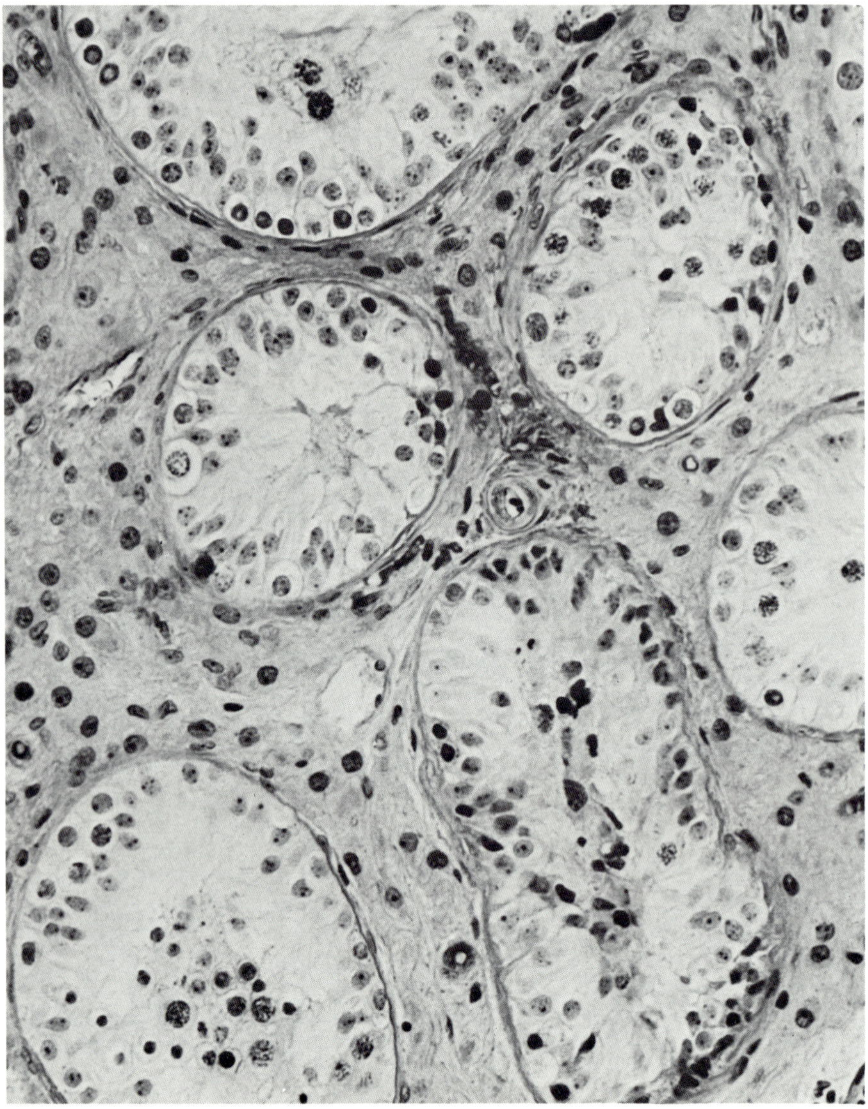

Fig. 3. (x63.) Testicular biopsy specimen following HCG therapy Definite increase in tubular diameter. Spermatogenesis has been stimulated.

at which time his plasma testosterone level was 0.02 μg %. His body height increased 5/8" during HGH therapy. Thereafter his treatment consisted of HCG for ten weeks, then combined HGH and HCG for twenty weeks and finally HCG plus HMG for seven months. His third testicular biopsy specimen obtained after his combined HCG-HGH therapy (Tables 3 and 4) revealed active spermatogenesis (Fig. 3) which had progressed to the Sc spermatid stage. The mean tubular diameter had now increased to 98.8μ. Maturation of his interstitial cells into Leydig cells was evident and his plasma testosterone titer was 1.17 μg %.

There was no evidence in this patient that HGH had any effect on his testicular status. However these results do not reject the possibility that HGH might supplement the action of FSH and LH during testicular maturation in normal puberty.

ACKNOWLEDGEMENTS

These studies supported in part by NIH grants AM05161 and AM05436 and AEC contract AT(45-1)-2225-T6.

REFERENCES

1. Paulsen, C.A., The Testis, In Textbook of Endocrinology, ed. Williams, R.H., 4th edition, W.B. Saunders Co., Philadelphia, 1968.
2. Rosemberg, E., In Gonadotropins 1968, ed. Rosemberg, E., Geron-X, Inc., Los Altos,Calif. p 426, 1968.
3. Crooke, A.C. and Butt, W.R. J. Obstet. Gynaec. Brit. Comm., 66: 297, 1959.
4. Albert, A., J. Clin. Endocr. 29: 1504, 1969.
5. Paulsen, C.A., ed., Estrogen Assays in Clinical Medicine, University of Washington Press, Seattle, 1965.
6. Paulsen, C.A., In Proceedings of the Sixth Pan American Congress of Endocrinology, Mexico City 1965, Amsterdam, Excerpta Medica Foundation, p. 212, 1966.
7. Paulsen, C.A., In Gonadotropins 1968, ed. Rosemberg, E. Geron-X, Inc., Los Altos, Calif. p 491, 1968.
8. MacLeod, J., Pagianos, A. and Ray, B., Fertil. Steril., 17; 7, 1964.
9. deKretser, D.M., Thesis, M.D., Monash University, Melbourne, Australia, 1969.
10. Rosemberg, E., Mancini, R.E., Crigler, J.F. and Bergada, C., In Gonadotropins 1968, ed. Rosemberg, E., Geron-X, Inc., Los Altos, Calif., p 527, 1968.
11. Bardin, C.W., Ross, G.T., Rifkind, A.B., Cargille, C.M. and Lipsett, M.B., J. Clin. Invest., 48: 2046, 1969.
12. Paulsen, C.A., Gordon, D.L. Carpenter, H.M., Gandy, H.M. and Drucker, W.D., Recent Progr.Hormone Res., 24: 321, 1968.
13. Kohler, P.O., Ross, G.T. and Odell, W.D., J. Clin. Invest., 47: 38, 1968.

14. Yen, S.S.C., Llerena, O., Little, B. and Pearson, O.H. J. Clin. Endocr., 28: 1763, 1968.
15. Rizkallah, T., Gurpide, E. and Vande Wiele, R.L., J. Clin. Endocr., 29: 92, 1969.
16. Midgley, A.R. Jr., Endocrinology, 79: 10, 1968.
17. Mayes, D. and Nugent, O.A., J. Clin. Endocr., 28: 1169, 1968.
18. Albert, A., Underdahl, L.O., Green, L.F. and Lorenz, N., Proc. Staff Meeting Mayo Clinic 28: 698, 1953.

DISCUSSION

MACLEOD: Dr. Paulsen, in your studies with long-continued administration of HCG in eunuchoid patients in whom you observed some degree of maturation of spermatogenesis, have you taken into account the FSH-like activity contained in HCG?

PAULSEN: Yes, we have to consider that HCG has several effects on the germinal epithelium. One is by stimulating endogenous testosterone secretion. The other may relate to a direct action on the germinal epithelium by the FSH property of HCG. What we need is comparable data as to the effect of HLH on the immature testis.

ROSEMBERG: The amount of FSH activity intrinsic to the HCG molecule could be estimated and this will be negligible in the studies reported here.

DICZFALUSY: Making an approximation, I think it is fair to say that in most HCG preparations the FSH-like activity corresponds to 1 IU for every 1,000 IU of HCG. Hence, this amount of FSH will not really have any effect.

ROSS: Dr. Paulsen, when you report detecting no follicle-stimulating hormone activity in the urine of these eunuchoidal patients, what quantity of urine in relationship to the 24-hour output have you injected per animal? What is the nature of the extract which you used: fraction A, B, C? I ask these questions to emphasize the difference between "failure to detect" and "total absence" of activity.

PAULSEN: I tried to be careful by stating that the urinary gonadotropins were "undetectable" as opposed to "absent". In general we inject a 12-hour aliquot per assay animal. We have not defined the small amounts of urinary gonadotropins which may be present in these patients. All we can state is that there is less gonadotropin excreted in these patients than is present in normal adult males. We use fraction A for our assays.

EFFECT OF URINARY FSH AND LH ON THE TESTICULAR FUNCTION IN HYPOGONADAL PATIENTS

Roberto E. Mancini

Centro de Investigaciones sobre Reproduccion.
Facultad de Medicina, Paraguay 2155, Piso 10,
Buenos Aires, Argentina

INTRODUCTION

The effects of human chorionic (HCG), pregnant mare serum (PMS) or other animal pituitary gonadotropin preparations on the development of spermatogenesis in prepuberal and postpuberal cases of hypogonadotropic hypogonadism have generally been disappointing (1-5). Although it has long been admitted that large doses and long term administration of HCG clearly stimulate the development and function of Leydig cells together with the appearance of secondary sexual signs, some discrepancies still remain with regard to its effect on the germinal epithelium and connective tissue structures of the tubular wall. It seems that only those cases with previous histological evidence of advanced meiotic process may respond successfully with production of spermatozoa (6,7). On the other hand, gonadotropins of animal origin seem to be able to stimulate weakly both Leydig and germinal cells; this restricted action may be imputable to the long known induction of antigonadotropins (1,3). However, results obtained in similar hypogonadal conditions seem to be more encouraging, with the use of human urinary menopausal (HMG) and pituitary gonadotropins (HPG) administered singly or combined with HCG. Their human origin and both FSH and LH activity are the main advantages of these preparations. It is now generally agreed that HMG or HPG alone may effectively stimulate the spermatogenic process in hypogonadotropic subjects, but that completion of spermatogenesis is achieved when full development of Leydig cells is produced by the addition of HCG (8-15). Consequently, the contention at present is in favor of the simultaneous need for FSH-LH and an excess of LH for the development of interstitial and seminiferous tubule structures.

In spite of this considerable progress in the understanding of the hormonal regulation of the spermatogenic process several points still remain to be clarified: a) The separate action of different doses and lengths of treatment of highly purified preparations of FSH and of LH. b) The effect of the successive or simultaneous administration of both hormones in different ratios. c) Cell stages reached by germinal and Sertoli cell populations in the qualitative progression of the spermatogenesis induced by FSH or LH. d) The extent to which Leydig cell differentiation and function is necessary for germinal, Sertoli cell and tubular wall structure development. e) Whether regression of peritubular hyalinization is under the direct control of FSH or LH or is correlated with Leydig or germinal epithelium stimulation.

This rather ambitious program of study was made possible with the collaboration of Dr. P. Donini (Serono Foundation, Rome) who provided the purified preparations of human urinary FSH and LH, Drs. O. Vilar and A. Perez Lloret, who performed histological studies and Drs. C. Bergada, J. Reforzo Membrives, A. Arguelles, M. Molosnick and J.C. Lavieri (Buenos Aires School of Medicine) who carried out the endocrine studies of the patients. In the present report, emphasis will be placed on the microscopical changes of the gonad. More detailed results concerning clinical data, hormonal assays and electron microscopic observations of testis will be published elsewhere.

The specifications of the FSH and LH urinary preparation were as follows: FSH: 1255 I.U./mg of the 2nd. IRP-HMG; LH contaminant: 3.3 I.U./mg of the 2nd. IRP. LH: 1025 I.U. per ampoule/2nd. IRP. FSH contaminant: 39.9 I.U./ampoule. The strength of both preparations was verified by the Steelman and Pohley and the O.A.A.D. methods and the radioimmunoassay according to Donini et al. (16). As it was estimated that 74 $\pm$ 4-5 days are required for the development of spermatogonia to the level of spermatozoa (17), FSH and/or LH were given to our groups of patients for three or four months. Biopsies of the testes and urinary steroid determinations were made before and at the end of each course of treatment. The evaluation of the histological changes induced by both gonadotropins was based on cell count according to previous work (18,19), where a detailed description of the various types of spermatogonial, Sertoli and Leydig cells was made. However, as the aim of the present study was to establish the effect of these hormones on the cell population of the three main phases of spermatogenesis, the spermatogonial cells (mitotic included), the spermatocytes and the spermiogenic cells (spermatids and spermatozoa) were considered separately. The estimation of the variations in the relative number of germinal and Sertoli cells was made by cell count in 20 approximately circular transverse sections of seminiferous tubules for each specimen. Calculations of the average number of each cell type per one tubular cross section were made and statistically verified by the "t" test. The diameter of the seminiferous tubules, excluding the basement membrane, was also measured in 30 transverse sections, expressed as an average and statistically verified by the "t" test. Changes in the wall of seminiferous tubules were estimated as disappearance of peritubular hyalin material and its replacement by normal fibrillar structures. With reference to the intertubular spaces, the fibroblast-like cells as precursor Leydig cells and the immature, mature and degenerating types of Leydig cells were estimated applying a differential count over 200 cells of this cell population and statistically verified by the binomial distribution (20).

In the following text the results obtained in the induction or recovery of spermatogenesis in prepuberal and postpuberal hypogonadal patients treated with urinary FSH and/or LH will be summarized. These findings will also be compared with those published by others who have used preparations of HMG or HPG containing different ratios of FSH and LH activities.

I - FSH AND LH IN THE INDUCTION OF SPERMATOGENESIS IN PREPUBERAL HYPOGONADOTROPIC HYPOGONADISM

Several reports have dealt with the action of gonadotropin preparations containing variable FSH-LH ratios in cases with classical signs of eunuchoidism, undetectable or low levels of urinary gonadotropins and a variety of steroids. Testicular biopsies showed in these cases the very well known histology of an immature or prepuberal gland i.e., tubules of small diameter containing only spermatogonia and various degrees of immature Sertoli cells; occasionally some leptotene, zygotene or pachytene spermatocytes were seen. Correspondingly the tubular wall is thin and simple and does not show the complex organization of the well developed tubules of normal adult testes as is seen under the light and electron microscope (21,22). Different spermatogonial cell types may appear as well as some unidentified intermediate forms, but few cytological studies have been made at the electron microscope level (23,24). It is difficult to explain the finding, in some of these eunuchs, of a moderate peritubular hyalinization which mimics that present in postpuberal hypogonadism (23,24). Finally the intertubular spaces are filled with so-called fibroblast-like cells, known as the precursors of immature and mature Leydig cells (19); however, the erratic presence of the latter cells cannot be excluded in all cases.

Based on the existence of an infantile testis and on the theoretical absence of gonadotropins, the eunuchoidal condition has been considered a suitable one to verify the effect of exogenous gonadotropins in the initiation or induction of spermatogenesis. Therefore, in previous publications, an HMG preparation with an FSH-LH ratio equal to unity or favoring FSH, given at a daily dose of 24 to 60 I.U. of FSH for several months has induced, in some cases of eunuchoidism, an increase in tubular diameter, differentiation of Sertoli cells, increase in the number of spermatogonial cells and development of a few spermatocytes; no changes were observed in the preexistent peritubular hyalinization, no development of Leydig cells and no ostensible modification in the urinary androgen assays (11). With 12.5 I.U. of FSH contained in another HMG preparation of unknown LH activity, administered three times weekly for three months, no modifications could be observed in the testis biopsy, in the steroid hormonal assays or in sexual signs (9). In some other cases, daily doses for six and one half weeks of HMG (27.3 to 81.9 I.U. of FSH and 42.5 to 127.5 I.U. of LH) had no effect on testicular histology or steroid levels (8). Doses of 225 I.U. of FSH per week (HMG containing equal amounts of FSH and LH) for 17 weeks produced no results in any of the histological, clinical or hormonal parameters (12) and the same is true of another case treated for 22 weeks with a weekly dose of 750 I.U. of FSH contained in an HMG preparation in which LH activity was not known (13). In another two cases 180 I.U. of FSH (HPG containing an FSH-LH ratio of 1:2) given three times a week for four or five months, resulted in an increase in tubular diameter and of spermatogonial and Sertoli cells, but no changes were seen in tubular wall thickness or in Leydig cell development (7).

In our studies the separate, successive and simultaneous effects of FSH and LH on the testes of similar cases of hypogonadotropic hypogonadisms were considered. Three groups of eunuchs each of three patients, aged from 18 to 25, were treated with the purified urinary FSH and LH already described. In the first and second groups the separate action of both hormones was investigated.

In the first group a weekly dosage (divided into three doses) of about 300, 500 and 800 I.U. of FSH (LH contaminant in the total dose given varied from 9 to 22 I.U.) was given to the first, second and third patients respectively for 12, 14 and 16 weeks. By comparing the biopsies, irrespective of the dose and length of time of administration of the hormones, an increased number in the population of Sertoli cells was observed with a marked predominance of the mature forms over the precursor cell types. No significant changes were detected in the diameter of the seminiferous tubules or in spermatogonial cells and primary spermatocytes. The preexistent normal structures of the tubular wall or the peritubular hyalinization remained the same as did the fibroblast-like cells of the intertubular spaces. In the second group of patients, treatment was scheduled with approximately the same amount of LH (FSH contaminant in the total dose varied from 123 to 383 I.U.) and duration of treatment in each one of the three patients. As with FSH, an increased number of Sertoli cells with a higher proportion of the mature types was seen in two cases, being less clear in the remaining one. Only in the patient who received the highest dose of LH was there in addition a slight increase in the number of spermatogonial cells, which was coincident with an increased population of fibroblast like cells and the appearance of few immature and mature types of Leydig cells. In no case could clear modifications of seminiferous tubule diameter be observed nor development of tubular wall structures or regression of peritubular hyalinization.

In a following step of our studies the successive effects of both hormones was investigated. Two patients of the first group who had been treated with FSH at low and high doses were subsequently treated with the same amount of LH during the same period of time, 12 and 16 weeks respectively. Similarly, another two patients of the second group treated with low and high doses of LH were subjected without interruption to another course of the same doses of FSH during the same length of time. By comparing in the same patient the biopsy after LH with the previous one after FSH, the following was seen: a) Slight increase in the number of spermatogonial cells. b) No change in the number of spermatocytes but more maturation of Sertoli cells. c) Slight increase in the tubular diameter, decrease in the peritubular hyalinization and development of immature and mature types of Leydig cells. d) No change in the level of urinary steroids. These effects were specially seen in the case given the higher dose of LH. In the patients of the second group treated with FSH preceded by LH the comparison of both biopsies showed: a) No changes in spermatogonial or spermatocyte cells. b) Increased maturation of Sertoli cells. c) No major changes in the diameter of seminiferous tubules, in the peritubular hyaline material or in the character of tubular wall structures. d) Disappearance of the already developed Leydig cells and reappearance of fibroblast like cells. e) Levels of urinary steroids remained the same.

In the third group of patients, the simultaneous action of both gonadotropins was tried. The first patient was given a weekly dose of 800 I.U. of FSH and 200 I.U. of LH for 16 weeks. The second subject during the same period received 400 I.U. per week of both FSH and LH. A weekly dose of 800 I.U. of LH plus 200 I.U. of FSH was administered to the third patient. When comparing the biopsies, the first case showed similar results to those obtained in the patients of the first group treated with FSH alone. In the second patient there was a moderate increase in spermatogonial cells, development of earlier stages of primary spermatocytes, maturation of Sertoli cells, increase in tubular diameter together with slight regression of peritubular hyalinization, appearance of a small number of immature and mature Leydig cells but no striking modification in the urinary steroids. The third patient showed a higher increase in spermatogonial cells, a marked maturation of Sertoli cells, development of primary spermatocytes up to the pachytene stage, increase in tubular diameter, a slight development of tubular wall connective tissue structures and higher levels of urinary steroids.

II FSH AND LH IN THE RECOVERY OF SPERMATOGENESIS IN POSTPUBERAL HYPOGONADOTROPIC HYPOGONADISM

Previous reports have pointed out the simultaneous need of both HMG and HCG preparations for the recovery and maintenance of spermatogenesis in hypogonadotropic hypophysectomized patients (15,25). The influence of the amount of pituitary gland removed, the persistence of some pituitary functions and the time which elapsed after operation upon the extent of the regression of germinal epithelium and Leydig cell population, have been discussed (15,25). It was also reported that patients showing in their control biopsies not only Sertoli and spermatogonial cells but also primary spermatocytes may respond better than those having only the first two types of cells (25). Moreover HMG, with a FSH-LH ratio equal to unity in weekly doses of 200 to 300 I.U. may recover spermatogenesis up to the spermiogenic phase, while the addition of HCG at a weekly dose of 2000 I.U., may induce production of spermatozoa after three or four months treatment (15,25).

In the present report the separate or successive effect of purified preparations of urinary FSH and LH were studied in two adult hypophysectomized patients aged 28 and 33. The operations were performed seven and ten months respectively before the testicular biopsies and hormonal assays were made. Histological study showed small hyalinized seminiferous tubules, with only spermatogonial cells, mature Sertoli cells with signs of nuclear atrophy and absence of Leydig cells. Urinary gonadotropins and steroids were undetectable or very low. The first patient was initially treated with a weekly dose of 800 to 1000 I.U. of FSH for 16 weeks; after withdrawal of the hormone the same amount of LH was given during the same period. The second patient was similarly treated but first with LH and afterwards with FSH.

By comparing biopsies taken before and after treatment, no change was visible in any of the testicular structures of the first patient treated with FSH; the exception being that the morphological nuclear abnormalities previously observed in Sertoli cells tended to disappear. No change was induced in the level of urinary steroids. In contrast, the subsequent course of LH in the same patient provoked a slight increase in the spermatogonial cells, appearance of primary spermatocytes, morphologic recovery of nuclei of Sertoli cells, partial regression of hyalinization, slight enlargement of tubules and development of a few immature and mature Leydig cells. No substantial change was detected in the level of urinary steroids. In the second patient the first course of treatment with LH induced similar changes as those described in the first patient but a subsequent course of FSH showed the disappearance of all the stimulatory effects achieved with that hormone; the exception being those induced in the Sertoli cells which persisted.

III COMMENTS

It is evident that the discrepancies in the results obtained in patients with hypogonadotropic eunuchoidism may be attributable to several factors, the most important being the variable potencies of both FSH and LH activity in the gonadotropin preparations used. Different doses and duration of treatment, the variable degree of susceptibility of testes to the hormones and the incompleteness of the histological examination of the biopsies also play a part. Nevertheless, taking into consideration the more detailed microscopical studies of the testis, it may be accepted that HMG with a FSH-LH ratio equal to unity or slightly favoring LH, administered in weekly doses of about 300 I.U. for several months, may provoke enlargement of tubules, increase the number of spermatogonial and Sertoli cells, but does not apparently modify the interstitial cell population or the clinical signs and steroid hormonal assays.

Assuming that the testicular response might be dose dependent, we have used in our studies on cases of prepuberal hypogonadism, different doses and lengths of treatment with FSH and LH. The fact that all cases had approximately a similar degree of undeveloped germinal epithelium and Leydig cells, enabled us to evaluate on a uniform histological background the action of both hormones on the stimulation of different phases of spermatogenesis.

Bearing in mind that differences in the individual response to the gonadotropins may exist in eunuchoidal patients, our results indicate that purified urinary FSH alone given in doses from 300 to 800 I.U. for several months is able to increase the number and induce a maturation process in the Sertoli cells; this interesting change includes the development of nuclear structures, mainly the nucleoli which are related to the synthesis of RNA. The absence of apparent changes in spermatogonial cells suggest that this hormone is incapable of initiating or inducing spermatogenesis. This predominant effect on Sertoli cells appears to depend only on the FSH activity as the amount of LH contaminant is negligible. This finding is also in accordance with those reported by others who have used HMG preparations rich in FSH activity (11). Moreover, an increased number of Sertoli cells have been induced in the prepuberal period of the lamb by injecting pituitary ovine FSH (26); hypertrophy of these cells was also obtained after intratesticular injection of the same hormone in the rat (27). Using immunohistochemical techniques, a selective accumulation in Sertoli cells of the rat was reported with light and electron microscopic studies after intravenous injection of native or labelled FSH; participation of vesicles and lysosome-like bodies in the uptake of the hormone was evident (28,29). Lack of effect on the remaining structures of the testis and on the urinary steroids favor the idea of a direct type of action of FSH upon Sertoli cells. The earlier contention that this cell plays a role in the spermatogenic process appears backed not only by its participation in the intratubular diffusion of serum proteins (30) but also by the fact that during normal puberty, advanced meiosis and spermiogenesis are accompanied by the maturation of Sertoli cells (31). This latter effect appears also reflected histologically in immature testicles of prepuberal boys subjected to the effect of HMG (32). It has been said that these cells reach a high glycogen content and show enzymes related to carbohydrate metabolism, especially at puberal ages (32,33). All these data strongly suggest that the development and function of the Sertoli cells may be under gonadotropic control and also that they may act as an intermediate site of FSH storage for the ultimate action on the spermatogenic process. The nature of this phenomenon will undoubtedly require biochemical studies at molecular biological level.

With regard to the effect of LH, it is interesting to note that the same doses and period of administration (contaminant of FSH was low) as that of FSH showed a similar effect on Sertoli cells but none on the remaining structures of the testis. The fact that only the highest dose of LH induced in addition an increment in spermatogonial cells coinciding with a slight development of interstitial Leydig cells, suggests but does not prove that LH might have a direct effect on Sertoli cells and an indirect one on spermatogonial cells mediated by Leydig cells. This dual action of LH which would indicate that this hormone may initiate spermatogenesis, is also supported by long experience in the use of large doses of HCG alone which induces spermatogenesis up to the pachytene stage, differentiation of Leydig cells, secretion of steroids, enlargement of tubular diameter and regression of hyaline material in hypogonadotropic eunuchoidal patients (6,8,32). The same results were obtained in prepubertal boys similarly treated (34). However, the view that the direct effect of LH might also be mediated by some activated function of the intertubular fibroblast-like cells cannot be discarded.

The successive use in our studies first of FSH and then of LH or vice-versa points to the lack of an additive effect of both hormones, except in the maturation of Sertoli cells. However, it should be noted that the higher doses of LH can preserve the beneficial action achieved by previous treatment with FSH, to which a stimulating effect on spermatogonial cells and appearance of Leydig cells is added. On the other hand, the inefficiency of FSH, with the exception of its effect on maturation of Sertoli cells, to preserve the stimulating action of previously administered LH was evident. These findings, which may merely reflect the separate specific action of each hormone on the testis, not only verify the more striking effect of LH but also demonstrate the simultaneous action of both hormones. This problem as faced in our studies suggests that similar or even lower doses of both gonadotropins administered for an identical period of time reinforced the separate effect of each, which does not apparently occur if an excess of FSH is given. Moreover, a higher ratio favoring LH (1:3), during similar periods of time, resulted in an efficient initiation and progression of spermatogenesis at least up to the pachytene stage, together with remarkable maturation of Sertoli cells, enlargement of tubules, regression of hyalinization, development of tubular wall structures and differentiation of Leydig cells. As has been proved, a much longer period of administration with even higher doses of LH given in the form of HCG together with lower dose of HMG may induce a complete spermatogenesis in hypogonadotropic eunuchoids (7,8,10). The necessity of FSH for further advance of meiosis is backed by those cases successfully treated first with large doses of HCG with resultant progression up to primary spermatocytes to which HMG was added (8,32,35). The fact that only higher doses of LH may influence the tubule wall structure development is backed by the specific localization of intravenously injected labelled LH, not only in both types of Leydig cells (28,36) but also in peritubular fibroblasts and less clear in Sertoli cells (28,29). This would rather suggest the existence of a direct effect of LH on Sertoli cells and tubule wall structures and an indirect and stronger one on germinal cells mediated by secretory Leydig cells. Consequently, the possibility that FSH together with LH may act directly and at the same time on seminiferous tubules and that a certain amount is essential for this effect could not be ruled out.

Whether or not some degree of Leydig cell function is necessary for full tubule development in the human being has not yet been definitely proved. However, and opposed to some reported data (37), it has been demonstrated that in the human testis during puberal maturation, spermatogenesis may start in the absence of Leydig cells but in the presence of their precursors such as fibroblast-like cells, but the full meiotic and subsequent spermiogenic processes are accompanied or may be preceded not only by development of mature Sertoli cells, but also by secretory Leydig cells (18,19,31). That Sertoli cells may be subjected to gonadotropin control paralleled with Leydig cells is supported by our findings on the simultaneous stimulation exhibited by both cells when the high dose of LH alone was used. Although Leydig cell activity is needed for germinal cell development, whether the same may be true for Sertoli cell function is at present a matter of mere speculation.

Results obtained in postpuberal hypogonadal patients confirmed those obtained in hypogonadotropic eunuchoids with respect to the impossibility of using low or high doses of FSH of LH alone or in successive administration to recover the spermatogenesis in adult hypophysectomized subjects; it also corroborates the predominant effect of FSH and LH in repairing the Sertoli cells and the more extended action of higher doses of LH. As happens with hypogonadotropic eunuchoid patients, this latter hormone seems to be capable of producing recovery in the germinal epithelium by stimulating the spermatogonial cells which then pass on to the meiotic phase. However, this cell progression as well as the regression of hyalinization and enlargement of tubules, is concomitant with the appearance of immature and mature Leydig cells. It would then appear likely that smaller doses of LH would have been ineffective in bringing about such changes, but would selectively affect the Sertoli cells. This is also supported by the administration in the same patients of much larger doses of HCG alone for the same periods, which resulted in more intense stimulation of germinal cells up to the pachytene stage, together with marked development of mature Leydig cells (25). Although these studies also showed the need for simultaneous use of FSH and LH with an excess of LH, it has been claimed that in eunuchs, HMG containing FSH and LH in equal amounts, administered for about three months, stimulates germinal cell progression up to the advanced meiotic or even the spermiogenic phases. However, Leydig cell differentiation and regression of hyalinosis were poor in these cases, and addition of HCG induced the completion of both cell populations, bringing about a normal condition of the tubular wall structures (15,25). The need for a much longer treatment in eunuchs might be due to the fact that induction of spermatogenesis would require the participation of more complicated cellular and hormonal mechanisms, like those which are present during normal puberal development. In hypophysectomized patients the gonad undergoes atrophy to a variable degree, but gonadotropins and spermatogenesis are present before operation.

Therefore the results obtained in both conditions would indicate that administration of both FSH and LH in a ratio equal to unity is not effective, a higher LH-FSH ratio and duration of treatment being required. Coincidentally it has been shown in hypophysectomized rats that FSH stimulates Sertoli cell development but only both hormones establish complete spermatogenesis (38). A FSH-LH ratio favorable to LH is required for the recovery of spermatogenesis, and the "gametogenic" action of LH includes some stimulation of Leydig cells, which may not appear reflected by changes in the adnexal glands (39).

Current studies on adult hypophysectomized patients given testosterone propionate alone or simultaneously treated first with HMG and HCG and then with HMG plus testosterone propionate at weekly doses of 50 to 200 mg, seem to indicate that the beneficial effect of LH given in HCG cannot be replaced by the androgen. By comparing the biopsies taken after a second course of treatment with those after HMG plus HCG where recovery of all testicular structures could be seen, a regression of spermatogenesis up to primary spermatocytes or even spermatogonia, atrophy of Leydig cells and reappearance of peritubular hyalinization was detected (40). These findings are in marked contrast with previous ones as regards the maintenance of spermatogenesis with testosterone in hypophysectomized rats (38,41) and resemble those obtained in adult normal subjects treated with high doses of androgens with resultant inhibition of pituitary gonadotropins, increase in estrogens and atrophy of the testes (42).

With regard to the effect of FSH and LH on the tubular wall structures it was postulated that peritubular hyalinization is a nonspecific process consequent to spermatogenic failure (43), or that it damages secondarily the seminiferous epithelium (44) or that there is an apparent synchronization between hyalinization and regression of germinal epithelium and Leydig cells (25). Histochemical and ultrastructural studies of this process have been made in adult hypophysectomized patients (45) and results obtained seemed to be similar to those observed in our group of eunuchs. In adult normal subjects the seminiferous tubule wall is mainly composed of an acellular basal lamina adjacent to the germinal epithelium and an outer cellular layer in which fibrils arranged in compact bundles and flattened cells are present (22). Immunochemical analysis of this structure revealed the existence of two classes of glycoprotein complexes, one corresponding to collagen and the other to reticulin substance (46). When peritubular hyalinization develops the basal lamina appears dissagregated in some areas. The underlying cellular layer increases in thickness, the cells exhibit regressive changes, and a deposition of an amorphous substance appears in between the fibrils, which show absence of characteristic electron density and cross striation. After HCG or HMG plus HCG administration, the thickness of the tubular wall tends to diminish, the cells recover their normal aspect, the amorphous substance disappears and normal cross striated fibrils reappear. That this effect is due to LH and not to FSH is confirmed in our group of eunuchs as shown above. As only the higher dose of LH was able to induce such changes, and assuming that peritubular cells are responsible for the production and maintenance of tubular wall structures, it is postulated that in this condition developing Leydig cells may influence the function of peritubular cells. However the theory that some other stimulated adjacent cells,like Sertoli cells, may participate in this phenomenon could not be discarded.

CONCLUSIONS

Based on our present and previous studies on the separate, successive and simultaneous effect of human urinary gonadotropins in prepuberal and postpuberal hypogonadism, the following is proposed: 1) Neither the separate nor the successive administration of FSH and LH may stimulate the germinal epithelium adequately. 2) Both FSH and LH are needed simultaneously for a long time and with a higher LH-FSH ratio for the induction or the recovery of spermatogenesis. 3) Low or high doses of FSH or a low dose of LH only induce hyperplasia and maturation of Sertoli cells in the testis of hypogonadotropic eunuchoids and repair of these cells in hypophysectomized patients. 4) As doses are increased LH stimulates the intertubular fibroblastic cells and might initiate spermatogenesis through the proliferation of spermatogonial cells which then proceed to the next meiotic phase until pachytene. At this stage FSH might participate in the further progression of meiosis. 5) An excess of LH with subsequent Leydig cell development and steroid secretion would be required for full maturation of Sertoli cells to reach the spermiogenetic phase and the completion of spermatogenesis. 6) Leydig cell function, by influencing the development of tubular wall connective tissue structures or the regression of hyalinization, might contribute to the enlargement of seminiferous tubules. 7) Nevertheless, it is hard to say if this hypothetical interpretation of the relationship between gonadotropins and spermatogenesis in the hypogonadotropic hypogonadal subjects, has its equivalent in the events that take place during normal development of the testis.

ACKNOWLEDGEMENTS

This work was supported by a grant from The Population Council, Inc., New York.

REFERENCES

1. Jailer, J.W. and Leathem, J., Proc. Soc. Exp. Biol. Med., *45*: 506, 1940.
2. Heller, C.G. and Nelson, O.W., J. Clin. Endocr., *8*: 345, 1948.
3. Maddock, O.W., J. Clin. Endocr., *9*: 213, 1949.
4. Hurxtal, L.M., Bruns, H.J. and Mussulin, M., J. Clin. Endocr., *9*: 1245, 1949.
5. Bartter, F.C., Sniffen, R.C., Simmons, F.A. and Albright, F., J. Clin. Endocr., *12*: 1532, 1952.
6. Nelson, W., J. Urology, *69*: 325, 1953.
7. Crooke, A.C., Davies, A.G. and Morris, R., J. Endocr., *42*: 441, 1968.
8. Paulsen, A., *In* Gonadotropins 1968, ed. Rosemberg, E., Geron-X, Inc. Los Altos, California, p. 491, 1968.
9. Lytton, B. and Kase, N., New England J. Med., *274*: 1061, 1966.
10. Johnsen, S.G., Acta Endocr. (Kobenhavn), *53*: 315, 1966.
11. Johnsen, S.G. *In* Gonadotropins, 1968, ed. Rosemberg, E., Geron-X Inc. Los Altos, California, p. 515, 1968.
12. Lunenfeld, B., Mor, A. and Mani, M., Fertil. Steril., *18*: 581, 1967.
13. Martin, F.I.R., J. Endocr., *38*: 431, 1967.
14. Gemzel, C. and Kjessler, B., Lancet, *1*: 644, 1964.
15. McLeod, J., Pazianos, A. and Bronson, R., Fertil. Steril., *17*: 7, 1968.
16. Donini, P., Puzzuoli, D., D'Alessio, I., Bergesi, G. and Donini, S., *In* Gonadotropins, 1968, ed. Rosemberg, E. Geron-X Inc. Los Altos, California, p 37, 1968
17. Heller, C.G. and Clermont, Y., Recent Progr. Hormone Res., *20*: 545, 1964.

18. Mancini, R.E., Narbaitz, R. and Lavieri, J.C., Anat. Rec., 136: 477, 1960.
19. Mancini, R.E., Vilar, O., Lavieri, J.C. and Andrada, J.A., Amer. J. Anat., 112: 2, 1963.
20. Dixon, W. and Massey, F.J., In Introduction to Statistical Analysis, McGraw-Hill Book Co. Inc. New York, p. 258, 1957.
21. Mancini, R.E., Vilar, O. and Perez del Cerro, M., Acta Physiol. Latino Americana, 14: 382, 1964.
22. Ross, M.H., Amer. J. Anat., 121: 523, 1967.
23. Conti, C. and Fabrini, A., In Atti Congr. Soc. Med. Inter. Edizioni L. Pozzi, Roma, p. 104, 1968.
24. DeKretser, D.M., Virchow Arch. (Zellpath), 1: 283, 1968.
25. Mancini, R.E., Seiguer, A.C. and Perez Lloret, A., J. Clin. Endocr. 29: 467, 1969.
26. Courot, M., J. Reprod. Fertil., 89: 2, 1967.
27. Murphy, H.D., Proc. Soc. Exp. Biol. Med., 118: 1202, 1965.
28. Mancini, R.E., Castro, A.E. and Seiguer, A.C., J. Histochem. Cytochem., 15: 516, 1967.
29. Castro, A.E., Seiguer, A.C. and Mancini, R.E., Proc. Soc. Exp. Biol. Med., 1970 (in press).
30. Mancini, R.E., Vilar, O., Alvarez, B. and Seiguer, A.C., J. Histochem. Cytochem., 13: 376, 1965.
31. Mancini, R.E., Rosemberg, E., Cullen, M., Lavieri, J.C., Vilar, C., Bergada, C. and Andrada, J.A., J. Clin. Endocr., 25: 927, 1965.
32. Rosemberg, E., Mancini, R.E., Crigler, J.F. and Bergada, C., In Gonadotropins 1968, ed. Rosemberg, E., Geron-X Inc., Los Altos, California, p 527, 1968.
33. Fabrini, A., Re, M. and Conti, C., J. Endocr., 43: 499, 1969.
34. Bergada, C. and Mancini, R.E., (In press).
35. Heller, C.J., In Estrogen Workshop Conference, ed. Paulsen, A., University of Washington Press, Seattle, p. 276, 1965.
36. De Kretser, D.M., Catt, K.J., Burger, H.G. and Smith, G.C., J. Endocr., 43: 105, 1969.
37. Johnsen, S.G., Acta Endocr. (Kobenhavn), 66: 1, 1962.
38. Lostroh, A.J., Endocrinology, 85: 438, 1969.
39. Woods, M.C. and Simpson, M.E., Endocrinology, 69: 91, 1961.
40. Mancini, R.E. and Perez Lloret, A., Acta Europea Fertil., 1970 (in press).
41. Nelson, W.O. and Merckel, C., Proc. Soc. Exp. Biol. Med., 36: 825, 1937.
42. Heller, C.G., Nelson, W.O., Hill,I.B., Henderson, B., Maddock, E., Junck, E.C., Paulsen, A.C. and Mortimore, G.E., Fertil. Steril., 1: 415, 1950.
43. Nelson, W.O. and Heller, C.G., J. Clin. Endocr., 5: 13, 1945.
44. Johnsen, S.G., Acta Endocr. (Kobenhavn), 124: 17, 1967.
45. Mancini, R.E., Seiguer, A.C. and Perez Lloret, A., In Gonadotropins 1968, ed. Rosemberg, E., Geron-X Inc., Los Altos, California, p. 503, 1968.
46. Denduchis, B., Gonzalez, N., Lustig, L. and Mancini, R.E., Acta Europea Fertil., 1: 810, 1969.

THE EFFECTS OF URINARY GONADOTROPINS FOLLOWING HYPOPHYSECTOMY AND IN HYPOGONADOTROPIC EUNUCHOIDISM

John MacLeod[1]

Department of Anatomy, Cornell University Medical College, New York, N.Y.

I should like to present summaries of two new cases treated with gonadotropins. The first is that of a 28-year-old married man with two children who had undergone hypophysectomy for an infarcted adenoma of the pituitary. I saw him for the first time one and a half years after this operation. He had returned to the neuro-surgeon (Dr. Bronson Ray) because his wife desired another child. In the interim, he had been supported only by cortisone and thyroid. He had not received androgens. He complained of low libido, loss of ejaculate and of pubic, axillary and body hair. He could attain erections and orgasm after considerable stimulation. He had not experienced a spontaneous erection since the operation. It was ascertained that he had been under-active sexually during his married life and before the illness that precipitated the operation. The post-operative loss of libido therefore, had not bothered him unduly. He could not produce an ejaculate for examination in spite of erection and orgasm.

Since the desired end was to initiate a pregnancy for this couple, it was decided to put him immediately on the combined HMG-HCG regimen which had been successful in the first case reported by the author (1). The respective doses were HMG (Pergonal-batch 20714 75 IU FSH/2nd IRP - 75 IU LH/2nd IRP) and HCG (APL) 4000 IU (HCG Std) on alternate days. Prior to treatment a bilateral testicular biopsy was requested and obtained.

---

[1]Career Scientist, Health Research Council of the City of New York.

PRE-TREATMENT BIOPSIES

These biopsies (Figs. 1-7) showed all stages of spermatogenesis up to mature spermatozoa in selected tubules but a marked quantitative depletion at all levels. The nuclei of many of the spermatogonia (Figs. 1 and 2) appeared to be unduly large but were otherwise normal in appearance. The pachytene stage of the primary spermatocyte (Fig. 3), while present in many of the tubules, was not conspicuous. The early and late spermatids (Figs. 4 and 5) were numerically high in certain tubules. Mature spermatozoa apparently ready for exfoliation (Figs. 6 and 7) also were obvious although bizarre head-shapes were easily identifiable, particularly the so-called "tapering" forms (Fig. 7). It is of interest to note that when the first spermatozoa appeared in this man's ejaculate following treatment, a rather high percentage were of the tapering variety.

Peritubular fibrosis was absent in both testes except in a few of the peripheral tubules. The basement membranes were normal as were the tubular diameters. Complete maturation was more evident in the left testis.

The interstitial tissue in both testes was edematous (a characteristic noted in the testes of all the hypox subjects seen) and relatively acellular. True Leydig cells were not identified.

Although the total epithelium was depleted, the presence of all stages of spermatogenesis in selected tubules, 1½ years after operation, suggested that some degree of hormonal stimulation remained in this individual. The urinary gonadotropin assay prior to treatment, while very low (3 m.u./24 hours), did indicate some residual activity of hypophyseal tissue.

RESPONSE TO GONADOTROPINS

Twenty-eight days after the initiation of treatment, an acellular ejaculate of 1.4 ml was obtained. At 77 days, the ejaculate volume was 2.0 ml and an occasional sluggishly-active spermatozoon was seen. At 83 days, the volume again was 2.0 ml and there was a detectable sperm count of 2 million/ml with sluggish progression. A rather high percentage of these cells were of the "tapering" variety (Fig. 7), bicephalic forms were obvious as were spermatids. From about the 15th post-treatment day, the subject was again experiencing spontaneous erections.

At 111 days, a sperm count of 44 million/ml with excellent progression was recorded. The tapering and immature forms had reached a normal level and the sperm morphology in general was attaining a normal equilibrium which it was to maintain throughout the study as long as any spermatozoa were present in the ejaculate. The peak sperm count of 114 million/ml was reached at 150 days and the semen

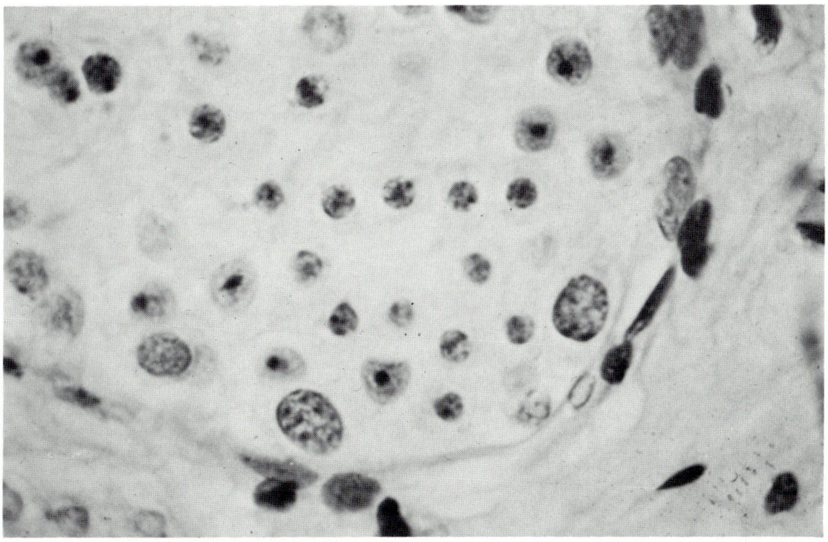

Fig. 1. Testicular Biopsy 1½ years after hypophysectomy. Large spermatogonia, early spermatids and Sertoli cells are conspicuous.

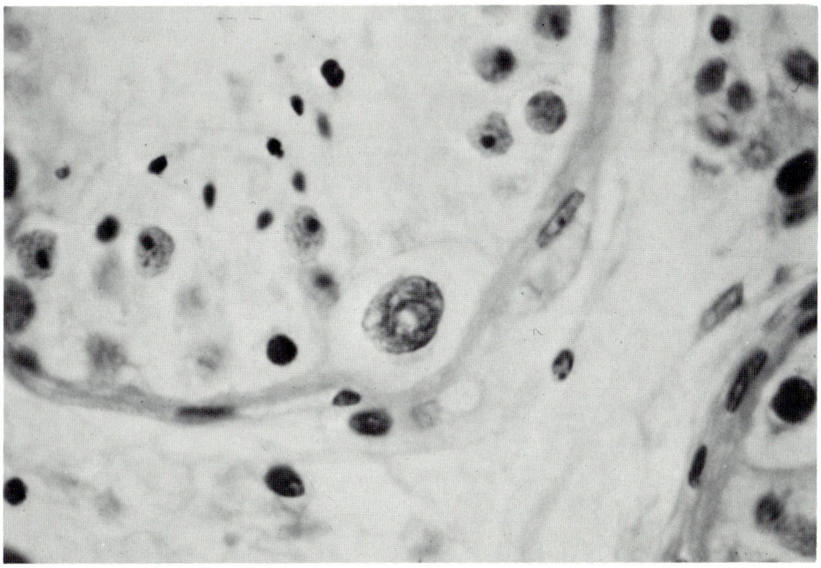

Fig. 2. Same biopsy. Megalo-type spermatogonium (note bulging of basement membrane). Late spermatids (probably spermatozoa) present.

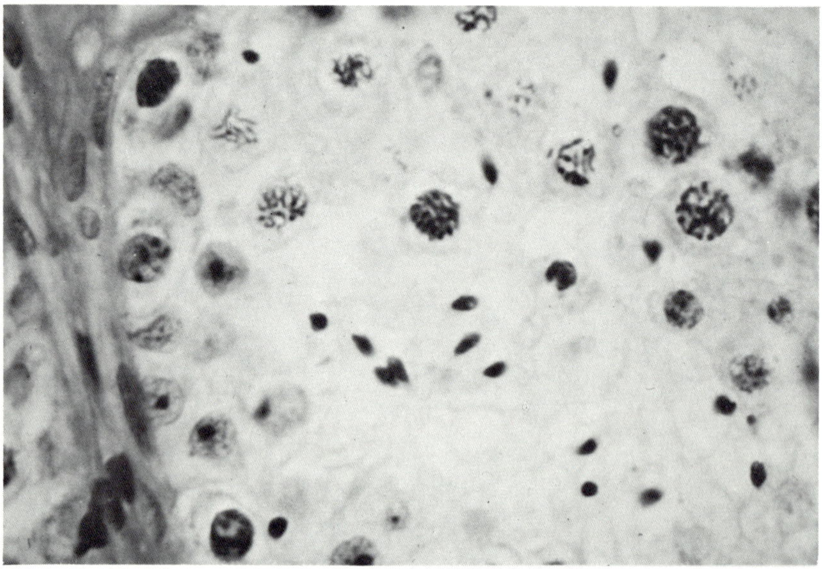

Fig. 3. Same biopsy. A few pachytene cells and spermatozoa are obvious.

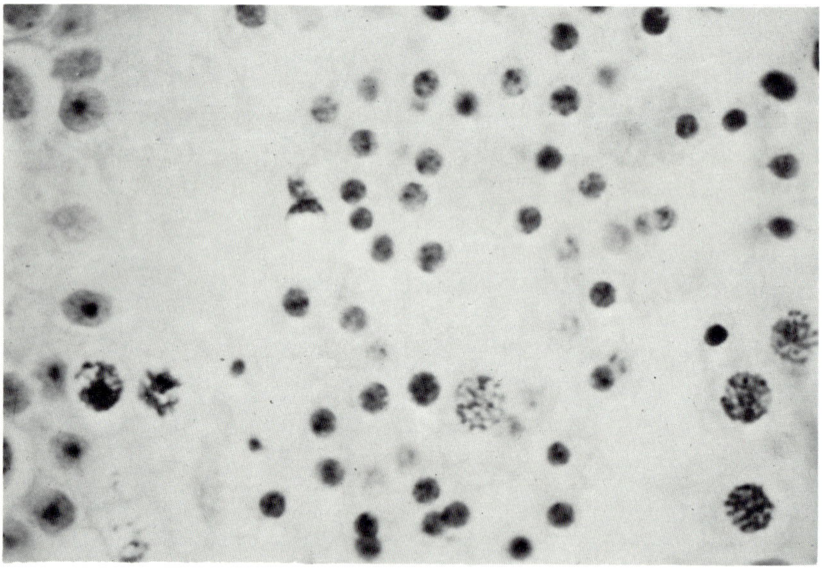

Fig. 4. Same biopsy. Good population of early spermatids.

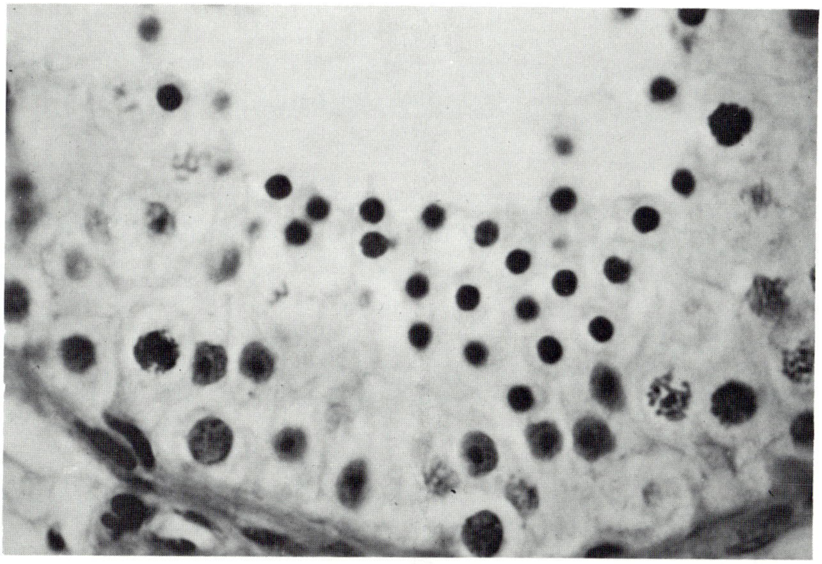

Fig. 5. Same biopsy. Middle and late stage spermatids.

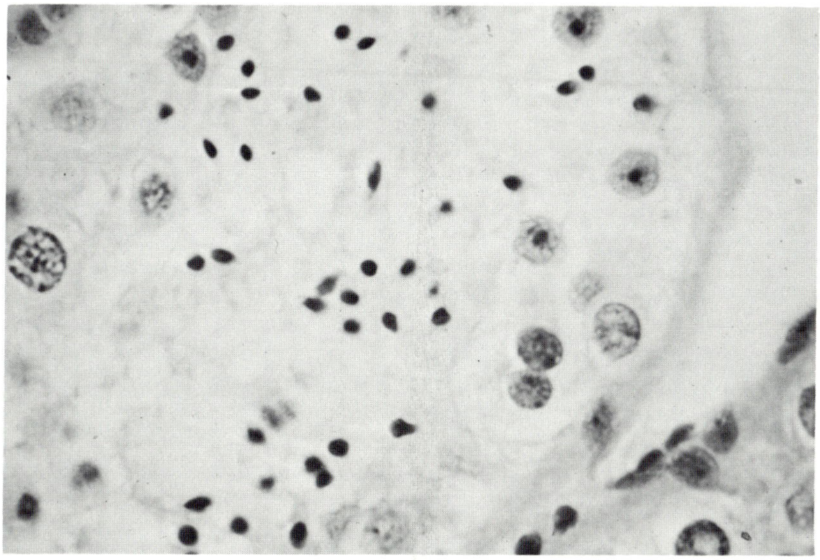

Fig. 6. Same biopsy. Late spermatids (probably spermatozoa) with bizarre head-shapes.

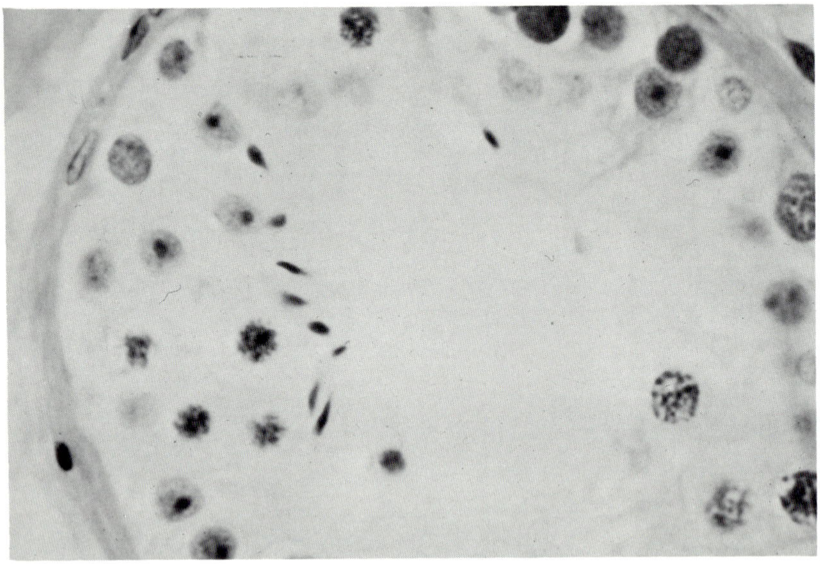

Fig. 7. Same biopsy. Tapering forms are conspicuous.

quality in general was excellent.

Unfortunately, at this stage and when a pregnancy could be expected, the patient informed me that his wife no longer wished for a child and had been on the contraceptive pill since she knew that spermatozoa had been found in the ejaculate.

The decision was made, therefore, to withdraw the Pergonal but to continue him on HCG for androgenic support. This approach added to the study in allowing us (1) to follow any involution of spermatogenesis if it occurred and (2) to determine if HCG alone would maintain spermatogenesis.

The second objective became most obvious within a few weeks at which time it was apparent that spermatogenesis was being maintained. The semen quality remained good at a level between 21 million and 54 million/ml for one year thereafter. In the interim, a decision to try for a pregnancy again was made by the couple. Conception occurred in the fourth cycle and a normal child resulted.

The patient refused a post-treatment biopsy but his semen quality was sufficient proof of good spermatogenesis.

With the pregnancy established and with the continued cooperation of the patient, androgen support in the form of HCG was withdrawn. We should note that from the early stages of HCG therapy in this subject, he had reported normal sexual vigor (for him), confirmed by his wife, and restoration of normal hair distribution.

Within 45 days after withdrawal of HCG, the ejaculate volume was reduced to 0.2 ml with only an occasional sperm present. At 59 days, only a drop of fluid was obtained. It appeared certain that involution of the reproductive tract again had occurred. At this point, testosterone enanthate (Delatestryl-200mg IM/biweekly) was given as a substitute for HCG in androgen support. After 84 days of this regimen, the ejaculate was not restored and the patient complained, as he had done after the withdrawal of HCG, of a feeling of lethargy.

He then was returned to HCG (2000 IU on alternate days). An ejaculate appeared within 30 days (1.4 ml) and at 51 days the volume was 2.2 ml. Spermatozoa were absent in both specimens. At intervals up to 6 months thereafter with continuation of HCG, the semen was examined. No cells of the germinal line were found at any time. In all other respects, the reproductive tract appeared normal. His sexual activity and general well-being were good.

DISCUSSION AND CONCLUSIONS

The salient features of this study are that 1) some degree of complete spermatogenesis remained 1½ years after hypophysectomy; 2) after complete restoration of spermatogenesis with HMG-HCG, this state could be continued for at least one year thereafter with HCG alone; 3) HCG alone could not re-initiate spermatogenesis after withdrawal of all gonadotropins and 4) testosterone could not replace HCG in restoring the ejaculate.

With regard to the first point, the urinary gonadotropin assay was positive at a low level which was enough, perhaps, to maintain a degree of spermatogenesis but not enough to support the Leydig cells and the more distal portions of the reproductive tract.

This conclusion gains support when considering point (2). The maintenance of normal spermatogenesis with HCG alone would mean that if normal function can be established with HMG-HCG, the FSH-like activity now known to be present in pregnancy urine extracts (2), coupled with small amounts of endogenous FSH, is enough to maintain spermatogenesis. In this regard, we agree with Johnsen (3) in that we can restore spermatogenesis in these subjects with smaller doses of gonadotropins than previously used and can maintain such function with minimal levels of FSH.

However, the maintenance level of FSH or FSH-like activity is not enough to re-initiate spermatogenesis even if large amounts of chorionic gonadotropins (LH) are given simultaneously. It would seem, therefore, that FSH does play an essential role in initiating spermatogenesis in the hypox subject.

Lastly, the failure in this case of testosterone to substitute for HCG in maintaining the ejaculate is not surprising. In another subject hypophysectomized for acromegaly, who refused testicular biopsies and attempts to restore his fertility, testosterone enanthate failed to maintain sexual vigor and ejaculate over extended periods. The replacement of testosterone with HCG fully restored the ejaculate and his masculinity within 30 days but did not return sperm to an ejaculate which, prior to operation, had shown excellent cellular quality. We found the same to be true in the following case of hypogonadism.

CASE 2 - HYPOGONADOTROPIC HYPOGONADISM

The patient, a medical resident 25 years old and married for 18 months, presented himself with a semen specimen because of infertility. The facies and general physical appearance suggested hypogonadism. The voice was high-pitched and while scalp hair was luxuriant, temporal recession was not present. Shaving was infrequent. While he was reluctant to admit that he had considered himself as hypogonadal, he remembered having been given methyl testosterone at about age 14 for retarded pubertal development. He did not continue this treatment nor did he take androgens at any time thereafter. His sexual activity prior to marriage was low. He did not recall spontaneous erections and ejaculations. In his marriage and with adequate stimulation he could perform intercourse once or twice weekly. The semen specimen he brought was obtained by masturbayion after one week of continence. The ejaculate volume was extremely low (0.30ml), a few spermatozoa of normal morphology but sluggish motility were present. Eleven days later, a second specimen of even lower volume (0.10ml) was seen which contained an occasional spermatozoon. He was then referred to Dr. Melvin Horwith and the endocrinology department.

Unfortunately, the patient did not consult him for some time thereafter. The case history does not record a physical examination until the patient had been on HCG (5000 IU on alternate days) for 22 days. A pre-treatment biopsy was not obtained. The first complete physical confirmed the hypogonadism, the testes being on the small side (3 cm x 1.5 cm) but firm. The penis was considered to be normal in size. Body hair distribution was normal but axillary, pubic and extremity hair were only moderate. Breast tissue was prominent but obvious gynecomastia was not recorded. Facial acne, never present in the past, was already apparent after 22 days of HCG. Gonadotropin levels prior to treatment, determined by radioimmunoassay, were detectable but low. Plasma testosterone was 0.02 mμg%.

After 22 days of HCG treatment, the ejaculate volume was appreciably greater (1.0ml) but virtually devoid of spermatozoa. At 50 days (7-31-68) the ejaculate volume had increased to 3.0ml with an occasional sperm and a fructose concentration of 90 mg%. The voice pitch was markedly deepened, facial acne was prominent and shaving had become more frequent. The patient's sexual drive and aggressiveness had increased. Thereafter, neither he nor a semen specimen was seen for six months but a bilateral testicular biopsy was obtained four months after the initiation of HCG. The germinal tissue in both testes contained an abundant population of normal spermatogonia and all levels of spermatogenesis and spermiogenesis were obvious. Ample evidence of mature spermatozoa was seen in many tubules but the epithelial appearance in general was highly disorganized. A considerable amount of premature exfoliation of middle and late spermatids into the tubular lumens had taken place. Peritubular fibrosis was absent in tubules of normal diameter and the basement membranes were not thickened. Leydig cells were present in normal interstitial tissue. Both testes were essentially similar. The findings could be interpreted as quantitatively good but disorganized germinal function. On the basis of the biopsy alone more spermatozoa could have been predicted in the ejaculate than had been found. The question remained, too, that the long course of HCG which preceded the biopsy may have stimulated maturation in the germinal epithelium.

Following the biopsy his physician withdrew HCG and substituted clomiphene citrate. He remained on this regimen for six weeks during which his sexual drive and feeling of well-being waned considerably. At the end of the clomiphene therapy gonadotropin was detectable by radio immunoassay but low. HCG therapy was resumed on 1-6-69. A semen specimen 52 days later (2-24-69) showed a volume of 2.4 ml, no spermatozoa and 290 mg% fructose. Pergonal therapy was begun on 3-18-69 (75 IU FSH - 75 IU LH) on alternate days with continuation of HCG (4000 IU three times weekly). Thirty-six days later, in an ejaculate of 3.5 ml, a sperm count of 4 million/ml was recorded, 85 percent showing excellent progression. The sperm morphology was disturbed. On the 52nd day of therapy the count reached 10 million/ml and on the 65th day, in a volume of 4.6ml, the count remained at the same level. The sperm motility continued to be excellent and the sperm morphology had stabilized in a reasonably good pattern. The count level on this date was the highest attained. Thereafter and until the Pergonal was discontinued the sperm count ranged from 8 to 10 million/ml. A pregnancy occurred about 123 days after Pergonal was begun or 87 days after the first obvious sperm count and good motility was found in the post-Pergonal ejaculate.

Pergonal was withdrawn 14 days after the pregnancy was confirmed, the HCG being continued at a reduced level of 2000 IU three times weekly.

At the time of writing, 127 days after withdrawal of Pergonal, the total sperm count level of approximately 30 million has been maintained, accompanied by excellent sperm motility, for this period. The highest total sperm count achieved by the combined HMG-HCG therapy was only 46 million, the mean total being approximately 33 million. HCG alone, therefore, has kept up the sperm count level for at least 127 days.

In contrast to the findings of others (2) in similar hypogonadotropic subjects, in this patient, we could not elevate the extremely low sperm counts in the pre-treatment ejaculate with the long continued use of HCG alone. However, the expected pubertal changes and higher ejaculate volumes were readily induced by the same therapeutic approach.

The addition of HMG to the HCG regimen promptly (36 days) produced the first sperm count elevation in the ejaculate and the initiation of excellent sperm motility. But continuation of this combined therapy for another 100 days did not push the sperm count beyond 10 million/ml. Paulsen (2) and Johnsen (3) have recorded similar failures in hypogonadotropic enuchoids.

The pregnancy probably occurred at a sperm count level between 5 and 10 million/ml but we should emphasize that the sperm motility was excellent. We have furnished evidence elsewhere (4) that pregnancies can be expected at these low count levels provided sperm motility is good.

ACKNOWLEDGEMENTS

The research was supported by Grant HD-00481 from National Institutes of Health. I am grateful to C.R. Thompson of the Cutter Labs. for the Pergonal and to Dr. John Jewell for the APL used in all subjects in these experiments.

REFERENCES

1. MacLeod, J., Pazianos, A. and Ray, B.R., Fertil. Steril, 17: 7, 1964.
2. Paulsen, C.A., Clin. Endocr., 2: 509, 1968.
3. Johnsen, S., In Gonadotropins 1968. ed. Rosemberg, E., Geron-X, Inc. Los Altos, Cal., p. 515, 1968.
4. MacLeod, J., Fertil. Steril., 20: 545, 1969.

DISCUSSION

JOHNSEN: At the gonadotropin meeting in 1968 (Gonadotropins, 1968, E. Rosemberg, ed. Geron-X, Inc., Los Altos, California) in Vista Hermosa, Mexico, I reported a case of a male having been deprived of pituitary function for nine years. We administered HCG to this patient but we did not observe the presence of spermatozoa. Then the patient received HMG and HCG. We observed spermatozoa up to 20 million per total count. His wife became pregnant and delivered a normal child. Therefore, we stopped HMG treatment and continued with HCG alone to maintain his sexual function. Exactly as Dr. MacLeod has pointed out, spermatogenesis continued and has continued ever since, for nearly two years, at the level of 40 to 70 million of total sperm count. On HCG alone his wife became pregnant for the second time and delivered his second son.

MACLEOD: I have nothing to add to what Dr. Johnsen has said. In our first case, the biopsy prior to treatment showed all stages of spermatogenesis; testosterone levels were extremely low, and there was no evidence of Leydig cell activity.

JOHNSEN: In my patient we observed only spermatogonia in nearly all tubules and in a few tubules a very limited number of spermatocytes.

E. STEINBERGER: If we make the assumption that HCG does stimulate testosterone secretion, then our discussion seems to indicate that in the human, the situation may be similar to that of the rat, namely that the initiation of spermatogenesis may require different hormonal milieu than the maintenance of spermatogenesis. Apparently spermatogenesis can be maintained with HCG or testosterone.

MACLEOD: I think that the situation is quite different in the rat. Dr. Clermont pointed out that in the testis of hypophysectomized rats there is apparently no diminution in the spermatogonial population whereas in the human male there is no question at all that following hypophysectomy there is a very severe depletion in the spermatogonial cell population.

LUNENFELD: I think you should have added, Dr. MacLeod, that it is not possible to maintain spermatogenesis with testosterone alone.

PAULSEN: If there is general agreement that it is possible to stimulate spermatogenesis with HCG and HMG in the hypophysectomized male and then maintain spermatogenesis with HCG treatment alone, this points to factors present in patients with hypogonadotropic eunuchoidism other than just gonadotropin deficiency. We have been unable to maintain spermatogenesis with HCG alone in those patients except when there was evidence of effective endogenous FSH secretion. As Dr. Ross' group suggested, a double defect probably exists in some of the patients with hypogonadotropic eunuchoidism.

JIRASEK: I would like to raise a question which remained entirely out of consideration, that is the sex of offspring of the hypophysectomized males. What was the sex of offspring of the hypophysectomized or hypogonadotropic eunuchoid males who received gonadotropin therapy?

JOHNSEN: Two boys.

MACLEOD: One boy so far. One miscarriage, and one still in utero.

PAULSEN: Three pregnancies. Patient J. P.'s wife had two sons. Patient M. S.'s wife had a girl.

CHAPTER VII

GONADOTROPIN THERAPY

SECTION 2: TREATMENT OF ADULT SEMINIFEROUS TUBULAR FAILURE

ASSESSMENT OF GONADOTROPIN THERAPY IN INFERTILE MALES

P. Troen, T. Yanaihara, H. Nankin, T. Tominaga,

and H. Lever

Department of Medicine, Montefiore Hospital and
University of Pittsburgh School of Medicine

Although human follicle-stimulating hormone (FSH) has been demonstrated to be effective in the initiation or restoration of human spermatogenesis (1), its use in the treatment of male infertility has had variable results (2). Various reports indicate that FSH has no effect on steroid biosynthesis in the testis (3,4) while others suggest a stimulating effect on testosterone and estrogen production (5). The present investigation was carried out to test the effect of a human FSH preparation on males with infertility of varying pathogenesis. In addition to following the response of the sperm count, the study included assay of pituitary and gonadal hormones in blood and urine and investigation of biosynthetic pathways in small amounts of testicular tissue obtained at biopsy. Criteria were sought for grouping infertile patients in relation to response to therapy.

MATERIALS AND METHODS

Pertinent data on the 11 patients studied are summarized in Table 1. Human memopausal gonadotropin (HMG - supplied by Cutter Labs. as Pergonal) was administered intramuscularly from ampules containing 63 to 85 I.U. (2nd IRP) FSH and 62 to 123 I.U. (2nd IRP) luteinizing hormone (LH). Human chorionic gonadotropin (HCG - supplied by Ayerst Labs. as A.P.L.) was administered intramuscularly three times weekly in doses of 5,000 I.U.

Seminal fluid was collected by masturbation after 2 days of abstinence. Volume, duplicate sperm counts and motility were determined within one hour of collection of the sample.

Serum FSH and LH levels were determined by double antibody

TABLE 1

CLINICAL MATERIAL

Pt. (Age)	Clinical Data	Testicular Biopsy	Clinical Response to Rx
L.R. (33)	Fertile 5 yrs. ago; infertile 4 yrs; testes: 4.0 cm	Disorderly spermatogenesis; sloughing; no arrest; ? decreased Leydig cells	Moderate weight gain on high dose HMG
R.D. (29)	Infertile 2 yrs; exposure to high temp 8 yrs ago; testes 3.5x2.0 cm	Focal disorderly spermatogenesis; slight sloughing, no arrest; Leydig cells normal	No change
M.R. (27)	Infertile 5 yrs; left varicocele; testis: R 4.5x2.0 cm L 3.0x2.0 cm	Arrest at 1° or 2° spermatocyte; marked tubular variation; ? decreased Leydig cells	No change
B.G. (32)	Infertile 2 yrs; testes: 4.5 cm	Arrest at spermatocyte; disorderly with slough; Leydig cells normal	Gynecomastia during HMG and HCG
W.J. (25)	Infertile 1 1/2 yrs; testes: 4.0x2.5 cm	Arrest at spermatogonium or 1° spermatocyte; sloughing; ? Leydig cells increased	Gynecomastia after HMG and HCG
L.B. (33)	Fertile (?) 13 yrs. ago; infertile 11 yrs; testes: 4.0 cm	Arrest at 2° spermatocyte; ? decreased Leydig cells	No change
R.A. (38)	Infertile 3 yrs; X-ray to penis 7 mos. ago; testes: 3.5x2.0 cm	Peritubular hyalinization; tubular epithelium chiefly Sertoli cells; ? Leydig cells increased	No change
I.L. (25)	Infertile 6 mos; testes: 2.8x1.5 cm, soft	Peritubular hyalinization; tubular epithelium chiefly Sertoli cells; Leydig cells normal	No change
E.G. (30)	Infertile 2 1/2 yrs; testes: 4.0 cm	Arrest at spermatogonium or 1° spermatocyte; slough; decreased Leydig cells	No change
P.W. (24)	Prepubertal; testes: 1.0x0.5 cm	Immature tubules; absent Leydig cells	Pubertal changes with HCG; regression on HMG alone
S.J. (28)	Prepubertal; testes: 1.5x1.0 cm	Immature tubules; almost absent Leydig cells	Pubertal changes with HCG; regression on HMG alone

radioimmunoassay (6) utilizing reagents provided by the Endocrine Study Section and National Pituitary Agency (7). Samples were assayed in duplicate in a single FSH and LH assay respectively.

Serum testosterone analyses were performed by Bio-Science Laboratories (8) using the technique of competitive protein-binding radioassay following extraction and chromatography. Urinary 17-ketosteroids and 17-ketogenic steroids were measured by the methods of Drekter et al. (9) and Metcalf (10) respectively.

Urinary estrogens were measured using the Brown (11) and Ittrich techniques (12) modified to extend the sensitivity of the method to 0.10 μg. Urinary estrogen production rates were determined following intravenous infusion of approximately 2.0 μc of ^{14}C-estradiol or ^{3}H-estrone (13,14).

Organ cultures of testicular biopsy tissue were performed for 48 hours using 3-6 mg of tissue with radioactive precursors ^{3}H-dehydroepiandrosterone (0.25 mc/0.005 mg) and ^{14}C-pregnenolone (0.05 mc/0.302 mg). Radiochemical homogeneity of metabolites was demonstrated on countercurrent distribution and by recrystalliaation to constant specific activity.

RESULTS

1. Testicular Histology

Repeat biopsies were performed on the patients with hypogonadotropic eunuchoidism (P.W. and S.J.) after therapy with HMG and HCG. P.W. showed the appearance of mature Leydig cells plus increase in tubule size with spermatogenesis to the primary and secondary spermatocyte level and, in several foci, spermatids. There was no associated increase in testis size. Repeat biopsy on S.J. showed a mature tubule pattern with mature Leydig cells. Spermatogenesis was present progressing to mature spermatozoa. Clinical evidence of tubular maturation was an increase in testis size to 2.3 x 1.5 cm during HMG therapy.

2. Seminal Fluid Examination

The findings on examination of seminal fluid during the course of gonadotropin therapy are indicated in Table 2. Despite the improvement after therapy in the histologic picture of P.W. and S.J., no spermatozoa appeared in the ejaculate. Treatment with HCG was required for measurable seminal fluid to be present. Of the three patients with sperm counts below 1 million per ml, patients I.L. and L.B. showed no change with therapy. The sperm count of E.G. increased on HMG therapy but the suggested improvement did not continue with the addition of HCG to HMG therapy.

TABLE 2
RESPONSE OF SPERM COUNT TO GONADOTROPIN THERAPY

Patient	Treatment: HMG (amp/week)	Treatment: Duration (weeks)	No. of Samples	Seminal Fluid Analysis: Ave. Vol. (cc)	Seminal Fluid Analysis: Ave. Count (10^6/cc)	Range (10^6/cc)	Ave. Motility %
L. R.	0	14	6	3.6	3.7	2.5-4.6	35
	3	19	9	3.8	8.0	1.3-17.4	20
	6	16	8	4.3	17.7	5.1-45.4	30
	14	43	8	3.7	11.0	1.4-44.2	30
	14 + HCG	31	7	4.4	9.8	4.5-30.1	15
	0	30	1	4.5	2.5		<10
R. D.	0	4	3	2.6	6.5	5.5-8.2	40
	3	8	5	2.1	8.4	1.6-15.7	35
	5	13	10	2.5	8.3	1.4-27.9	30
	10	4	3	2.3	7.6	1.9-18.0	25
	0	4	2	1.9	6.8	5.5-8.1	35
M. R.	0	26	4	4.1	4.7	3.8-5.6	40
	3	10					
			4	2.3	18.8	6.5-40.4	50
	6	3					
	14	4	1	3.2	10.7		60
	0	21	1	3.5	9.9		90
B. G.	0	9	9	4.8	12.4	4.7-44.5	30
	3	16	5	4.8	4.8	2.0-9.8	25
	6	13	9	4.7	11.1	4.6-17.5	30
	14	22	7	5.5	9.0	3.7-14.3	15
	14 + HCG	20	3	6.1	7.1	3.3-9.6	35
W. J.	0	17	7	6.8	2.5	0.6-11.0	15
	3	13	8	7.5	1.7	0.1-3.1	10
	6	9	5	7.7	1.6	0.1-3.7	25
	6 + HCG	7	4	8.1	2.2	0.1-4.2	10
L. B.	0	4	2	2.4	0		
	3	30	3	1.3	0		
R. A.	0	17	8	1.7	2.4	0.5-7.9	30
	3	16	4	2.0	2.3	0.5-7.0	30
I. L.	0	2	2	2.8	0.2	0.1-0.3	5
	3	10	2	2.7	0.4	0.1-0.7	5
E. G.	0	6	3	2.7	0.5	0.37-0.73	60
	14	21	3	4.2	3.0	2.3-4.3	60
	14 + HCG	6	1	4.0	0.63		40
	0	6	2	3.8	1.2	0.9-1.5	50
P. W.	0			0			
	HCG	28	2	0.5	0		
	0	40		0			
	14	17		0			
	14 + HCG	8	2	0.5	0		
	6 + HCG	8	1	0.5			
S. J.	0			0			
	HCG	26	2	0.75	0		
	0	22		0			
	14	17		0			
	14 + HCG	13	2	1.5	0		
	5 + HCG	5	1	1.0	0		

Four patients, B.G., R.D., R.A. and W.J. with initial average sperm counts from 2.4 to 12.4 million per ml showed no improvement in sperm count on varying treatment regimens of up to 14 ampules of HMG per week. The addition of HCG to HMG in B.G. and W.J. also yielded no improvement.

From initial average sperm counts of 3.7 and 4.7 million per ml, L.R. and M.R. had increased counts on HMG therapy. There was no further increase at the highest HMG dosage or with added HCG (patient L.R.). No patient's wife became pregnant during the treatment program.

3. Serum Gonadotropin Levels

Before therapy, P.W. and S.J. had low total urinary gonadotropin excretion and E.G. had normal gonadotropin excretion by bioassay. In Table 3 the values for serum FSH and LH by radioimmunoassay are given. Levels of gonadotropin were determined after a minimum of 17 days and an average of 84 days on a given treatment schedule. The time from last injection of HMG to collection of blood for assay was 34 hrs. at the dosage of 3 ampules per week, 24 hrs. at 6 ampules per week and 14 hrs. at 10 and 14 ampules per week.

I.L. and R.A. twice had elevated baseline FSH values. Both patients had testicular biopsy pictures characterized by loss of germinal epithelium with preservation of Sertoli cells and peritubular hyalinization. Baseline FSH values of the other six patients were in the normal range. Administration of three ampules of HMG per week resulted in increased FSH levels in B.G., R.D. and L. R., the three patients with the lowest pre-treatment levels. At 10 and 14 ampules per week, all patients studied showed further elevation of serum FSH reaching similar levels at the highest dosage of HMG. After cessation of therapy, serum FSH values fell, returning very closely to the pre-treatment values (R.D. and L.R.).

I.L. and R.A., in addition to elevated FSH levels, twice had values of LH which seemed abnormally high. The exact degree of LH elevation was not determined. The baseline serum LH values of the other patients were in the normal range. Treatment with HMG resulted in no consistent alteration of serum LH for all patients, although B.G. showed a progressive decrease in serum LH. The varying content of LH in different lots of the HMG preparation appeared to have no correlation with changes in serum LH.

4. Plasma Testosterone

Baseline plasma testosterone values showed a wide range from 242 ng% (L.B.) to 540 ng% (R.D.) with the majority of patients

TABLE 3

VALUES OF BLOOD FSH, LH AND TESTOSTERONE AND URINARY 17 KETOSTEROIDS AND 17 KETOGENIC STEROIDS IN RELATION TO GONADOTROPIN THERAPY

Patient	HMG (amp/wk)	FSH (mIU/ml)	LH (mIU/ml)	Testosterone (ng/100 ml)	17-KS (mg/24 hr)	17-KGS (mg/24 hr)
L. R.	0	2.1	5.0	486	13.9	12.4
	3	3.9	3.3	336	14.6	14.3
	6				14.1	14.2
	14	8.2	6.9	644	14.9	15.2
	14	6.6	7.6	413		
	14 + HCG	6.4	>14.0	1330	17.4	15.7
	0	3.1	3.9	387	15.5	17.1
R. D.	0	2.1	5.9	540	16.8	16.2
	3	3.8	7.5	408	16.6	16.6
	10	5.3	5.2	339	17.6	18.6
	0	2.9	5.7	444	15.4	14.8
M. R.	0	5.2	5.1	324		
	0	4.6	2.9	310	15.7	13.4
	0	5.1	2.9	239		
	3	5.4	10.1	267	14.6	12.2
	6				16.7	15.2
	14	7.1	5.4		15.8	11.1
	0			248		
B. G.	0	3.0	12.2	255	13.0	9.6
	3	5.0	9.4	222	14.2	14.7
	6				11.3	12.7
	14	7.7	8.3	162	13.4	12.4
W. J.	0			370	20.3	16.7
	3	5.7	5.2	388	23.4	19.0
	6	6.1	11.9	478	20.6	18.9
	0	5.7	9.4	412		
L. B.	0	6.6	5.1	242	9.8	19.6
	0	7.0	6.6	239		
R. A.	0	21.1	>14.0	439	17.3	17.4
	3					
	0	22.6	>14.0	410	13.7	15.8
I. L.	0	17.5	>14.0	374	12.4	15.9
	0	22.2	>14.0	430		
	3				11.0	10.9

Normal Values:

Serum FSH: mean 3.6 mIU/ml; range 1.6 - 8.25
Serum LH: mean 4.9 mIU/ml; range 2.3 - 15
Plasma testosterone: range 400 - 1200 ng/100 ml
Urinary 17-ketosteroids: range 5 - 25 mgm/24 hrs
Urinary 17-ketogenic steroids: range 5 - 21 mgm/24 hrs

Average values during treatment period are given for 17-KS and 17-KGS having values at or below 400 ng% (Table 3). None of these patients had clinical androgen deficiency. In two patients with low plasma testosterone (L.B. and M.R.) there was a suggestion of decreased Leydig cells on biopsy. There was no correlation between plasma testosterone values and the sperm count.

During the several stages of HMG therapy, the plasma testosterone level had a variable course. In two patients (B.G. and R. D.), there was progressive decrease in plasma testosterone, associated in B.G. with a decreasing serum LH value. In contrast, the plasma testosterone of W.J. increased with therapy and was accompanied by a higher serum LH value. L.R. had an initial decrease of plasma testosterone and serum LH but then an increase in both values particularly when HCG was added to the therapy (15). In contrast, M.R. showed no correlation between changing values of LH and plasma testosterone.

5. 17-Ketosteroid and 17-Ketogenic Steroid Excretion

Values for 17-ketosteroid and 17-ketogenic steroid excretion were within the normal range without significant change during gonadotropin therapy. The lowest baseline 17-KS excretions observed were for L.B., who had the lowest plasma testosterone, and S.J. (5 mg/24 hrs.), a hypogonadotropic patient.

6. Urinary Estrogens

The excretion values for estrone (E_1), estradiol (E_2) and estriol (E_3) were similar to those reported for normal males (13, 14) except for a high pre-treatment value for estriol in R.D. (Table 4). During HMG therapy, estrogen escretion remained normal. Urinary production rates of estradiol, although higher in L.R. and R. D. toward the end of HMG therapy, were within the normal range before and during HMG therapy. One measurement of urinary estrone production rate during HMG therapy was also normal. The addition of HCG to the treatment of L.R. resulted in a marked increase both in excretion of each estrogen and in estradiol production rate (15).

7. Organ Culture of Testicular Biopsy Tissue

Following organ culture with ^{3}H-DHA and ^{14}C-pregnenolone, the incubating medium yielded 49% to 78% of the ^{3}H and 31% to 58% of the ^{14}C-radioactivity. Conversions to specific metabolites (as percent of recovered radioactivity) were calculated, without correction for losses, following recrystallization to constant specific activity (Table 5). The polar compounds in the neutral fraction as well as the water soluble (conjugated) fraction are under study.

The organ cultures showed a significant metabolism of added precursors to testosterone. Ready conversion of Δ^5 to Δ^4 com-

TABLE 4

URINARY ESTROGEN EXCRETION AND ESTROGEN PRODUCTION RATE DURING GONADOTROPIN THERAPY

Patient	HMG (amp/week)	Excretion (μg/24 hr.) Estrone	Estradiol	Estriol	Prod. μg/ Rate 24 hr. E_2	E_1	% Recovery Radioactivity Estrone	Estradiol	Estriol	Total
L. R.	0	5.10	0.74	2.03	13.5		9.0	5.6	5.7	20.3
	3	4.41	0.56	2.21	13.5		7.2	4.1	4.2	15.5
	14	4.64	0.43	1.78	9.6		9.4	4.4	4.9	18.7
	14	4.00	0.67	1.85	33.9		10.2	2.3	2.0	14.5
	14 + HCG	22.72	3.06	8.47	160.6		9.5	2.9	3.5	15.9
R. D.	0	3.90	0.84	12.90	19.0		6.4	4.5	5.4	16.3
	3	4.10	0.99	4.00	21.7		6.1	4.6	4.5	15.2
	10	3.10	0.54	0.84	31.5		9.5	5.6	1.4	16.5
	0	4.50	0.97	3.82	21.3		7.4	4.6	3.7	15.7
M. R.	0	2.84	0.58	2.01	17.3		6.3	3.2	6.1	15.6
	0	2.83	0.28	3.21	7.4		6.0	3.7	8.1	17.8
					13.8		6.1	4.3	7.3	17.7
	14	3.14	0.58	3.38		49.8	6.4	2.6	6.9	15.9
Normal values: mean		4.42	0.94	3.72	29	46.3	9.3	3.9	6.9	20.1
(Ref. 13, 14) S. D.		1.30	0.34	1.73	14.3	12.7	3.1	1.1	2.2	5.3

TABLE 5

RADIOACTIVE STEROIDS IDENTIFIED IN NEUTRAL FREE FRACTION FROM MEDIUM OF TESTIS ORGAN CULTURE USING PRECURSOR ^{3}H-DEHYDROEPIANDROSTERONE AND ^{14}C-PREGNENOLONE

Patient	M. R.			W. J.			R. A.			I. L.		
	^{3}H	^{14}C	$^{3}H/^{14}C$	^{3}H	^{14}C	$^{3}H/^{14}C$	^{3}H	^{14}C	$^{3}H/^{14}C$	^{3}H	^{14}C	$^{3}H/^{14}C$
Precursor (μc)	0.4	0.1	4.0	2.1	0.7	3.0	2.1	0.7	3.0	2.1	0.7	3.0
Recovery %	59.0	50.4	4.7	49.6	31.5	4.7	78.0	47.1	5.0	65.1	57.7	3.4
% Recovered Radioactivity												
Testosterone	40.1	3.3	57.9	6.7	3.9	8.2	53.0	3.1	85.2	59.2	16.9	11.9
Pregnenolone		7.3			31.7			1.2			19.4	
Progesterone		2.5			2.2			0.4			1.6	
17 OH-Preg.		--			1.0			--			0.3	
17 OH-Prog.		3.7			6.4			3.2			8.1	
DHA	1.4	--	--	8.8	0.7	59.5	1.2	--	--	19.2	0.3	227.6
Δ^{4}-A	0.5	0.9	2.6	1.7	2.9	2.8	--	0.5	--	0.7	0.6	3.9
Δ^{5}-A	2.2	--	--	11.8	--	--	2.0	--	--	0.7	--	--
Polar	4.1	16.1	1.2	42.2	53.3	3.8	4.7	30.7	0.8	6.0	31.3	0.6

(-) not identified

17-OH-Preg = 3β, 17α-dihydroxypregn-5-en-20-one
17-OH-Prog = 17α-hydroxypregn-4-ene-3, 20-dione
DHA = 3β-hydroxyandrost-5-en-17-one
Δ^{4}-A = androst-4-ene-3, 17-dione
Δ^{5}-A = androst-5-ene-3β, 17β-diol

pounds took place. The higher $^{3}H/^{14}C$ ratio for testosterone than for androstenedione suggested that a significant portion of the testosterone arose from DHA by a pathway other than through androstenedione (16). We are continuing studies of these pathways (17).

No correlation was noted between patterns of conversion of steroids in these organ cultures and sperm counts, levels of plasma testosterone or serum gonadotropins, or response to HMG therapy.

DISCUSSION

The 11 infertile males in this study include a wide range of abnormalities of testicular histology and function. Four groups of patients can be separated. 1. The two hypogonadotropic patients, following combined HMG and HCG therapy, showed a histologic response of the testis, but there was no correction of the azoospermia. In these patients with a presumably responsive condition (1,4), the incomplete results may be due to a combination of factors including duration of therapy, dosage and ratio of FSH/LH therapy. 2. Three normogonadotropic patients with disorderly spermatogenesis or spermatogenic arrest had increased sperm counts during HMG therapy, but remained at oligospermic levels. Whether this reflects the limit of responsivenesss or inadequate knowledge concerning effective treatment regimens in not known. 3. Four other normogonadotropic patients showed no increase in sperm count on HMG therapy. They were not distinguishable from the previous three patients by such criteria as histologic appearance of the testis or the preliminary data on response to therapy of serum gonadotropin, plasma testosterone or urinary estrogen excretion and production rates. 4. Two hypergonadotropic patients showed no response to less intensive treatment programs. These patients would appear to be unlikely to respond to exogenous HMG therapy because the endogenous FSH is at a level higher than that produced by treatment.

Under the time relations of injection and venipuncture used here, levels of serum FSH remained within the range for normal adult males although they increased during HMG therapy. Attempts to improve spermatogenesis in normogonadotropic males by use of additional FSH stimulation may require levels of serum FSH above the normal range. Monitoring of serum FSH levels during therapy is suggested for future treatment programs. It is not known whether continuous high levels or intermittent peaks of FSH would be effective in stimulating spermatogenesis. Further information concerning the half-life of injected HMG (18) may help to establish optimal time-dose relationships.

The finding of low plasma testosterone values in association with oligospermia but normal secondary sex characteristics warrants further study. The possibility of a dissociation between levels of circulating testosterone required for spermatogenesis and levels required for secondary sex characteristics would have therapeutic significance. The question of possible interaction between germinal epithelium and Leydig cells in maintaining normal steroid biosynthetic activity is again raised.

The significance of the changes noted in plasma testosterone during HMG therapy is not clear. A direct relation to changing serum LH levels is suggested in some of the patients but other patients showed no correlation. The finding of high LH values with low normal plasma testosterone values in two patients suggests altered testis responsivenesss to circulating LH.

The administration of HMG despite its content of LH did not result in any consistent change in serum LH values. This may be due to the shorter half-life of LH compared to FSH (19,20). There was no clinical indication of physiologic LH activity of the administered HMG in the hypogonadotropic patients and no evidence for testis stimulation as measured by estrogen excretion or production. The plasma testosterone levels varied during treatment, but, as indicated above, there was no consistent pattern of increased LH nor did the plasma testosterone rise above mid-normal levels until HCG was added.

The possibility of abnormalities of steroid biosynthesis being associated with disorders of spermatogenesis suggested the study in vitro of testicular tissue from infertile males (21). Using an organ culture technique, small amounts of tissue(3-6 mg), as would be obtained with conventional biopsy procedures, have now been used for investigation of steroid metabolism in these patients. Conversion of pregnenolone to testosterone with identification of various intermediates has been demonstrated. Studies are in progress concerning pathways, response to stimulation and comparison with tissue with normal spermatogenesis.

ACKNOWLEDGEMENTS

This research was supported in part by U.S.P.H.S. Grant AM-08375 and the B.F. Anathan Fund. The technical assistance of Miss Harriet Savasten, Miss Linda Kuntz, Mrs. Lisa Paraska and Miss Masumi Kubomoto is gratefully acknowledged. The assistance of Dr. Harvey Mendelow in obtaining and examining the testicular biopsies is appreciated.

REFERENCES

1. Mancini, R.E., Seiguer, A.C. and Lloret, A.P. J. Clin. Endocr., 29: 467, 1969.
2. Lunenfeld, B., Goldman, B. and Shalkovsky, R. In Progress in Endocrinology, ed. Gual, C., Excerpta Medica Foundation, Amsterdam p 1044, 1969.

3. Mroueh, A., Lytton, B. and Kase, N. J. Clin. Endocr., 27: 53, 1967.
4. Paulsen, C.A., In Estrogen Assays in Clinical Medicine, ed. Paulsen, C.A. Univ. of Washington Press, Seattle, p.274, 1965.
5. de Kretser, D.M., Taft, H.P., Brown, J.B., Evans, J.H., and Hudson, B. J. Endocr., 40: 107, 1968.
6. Odell, W.D., Ross, G.T., and Rayford, P.L., J. Clin. Invest., 46: 248, 1967.
7. Albert, A., Rosemberg, E., Ross, G.T., Paulsen, C.A. and Ryan, R.J., J. Clin. Endocr., 28: 1214, 1968.
8. Demetriou, J.A. et al. Clin. Chem., to be published.
9. Drekter, I.J., Heisler, A., Scism, G.R., Stern, S., Pearson, S. and McGavack, T.H., J. Clin. Endocr., 12: 55, 1952.
10. Metcalf, M.G., J. Endocr., 26: 415, 1963.
11. Brown, J.B., Advances Clin. Chem., ed. Sobotka, H., Academic Press, New York, Vol. 3, p. 157, 1960.
12. Salokangas, R.A.A. and Bulbrook, R.D., J. Endocr., 22: 47, 1961.
13. Crowell, G.G., Turner, M.E., Jr., Schmidt, F.H., Howard, C.M. and Preedy, J.R.K., J. Clin. Endocr., 27: 807, 1967.
14. Eren, S., Reynolds, G.H., Turner, M.E., Jr, Schmidt, F.H., Mackay, J.H., Howard, C.M. and Preedy, J.R.K. J. Clin. Endocr., 27: 819, 1967.
15. Lipsett, M.D., Wilson, H., Kirschner, M.A., Korenman, S.G., Fishman, L.M., Sarfaty, G.A., and Bardin, C.W., In Recent Progr. Hormone Res., ed. Pincus, G. Academic Press, New York, Vol. 22, p. 245, 1966.
16. Perez-Palacios, G., Lamont, K.G., Perez, A.E. and Jaffe, R.B., J. Clin. Endocr., 29: 786, 1969.
17. Yanaihara, T. and Troen, P., Proc. Central Soc. Clin. Res., 42: 122, 1969.
18. Rosemberg, E., Joshi, S.R., and Nwe, T.T., In Gonadotropins 1968, ed. Rosemberg, E. Geron-X, Los Altos, California, p. 139, 1968.
19. Yen, S.S.C., Llerena, O., Little, B., and Pearson, O.H., J. Clin. Endocr., 28: 1763, 1968.
20. Stevens, V.C., J. Clin. Endocr., 29: 904, 1969.
21. Danezis, J.M., Fertil. Steril., 17: 488, 1966.

DISCUSSION

HUDSON: Dr. Troen commented that his patients exhibited low levels of plasma testosterone. I think that this is a relevant question in view of Dr. Heller's presentation. What does Dr. Troen regard as the lower extreme of the normal range in his laboratory? Among our own group of infertile men without hypogonadotropic syndromes, the only patients who consistently show abnormalities in levels of plasma testosterone are those patients with the Sertoli cell only syndrome. In 25% of these patients, the plasma levels of testosterone are less than

300 ng/100 ml of plasma, which we regard as significantly lower than normal. Oligospermic patients with germinal cell arrest rarely show abnormalities in testosterone secretion, clinically or chemically.

TROEN: We consider the low limit of the normal range to be 400 ng/100 ml. The patients referred to had values of plasma testosterone as low as 240 ng/100 ml.

E. STEINBERGER: Dr. Troen, in the incubates with ^{14}C pregnenolone and tritiated DHA you found the ratio of tritium to carbon to be greater in testosterone than in androstenedione. You interpreted these findings as indicating that the pathway does not go via androstenedione?

TROEN: Yes, in the organ culture studies, we incubated ^{3}H dehydroepiandrosterone and ^{14}C- pregnenolone and found that the tritium/^{14}C ratio of the recovered testosterone was greater than that for androstenedione suggesting therefore that a significant portion of the testosterone arose from DHA by a pathway other than through androstenedione. As we indicated in discussion earlier during this meeting additional data indicate this is via Δ^5-androstenediol.

ASSESSMENT OF GONADOTROPIN THERAPY IN MALE INFERTILITY

Carl Schirren and Joseph O. Toyosi

Andrology Department, University Clinic for Skin Diseases
Hamburg-Eppendorf, Bundesrepublik Deutschland

The treatment of male subfertility has involved several different gonadotropin preparations. We shall describe our experience with the following: a) Pregnant mare serum (PMS), b) Human chorionic gonadotropin (HCG), c) Human menopausal gonadotropin (HMG), d) Human hypophyseal gonadotropin (HHG) and e) various combinations of these agents.

Emphasis will be laid on the influence of these gonadotropins on the seminal fluid (sperm count, sperm morphology and sperm motility). Our studies were carried out between the years 1953 and 1969 and involved 449 cases. (See Table 1).

Table 1. Survey of Patients Treated with Gonadotropins.

PMS		
Oligospermia	284	
Hypozoospermia	79	
Hypokinesis	58	
		421 cases
HMG and HCG		
Oligospermia	26	
Azoospermia	1	
		27 cases
HHG and HCG		
Azoospermia	1	1 case
Total		449 cases

Until recently, the most widely used gonadotropin preparation for male subfertility was PMS. PMS was first used by Tonutti (1). Although PMS is placental in origin, it primarily exerts a follicle stimulating hormone (FSH) action rather than an interstitial cell stimulating hormone (ICSH) action. Tonutti concluded that ICSH has no direct or indirect influence on spermiogenesis when used to stimulate testicular function following hypophysectomy. He also concluded that the presence of FSH was necessary for maturation from primary spermatocytes to secondary spermatocytes.

The first consideration was the influence of PMS on sperm morphology. PMS was initially administered at the dose rate of 1,000 I.U. twice weekly for six weeks. Recently the dosage rate has been increased to 2,000 I.U. twice weekly for three weeks because of the antigonadotropic effects of PMS. The results obtained are summarized in Table 2. There was a mean increase of 11% in the number of normal structured sperm. A corresponding decrease of 4.9% was observed in the "changed middlepart" sperm. Both the mean sperm count and the motility increased. Data derived from an additional 151 cases are summarized in Table 3. An improvement in the three important factors, i.e., motility, morphology and sperm count was noted.

Table 2. The Effect of PMS on Human Spermatozoa (1,000 I.U. PMS twice weekly for 6 weeks) (72 cases)

Morphology								Sperm	Motility		
a	b	c	d	e	f	g	h	Count	I	II	III
before PMS:											
44.2	10.8	0.66	17.5	14.5	3.1	1.7	2.1	41.1	39.4	15.7	44.9
after PMS:											
55.7	7.7	0.11	12.6	14.4	3.1	2.0	4.4	82.1	52.0	14.0	34.0

a: normal sperm, b: small head, c: giant head, d: changed middlepart, e: double head, f: malformed head, g: phantom, h: abaxial implantation, Sperm Count: (in millions/ml.), I: high motility, II: moderate motility, III: immotile.

Table 3. The Effect of PMS on Sperm Count, Motility and Morphology in Patients with Subfertility (151 cases).

Group (millions/ml) (cases)	Before/After Treatment	Motility (%)	Morphology normal (%)	Sperm Count millions/ml.
1 -10	before	48	48.3	4.3
(16)	after	52	61.2	20.2
11-20	before	35	53.6	13.6
(29)	after	55	54.1	25.5
21-30	before	56	67.3	26.9
(28)	after	65	72.3	62.8
31-40	before	54	68.2	34.5
(39)	after	59	70.0	42.8
41-60	before	53	71.7	41.4
(18)	after	66	74.9	63.4
hypokinesis	before	39	36.1	131.2
(21)	after	47	60.0	120.0

From our experience with PMS, the following points are worthy of note: 1) treatment with PMS in the human is risky because of antihormone production. When used we recommend 2,000 I.U. twice weekly for a limited period of three weeks. 2) With careful patient selection, PMS alone will usually improve sperm count, sperm motility and sperm morphology. 3) We have modified our PMS treatment by adding androgen (2). The addition of testosterone augments the PMS and to a certain extent maintains the achieved result for longer periods of time. We recommend Mesterolone at a daily dosage of 20 mg for five months.

We believe that by using the guidelines of PMS therapy our treatment can be improved by using homologous gonadotropins. To date, we have treated 27 patients with HMG, 21 with Humegon and 6 with Pergonal.

HMG treatment was given to 20 males using a dosage of 500 I.U. (IRP= 75 I.U. FSH) thrice weekly for 12 weeks. In another group (6 patients) the weekly dose was doubled. The results of these studies are seen in Fig. 1.

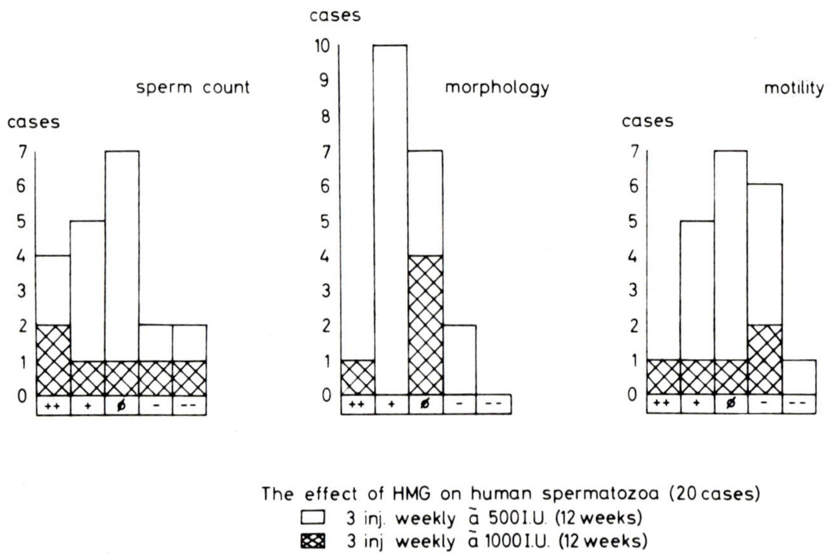

Fig. 1. An improvement in sperm morphology only is seen; the sperm count increases slightly, no change in sperm motility. Between the dosage of 500 I.U. and 1,000 I.U. there is no difference in the results obtained. ++: important improvement (>50%), +: moderate improvement (11-49%), Ø: no change ($\pm$ 10%), -: moderate decrease (11-49%), --: important decrease ($\geq$ 50%).

Table 4. Clinical Data of Six Patients Treated with HMG + HCG

No.	Year of Birth	Testes Volume	Diseases in Anamnesis	Urinary Gonadotropins (FSH-I.U.)
1	1925	normal (soft)	Ø	6.6
2	1930	normal	hepatitis diphtheria	6.6
3	1937	normal	tonsillectomy	13.2
4	1927	normal	Ø	6.6
5	1932	normal	Ø	26.4
6	1931	normal	Ø	26.4

Table 4 shows the clinical data of patients treated with HMG and HCG alternately (Pergonal and Choragon). In three cases the gonadotropin content in urine was low, in the other cases the levels were normal. The sperm counts differed between below 3 million/ml. and 12.3 million/ml. before the hormone treatment. The control spermatogram after three months of treatment shows an improvement of sperm count in one case only, in the other five cases the sperm count diminished or remained unchanged. The morphology and motility remained unchanged in all cases. In one case we noted gynecomastia during the treatment, and the hormone treatment was interrupted because of swollen and painful breasts.

The last case in this study was a 33-year old man with a clinical diagnosis of azoospermia. The histological picture shows germinal cell arrest (Case 2 Tables 4 and 5). HMG (Humegon) can produce sperm in the ejaculate but no motility. Later HHG was administered for 10 days at a dosage of 500 I.U. daily. In connection with this treatment we also injected 5,000 I.U. HCG daily for 10 days. The spermatogram of this patient remained unchanged.

Table 5. Effect of HMG/HCG on Human Testis

No. (Diagnosis)	Testicular Biopsy Tubule Diameter (μ)	Sperm Count (mill/ml)		Morphology (% normal)		Motility (%)		Side Effects
		a*	b†	a*	b†	a*	b†	
1 (O)	144-180	6	< 3	30	40	30	40	∅
2 (A)	108-180	0	< 3	0	0	∅	∅	∅
3 (O)	108-216	11.4 12.3	19.5	70	65	70	65	gyneco-mastia
4 (O)	120	6.8 7.2	5.0	45	40	40	40	∅
5 (O)	95	5.4 6.2	< 3.0	45	49	40	40	∅
6 (O)	145	11.4 9.7	10.2	35	40	40	45	∅

a*: before treatment, b†: after treatment for 3 months,
(A): azoospermia, (O): Oligospermia.

The hormone status in his urine showed an increase in 17-ketosteroids, estrogens, pregnanediol and gonadotropins.

Table 6. Effect of HMG, HHG and HCG in Azoospermia

Date (1963)	Treatment	Spermatogram	Hormone Status in Urine a*	b**	c †	d ††
22.1	HMG (Humegon) 75 I.U. 3 x weekly for 12 weeks	azoospermia				
13.6		some sperms	11.06	20.9	1.70	6.6
20.8	HHG+ (500 I.U. daily for 10 days)	some sperms				
1.10		some sperms	14.0	35.2	1.92	26.4
10.10	HCG (5,000 I.U. daily for 10 days).	some sperms	14.2	34.8	1.90	26.4

\+ : Sponsored by G. Bettendorf.

a*: 17-ketosteroids in mg., b**: estrogens in μg, c † : pregnanediol in mg, d ††: gonadotropin in mouse U.U.

The application of HMG is limited. This opinion is supported in the literature (3-7). This treatment is mainly for hypogonadotropic hypogonadism. Even in this disease it is not possible in all cases to produce an improvement in the sperm factor. According to Lunenfeld (4) the following criteria are important if a positive reaction of the seminiferous tubules is to be obtained: a) tubule diameter from 50 to 70 μ , b) germ cells with Sertoli cells, spermatogonia and spermatocytes , c) hypogonadotropin content in urine.

CONCLUSION

The treatment of the subfertile male having oligospermia and hypokinesis with gonadotropin preparations should not be compared with the use of these agents in men following hypophysectomy. In the latter gonadotropin therapy is highly successful.

Since the causes of oligospermia are quite extensive, therapy is difficult at the present time. Now that human gonadotropin material is available it is imperative that our diagnostic capabilities are improved. Prior to treatment, it is important to measure the endogenous gonadotropin levels and examine a testicular biopsy specimen. We do not support the notion that repeated testicular biopsies are necessary during treatment. We hold the view that the testes are vulnerable to repeated operations and that permanent damage may result. The spermatogram affords an insight into the effectiveness of gonadotropin preparations after a longer period of observation.

Since our experience with HMG, alone or in combination with HCG, is somewhat limited, we cannot give a positive prognosis. It is possible that with a thorough selection and examination of the patients, better results could be achieved.

REFERENCES

1. Tonutti, E., Z. Urol. 11, 1955.
2. Schirren, C., Internist (Berlin) 8:2, 1967.
3. Johnsen, S. G., and Christiansen, P., In Gonadotropins 1968, ed. Rosemberg, E., Geron-X, Inc., Los Altos, California, p 516, 1968.
4. Lunenfeld, B., Goldman, B., and Ismajovich, B., In Gonadotropins 1968, ed. Rosemberg, E., Geron-X, Inc., Los Altos, California, p 513, 1968.
5. Mancini, R. E., Seiguer, A. C., and Levret, P., In Gonadotropins 1968, ed. Rosemberg, E., Geron-X, Inc., Los Altos, California, p 503, 1968.
6. Paulsen, C. A., In Gonadotropins 1968, ed. Rosemberg, E., Geron-X, Inc., Los Altos, California, p 491, 1968.
7. Rosemberg, E., Mancini, R. E., Crigler, J. F. and Bergada, C., In Gonadotropins 1968, ed. Rosemberg, E., Geron-X, Inc., Los Altos, California, p 527, 1968.

ASSESSMENT OF GONADOTROPIN THERAPY IN MALE INFERTILITY

B. Lunenfeld and R. Shalkovsky-Weissenberg

Institute of Endocrinology, Tel-Hashomer Government Hospital, Israel and Department of Life Sciences, Bar-Ilan University, Ramat-Gan, Israel

Male infertility may be produced by genetic, mechanical, infectious, inflammatory or hormonal causes. Correct diagnosis is essential before any therapy is started. In this presentation we will analyze and discuss therapeutic results only in such cases where infertility was presumably due to hormonal factors.

In order to evaluate correctly the results of hormonal therapy in male infertility, it was found necessary to summarize existing knowledge on the hormonal control of testicular function.

Hypophysectomy causes morphological changes in Leydig cells and Sertoli cells as well as atrophy of androgen-dependent parts of the male reproductive system (1-4).

It is universally accepted that Leydig cell proliferation and function is under the control of ICSH (interstitial cell stimulating hormone). This is also evidenced by the fact that administration of ICSH or HCG (human chorionic gonadotropin - biological activity similar to ICSH) promotes excessive Leydig cell function (5), and that fluorescein-labelled ICSH is selectively localized in Leydig cells (6). It seems clear that the main secretory product of the testis is testosterone and that this is produced mainly by the Leydig cells.

Several pathways of testosterone biosynthesis have since been proposed (7). Furthermore, it has been shown that the secretion of the Leydig cells is stimulated by ICSH and HCG and is suppressed by the administration of androgen and estrogen (8).

Gonadotropins also have a particular action on supporting cells (immature Sertoli cells). Courot (9) showed that in the impuberal lamb the number of supporting cells was reduced by almost half of the initial control within a few days following hypophysectomy. The supporting cells which survived hypophysectomy were not transformed into Sertoli cells. Vilar (10) showed that following hypophysectomy in the rat the Sertoli cells became smaller, atrophic and the amount of cytoplasm of these cells decreased. Sertoli cells seem to present the first target of gonadotropic action in the seminiferous tubules; therefore they may have an important role in spermatogenesis. Mancini (6) demonstrated that fluorescein-labelled FSH (follicle stimulating hormone) appears mainly in Sertoli cells, while the labelled ICSH is selectively localized in Leydig cells. This finding shows that Sertoli cells are influenced by gonadotropins.

It has been postulated by de Robertis et al. (11,12) that in amphibians ICSH provokes release of spermatozoa from Sertoli cells; this has been further clarified in electron microscope studies by Burgos et al. (4). Furthermore, Burgos et al. showed in preliminary experiments with male hamsters that a similar mechanism may exist in mammals, i.e. that ICSH may be responsible for sperm release from the Sertoli cells. On the basis of these studies the authors postulated that the Sertoli cell cytoplasm is a target for ICSH activity; the cytoplasmic swelling and the unfolding of the apical recesses which is accompanied by the release of spermatozoa in the hamster was considered by these authors as the counterpart of ovulation.

Hypophysectomy also causes an arrest in spermatogenesis in practically all mammalian species (3). The exact role of gonadotropins on the germinal epithelium is still debated. Some authors (2,13,14) claim that gonadotropins act on the first stages of spermatogenesis. Steinberger and Duckett (15) concluded that the progression of type A spermatogonia to late stages of pachytene spermatocytes may not require hormonal factors. Smith (16), Crooke and Gilmour (17) and Tonutti (18) believe that gonadotropins act on spermatogenesis at the late stages of meiotic division of the primary spermatocytes. Clermont and Morgentaler (19) stated that, in the hypophysectomized rat, the process of spermatogenesis may proceed as far as step 7 of spermiogenesis. Lostroh et al. (20) observed spermatogonia as well as primary spermatocytes in the tubules of hypophysectomized male rats even six months after operation. Since these authors came to the conclusion that after "complete" hypophysectomy residual gonadotropic activity might be present, they attempted to neutralize this activity with antisera to ovine ICSH; this resulted in further atrophy of the testes, but degenerating spermatocytes and mitosis of spermatogonia, although infrequent, were still observed.

The same author (21) demonstrated that administration of ICSH to hypophysectomized animals elicited an increase in the population of young primary spermatocytes. Spermatogonia in mitosis were much in evidence, but no spermatids were observed. Since hyperplasia of Leydig cells was noted, and since the functional activity of these cells was demonstrated by increased weight of seminal vesicles and ventral prostate, one cannot conclude from the experiment whether the spermatogenic activity seen was due to the ICSH or to the androgens produced by the interstitial cells through ICSH stimulation. Injection of FSH to hypophysectomized rats initiated an extensive and orderly repair of a large number of seminiferous tubules; most tubules contained several rows of primary spermatocytes in addition to young spermatids. Although from these results one could claim that FSH stimulated the formation of spermatocytes, it is unfortunate that the FSH preparation used was probably contaminated with ICSH. This becomes evident from the fact that, although the interstitial tissue was still deficient, it showed signs of stimulation over and above that of the controls. Lostroh's experiments, therefore, are not conclusive as to the selective role of FSH, ICSH and testosterone on the first stages of spermatogenesis in the mature hypophysectomized rat.

Cutly and Cutly (22) showed that spermatogenesis in the testes of hypophysectomized rats can be maintained with testosterone propionate. The testes of hypophysectomized testosterone-injected animals did not differ histologically from those of the normal controls.

The above mentioned experiment demonstrated that hypophysectomy of the mature animal will severely affect spermatogenesis and spermiogenesis and indicates clearly the necessity of circulating gonadotropins to maintain normal testicular function. The authors could not conclusively pinpoint any particular stage in the process of hormonal restoration of spermatogenesis.

The study of mechanisms controlling initiation of spermatogenesis was hampered by the fact that hypophysectomy at birth or in early infancy was practically impossible, since such young hypophysectomized animals either die or are killed and abandoned by their mothers. Moreover, by its very nature hypophysectomy may lead to inconclusive results due to deprivation of other vitally important pituitary hormones. Steinberger and Duckett (15) thus attempted to suppress gonadotropic activity by injecting estradiol from birth. In rats receiving estradiol daily from birth spermatogenesis commences, and at the age of 15 days the testes show progression of spermatogenesis similar to that of normal uninjected controls (23). However, the pachytene spermatocytes are unable to complete the meiotic division and degenerate at diakinesis. In testes of 60 and 90 day old rats the tubules contain Sertoli cells, spermatogonia and only occasional spermatocytes.

These results suggest that in the absence of gonadotropins and additionally in the secondary absence of testosterone production, the initial wave of spermatogenesis commences at puberty. However, the spermatocytes are unable to complete the reduction division. The question arises whether estrogen administration blocks gonadotropic release and therefore the few spermatocytes found after estrogen administration in the adult animal may be due to small amounts of gonadotropins released. Furthermore, one would have to exclude a direct effect of estrogens on the testes.

The purpose of our investigation was to elucidate the factors governing testicular development and initiation of spermatogenesis. This includes the hormonal requirements in spermatogenesis and spermiogenesis, as well as the conditions which lead to normal sperm formation. An experimental approach to the above mentioned problem was to compare animals deprived of gonadotropins from birth to normal littermates, at different stages of testicular development. A continuous deprivation of circulating endogenous gonadotropins in mice, from birth onwards, is made possible by the continuous administration of antisera to rat gonadotropin (24).

From Table 1 it can be seen that there was no significant difference in testicular development during the first week of life. At the age of 14 days the difference between the control and the gonadotropin-deprived animals is apparent inasfar as the number of spermatogonia and spermatocytes is significantly reduced in the experimental animals.

During the third week of life the first spermatids could be in some of the tubules. In the experimental animals no tubules containing spermatids were found (for each testis at least 50 cross - sections were examined). The number of spermatogonia and spermatocytes in the gonadotropin-deprived animals remained significantly reduced. The mean diameter of the tubules of the experimental animal was significantly smaller than the control.

In the fourth and fifth weeks of life spermatids in the normal animals became abundant, and a mean of 102 per tubule could be counted on day 30. In the gonadotropin-deprived animals spermatid formation was totally inhibited, and the number of spermatogonia and spermatocytes in the gonadotropin-deprived animals remained similar to the numbers found on day 14, and these were significantly less than in the control animals. Whereas the mean total number of cells of the germinal layers increased continuously up to day 30 in the control animals, no change was observed in the gonadotropin-deprived animals. It can therefore be concluded that in the absence of gonadotropins during puberty, spermatid formation ceases and there is no increase in the total number of cells of the germinal layers from day 14 onwards. The increase of spermatogonia and their transformation to spermatocytes from day 7 to day 14 in the antiserum-treated animals cannot yet be interpreted (Table 1).

When gonadotropin-deprived animals received substitution of FSH + ICSH, a spermatogenic pattern similar to that of the normal was

Tabl[illegible]

EFFECT OF GONADOTROPIN DEPRIVATION AND SUBSTITUTION ON TESTICULAR DEVELOPMENT IN MICE

Age (days)	Treatment	Spermatogonia Mean	P	Spermatocytes Mean	P	Spermatids Mean	Total mean	Sertoli Mean	Tubule Diam. Mean μ	Wt. of Testes as % of body wt.
		Mean No. of Cells Per Tubule Cross Section and (S.D.)								
7	NRS*	5.0 (1.0)	< 0.05	0		0	5.0	22 (3.0)	45.0	-
7	ARG**	3.2 (2.1)		0		0	3.2	23 (2.8)	40.5	-
14	NRS	25.0 (9.8)	< 0.0025	20.4 (6.9)	< 0.01	0	45.4	20.4(5.1)	72.0	0.35
14	ARG	15.0 (5.2)		14.1 (6.1)		0	29.1	20.5(7.8)	66.6	0.14
19	NRS	28.6 (10.3)	< 0.01	38.0 (3.9)	< 0.005	7.6	74.2	14.8(7.3)	117.0	0.44
19	ARG	12.6 (4.3)		12.4 (5.4)		0	25.0	19.8(3.0)	33.6	0.17
25	NRS	52.0 (10.0)	< 0.005	40.2 (15.8)	< 0.005	33	125.2	12.0(3.0)	132.0	0.30
25	ARG	18.3 (8.0)		14.0 (5.0)		0	32.3	17.0(5.0)	54.0	0.15
30	NRS	47.3 (26.8)	< 0.005	54.0 (9.0)	< 0.005	102	203.3	15.4(4.4)	140.0	0.55
30	ARG	11.0 (5.5)		14.2 (5.6)		0	25.2	17.2(4.5)	66.0	0.20
25	ARG+HMG	65.0 (31.9)		72.1 (23.0)		48.0(46.0)	185.1	20.2(6.7)	90.0	1.30
25	ARG+HCG	26.6 (9.1)		25.8 (5.9)		31.5(22.0)	83.9	12.3(3.4)	68.0	0.35
25	ARG+FSH	32.7 (13.8)		33.0 (12.5)		8.0(6.6)	73.2	14.2(4.8)	66.0	0.50

* Normal rabbit serum. ** Anti-rat gonadotropin.

obtained. Antiserum to rat gonadotropins, together with non-cross-reacting human FSH qualitatively restores spermatogenesis up to the spermatid stage, although quantitatively less spermatids are found than in the normal littermates. It is of interest that HCG in the presence of anti-rat gonadotropins permitted the meiotic process to progress to completion, as shown by the occurrence of spermatids (Table 1).

It is interesting to note that when Steinberger and Steinberger (25) cultured testes from five day old rats, only differentiation up to the pachytene stage of meiosis was shown to take place in vitro in the total absence of hormones. This seems to be in accordance with our in vivo results in mice up to the age of 14 days, where spermatogonia proliferated into pachytene spermatocytes in the absence of gonadotropins.

The effect of hypophysectomy in men was investigated by several authors. Mancini et al. (5) examined testicular biopsies in men one month to six years after hypophysectomy. When examining the biopsies, the authors found that the extent of regression of the seminiferous epithelium, tubular wall and interstitial cells were of different degrees. Some biopsies were characterized by Sertoli cells, almost complete spermatogenic line, slight hyalinization of the tubular wall and an appreciable number of Leydig cells. In other biopsies the tubules contained Sertoli cells and primary spermatocytes up to the pachytene stage, moderate hyalinization of the tubular wall and a low number of Leydig cells. There was a correlation between the time elapsing after operation and the degree of involution of the testes, indicating that the degenerative process took from a few weeks to several years. The authors found that PMSG (pregnant mare serum gonadotropin) and HCG treatment acted upon increase of spermatogonial cells, thus giving rise to primary spermatocytes. HMG (human menopausal gonadotropin) caused a further augmentation of testicular function, and combined therapy of HMG and HCG caused a significant stimulation of all types of cells, especially from the spermatocyte onward, and even up to spermatozoa. It also caused a marked increase in the number of mature Leydig cells.

Restoration of spermatogenesis in a hypophysectomized patient with HMG was reported by MacLeod et al. (26,27). Treatment of this patient was started when the process of involution of the seminiferous tubules was virtually complete, except for the presence of a few primary spermatocytes at the pachytene stage.

After 67 days of daily HMG injections, testicular biopsy revealed that maturation had occurred close to the stage of exfoliation of spermatozoa into the lumen. However, this stage of maturation was achieved only in some of the tubules. A testicular biopsy, performed 100 days after initiation of therapy, demonstrated a fully quantitative restoration of spermatogenesis. There was no evidence of

Leydig cell proliferation or successful ejaculation by the patient, and blood testosterone was exceedingly low. This indicated that the ICSH content of HMG was insufficient for the restoration of the interstitial tissue. This seems to imply that spermatogenesis and spermiogenesis can proceed without any morphological or biochemical evidence of Leydig cell proliferation and function. This should not be surprising, since Pasqualini and Bur (28) and Johnsen (29) have discussed the so-called "fertile" eunuchs, a condition of tubular development and spermatogenesis with complete absence of Leydig cells.

Fifty-one days after initiation of combined HMG and HCG therapy, a measurable volume of seminal plasma was obtained in which the sperm count was 60,000,000 per ml. According to this study, it would appear that daily HMG (200 IU FSH + 200 IU ICSH) is sufficient to restore spermatogenesis and spermiogenesis within 100 days, but contains insufficient ICSH to detect any stimulation of Leydig cells.

Mancini et al. (5), studying hypophysectomized subjects aged 18 to 63, demonstrated that HCG was capable of stimulating Sertoli cells, increasing tubular size and causing maturation of germinal epithelium up to pachytene stage, regression of "hyalinization" and proliferation of Leydig cells. HMG (75 IU FSH+ 75 IU ICSH), similar to HCG, not only provoked growth of seminal tubules and maturation of Sertoli cells, but also advanced proliferation of germinal epithelium with the production of spermatids and occasional spermatozoa.

HMG + HCG significantly reinforced the effect of HMG alone on the production of spermatids and spermatozoa. However, within the 74 $\pm$ 5 days of this treatment regime, the quantitative level of spermatogenesis and spermiogenesis seen in normal adult patients was not reached. These authors also demonstrated that testosterone, given together with gonadotropins, had an inhibitory effect on the response to HMG therapy.

This study seems to confirm the earlier work of MacLeod et al. (26,27), in which HMG + HCG restored spermatogenesis in a hypophysectomized patient. The qualitative resemblance but quantitative difference between these two groups of authors might be due to the different amounts of HMG administered (MacLeod et al., 200 IU FSH + 200 IU ICSH; Mancini et al., 75 IU FSH + 75 IU ICSH).

The partially hypophysectomized patient of Gemzell and Kjessler (30) showed a pre-treatment biopsy with spermatogenic activity up to early spermatid stage. After three weeks of human pituitary gonadotropin (HPG) therapy, spermatozoa could be seen in the ejaculate. After 13 weeks of treatment, the number of spermatozoa in the ejaculate rose to 72,000,000 per ml. In this study all stages of the first meiotic division and the metaphase of the second meiotic division, together with immature spermatids, could be demonstrated prior to HPG treatment. The authors therefore claim, in contradiction to MacLeod, that spermatogenesis was independent of gonadotropic stimulation and that the effect of HPG was specific for spermiogenesis.

However, it could be argued that if this patient was only partially hypophysectomized, enough gonadotropic activity could have been present to prevent complete involution of the germinal epithelium, but not sufficient for the final stages of maturation. With HPG therapy, spermiogenesis was rapidly restored and sperm appeared in the ejaculate within only 21 days of treatment. The effect of HPG on the earlier stages of sperm production (i.e. spermatogenesis) may be indicated by the steady increase in sperm counts up to the 13th week of treatment. The full restoration of sperm production by HPG alone indicates either a higher ICSH content of this preparation or the presence of endogenous ICSH.

The results of these earlier investigations can therefore be interpreted as showing the need for both FSH and ICSH in order to completely restore spermatogenesis after partial or complete gonadotropic deprivation. There is no conclusive evidence that any stage of spermatogenesis in man may be independent of gonadotropic stimulation.

It must be realized that data on restoration of spermatogenic activity with human gonadotropic preparations after partial or complete gonadotropic deprivation does not necessarily imply that a response can be obtained in immature testes of children or eunuchoids with complete or partial lack of gonadotropins. It might be that gonadotropin therapy promotes spermatogenesis only in the previously stimulated germinal epithelium.

After administration of HMG (16-75 days) to four children aged six to seven years with unilateral cryptorchidism, Rosemberg et al. (31) demonstrated maturation of Sertoli cells and a significant increase in spermatogonial cells, as well as maturation of germinal epithelium up to primary spermatocytes.

Bergada and Mancini (32) compared the differential effects of pregnant mare serum (PMS), HCG, PMS followed by HCG, and HMG + HCG in 17 children aged six to nine years with unilateral cryptorchidism. In the HMG-HCG therapy group, a greater increase in tubular size, as well as a greater stimulation of the germinal epithelium, was provoked compared to the other therapeutic regimes. No regime provoked maturation beyond the spermatocyte stage. Sertoli cell maturation and Leydig cell proliferation were found both with HMG + HCG as well as with PMS + HCG. The authors conclude that both FSH and ICSH-like activity might be necessary for initiation of spermatogenesis.

Furthermore, data has now accumulated on the effect of human gonadotropins on adult eunuchoidal men. Heller (33) treated a eunuchoidal male first with HCG and then with HCG and HMG simultaneously. Eight weeks after the latter treatment, testicular biopsy showed complete spermatogenesis. Davies (34) treated a hypogonadotropic eunuchoid with HPG, 600 mg eq. of the International Reference Preparation (IRP HMG) three times weekly. After four months, increase of testicular size and enlargement of tubules was seen. The dose was then increased to 2000 mg eq. IRP HMG three times a week for two more months and a still greater increase of testicular size was noted; there was no maturation of the germinal epithelium nor were any Leydig cells seen. When 12,000 IU of HCG was added to this regime for another four months, Leydig cells were prominent and spermatozoa were found in a testicular biopsy. One month later spermatozoa appeared in the ejaculate.

Martin (35) demonstrated in a patient with an apparently isolated deficiency of pituitary gonadotropins and with a testicular biopsy showing only spermatogonia and isolated spermatocytes, that prolonged therapy with HCG (12 months) did not modify testicular morphology significantly. There were still only two or three layers of cells within the tubules, although mitosis was more frequent and more obvious. No spermatids or spermatozoa were found. In contrast, interstitial cells were much more numerous and obvious, and there was a slight increase in the fibrous elements of the interstitial tissue. After HPG (500 IU FSH twice weekly) + HCG (1,000 IU once a week) for 61 days, motile, morphologically normal spermatozoa were seen in the ejaculate. The sperm count rose steadily and reached a level of 25,000,000 per ml eight months after treatment.

Johnsen's extensive study (36) of two adult men with severe hypogonadotropic hypogonadism with infantile testes treated with HCG for 23 and 6 months respectively, revealed the development of secondary sex characteristics and probably stimulation of tubular diameter. HMG treatment alone, following the HCG regime, did not significantly modify testicular morphology, except that in both cases the number of Sertoli cells per tubule increased (28.5 ± 6.4 to 39.4 ± 9.7; 38.9 ± 10.9 to 51.8 ± 20.8). The combined HMG-HCG regime for 12 and 9 months respectively induced a complete gonadal maturation in both cases.

Paulsen (37) studied five hypogonadotropic hypogonadic eunuchoids. From his study it seems that HMG alone for up to six weeks stimulated increase of tubular diameter in two out of three cases, an increase of mean cell count in one out of three cases, but without significant maturation of the germinal cell epithelium. For two cases who received HCG alone for 42 to 56 weeks, Sertoli and Leydig cell maturation were stimulated; in one patient the proliferation advanced to Sd spermatids, and in the other only up to the stage of pachytene spermatocytes, and varying degrees of germinal cell maturation were noted.

Two of the patients who initially received HMG therapy alone were subsequently treated with HCG for 20 to 25 weeks. One of these patients showed germinal cell maturation to the Sd spermatid and the other patient remained unresponsive. In the one patient who received HMG, followed by HCG, and finally HMG + HCG therapy, full spermatogenesis and spermiogenesis were obtained, and an occasional sperm was encountered in the ejaculate. Of the two patients who initially received HCG and subsequently received HMG + HCG, one responded with full spermatogenic and spermiogenic stimulation with 13.6 million sperm in the ejaculate, and the second showed only pachytene spermatocytes.

Lytton and Kase (38) studied a 19 year old primary panhypopituitary hypogonadic male after partial evacuation of a craniopharyngioma and radiation therapy, whose testicular biopsy revealed fetal type testes with germinal arrest and absence of Leydig cells. After the administration of HMG (12.5 IU FSH three times a week for three months), no changes were observed in either gonad or secondary sexual characteristics. He was then given HCG (2000 IU three times a week for some six and a half months). Secondary sex changes developed and a testicular biopsy revealed an increase of interstitial cells and germinal epithelium stimulation to the stage of spermatids. He was then given a combined HMG-HCG regime (12.5 IU HMG + 2000 IU HCG) three times a week for another two months. A testicular biopsy at that time revealed marked focal areas of mature tubules, showing the presence of spermatozoa.

Therefore it can be noted that in most cases(eight out of nine patients)the combined HMG-HCG therapy induced complete gonadal maturation (Table 2).

Table 2

		Patient	Complete Gonadal Maturation
Heller (33)	1965	1	1
Davies (34)	1965	1	1
Paulsen (37)	1965	3	2
Lytton and Kase (38)	1966	1	1
Johnsen (36)	1966	2	2
Martin (35)	1967	1	1

The demonstration that combined HMG-HCG treatment can induce complete gonadal maturation in some patients has been confirmed by Joel (39) who induced complete gonadal maturation in three cases of azoospermia whose pre-treatment testicular biopsies revealed the presence of spermatogonia. (No effect was found in eight other cases whose pre-treatment biopsies showed tubules with only Sertoli cells). Furthermore, Lunenfeld et al. (40) demonstrated that in all six cases of hypogonadotropic azoospermic males whose pre-treatment biopsies revealed infantile testes with mean tubular diameter of 50 to 70 μ containing Sertoli cells and cell elements up to various forms of spermatogonia, complete gonadal maturation could be obtained within 80 to 190 days of combined therapy. Five out of 15 patients who had tubules of normal or near-normal size (170 to 250 μ) with normal, moderate, or thickened walls, containing spermatogonia, Sertoli cells and, in some tubules, occasional spermatocytes, had normal sperm counts after HMG-HCG treatment. Based on the knowledge of the length of the spermatogenic cycle, treatment was given for 80 to 144 days in this group of patients.

Sixteen out of the 17 patients who had tubules of normal or near normal size and which contained only Sertoli cells were unresponsive to therapy. This may be explained by the fact that no spermatogenic response can be expected in the absence of cellular elements pertaining to the germinal line. Since biopsy material might not represent the status of all the tubules, patients diagnosed as having a "Sertoli-only cells" syndrome might actually have mixed forms. In such cases gonadotropic therapy may be beneficial therapeutically or it may at least serve as a diagnostic tool.

In a different series of patients showing normal tubules which contained spermatogonia, treatment was continued without any fixed time limitation (75 IU FSH + 75 IU ICSH + 2500 IU HCG; three times per week). One patient responded after 17 months with occasional spermatozoa in the ejaculate; a month later a normal sperm count was obtained and his wife became pregnant. Three other patients responded after 12 to 15 months of treatment, and the remaining patients are still under therapy.

It can be speculated that administration of human gonadotropins may stimulate spermatogenesis in hypogonadotropic oligospermic men and also in oligospermic patients with a hyposensitive response to normal gonadotropic stimulation, thus improving the sperm count and/or quality.

Treatment with various gonadotropic preparations with FSH and ICSH activity have been used in males with primary spermatogenic disorders, but the results have been variable and, on the whole, unsatisfactory (see Tables 3 and 4).

These unsatisfactory results can be explained by the relative lack of knowledge of other pathological conditions, besides gonadotropin deficiency, which lead to oligospermia (e.g. varicocele, infection, inflammation, genetic conditions), and the lack of data on the relationship between dose and scheme of gonadotropic treatment and the spermatogenic response.

Table 3

Results of Gonadotropic Treatment in Group I (Severe Oligospermia 0.1 - 10 x 10^6/ml.)

Author	No. of Cases	Improvement from I to II	Improvement from I to 20-30 x 10^6/ml	Improvement from I to > 30 x 10^6/ml	No. of Pregnancies
Schoysman (41)	4	1	1	0	2
Lytton and Mroueh (42)	9	1	0	1	0
Abelli and Falagario (43)	6	2	0	0	2
Cittadini and Quartaravo (44)	11	5	1	1	1
Polishuk et al. (45)	9	1	2	1	1
Mroueh et al. (46)	4	0	0	0	0
Danesis and Batrinos (47)	9	2	1	0	1
Debiasi and Misurale (48)	8	1	0	2	1
De Kretser et al. (49)	2	1	0	0	0
Makler et al. (50)	9	1	2	2	1
Lunenfeld et al. (40)	27	6	0	8	1

Table 4. Results of Gonadotropic Treatment in Group II (Moderate Oligospermia 10-20 x 10^6/ml.)

Author	No. of Cases	Improvement from II to >30 x 10^6/ml	No. of Pregnancies
Schoysman (41)	4	2	0
Lytton and Mroueh (42)	9	6	2
Abelli and Falagario (43)	26	9	7
Cittadini and Quartaravo (44)	2	2	0
Polishuk et al. (45)	5	1	0
Mroueh et al. (46)	2	1	0
Danesis and Batrinos (47)	1	1	1
Debiasi and Misurale (48)	7	4	2
De Kretser et al. (49)	0	0	0
Makler et al. (50)	2	2	1
Lunenfeld et al. (40)	24	12	4

It should be noted that the mechanisms by which FSH and ICSH or HCG effect spermatogenesis, spermiogenesis or release of sperm and contribute to the normal behavior of the sperm and its motility are poorly understood. The role that the FSH/ICSH ratio may play in any one of these processes is still unknown. It can be speculated that these processes are regulated by a feedback mechanism between the pituitary and the testes, as well as by an interplay between the two major testicular components, the Leydig cells and the germinal epithelium.

It can be expected that when oligospermic conditions are defined and separated into specific categories and when the pathological mechanism leading to each condition is better understood, certain groups will be found which would benefit from individually adjusted gonadotropic treatment.

When treating female patients, ovarian response to gonadotropins will be reflected by changes in cervical mucus, in vaginal smear and the endometrial epithelium as well as by levels of ovarian steroids in body fluids.

In the male the steroid excretion pattern of Leydig cells is not directly correlated to spermatogenic activity. Furthermore, the ovarian cycle is relatively short (follicular ripening is approximately 15 days), whereas in the male the spermatogenic cycle is approximately 70 days. Sperm analysis and quantitative histology of testicular biopsies are the only practical tests now available to indicate, although late, the testicular response to gonadotropic stimulation. Due to the delay in appearance of response, these tests cannot be used for simultaneous monitoring of treatment in males.

In female patients the daily dose requirements to induce ovulation vary from 75 IU to 375 IU FSH and ICSH daily, and the mean daily dose was 188 IU FSH and ICSH. Most authors reporting on the use of gonadotropins in males administered dosages significantly lower than have been used for the induction of ovulation. Thus it is not surprising that in the absence of basic information about the physiological requirement of gonadotropic hormones at different stages of the spermatogenic cycle and in the absence of clinical indices for monitoring treatment, the results obtained so far are unsatisfactory.

Before a final evaluation of the use of gonadotropins in oligospermic men can be attempted, it would only be fair to administer to a sufficiently large group of well defined patients the daily mean dose of gonadotropins which was sufficient to induce ovulation in females. The analysis of such a study would probably produce a guideline for empirical treatment.

Treatment with gonadotropins must remain empirical until appropriate parameters reflecting responses suitable for monitoring treatment become available.

ACKNOWLEDGMENT

This study was supported in part by Ford Foundation Grant No. 67-470.

REFERENCES

1. Greep, R. O., Fevold, H.L. and Hisaw, F.L., Anat. Rec., 65: 261, 1936.
2. Greep. R.O. and Fevold, H.L., Endocrinology, 21: 611, 1937.
3. Greep, R.O. In Sex and Internal Secretion, 3rd ed., ed. Young, W.C., Williams and Wilkins, Co., Baltimore, Maryland, Vol. 1, p 240, 1961.
4. Burgos, M.H., Vitale-Calpe, R. and Russo, J. In Gonadotropins 1968, ed. Rosemberg, E., Geron-X, Inc., Los Altos, California, p 213, 1968.
5. Mancini, R.E., Siegueur, A.G. and Perez Lloret, A. In Gonadotropins 1968, ed. Rosemberg, E., Geron-X, Inc., Los Altos, California, p 503, 1968.
6. Mancini, R.E., J. Histochem . Cytochem., 15: 516, 1967.
7. Samuels, L.T., Uchikawa, T. and Huseby, R.A. In Endocrinology of the Testis, Ciba Foundation Colloq. Endocr., eds. Wolstenholme, G.E.W. and O'Connor, M., J. & A. Churchill, London, Vol. 16, p 211, 1966.

8. Hudson, B., Coghlan, J.P. and Dulmanis, A. In Endocrinology of the Testis, Ciba Foundation Colloquia on Endocrinology eds. Wolstenholme, G.E.W. and O'Connor, M., J. & A. Churchill, London, Vol. 16, p 140, 1966.
9. Courot, M., J. Reprod. Fertil. Suppl. 2: 89, 1967.
10. Vilar, O. In Gonadotropins 1968, ed. Rosemberg, E., Geron-X, Inc. Los Altos, California, p 205, 1968.
11. De Robertis, E.D.P., Burgos, M.H. and Breyter, E., Rev. Soc. Argent. Biol., 4: 21, 1945.
12. De Robertis, E.D.P., Burgos, M.H. and Breyter, E., Proc. Soc. Exp. Biol. Med., 61: 20, 1946.
13. Greep, R.O., Van Dyke, H.B. and Chow, B.F., Anat. Rec., 78:88, 1940.
14. Albert, A. In Sex and Internal Secretion, 3rd ed., ed., Young, W.C., Williams and Wilkins, Baltimore, Maryland, 1961.
15. Steinberger, E. and Duckett, G.E., J. Reprod. Fertil., Suppl. 2: 75, 1967.
16. Smith, P.E., Amer. J. Anat., 45: 205, 1930.
17. Crooke, A.C. and Gilmour, J.B., J. Path. Bact., 47: 525, 1938.
18. Tonutti, E., Z. Zellforsch, 32: 495, 1943.
19. Clermont, Y. and Morgentaler, H., Endocrinology, 57: 369, 1955.
20. Lostroh, A.J., Johnson, R. and Jordan, C.W., Acta Endocr. (Kobenhavn) 44: 536, 1963.
21. Lostroh, A.J., Acta Endocr. (Kobenhavn) 43: 592, 1963.
22. Cutly , E. and Cutly, E.C., Endocrinology, 26: 503, 1940.
23. Steinberger, E. and Duckett, G.E., Endocrinology, 76: 1184, 1965.
24. Lunenfeld, B. and Eshkol, A. In Gonadotropins 1968, ed., Rosemberg, E., Geron-X, Inc., Los Altos, California, p 197, 1968.
25. Steinberger, A. and Steinberger, E., J. Reprod. Fertil., Suppl. 2, 117, 1967.
26. MacLeod, J., Pazianos, A. and Ray, B., Lancet, 1197, May 30, 1964.
27. MacLeod, J., Pazianos, A. and Ray, B., Fertil. Steril., 17: 1, 1966.
28. Pasqualini, R.A. and Bur, G., Fertil. Steril., 6: 144, 1955.
29. Johnsen, S.G., Acta Endocr. (Kobenhavn) Suppl., 66: 1, 1962.
30. Gemzell, C. and Kjessler, B., Lancet, 644, March 21, 1964.
31. Rosemberg, E., Mancini, R.E., Crigler, J.F., Jr., and Bergada, C. In Gonadotropins 1968, ed., Rosemberg, E., Geron-X, Inc., Los Altos, California, p 527, 1968.
32. Bergada, C. and Mancini, R.E. , J. Reprod. Fertil., in press.
33. Heller, C.J. In Estrogen Workshop Conference, ed. Paulsen, C.A., University of Washington Press, Seattle, Washington, p 276, 1965.
34. Davies, A.G., Proc. Roy. Soc. Med., 58: 580, 1965.
35. Martin, F.I.R., J. Endocr., 38: 431, 1967.
36. Johnsen, S.G., Acta Endocr. (Kobenhavn) 53: 315, 1966.
37. Paulsen, C. A. In Proc. of Med. VIth Pan-American Congress of Endocrinology, Mexico City, 388, 1965.
38. Lytton, B. and Kase, N., New Eng. J. Med., 274: 1061, 1966.

39. Joel, C.A., Harefuah, 71: 281, 1966.
40. Lunenfeld, B., Mor, A. and Mani, M., Fertil. Steril., 18: 581, 1967.
41. Schoysman, F., Bulletin de la Societe Royale Belge de Gynecologie et d'Obstetrique, 34: 399, 1964.
42. Lytton, B. and Mroueh, A., Fertil. Steril., 17: 696, 1966.
43. Abelli, A. and Falagario, M., Attualita Ostet. Ginec., 12: 723, 1966.
44. Cittadini, E. and Quartaravo, P., Agg. Ost. Gin. Palermo, 1, 1966.
45. Polishuk, W.Z., Palti, Z. and Laufer, A., Fertil. Steril., 18: 127, 1967.
46. Mroueh, A., Lytton, B. and Kase, N., J. Clin. Endocr., 27: 53, 1967.
47. Danesis, J.M. and Batrinos, M.L., Fertil. Steril., 18: 788, 1967.
48. Debaisi , E. and Misurale, F., Monit. Ost. Ginecol. Endocr. e del Metab., 38: 5, 1967.
49. DeKretser, D.M., Taft, H.P., Brown, J.P., Evans, J.H. and Hudson, B., J. Endocr., 40: 107, 1968.
50. Makler, A., Paldi, A., Peretz, A. and Barzalai, D., Harefuah, 75: 102, 1968.

DISCUSSION

A. STEINBERGER: Dr. Lunenfeld, you were somewhat concerned about not getting an increase in numbers of Sertoli cells in the 14-day or older mouse when treated with antigonadotropic sera. I would like to point out that in the rat, the Sertoli cells completely cease to divide after about the 13th day of life. We did a study with a ^{3}H thymidine pulse at various ages and found that the percent of labelled Sertoli cells decreases from about 30% at birth to zero at about 13 days of age. Similar results were also obtained in culture. Considering that in the mouse, spermatogenesis takes only about 36 days as compared with about 48 days in the rat, I would assume that the Sertoli cells stopped dividing in the mouse even earlier. Once the Sertoli cells stop dividing nothing seems to be able to stimulate their division and increase their number.

ROSS: Dr. Lunenfeld, is it true that testicular weight expressed as a function of body weight remained constant over the period of 14 to 30 days in animals treated with antigonadotropic serum? Were these animals gaining weight during this period?

LUNENFELD: The weight increase in these animals was normal. We consider this information as indicative that the antiserum is not contaminated with anti growth hormone.

ROSS: How do you account for the gain in gonadal weight if the antigonadotropic serum was entirely effective in neutralizing endogenous gonadotropin?

LUNENFELD: We said that the testis weight as a percentage of the animal weight did not increase. Absolute testis weight increased but this can be expected for growing animals. A general weight increase does not have to be gonadotropin dependent.

ROSS: If you had eliminated gonadotropic activity by hypophysectomizing these animals would you have expected the gonads to increase in weight?

LUNENFELD: To my knowledge hypophysectomy at birth has never been attempted. Furthermore, hypophysectomy would deprive the animal also of growth hormone and other functions. In this experiment we intended to deprive the animal only of gonadotropic hormones.

CLERMONT: Concerning the Sertoli cells in growing rats, we found them proliferating until about 20 to 21 days of age.

E. STEINBERGER: Dr. Lunenfeld, I think that your experiments are exceedingly interesting because this approach permits us to examine the effect of gonadotropin deprivation on spermatogenesis in the presence of the pituitary. Experiments using ablation of the pituitary have many drawbacks. However, we should not forget that in the type of experiments you reported we are looking only at the mechanisms concerned with initiation of spermatogenesis rather than maintenance, and I think these are different. Furthermore, I wish you had done a quantitative analysis of the germinal epithelium using slightly different techniques which would have given us more precise information.

LUNENFELD: This was a progress report of an experiment which is still going on. All the material will be analyzed. I am sure that more information will be derived from this experiment at its final stage.

HUDSON: Dr. Lunenfeld, was the anti-rat gonadotropin an antiserum to crude pituitary extract or specifically to LH or FSH?

LUNENFELD: This was an antiserum prepared to a gonadotropin extract obtained from rat pituitary glands. It neutralizes both FSH and LH activity. The characteristics of this antiserum were published in Acta Endocrinology, 1967, 59: 311.

ROSEMBERG: Could we turn our attention to a discussion of gonadotropin therapy in males with idiopathic oligospermia and assumed normal pituitary function?

GENERAL DISCUSSION: Treatment of Male "Infertility"

JOHNSEN: We have tried to select a group of men in whom we had every good reason to believe that the cause of oligospermia was an FSH deficiency. We think that we can select these patients from the characteristics of their testicular biopsy. We also perform FSH assays. With respect to dosages used in the treatment of male infertility, we know fairly well how much FSH is excreted in the urine. Hence it is possible to calculate how much FSH will have to be administered to replace the amounts of FSH secreted by the pituitary in the normal male. We proceeded along this line. Despite the fact that we treated men with an assumed hormonal deficiency, which was substituted by the administration of HMG, we did not observe the desired results. However, it is conceivable that the FSH dose administered (160 IU 2 to 3 times per week) was not sufficient.

LUNENFELD: I think that we cannot use the comparative amount of gonadotropin excreted in order to set up dosages. We have to take into account also the half-life and the transport of the hormone from the site of injection to the target organ. Dr. Ross has informed me that their data related to pituitary production of FSH in normal women during the follicular phase of the cycle range from 200 to 800 IU per day. They do not have comparable data on normal men.

TROEN: I think the point is to distinguish, as we know in clinical medicine, between physiologic and pharmacologic doses. I think it should be quite apparent that there are at least two possibilities in the approach to therapy: one would be to replace an amount of gonadotropin that the body lacks, but with an otherwise responsive end organ. It is clear that this approach has not been successful in a large number of normogonadotropic males. Another possibility open to us is to give pharmacological doses of HMG which we know to be an effective agent. The dosage of HMG that we have given was not in excess of that which we would expect to be normally produced either by our knowledge of production rates or by studying blood levels. Therefore, my suggestion is to give larger doses in order to attempt to achieve a pharmacological action upon the germinal epithelium.

E. STEINBERGER: I fully agree with Dr. Troen. The fact is that one of the most important problems is the ability to make a proper diagnosis and to understand the pathophysiology. If we had the means to establish the pathophysiology of each testicular abnormality seen in our offices, we could offer therapy in a rational fashion either by replacement therapy or using gonadotropins in pharmacologic dosages. Therefore, I think that it is of extreme importance to learn how to diagnose the various types of testicular disorders.

PAULSEN: Dr. Steinberger, you indicated previously that good results were achieved with HMG therapy in two patients. One was an example of hypopituitarism while the second patient had primary testicular disease with normal pituitary function. Would you please repeat the details with respect to the second patient? We could then try to characterize those patients who might respond favorably to HMG therapy.

E. STEINBERGER: I think this particular patient was an example of abnormal steroid biosynthetic activity in the testis. While the biosynthesis of steroids was proceeding, a large amount of the material was shunted to a biologically inactive steroid (pregnenolone and androstenediol). By increasing the total biosynthetic activity of the Leydig cells, using pharmacologic doses of gonadotropins, we increased the total steroid synthesis and thus also increased the testosterone output. I would assume that gonadotropins were responsible for the effects observed.

ROSEMBERG: From the experimental evidence presented during this meeting, it seems that initiation of spermatogenesis may be accomplished by the use of mixtures of FSH and LH with a ratio favorable to LH. Would you agree, Dr. Lunenfeld, that, if we were to have a preparation of gonadotropins with a mixture of FSH and LH, with a ratio favorable to LH, this type of preparation will give better clinical results. Of course, we should have to consider the type of patient to be treated with such mixtures.

LUNENFELD: Dr. Rosemberg, why would you think it worthwhile to add to the Pergonal preparation a high amount of LH? I think it would be just as good to use the existing Pergonal preparation and inject HCG simultaneously, in the specific amounts necessary for each patient, monitored by testosterone levels.

ROSEMBERG: I think this is of practical importance. Dr. Donini can tell us how easy it is for him to prepare an LH:FSH combination in an HMG preparation with an LH:FSH ratio of 3 to 1, for example. Would it be just the same, Dr. Donini, to add HCG instead of increasing the amount of urinary LH in it?

DONINI: I think that for some small clinical trials, it would be possible to prepare ampoules with a ratio of LH to FSH of 3 to 1 for example, but it would be difficult to have available such an amount of LH for large clinical trials.

PAULSEN: I fail to see where there is any data to suggest that we need more LH in the patient with adult seminiferous tubule failure. It appears that we have to explore the effect of FSH in those patients who do not exhibit a disturbed biosynthetic pathway and who are androgenically normal. Furthermore, we need to study the pharmacologic effect of FSH on the abnormal germinal epithelium.

ROSEMBERG: If we accept the theoretical implication that the local effect of testosterone is very important, then, if a preparation with a higher amount of HCG is administered, the amount of testosterone secreted by the Leydig cells will be increased. This may be necessary.

TROEN: I stressed the finding, which to us was surprising, of low values of plasma testosterone in patients who are otherwise clinically normal, to point out that there is great variation in patients. To try to make the right combination of FSH and LH in advance might therefore be difficult. More to the point would be to obtain a complete profile of each and every patient with regard to what his actual function may be, to find out how this may vary from whatever norms we may have and then apply the proper therapy.

E. STEINBERGER: I agree with Dr. Troen. However, it is possible that some patients may exhibit local "intratesticular" androgen deficiency. Thus circulating levels and production rates of testosterone may not necessarily tell us whether in these patients the levels of testosterone at the target cell are adequate.

HELLER: May I remind you that we already have a circumstance in the human where we can increase LH, FSH and testosterone and concomitantly increase spermatogenesis. This is accomplished by the administration of clomiphene. We have all three hormones elevated, so I do not think you should abandon the idea that LH may not be important in this mixture.

PAULSEN: One final comment about HCG administration. We have gone through some 20 years of clinical studies which have dealt with treating oligospermic males with HCG. I have not seen any evidence to indicate that this has been beneficial.

ROSEMBERG: These were high doses of HCG.

PAULSEN: Not necessarily so. Many investigators have administered small doses of HCG. In some instances HCG alone and in other instances HCG plus exotic substances such as liver extract were administered.

MACLEOD: The emphasis during this discussion has been placed on evaluating the response to pharmacologic doses of HMG. I would prefer the contrary, let us say administering 15 instead of 75 IU. Some of the evidence presented today indicated that high dosages of FSH were not necessary.

LUNENFELD: Dr. Heller, I think that it was shown earlier during this meeting by Dr. Ross that in hypogonadotropic patients clomiphene had no effect on FSH and LH levels. Dr. MacLeod, have you any evidence that with 15 IU of FSH you can obtain any response or is this speculation in your part?

MACLEOD: No, I have no direct evidence. All I know is that a 75 IU dose produced full spermatogenesis in the hypogonadotropic male. Indeed I think that we are giving too much in view of the fact that one can maintain spermatogenesis with what we presume to be extremely low levels of FSH. Therefore, I would prefer to start at much lower levels of FSH in hypophysectomized male subjects.

E. STEINBERGER: I have to be the devil's advocate and re-emphasize Dr. MacLeod's statement. There is some evidence in the lower species which supports his comments considering the possible damaging effect of high levels of gonadotropins. There is a paper by Dr. Dorner showing the damaging effect of high doses of FSH in the rat. We have found high doses of PMS to be damaging to spermatogenesis. Thus, we should keep our minds open to the possibility that overdosing with gonadotropins may produce a result opposite to the one we desire.

ROSEMBERG: We are forgetting that comparison with animal experiments is not absolutely fair in this situation. Animals do not have ovaries or testes which have been exposed to any damage and they differ from patients having some sort of defect in the ovaries or testes. We are administering pharmacological doses to female patients who do not ovulate on their own. They may secrete endogenous FSH and LH but the end organ does not function. In the infertile male there is a defect in testicular function. Hence, the consideration of dosage should be related to the type of end organ which has to be treated.

JOHNSEN: Dr. Lunenfeld requested me to indicate the characteristics of the testicular tissue in hypopituitarism (FSH deficiency) in adult males. There is a greater or minor inhibition of spermatogenesis at the spermatid level so that, in the score count method, the majority of the figures will be placed at steps 8, 7 and 6 without finding any signs of degenerative processes, such as hyalinization: Finally, there will be no Leydig cell hyperplasia.

LUNENFELD: I think that we could summarize the problem in the following way. There seems to be no controversy as to our first task which is to correctly diagnose the patient for gonadotropic therapy. Unfortunately to date we have no clear cut way to arrive at the proper diagnosis. Some of the participants presented improved ways for selection of patients for HMG therapy; 2) I think all of us agree that more experimental work is needed to elucidate the specific pathological mechanism leading to oligo or azoospermia; 3) I believe that we do not have the right to deprive a patient of possible benefits which could be derived from gonadotropin therapy. Consequently, the "empirical" choice of patients as well as improvement of methods for monitoring gonadotropic therapy has to be continuously revised as new data become available. I do believe that we are administering low doses of gonadotropin. With respect to monitoring gonadotropin therapy, I again suggest that the testosterone level has to be kept slightly above normal. We also have to consider that hypogonadotropinism may be due to either too low endogenous gonadotropin production or, that the target cell may be relatively insensitive to endogenous gonadotropin stimulation. Such patients may need larger dosages of HMG because endogenous gonadotropins which appear to be normal may be insufficient. Furthermore, sperm counts, especially in oligospermic patients, vary. A sufficient number of pre-treatment sperm examinations are necessary to assess a possible response to gonadotropic therapy. Lastly it must be emphasized that not all testicular pathology is of an endocrinological nature and that gonadotropic therapy cannot be expected to be of value in all conditions of testicular dysfunction.

CONCLUDING REMARKS

Although many topics were discussed during this three-day meeting, it is evident that a Workshop Conference cannot be all inclusive in its scope. In this regard, it should be noted that less established genetic factors influencing male fertility were considered rather than entities caused by sex chromosomal aberrations. It was also beyond the scope of this Conference to include a discussion on the surgical treatment of disorders leading to testicular dysfunction such as cryptorchidism or varicocele.

The main thrust was directed toward placing present concepts and hypothesis in a more appropriate perspective and in presenting newer material which in some instances was embryonic in nature. Finally, it was intended to blend the above with established data so that guidelines for future investigations could be set forth.

Eugenia Rosemberg

C. Alvin Paulsen

INDEX

F

G

H